Praise for previous edit
How to Care for Aging Parents

"Indispensable!"
—AARP

"A compassionate guide of encyclopedic proportion."
—*The Washington Post*

"One of the most insightful books on this subject."
—*Chicago Tribune*

"Full of insight and great coping strategies for any situation."
—*New York Daily News*

"A smart, compassionate, and timely book
for every child who must care for an aging parent."
—*The Seattle Times*

"A thoroughly researched, well-organized, and comprehensive manual."
—*Library Journal*

"The bible of elder care."
—*ABC World News*

"Morris's book may contain the most valuable
advice anyone in that situation can get."
—Associated Press

"A comprehensive resource for providing help with difficult decisions."
—*Ladies' Home Journal*

"A work of great value, written with sensitivity and wisdom . . .
It fulfills an obvious need better than anything I've seen. . . .
This book deserves enormous circulation."
—Sherwin B. Nuland, M.D.

"This is a tremendous work . . . truly excellent.
It will be a great help to many people."
—Ronald Miller, M.D.

How to Care *for* Aging Parents

3RD EDITION
Completely Revised and Expanded

A One-Stop Resource for All Your Medical, Financial, Housing, and Emotional Issues

VIRGINIA MORRIS

Foreword by Jennie Chin Hansen,
CEO, the American Geriatrics Society and Health in Aging Foundation

WORKMAN PUBLISHING • NEW YORK

Library of Congress Cataloging-in-Publication Data is available.

ISBN 978-0-7611-6676-4

Cover photograph © by Mara Lavitt

Workman books are available at special discounts when purchased in bulk for premiums and sales promotions as well as for fund-raising or educational use. Special editions or book excerpts can also be created to specification. For details, contact the Special Sales Director at the address below, or send an email to specialmarkets@workman.com.

Workman Publishing Company, Inc.
225 Varick Street
New York, New York 10014-4381
workman.com

WORKMAN is a registered trademark of Workman Publishing Co., Inc.

Printed in the United States of America
First printing January 2014
10 9 8 7 6 5 4

To
Dr. John McLean Morris
(1914–1993)

In your living, you taught me about
courage, determination, philanthropy, and truth.
In your dying, you taught me about love.
I will miss you, always.

Many Thanks

At the end of one of his comedy shows, Steve Martin said to his audience, "You've been great and I'd like to thank each and every one of you." He then proceeded to point to people in the audience saying, "Thank you, thank you, thank you, thank you, thank you, thank you, thank you . . ."

I, too, would like to thank each and every person who helped create this book—the scores of doctors, lawyers, researchers, advocates, and social workers who generously shared their experience, insights, and time; the various experts at groups like the Alzheimer's Association, the National Institute on Aging, and AARP, who fielded my questions with patience and thoroughness; and most of all, the hundreds of caregivers who opened their hearts and homes, and shared their joys and sorrows with me. To each and every one of them, I am grateful. But because it is impossible to thank so many individuals here, I have limited my acknowledgments to a few essential players who made this, the third edition of the book, possible.

First and foremost, several people not only took the time to respond to a stream of questions from me, but also reviewed chunks of the manuscript. Amazing. Thank you, thank you, thank you to Dr. Margaret Drickamer, professor of medicine, University of North Carolina, and professor emeritus, Yale School of Medicine; Timothy Casserly,

elder law attorney at Burke & Casserly; Robyn Grant, director of public policy and advocacy at the National Consumer Voice for Quality Long-Term Care; and Julie Gray, past president, National Association of Professional Geriatric Care Managers.

Many thanks also to Dr. Marie Bernard, deputy director of the National Institute on Aging; Laurie Orlov, industry analyst at Aging in Place Technology Watch; Dr. Bennett Blum, geriatric psychiatrist and elder abuse expert; Janice Nadeau, psychologist and author of *Families Making Sense of Death*; and Julie Hall, estate professional.

Of course, a veritable army of people at Workman Publishing literally made this book. Thanks to my editor, Margot Herrera, who mysteriously stays calm in any storm, and much appreciation to Mary Wilkinson, Carol White, Janet Vicario, Ariana Abud, and John Jenkinson.

As always, the best must be saved for last. Thank you to my wonderful husband, Bob Plumb, who saw me through (and put up with me through) every step of this project; to Jack and Emma, who are absolutely the best children in the world and heroically handle a mom on a deadline (which is a pretty scary thing); and my four siblings, who are not only family, but better yet, my friends.

To each and every one of you, thank you.

Contents

Foreword by Jennie Chin Hansen xi

Introduction: Something Unexpected xiii

1   First Things First 1
Ten Survival Tips • Critical Conversations • Gathering Vital Documents
• Exploring the Options • Getting Organized • When You Can't Be There

Adapting to New Roles

2   Your Parent and You 22
A Changing Relationship • When They Won't Listen • Defusing Old Struggles
• Coping Day to Day • Exceptionally Difficult Parents

3   Caring for the Caregiver 41
Setting Limits • Emotional Minefields • 12 More Steps to a Healthy Mind-Set
• The Male Caregiver

4   The Inner Circle 60
Working with Siblings • Compensating the Caregiver • A Family Meeting
• Significant Others • Time for Kids • Multilayer Sandwiches • Careers and Caregiving

The Golden Years

5   A Healthier Body 82
In the Gym • The ABCs of Diet • The Liquor Cabinet • Up in Smoke

6   A Happier Soul 96
The Quest • Family and Friends • Spiritual Fulfillment • Reminiscing •
Volunteering and Working • Involved and Active • Dating, Sex, and Marriage

Life at Home

7   Tips for Daily Living 114
Safety First • Monitors and Alert Systems • Preventing Falls • Room-by-Room
Modifications • Bathing and Grooming • Dressing • What's for Dinner? •
In the Driver's Seat • Gadgets and Gizmos

8 Getting Help 147

Assessing the Need • Family and Friends • Community Services
• Geriatric Care Managers

9 Paid Help at Home 159

In-Home Care • The Hiring Process • From Day One • Managing the Troops
• When There Is Trouble • Respite Care

The Halls of Medicine

10 Rx for the Elderly 180

The Age Difference • Finding a Doctor • A Wellness Visit • A Geriatric
Assessment • A Personal Health Record • An Informed Advocate •
Complementary and Alternative Medicine

11 The Body Imperfect: Part I....................... 196

A Muddle of Medications • Vision • Hearing • Sleep • Temperature Regulation
• Dehydration • Skin Care • Arms, Legs, and Feet • Teeth and Mouth

12 The Body Imperfect: Part II 233

Bones and Joints • Incontinence • Constipation • Other Digestive Disorders •
Anemia • Diabetes

13 Matters of the Mind............................... 259

Depression • Delirium • Anxiety Disorders • Delusions and Hallucinations
• Hypochondria

14 In the Hospital...................................... 274

Avoiding It • Choosing a Hospital • Admission • Following His Wishes •
Tests, Surgery, and Treatments • At the Nurses' Station • Providing Comfort
• When You Are Far Away • Hospital Dangers • Resolving Disputes •
Preparing for Discharge • Bills, Bills, Bills

Handling the Paperwork

15 Paying the Way 302

Talking About Money • First Steps • Dipping into Your Own Funds •
Financial Planning • Benefits and Discounts • Getting Cash Out of a Home
• Tax Tips • Professional Help

16 Avoiding Fraud 325
Who's at Risk? • Common Scams and Scoundrels • Preventing Exploitation
• Signs of Trouble • What to Do

17 Paying for Health Care 337
Medicare • Medicaid • Long-Term Care

18 Legal Issues 359
Where There's a Will . . . • Power of Attorney • Advance Directives • Trusts
• Reducing Estate Taxes • Probate • A Question of Competence • Legal Help

Home Away from Home

19 Moving Out, Moving In 384
Launching the Discussion • Is It Time to Move? • Should Mom Move Closer?
• Should Dad Move In? • Under One Roof • Separate Quarters

20 An Array of Housing Options 401
Roommates and Shared Housing • Congregate Housing • Retirement
Communities • Senior Apartments • Foster Homes • Assisted Living • Continuing
Care Retirement Communities

21 A Good Nursing Home 415
The Decision • Starting the Hunt • What to Look For in Any Facility •
Getting In • Admission • Who Pays?

22 Making the Move Work 434
Moving Day • A Plan of Care • Visiting • Being an Advocate • Long-Distance
Caregiving • When Trouble Brews • Is This Move Working?

When They Forget

23 The Aging Brain 454
What Is Normal? • Mild Cognitive Impairment • Dementia • Getting Tested •
Alzheimer's Disease • Vascular Dementia • Lewy Body Dementia • Dealing with
the Diagnosis • Treating Dementia

24 Living with Dementia 477
Helping Your Parent • Helping Yourself

25 Managing Day to Day............................ 493
Hygiene and Dressing • Incontinence • Eating • Communication • A Sense
of Time • Other Challenges • Problem Behaviors • Psychotic Symptoms •
Late-Stage Dementia

The Last Good-bye

26 Nearing the End.................................. 524
Well in Advance • Making Decisions • Your Parent's Perspective •
Communicating • Caring for Your Parent Now • Taking Care of Yourself
• Care at Home • Hospice Care • In the Hospital • What Death Looks Like
• The Moment After

27 The Aftermath 552
A Funeral Director • The Obituary • Planning a Funeral • Taking Care of Business
• Dividing Possessions

28 Good Grief 567
Facets of Grief • Caregiver Grief • Growing from Grief • The Surviving Parent
• Children and Grief

A Final Note

29 You're Next..................................... 584
Talk About It • Paying for Old Age • A Question of Where • Your Body •
Your Mind • Your Life

Resources

Useful Organizations....................................... 607
Caregiver's Organizer 635
Index... 654

Foreword

by *Jennie Chin Hansen,*
CEO, the American Geriatrics Society and
the Health in Aging Foundation

In 1984, my 74-year-old father had a debilitating stroke that left him unable to continue caring for my mother, who had severe heart disease. At the time, my parents lived in Boston. I was widowed and raising my seven-year-old son in San Francisco. I knew what I wanted to do: I wanted to bring my parents to California to live with me and my son.

I first brought my mother. And when my father was strong enough to make the trip, I was able to bring him to live with us, too. I'll never forget that first night. As I helped my parents into bed, I felt that, if either or both of them died the next day, it would be all right, because I had finally been able to bring them together for the first time in seven months.

With the right care and therapy, my parents' quality of life improved. My mother lived for three more years, and my father lived another five wonderful years that were spent getting to know his grandson.

Caring for an older parent is one of the most demanding and one of the most deeply rewarding things you'll ever do. I know this from both personal and professional experience. I'm the CEO of the American Geriatrics Society and a past president of the AARP. As a nurse and systems developer, I enjoyed years of caring for older people and partnering with other health care providers to create innovative programs that enabled older adults to remain in their homes and communities as long as possible. And of course I had the wonderful privilege of caring for my parents at the end of their lives.

Thanks to decades of breakthroughs in public health, nutrition, and medicine, an unprecedented number of adults are now living into their 80s, 90s, and longer. Odds are you have an elderly parent or parents who need assistance. You also may be raising children or caring for grandchildren. And chances are you're a Baby Boomer. The oldest of us Boomers started turning 65 in 2011 and have now officially reached "retirement age." Yet surveys find that few Boomers are planning to stop working any time soon. So a big question for many of us is: How can we give Mom and Dad the care they need, take care of our own health, and juggle our jobs and other responsibilities?

The answer to this difficult question is: with help.

There is simply no way to do it all on your own. The book you're reading provides essential information that can point you toward the help you need. It's easy to understand, painstakingly researched, and comprehensive. Best of all, it's warmly empathetic. An award-winning writer, Virginia Morris understands the terrain, because she's covered it herself—she, too, cared for her parents through the end of their lives.

One of the many things I like about this book is how respectful it is of older people. In the very first chapter, it addresses one of the most difficult parts of caring for a parent: helping Mom and Dad realize that they need assistance. After spending 20 years or so helping you grow up, it's understandably hard for them to switch roles. Morris offers advice for making that easier.

You can read the chapters of this book in virtually any order, but I suggest you read Chapter 3, "Caring for the Caregiver," first. Taking care of an older parent is a labor of love, but it's also complicated, time consuming, demanding, and physically and emotionally draining. To take care of your mother or father, you *must* take care of yourself too.

I also recommend reading Chapters 10 and 11 early on—they do a great job of explaining how to work with your parent's health care providers to reduce risks of medication side effects and interactions. These are common and often harmful for older people. Morris explains that providing health care for older adults with multiple health problems is, by necessity, a "team" undertaking that involves physicians,

nurses, pharmacists, and other care providers—led, typically, by the patient's primary care physician: "One doctor should keep track of all of her ailments and medications . . . and coordinate her care so that treatments for one problem don't aggravate another."

Chapter 14—which covers what to do when your parent is hospitalized—provides the right amount of information so you know what to do when the time comes, but not so much that you're overwhelmed. From choosing a hospital through discharge and follow-up, Morris explains what to do and what questions to ask.

The hardest chapter to read is, as you might expect, the chapter called "Nearing the End." (You may want to read it in installments for this reason.) Along with information in Chapter 18—which focuses on essential legal matters such as power of attorney and advance directives—this chapter can help ensure that your parent's wishes are honored at the end of life. Just as important, the chapter addresses your feelings and needs as your parent's life draws to a close.

From that first conversation to the last, Morris provides an invaluable guide for those caring for aging parents (or other family members or friends). I wish everyone who reads this book a meaningful experience as a caregiver, with all its rewards and challenges. And I encourage you to have conversations early and often with those for whom you're caring. They can be among the most poignant, clarifying, and affirming experiences of your life.

Introduction

✍

Something Unexpected

When I began researching the first edition of this book in 1991, there was no World Wide Web, no Google, not even Ask Jeeves. People caring for an aging parent had to hunt down information by telephone, often calling one organization after another as each person directed them to someone else.

Caregivers typically had overflowing piles of papers around the house because, after making these calls, they would receive a massive amount of mail—brochures, pamphlets, forms, and information sheets—all of which would be added to the heap. You couldn't throw anything out because who knew what you might need one day. (Not that you would ever find it, but you had to keep it just in case.)

By the time the second edition was released in 2004, caregivers could tap a mouse and, before the next blink, have facts about Medicare, a list of local nursing homes, or a summary of arthritis treatments. They could join a chat group and, without exposing their identities or getting up from the couch, share their stress and guilt with others.

Now as I wrap up the third edition, "aging in place" technology, intended to let your parent stay in his home and to ease your worries, is well on its way. Automatic pill dispensers will text you if your parent misses a dose; fall sensors will determine whether your mother actually slipped or simply lay down for a nap; health monitors will notify the doctor if your father's temperature spikes; and motion detectors will alert you if your parent didn't have his morning coffee (suggesting something is amiss because he always has his morning coffee).

We can keep tabs on our parents via video chat or webcam; monitor a confused parent's location with a GPS tracking device; organize a crew of caregivers with an online calendar and messaging system; and, in some areas, forgo the car ride because Mom can get virtual physical therapy, or "telerehabilitation," from home.

Technology is reshaping the world for caregivers.

Sort of.

Yes, we have information at our fingertips, but there's so darn much of it.

The Internet has become so overloaded with bad advice and websites that are covertly trying to sell us something that it can be mind-boggling, misleading, and, because it's so easy to get sidetracked, time consuming (which is oddly ironic—while life got easier, it also got busier).

And yes, we can monitor what time Dad had his lunch and took his meds, but knowing what a parent is doing every minute of every day can be exhausting. It's also not foolproof because, of course, webcams and motion detectors can't cover every square inch of a house, and it wouldn't be out of character for Dad to take a pill from the automatic dispenser and then, on the way to get some water, put it down and forget to swallow it.

The point is, we still have to wonder if Mom is lonely and depressed. We still have to fret about what this is costing. We still have to deal with a sibling who's in denial about a parent's abilities. Despite any technological advances, the substance of caregiving—the planning, the worry, the guilt, the cost, the family tension—hasn't changed all that much.

So the basic advice from the first edition of this book remains exactly as it was. Plan ahead. Take care of yourself, because this is a tough job and it can flatten you if you're not careful. And whenever possible, let your parent live life his way (even when it's not your way).

As for the websites and gadgets, take it easy. Stick to a few reliable websites (such as those listed at the end of this book), and as you peruse "aging in place" technology, know that the most effective tools are still the simplest ones:

handrails, grab bars, raised toilet seats, clear pathways, evenly distributed lighting, and the like.

At the end of the day, no matter how automated their homes may be, our parents need human contact. They need people in their lives, they need a sense of purpose, and on some fairly regular basis, they need us—not by video chat, not by text message, but in person.

Honestly, one of the most exciting shifts in the land of parentcare since the last edition is not all that well known, probably because it is not technological, but philosophical.

The premise is this: People who need care should have a say in what that care looks like.

So instead of Medicaid determining that it will pay for your father to have a home health aide for X hours each week, he can decide to spend that same money on a scooter and ramp or, in most states, to pay a family member to care for him instead of a stranger.

This philosophy of "person-directed care" (or "person-centered care") is being adopted by a growing number of nursing homes and other long-term care facilities, thanks to groups such as Pioneer Network, the Green House Project, and Eden Alternative.

Rather than stripping your parent of all control—dictating when he eats, what he eats, when he exercises, what time he goes to sleep, and even when he goes to the toilet—the nursing home lets your parent live, well, almost as he would if he lived on his own and made his own decisions. He wants ice cream at midnight? He can go right ahead and have it. He likes to sleep until ten? That's his prerogative. Was your mother an avid gardener? Then bring on the gardening gloves.

It's all about dignity, self-respect, and personal control—quite unlike the traditional nursing-home paradigm. This is a welcome change indeed. Look for it, ask about it, demand it.

On a personal note, when I started the first edition, I had two parents, neither one in need of care. Now I have none.

My father died when I was halfway through writing the original book. Although he was sick for many years, he didn't need assistance until the last four months of his life.

My mother, on the other hand, was in various stages of need and illness for more than 15 years. She had acute lung disease, which had a habit of turning a sniffle or some overexertion into acute pneumonia. And so she swung between living fully and dying imminently.

During her last decade and a half, she fell in love, traveled the world, played tennis, and studied art, Buddhism, and ethics. But between these joyous moments, I sat by her side in a multitude of hospitals, watching over her tiny body as doctors whispered the worst.

She lived many years longer than any of them expected, and it wasn't her lousy lungs that got her in the end. She had a stroke, partial paralysis, a frightening amount of weight loss, a bad fall, and, just when we thought the worst was over, cancer.

Her death two years ago was the last step of a long and exhausting journey into my own subject, my own field of expertise.

Yes, normally the experience comes first and the book second. Any author will tell you, write what you know. But I did it backward, partly because I was a medical writer and this was an issue that needed attention. Also, I have found that sometimes it's better to investigate issues that you haven't experienced. This way, you come to your subject clean, without all the passions, memories, and opinions that can shape the research and infiltrate the writing.

Most of what I have experienced over the last dozen years was in the book already, but a few things surprised me.

It turns out that I'm very bad at taking my own advice (such as *Take care of yourself, Don't own it all, Get others to help*). Like so many caregivers, I didn't realize how deeply it was affecting me and what terrible shape I was in until it was over, until I could finally release my drawn shoulders and cry.

How could I, the "expert," not be attuned to this? How could I make the very mistakes I regularly warn others to avoid?

I was musing over my failings when, one evening over dinner, a doctor friend complained that he had to be on call the next night. Although he didn't usually get called to the hospital, he explained that he couldn't relax, knowing that he might be.

That was it. That was the part of this job I hadn't expected, hadn't recognized, and couldn't really explain. Even when you're not juggling medications, or cleaning up vomit, or finding an aide to fill in, you are on call. You know that all is not right in the world, that disaster could strike at any moment, and that when it does, you will have to deal with it. And, whatever happens, you will feel responsible for it.

I had been on call for as long as I could remember, and it was this, perhaps more than all of the daily care, that had worn me out.

So I urge my readers more vehemently than before to share the work, get others involved, and be extraordinarily kind to yourself.

Another thing that surprised me was how important it is to jump off the merry-go-round occasionally. To do something unexpected or out of character. I just wish I'd done it more because these are the moments I now keep securely in my heart.

Let me share one small example. Toward the end of my mother's life my sister came to visit, and—as happens to so many caregivers—it struck me how pleasant her visits were. She and Mom would have a lovely lunch because, of course, this visit was special. They would talk and laugh, and my sister would leave saying how nice it was to spend time with Mom.

My time with Mom was spent organizing medications, consoling aides, handling bills, and driving her to appointments. She didn't get cleaned up *in preparation* for my visit because my visit was all about cleaning her up.

I wanted a taste of this "nice time with Mom" stuff.

The next day when I arrived, Mom immediately looked apologetically at a stack of mail that needed attention. She asked if I'd cut her fingernails and put some cream on her. And, oh, I needed to switch her physical therapy appointment.

I looked at her in bed and said, "Scootch over."

And thus we spent a gray afternoon lying in bed, arms intertwined, watching *An American in Paris*, melting over Gene Kelly, and singing along, despite our terrible voices. It was pure heaven. Throughout the movie, I could see our reflection in my iPad screen, her head leaning comfortably against mine.

I did feel bad that the mail and fingernails and appointments were ignored, but the guilt was infinitesimal compared with how great I felt about our afternoon together playing hooky.

Sometimes, you just have to live life and to heck with the other stuff.

I wish you luck with your parent's care. I hope this book gives you some helpful guidance, a lot of emotional support, and permission to occasionally do something completely unexpected.

VIRGINIA MORRIS
NOVEMBER 2013

Chapter 1

First Things First

Ten Survival Tips • Critical Conversations • Gathering Vital Documents • Exploring the Options • Getting Organized • When You Can't Be There

Most of us don't plan to take care of a parent. We don't set aside time or money for the task, or factor it in when thinking about retirement. For the most part, a parent's old age, and the needs and dilemmas that typically accompany it, seem to come out of nowhere.

The transition can come with a jolt—after a fall, a stroke, or a diagnosis—but more often than not the demands of parentcare slide slowly into our lives. Dad is a little hunched over, his step wobbly. Mom left the stove on and burned a pot. Again. The car has a new dent. Pill bottles line the sink.

Even then, some part of us clings to the hope that our parents will be all right and our services will not be needed. But with time come housing issues, money problems, medical complications, and questions, so many questions. *How do we stop her from driving? Is he eating properly? Can she be left alone? Who will take him to his doctor's appointment? Is that a new symptom? Will insurance cover this?*

We don't plan for it, but at some point we are in it, solving each crisis only to find another in its wake. We muddle through, day by day, juggling their lives, and ours.

No matter where you are in the process—whether you're just starting out, deeply enmeshed, or nearing the end—the most important thing you can do for your parent, and yourself, is this: Be prepared for what might come. Complete the paperwork, explore the options, discuss his wishes, create a plan. When using this book, after reading the sections that apply to your current situation, take a look at some issues that you are not yet dealing with—but may very well have to tackle one day.

Staying one day ahead, one question ahead, one chapter ahead will give you and your parent time to consider the options carefully. It will help ensure that your parent has choices and receives the best care possible. And just as important, planning ahead will mean far less work, less stress, and fewer headaches for you. It should even give you a little peace of mind.

Ten Survival Tips

Whether you are already deep in the trenches of parentcare or just beginning your journey, here are a few key tips for surviving the job. All of them are discussed in detail later in the book, but they are useful to know from the get-go.

1. ASSESS. If you are racing frantically, stop. Sit with yourself for a moment, be still, breathe deeply, unclench your jaw, and clear your mind. Now, using the most rational (and least emotional) corner of your brain, ask yourself: What really must be done and what can be deleted from your crowded to-do list? Once you know that, determine what has to be done by you and what can be done by someone else. Prioritize, and once you take an item off the list, let go of it.

2. ORGANIZE. Locate important documents. Keep a record of key contacts (doctors, aides, lawyers, pharmacist, and so on), passwords, and your parent's medical history in a document that you can access from your phone or other devices.

SIGNS THAT YOUR PARENT NEEDS HELP

If you aren't yet in the throes of caring for your parent, how do you know when to get involved? As this chapter makes clear, "sometime in the future" can become "today" quite suddenly, so don't delay. Have the conversations outlined here, and be sure your parent's legal and financial affairs are in order.

If that's all been done and your parent is living on her own quite well, be aware of signs of trouble, particularly any changes in her behavior, appearance, or habits. If you suspect something is off, get involved right away. It could be a sign of illness or depression, or a signal that a problem is imminent, such as a fall, car accident, or nutritional deficiencies. Talk with your parent and/or her doctor. Some clues that your parent needs help:

• She's unsteady. Is she wobbly on the stairs? Is her gait uneven? Does she get dizzy getting up from a chair? Or has she already fallen?

• His personal hygiene has fallen to the wayside. Is your parent skipping showers, forgetting to shave, looking unkempt?

• Your parent has gained or lost weight, which could be a sign of illness or depression, or an indication that she's having difficulty shopping and cooking.

• The house and yard are no longer maintained. Is your mother's beloved flower garden weedy, her usually clean house dusty, or the dishes piled up in the sink?

• Her personality has changed. Is your sweet mother suddenly critical or irritable? Your vocal father suddenly quiet and compliant?

• There's nothing to eat. Is there food in the refrigerator? Is it spoiled and moldy?

• The mail is unopened or bills are unpaid.

• She misses appointments, gets lost, forgets important information, or loses things.

• The car has dents, your parent has a traffic violation, or you simply don't feel safe letting your children in the car with Grandpa driving.

• Your parent no longer does things she used to enjoy. Has she stopped going to her bridge club, doing the crossword puzzle, or seeing her friends?

• The mail is suddenly full of new subscriptions, sweepstakes entries, and requests for donations. Or your parent has a new best friend. This could be a sign of fraud.

3. PLAN. Don't wait for a crisis. Get critical documents (power of attorney, health care proxy) signed. Talk with your parent and family about your parent's future care, housing, and finances. Hold a family meeting. Be a step ahead.

4. TAKE CARE OF YOURSELF. Be sure to get away from it all from time to time—physically, mentally, and emotionally. Make an effort to eat well, exercise, see friends, and rest. Caring for yourself will mean better care for your parent.

5. GET HELP. You do not have to—and should not try to—do it all. Get others involved, tap into community services, hire aides, and look into other housing options. Get help long before you think you'll need it.

6. COMMUNICATE. Keep lines of communication open—with your parent, doctors, aides, and especially your siblings. Talk with them about who will do what and how you can support each other. Consider ways to compensate a sibling who is doing the bulk of the work.

7. SHOW RESPECT. Despite the toll of aging and illness, your parent is still an adult and still your parent. As difficult as it might be sometimes, treat her with respect. Hear her views.

8. DUMP THE GUILT. Out. Gone. Finito. Finished. Enough of that. You are doing a good job.

9. PREPARE FOR THE END. Everyone will be focused on keeping your parent alive, which is natural, but this single-minded quest often makes people miserable. Question it. What does your parent want most (time, mobility, comfort, lucidity)? Be sure her goals are at the center of all decisions.

10. BE SPONTANEOUS. Do something with your parent that's fun and unexpected, something that has nothing to do with doctors, medications, or aides. In all your time of caregiving, this will be one of the moments you'll remember most fondly.

Critical Conversations

Although it can become too late quite suddenly, it is never too soon to talk to your parent and siblings about the future—her medical care, housing, finances, and personal needs. Obviously, if your mother is extremely sick and frail, these talks are urgent. But even if she is relatively healthy and independent, planning for the future is vital.

No one wants to deal with this. No one wants to imagine, much less discuss, a time when nursing homes or, God forbid, end-of-life decisions are necessary. It can be awkward and difficult to bring up, and also feel morbid or

depressing, or as if you're rushing your parent to a place no one wants to go.

And if you're already in the thick of it, who has the time? Your mother needs help getting meals, she's convinced the aide is a thief, and your siblings aren't helping out. How are you supposed to make plans for the future when the here and now is so pressing?

Or maybe you think the planning's been done. She has a will. She's signed all the legal documents. She plans on staying in her house. And you know very well that she doesn't want things "dragged out."

If only it were that simple. What happens when your mom is in the hospital and your dad is left on his own? What happens when your mother needs someone to bathe her, dress her, and feed her? What happens when the doctor turns to you and says, "Should we put her on a respirator?" Are you ready? Really?

Go ahead. Have the conversations. Don't put this off. Talk with your parent and, depending upon the situation, hold a family meeting to discuss your parent's current care and future needs. Assign jobs, sort out finances, and make plans for what sort of care he will need as he grows more frail.

For your parent, planning ahead ensures that he has a say in his future, it affords him more choices, and it gives him time to prepare for change. If your father is encouraged to think about the possibility of moving out of his house long before such a move is an issue, it will be easier for him to make the move if it does, one day, become necessary.

For you, planning means less work when your parent needs help (because plans are in place), it means you aren't always reacting to a crisis, and it means peace of mind.

Do it now because it is much, *much* easier to have these discussions when there is no dire problem at hand, when you are talking about some distant possibility, when it's a matter of "What if . . ." *Mom, what if one day you couldn't handle your own finances?*

Talk now; you'll be glad you did.

Your Reluctance

Admittedly, asking your father about his finances or anticipating a time when he can no longer take care of himself is not easy. You might have a relationship in which personal issues, particularly *his* personal issues, are not discussed. Raising them might upset a relatively comfortable balance.

If your parent is a domineering or protective force in your life, you risk losing—at least for a moment—the role of the child. And you could find yourself taking on a strange, and not particularly welcome, new role.

More difficult than anything else, such conversations force you and your parent to acknowledge openly that he very likely will decline, will need help, and is indeed mortal.

Certain subjects—money, death— might make you particularly uneasy. But the truth is that your parent probably shares your concerns, and your reluctance. In fact, your mother might be keeping quiet because she is worried about upsetting you. Breaking the silence might be awkward, but once everyone's gotten over the initial discomfort, it should be a welcome relief for all.

Keep in mind that talking about the worst-case scenarios won't make them come true, and refusing to talk about them won't make them go away. Ignoring the inevitable will only leave you unprepared for a crisis that will almost surely one day come.

Breaking the Silence

So how does one start such conversations? That will depend on the situation and your relationship.

If you are caring for a parent who is already quite frail or has a serious diagnosis, and questions are already hovering, you might just tackle this head-on. *Mom, given your health and what the doctor's told us, I think we need to talk about some things.*

If matters aren't pressing and you'd rather use a less direct approach, asking for advice is a good opener. Parents love to give advice. *Dad, Fred and I are saving for our retirement and I'm just wondering how you approached this. How much is enough? Do you worry about the cost of long-term care? Do you feel you saved enough?*

Or simply start by asking general questions about your parent's life—what she most enjoyed, what she wishes she'd done differently. Then, gradually move the conversation forward. What does she want out of the future? What does she worry about?

You can also start by talking about someone else's situation, such as a friend or family member who is elderly. How did the family handle it? What might have been done differently? What would your parent want to happen if she were in a similar situation?

If your parent cared for an elderly parent, ask how she handled certain matters, what was frustrating about it, and what was rewarding.

Or, use a magazine article or television show as a springboard. *I was reading an interesting article on new aging-in-place technologies. Have you heard anything about that, Mom?*

If launching this discussion face-to-face is too difficult, write down some questions for your parent. Tell her that these are some issues you are concerned about and ask her if she would think about them. Then plan a time to sit down with her and discuss them.

Listen

However you launch this conversation, start by listening, even when you have specific issues you want to discuss or firm convictions about what should be done.

You might be sure that your father needs to move into an assisted living

WHEN YOU TALK

- Pick a time when you and your parent are calm and rested, and when you won't be interrupted.

- Be careful not to dismiss your parent's concerns by suggesting that they are silly or by offering quick "solutions."

- Be open with the facts—a poor medical prognosis, a major financial hurdle, a less-than-optimal selection of housing options. Be gentle, but don't lie or hide information to protect your parent, as this will only hurt him in the long run.

- End each discussion before you or your parent becomes tired or overwhelmed.

- Leave the conversation open. One discussion breaks the ice, but these topics need to be revisited.

- If your parent changes the subject or makes it clear that she doesn't want to talk about something, be gentle. Let her know you are concerned and then, if the matter isn't dire, back off and try again another time.

facility, but for now, just ask questions. What does he worry about? What would ease his worries? How does he see this playing out? What does he still enjoy? What does he need from you?

And then listen. Really listen. Be open-minded to his views. You might assume that he's worried about his daily care but discover that he is most frightened about becoming a burden, losing people's respect, or being forgotten.

This is a whole new stage of life. Your parent is likely to have fears and hopes that he has never voiced before, ones that you haven't considered.

For example, you may want to talk about finances, but your parent may be so afraid of falling or he may be so mired in grief that he can't even think about money.

Once he's had a chance to talk (without interruption), let him know that you hear him. Repeating what he's said, using slightly different words, assures him that you get it. *I understand that seeing your grandchildren is the most important thing for you now.*

If you listen first, you will probably learn something, and your parent will be more likely to listen to your views, in turn.

What *Not* to Do

When you raise difficult subjects, avoid these common mistakes. Don't:

MAKE DECISIONS FOR HIM. Often, with all the best intentions, siblings have discussions and make decisions and then present a master plan to a parent. *Ben and I found an assisted living home near us. It's perfect. We've talked to a real estate agent about getting your house on the*

market, and he says we can make this happen before November.

There are few more effective ways of blocking any further conversation.

ARRIVE ARMED WITH PAPERWORK. Pages of legal documents and brochures about retirement homes will only overwhelm your parent. This first conversation is just an opener, not a homework session.

TREAT YOUR PARENT LIKE A CHILD (OR IMBECILE). No matter how sick or confused your parent might be, he is an adult. Don't talk down to him. Avoid the urge to nag or lecture.

TALK OVER TURKEY. Or birthday candles, or Christmas or Hanukkah presents. The holidays might be the only time you're all together, but you probably won't get a great response if you pull out a living will and pen while the pumpkin pie is making the rounds. If this is the only time you can talk, then give your parent a little notice and talk when the festivities are over.

What to Talk About

Here are a few major topics to get you started. All of these issues are discussed in detail in later chapters, including suggestions on how to talk about them. You won't be able to cover all of this in one sitting, most certainly. Discuss what you can, and come back to other topics later.

NEEDS AND GOALS. What does your parent most want out of her life now? What matters to her? What does she enjoy? What does she still hope to do?

It might be something grand—take a trip, finish a project, see a monument—or it might be something simple.

AVOID MAKING PROMISES

Even though you might believe fervently that you will never *ever* put your parent in a nursing home, you simply don't know what the future holds, either for your parent or for you. Your parent may become so ill that you cannot continue to manage her care. Your own life may change in such a way that you cannot give your parent the attention that you assumed you could.

Given such possibilities, don't put yourself in the position of having to break a promise; don't make it in the first place. If your parent asks you to promise that you will never put her in a nursing home, assure her that you will do whatever you can to avoid it and that you will never abandon her.

Can he bathe and groom himself? Can he get to the grocery store and prepare meals? Does he fall now and then or feel unstable? Can he keep track of bills and write checks? Is he still driving?

There are solutions to most issues (discussed throughout the book), but you can't help him if you don't know what the problems are.

Your parent might be embarrassed about certain issues. Probe gently. Assure him that most problems are common and manageable and that admitting to them doesn't mean you'll cart him off to a "home."

Perhaps your mom loves having lunch with a friend, talking with her grandchildren, watching the birds at the feeder, or listening to music. Or maybe your father wants to go trout fishing again, see a lake he loved as a child, or just tinker with some projects around his house.

Does he care more about staying in his home, being safe, or being near family? Does she want to continue to garden or play the piano wherever she lives?

All other conversations, about housing and finances and medical care, should be based on your parent's particular goals and priorities.

DAILY ACTIVITIES. Before you plan the future, sort out the present. How is your parent managing day to day? You will witness some of this, but ask him what he considers to be the biggest obstacles.

HOUSING. How does he feel about his current housing situation? Can changes be made to make life more manageable? What about the future? Where would he want to live if he could no longer live at home? What if it isn't possible for him to live with other family members? If he has to move, what is most important to him (staying in his hometown, proximity to you, the ability to keep a pet with him, climate)?

Even if your family has no interest in any sort of senior housing, consider all the options. Visit a few facilities. Living at home can be lonely and, unless there are ample resources or generous community services, unfeasible.

FINANCIAL AND LEGAL ISSUES. What are your parent's current financial needs and potential future needs? Can she meet these needs? Is she tapping into all the benefits and discounts for which she is eligible? Is she spending with abandon or saving so fiercely that it's dangerous? Is her insurance—including life, health, home, and auto insurance—adequate and current? Can she simplify her finances?

The biggest financial issue for most elderly people is the cost of long-term care. Medicare covers the majority of doctor bills, hospital bills, laboratory tests, and even a limited amount of nursing care, but it does not cover the kind of day-to-day care most elderly people eventually need—aides, companions, and homemakers, or extended care in a nursing home or other facility.

These bills can be astronomical. Such care can cost more than $80,000 a year, devouring what seemed like a comfortable nest egg. Those who have long-term illnesses or disabilities often have to pay out of pocket until they are broke, and then they go on Medicaid, the government's insurance for the poor. Consider how your parent and family might handle such expenses.

Also, has your parent executed all necessary legal papers, including a will, durable power of attorney, and advance directives? Is there anything she might do to protect her estate from excessive taxes or, if she has little savings, to get on Medicaid early?

MEDICAL CARE. Does your parent have a good primary physician whom she trusts? Does this doctor communicate with her other physicians and coordinate all of her care? Does he or she take her complaints seriously and pay attention to issues that are not life threatening but troubling nonetheless? Some doctors give short shrift to mild memory loss, incontinence, depression, stiff joints, and anxiety, even though these issues will make your parent's life (and yours) difficult.

If your parent couldn't make medical decisions for herself at some point, whom does she trust to do that for her? Has she legally named a health care proxy to make these decisions for her? Has she talked to that person in depth about her wishes?

What are your parent's goals concerning medical care? What should be considered when making medical decisions? What's most important to her—time, mobility, comfort, lucidity? Any time medical decisions are made, talk with the doctor and your parent

ON THE LOOKOUT FOR FRAUD

The elderly are conned *routinely*. Don't think for one minute that your parent is immune, no matter how smart, capable, or tough he might be.

Scams run the gamut from sweepstakes and lotteries, to reverse mortgages and investments, to aides, friends, and family members who tap into your parent's heart and checkbook.

The best prevention is to alert your parent to common scams and to be sure he isn't isolated because a lonely, worried, elderly person is the perfect target. See Chapter 16 for more on protecting your parent from being swindled and what to do when it happens.

about the goals of treatment, the likely outcomes, and other options for care.

END-OF-LIFE CARE. This is a tough subject to discuss, no doubt about it, but it is a crucial one. Don't ignore it because such discussions could save your family from untold agony and grief.

Despite any promises made or papers signed, many people die in pain, afraid, and hooked to machines. They die after agonizing medical treatments of questionable value.

Talk—really talk—to your parent about her medical state and wishes concerning aggressive medical care. Get her to sign a living will and health care proxy, but realize that these documents are just a starting point. Alone, they will not protect your parent from unwanted treatments and a painful death.

Don't accept vague (and not terribly helpful) comments like, "Don't drag it out" or "When I'm at that point, pull the plug." Push the conversation further.

What frightens your parent about dying? What level of pain, dependence, and disability would be unbearable? Is there a certain point after which she would no longer want life-sustaining medical care, such as a ventilator, artificial nutrition and hydration, or surgery? Would she prefer that treatments be focused instead on other goals, such as comfort, mobility, or lucidity? What does she think about hospice care?

Ask her doctor to describe various treatment options that might lie ahead, and the pros and cons of each. Help her get a realistic sense of what can be done and what can't.

Also, talk with your parent and the doctor about getting an "at-home" Do Not Resuscitate order or POLST (Physician Orders for Life Sustaining

CRUCIAL DOCUMENTS

Whatever else you do, be sure your parent has the following:

AN UPDATED AND VALID WILL. This ensures that his belongings (no matter how extensive or meager) will be allocated according to his wishes. A current will also reduces the likelihood of family conflict and complicated probate. And for a larger estate, a properly drafted will can reduce taxes.

A DURABLE POWER OF ATTORNEY. This authorizes someone to act on your parent's behalf, from signing checks to making housing choices, should he become incapacitated. Without one, your family might have to go to court to have a legal guardian named.

ADVANCE DIRECTIVES. These include a living will and a durable power of attorney for health care (also known as a health care proxy). The first outlines your parent's wishes concerning end-of-life medical care, and the second gives a trusted relative or friend the authority to make health care decisions for your parent when he cannot make them for himself.

BE PREPARED FOR AN EMERGENCY

If your parent has a medical condition or diagnosis that emergency crews would need to know about, make this information easily available.

Put essential medical and contact information, along with any living will, health care proxy, and advance medical orders in a clear plastic bag. Label the bag and tape it to the door of the refrigerator or the back of your parent's front door (where emergency crews will look for it).

In addition, get your parent a medical emergency bracelet that identifies him and provides critical medical information.

Treatment). Despite what TV shows suggest, cardiopulmonary resuscitation, or CPR—attempts to restore some function to the heart and lungs—is a brutal procedure. A sick, older person is unlikely to survive it or ever leave the hospital.

Once you know your parent's wishes, you may have to brace yourself to make some tough decisions and to fight a system that is focused on aggressive treatment.

For more on these documents and talking about end-of-life care, see pages 368 and 527.

Your Parent's Denial

When your parent is hiding behind denial or simply dodging the issues— *Oh, honey, why do you bring up such dreadful things? Everything is fine. Let's talk about something more pleasant*—grant her some of that protection. Be patient and try to understand her fears and the reasons why she might not want to face facts. Old age and the disability and dependence that often come with it are, obviously, difficult to accept. Denial and avoidance are natural responses.

> After my father died, I was very worried about my mom being able to handle her finances. My dad always took care of everything that had to do with money. I don't think my mother had ever even balanced the checkbook.
>
> I said to Mom over and over, 'Let's review your financial situation,' and I offered repeatedly to take care of her bills for her. She'd say, 'Brenda, don't worry about it. I'm fine.' And then she'd change the subject.
>
> Then my brother came to visit, and within a day he had Mom pulling out folders and showing him bank statements. By the time he left, she had handed over almost all of her financial stuff to him.
>
> I was stunned. I mean, I was glad to have it settled, but I was also a little annoyed. I'm an accountant. He's a teacher. I guess she feels that money is men's work.
>
> I probably should have thought to get him involved right from the start."
>
> —Brenda S.

Remind her that you care and want to be helpful, and then ask her to please think about the matter. You have planted a seed. She will surely give the subject some thought.

Give her a couple of weeks and then bring it up again. *Mom, I know this is difficult for you. But if we talk about these things, we can make sure that you get the kind of care you want.*

If you still are not successful, ask another family member or close family friend to talk with her. For whatever reasons, she may be more receptive to someone else.

You might also suggest that your mother talk with a member of the clergy, a social worker, a lawyer, or a doctor about certain matters. If that doesn't work, you might call these people and ask them to raise the subject with her. It's often easier for people to talk to and accept the advice of someone outside the family circle, especially if that person is a trusted professional.

If, no matter what you do, your parent remains steadfastly silent, talk with your siblings and prepare without her.

CHECKLIST: INFORMATION YOU WILL NEED

Documents, information, and items that you are likely to need:

❏ Names, addresses, and phone numbers of:

- doctors, dentists, pharmacist, and other medical providers and suppliers

- lawyers, financial advisers, accountants, and insurance agents

- banks, investment firms, and other financial institutions

- clergy members or religious organizations

- your parent's relatives, close friends, caregivers, and neighbors

❏ Medical history (illnesses, medications, treatments, allergies, immunizations)

❏ Certificates of birth, marriage, divorce/ separation, and citizenship

❏ Military/veteran's papers

❏ Driver's license and/or passport

❏ Your parent's will and any codicils (amendments) to the will

❏ Durable power of attorney

❏ Living will and power of attorney for health care

❏ Keys to his house, office, safe-deposit box, and post office box, as well as combination to any safe or lock

❏ Insurance policies (life, health, disability, homeowner's, and auto)

❏ Social Security, Medicare, and Medicaid numbers and identification cards

❏ A list of employers, dates of employment, and terms of employment

❏ Any business contracts or rental agreements

❏ Deed to his house or rental agreement

Gathering Vital Documents

As your parent grows increasingly frail, your family will need certain financial statements, contact information, and medical records. Locating these things when your parent can no longer guide you can be exceedingly difficult. Gather them—at least the most critical ones—now.

If your parent is infirm and you have to look for these papers without his help, start in the obvious places—a safe-deposit box, desk and bureau drawers, office files, and papers stacked on tables and in corners. If you have trouble locating certain documents, call your parent's lawyer, accountant, or anyone else who has had a hand in his financial or legal affairs. Look for leads such as bills, canceled checks, receipts, address books, and letters.

You might be able to track down some documents on the Internet.

❑ Deeds or titles to real estate, automobiles, boats, and other vehicles

❑ The location of any valuables (including anything hidden away)

❑ A list of all charge, debit, and banking cards

❑ Passwords, access codes, PINs

❑ Any automatic bill-paying or electronic transfer arrangements

❑ Appraisals of personal property

❑ Copies of federal and state tax returns from the past three to five years

❑ Receipts from property taxes and other large recent payments

❑ Burial and funeral instructions, if any

Your parent or you should make lists of the following (there is a "Financial Planner" on page 651 and at careforagingparents.com that will help you organize this material):

❑ Monthly bills (utilities, taxes, mortgage, insurance premiums)

❑ Your parent's assets, including the value of:

• savings, checking, money market, and retirement accounts

• stocks, bonds, and other securities

• real estate

• automobiles, boats, and other valuables

• business ownership and partnership agreements

• profit-sharing and pension plans

• trust agreements

• outstanding loans

❑ All debts, including mortgages and other loans, credit card balances, outstanding bills, and other liabilities

The Centers for Disease Control and Prevention website has a state-by-state list of offices to contact for vital records (cdc.gov/nchs/w2w.htm), as does the federal government's website (usa.gov). The Department of Veterans Affairs (va.gov) and the Social Security Administration (ssa.gov) also have useful information.

Insurance companies will often provide information about a policy even when the request comes from a family member of the insured. The Social Security office, former employers, and the local office of veterans' affairs might also be willing to send you information about pensions and other benefits.

Banks are not very open in these situations unless you have proper authorization or are dealing with a local bank where the manager knows your family. By law, banks can give out account information only to the owner of the account or the owner's legal proxy or guardian.

" During my mother's illness, I accumulated so much stuff—brochures from nursing homes, documents from lawyers, forms from Medicare, pamphlets from social service agencies. Every time I got something, I just tossed it into this giant box in my bedroom. Then whenever something came up, like when I wanted to get meals delivered to her while I was away, I would think, 'Oh yeah, I have something on that,' but I could never find it.

A friend came over one day and dumped out my box and started sorting through it. She spent the entire day organizing the whole mess.

That was the best thing anyone did for me during those two years. Not only could I find things quickly, but it made me feel better. I'd been feeling so out of control, and that gave me a little edge. It made an enormous difference."

—Terry B.

Exploring the Options

Don't wait until there is a crisis or you are completely frazzled to learn about community services and housing options. It will be too hard to do such research then, the options will be limited on short notice, and honestly, you should use such services long before you think you need them (because you need them long before you think you need them).

Starting Points

Your parent's doctor might know about some local services or should be able to direct you to someone who does. Friends who have been in a similar situation might also be helpful. Beyond that:

THE AREA AGENCY ON AGING is the best place to start. These agencies go by a medley of names—bureau on aging, council of senior services, commission on the elderly, and so on. You can find the one for your parent's town through the Eldercare Locator (eldercare.gov or 800-677-1116).

The agency will have information about many of the services, programs, and housing options available in your parent's community. Although you can get general leads from an agency's website, it's a good idea to call. A staff member should be able to answer specific questions about your parent's care.

LOCAL SENIOR CENTERS, COMMUNITY GROUPS, AND RELIGIOUS ORGANIZATIONS often offer or can refer you to local services, programs, volunteers, courses, and organizations.

A HOSPITAL'S DISCHARGE PLANNER or social services department is responsible for making sure that patients have the services they need when they leave the hospital. These caseworkers should know a great deal about the options in your parent's community. Some will offer guidance even if your parent is not in the hospital.

Be aware, however, that some hospitals have agreements with certain agencies and facilities, and thus the discharge planners might be biased.

EMPLOYEE ASSISTANCE PLANS at larger companies often provide information on eldercare. See what your workplace offers. Some can refer you to services in other areas, and others will put you in touch with a trained care manager who can guide you.

THE STATE LONG-TERM-CARE OMBUDSMAN'S OFFICE, which represents residents of nursing homes and their families, can give you information about local nursing homes and other types of housing for the elderly (ltcombudsman.org).

MEDICARE'S WEBSITE (medicare.gov) explains coverage and benefits and provides information about home care and housing options.

CAUTION ON THE WEB

Although there are a number of good websites on the topic of aging (see the ones listed in Useful Organizations on page 608), there are an abundance of useless ones and quite a few unsavory ones. Use the Internet with caution.

Care of the elderly is big business. Drug companies, insurance companies, medical supply companies, and others who are simply trying to sell something set up sites that appear to be reputable and unbiased—but aren't.

Several large sites that offer general caregiving help and free personal assistance get generous commissions for leading people to specific nursing and assisted living homes. Others tilt articles to appease advertisers. A good dose of skepticism should see you through.

A GERIATRIC CARE MANAGER can (for a price) assess your parent's needs and hook her up with local services or take over your parent's care almost entirely. You can find one through the National Association of Professional Geriatric Care Managers (caremanager.org).

ORGANIZATIONS FOR A PARTICULAR DISEASE often have local chapters that can direct you to services and programs near where you live. Some of these organizations are listed in the Resources section, starting on page 610. You can also get referrals to national organizations from the National Health Information Center (health.gov/nhic) or the National Rehabilitation Information Center (naric.com).

211. Many states have established human service information lines, which are contacted by dialing 211 (or visiting 211.org). Operators are trained to link people to social services and local programs.

Getting Organized

If you diligently write lists on scraps of paper and then misplace them, or if you're constantly remembering things that you shouldn't have forgotten in the first place, know that life is only going to get crazier now.

When a parent needs care, the reminders, names and numbers, appointments, bits of information, and to-do lists start pouring into your life like confetti. Organization is the only way you will survive this.

If you didn't start out organized, pull it together now. Really, an hour or two of work now will save you many hours and untold frustrations later. You'll find your own system, but here are a few possibilities to consider:

HAVE A PLAN B

If your parent depends upon one person for her care, have a contingency plan ready in case that person is suddenly unavailable. Be sure that someone can step in on short notice, or that your mother can go to a senior center, adult day care, someone else's house, or into a local senior residence for a temporary stay.

You don't want to be caught in dire straits when life takes an unexpected turn. And life with an elderly parent is apt to take unexpected turns.

❏ Once you have a master list of all essential names and phone numbers, create a "group" in your contact list that you can access from your phone, tablet, or a computer, anywhere at any time. (If your inner Luddite has kept you from such technology, do it the old-fashioned way, on a piece of paper or in an address book that you keep with you.) Have the most critical phone numbers on speed dial.

❏ Put your parent's medical information, passwords, and other critical information on a flash drive (that you carry with you) or in a document that can be accessed from any computer. A variety of apps allow you to do this, including Dropbox, Evernote, and Apple's Notes. Keep these files up to date!

❏ Set up an online calendar with all of your parent's appointments and schedule that others can access. There are many to choose among (Google Calendar, Yahoo Calendar, Apple's iCal, or Scrybe, to name a few.)

❏ Keep a log of your parent's medical care, either on the aforementioned calendar or in a separate document (see page 643). Include dates of treatments, when medications were started and stopped, instructions, and symptoms. Then you can tell a doctor when a symptom began or remind a nurse when a medication was started.

❏ Keep all other relevant information—documents, brochures, medical papers, and so on—in one location. Buy some folders and a file box, or an accordion file.

❏ Rather than scribbling errands on scraps of paper and leaving Post-its around the house, have a single to-do list that is accessible from your phone or computer.

❏ Download a scanner app to your cell phone so that you can scan important documents on the spot.

❏ Get your parent signed up for automatic deposits and automatic bill paying.

❏ If family and friends want to know the latest news, create a group email list, start a Facebook group, or use a web service such as CarePages (carepages .com) or Caring Bridge (caringbridge .org).

SIGNS THAT YOU NEED HELP

Don't wait for warning signs. If you are a primary caregiver, you need help. Period. Get siblings and other relatives, friends, volunteers, and professionals involved from the start.

Some signs that you need help urgently: You are angry, frustrated, short-tempered; not eating or eating constantly; not sleeping, unable to get out of bed; losing weight or gaining weight; sick, anxious, crying at odd moments; wishing you hadn't had that extra drink last night; or lashing out at your kids, your parent, your spouse, or anyone within earshot.

Contact the Eldercare Locator (eldercare.gov or 800-677-1116) to learn about local support services. Then use them.

WEBSITES THAT HELP YOU GET ORGANIZED

If a number of people are involved in your parent's care, sign on to a caregiver website. Although they are all a bit different—and evolving—the simplest ones let you organize contact lists and post news, photos, and messages. Most include a calendar where you can keep track of appointments and work shifts, and post tasks that need doing so others can volunteer to help. A few let you store medical and legal information, get updates from doctors (if they are inclined to use the site), and keep track of medications and symptoms.

These sites let everyone involved communicate about your parent's health, schedule, and needs. *Does anyone have a small shower seat? Can someone sit with Dad for a few hours on Friday night?*

Most sites have a free trial period and then charge some sort of fee. This is not a bad thing, as it generally means that they do not have advertisers, do not have a bias, and do not sell your information.

Of course, these sites are only as good as the people who use them. If people are diligent, then it's a great way to be sure others know what's what when you leave for a few days or to be sure that an aide gave Dad his evening pills.

It's a growing market, but here are a few sites to consider: Lotsa Helping Hands (lotsahelpinghands.com), Caring Bridge (caringbridge.org), CareZone (carezone.com), Saturing (saturing.com), and Tyze (tyze.com).

❏ Each time you call a home care agency, lawyer, or social worker, make a note about the call (on your incredibly organized calendar, perhaps), including the name of the person you spoke with and what you talked about, so you can refer to it later. *(But I spoke to Anne Preston on March 18, and she confirmed that the home health aide would start tomorrow.)*

❏ Whenever you make calls to agencies, doctors, and so on, have all the necessary information in front of you, with your questions written out. Otherwise, you may forget an important question and have to go through all the secretaries and recorded announcements again. When you get the information you're after, write it down so you can

relay it reliably to others. Get into the habit of asking for people's direct lines or extensions, and keep note of them.

❏ Confirm, confirm, confirm. It's better to confirm an appointment the week and/or day before than to find out that your father's physical therapist has taken an unscheduled vacation and his assistant forgot to cancel his appointments.

❏ Make copies of important papers—receipts, insurance claims, nursing home applications—before handing them over or putting them in the mail.

❏ If the days slip away from you try writing a detailed schedule to help you organize your time and use it more efficiently. You might not adhere to it precisely, but it will help structure your day so you are not constantly thinking, *I've got to get to the grocery store. I can't believe I forgot to call the Social* *Security office. Wasn't someone supposed to pick up Mom's walker?* The task—or the breather you so desperately need—will already be assigned to a time slot.

When You Can't Be There

If you live far away or are busy at work, you have to be extra organized. You must plan ahead because you don't have the luxury of responding immediately to a crisis. What are you going to do when you're at work, two hundred miles away, and you get a call that your father has taken a turn for the worse and needs help?

At least a third of all family caregivers care from afar. They live at least an hour away and usually four or more hours away. About half of caregivers work either full-time or part-time.

Not being with an elderly parent day in and day out can make life easier in some ways, but it increases the burden in others. The cost of travel, phone calls, and hired help can be hefty of course, but it's the worrying and guilt that can be unbearable. *Is she all right? How will I know if she isn't? Should I book a flight? Should I take time off from work?*

Forget the guilt trip, but do make the most of your visits. Now more than ever, organization and preparation are the keys to your success—and your survival.

Take another good look at what's been discussed so far in this chapter. Here are a few additional tips for organizing from a distance:

- Have all important phone numbers — doctor, lawyer, aides, and so on—with you at all times.

- Be sure that your parent, her doctor, and anyone involved in her care know how to reach you.

- Check out local services and facilities well in advance.

- Sign her up for any helpful services as soon as you think they might be of use.

- Establish a local support network. Make a list of friends, family, or neighbors who live near your parent. Let these people know of your concern. They can alert you to signs of trouble and help out in a crunch.

- Have the name and number of a local handyman. (A pipe just burst in your mother's house. Who are you going to call?)

- Leave a duplicate of your parent's house key (or code to a security system) with a trusted neighbor or friend, and/or hide one outside her house in case there is an emergency and someone needs to get in.

- Get your parent hooked up to the Internet so she can communicate with you and others. You can find laptops and tablets that are very simple. Also set her up with Skype or another video chat service. This way, you can see your parent as well as hear her, which will help you spot problems. You might connect while you cook or your family eats dinner so your parent can be a part of things. It's no work for you, and it will make her feel less isolated.

- Organize your visits in advance so you can accomplish as much as possible. If you need to meet with a doctor or lawyer, set up the appointment at least a month in advance, as their schedules fill quickly.

- When you are with your parent, try to identify possible problems. Is her gait unsteady? Has her weight, hygiene, or temperament changed? Are her bills piling up? Is her food spoiled? Is she getting out and doing things? Is she asking you to repeat yourself and forgetting important information? Be alert to signs of depression, infection, dementia, waning eyesight or hearing, and other ailments.

- Even though your life is busy, try to spend some time simply being with your parent, chatting, watching a movie, shopping, or just sitting quietly. A trip that's all business misses a critical element.

- Learn to distinguish real emergencies from unfounded complaints. It's okay to say that you can't come right now, that you were just there last week. Reassure her without feeling guilty.

(Be aware that unending complaints and requests for reassurance may be an early sign of dementia; if this is a new habit, talk to her doctor.)

- If your parent lives alone and doesn't get out much, see if a relative or friend will stop by occasionally. A local church, senior center, or religious organization might know of volunteers who can check on your parent. Or you can hire a companion. If your parent has in-home care or lives in a nursing home or other institution, it is still important that someone check in on her regularly.

- Buy your parent an emergency response system (see page 120) so she can get help immediately if she falls or is injured.

- Although the Internet is amazing, sometimes it's handy to have a copy of the phone book or yellow pages from your parent's hometown to look up a home care agency, say, or track down a particular doctor.

- When things get unwieldy (preferably *before* they get unwieldy), consider hiring a geriatric care manager, or find out if a local agency offers subsidized care management. A manager can assess your parent's needs, organize local services, handle emergencies, and keep you up to date.

- Above all, take care of yourself. Recognize and accept the limits of what you can do, and give yourself credit for all you are doing. Don't hesitate to ask for help or use community services. And get support from friends or a professional counselor to help you alleviate stress and guilt.

Adapting to New Roles

Chapter 2

Your Parent and You

A Changing Relationship • When They Won't Listen •
Defusing Old Struggles • Coping Day to Day • Exceptionally
Difficult Parents

Parent-child relationships are, to say the least, complex. Your father may be critical, distant, or domineering. Your mother may make you feel guilty, embarrass you, or smother you. The traits we dislike in them we fight in ourselves.

Long after we think we have outgrown the parent-child power dance, sometimes after years of therapy, a casual comment or a certain look can trigger a familiar surge of adrenaline.

When a parent grows frail and dependent, bonds can grow stronger, but tensions can also intensify. This is the paradox of parentcare. On one hand, the prospect of losing your parent makes this time precious. On the other hand, you are so entangled in each other's lives that problems are unavoidable. The issues on the table—her health, finances, housing—are laborious, painful, and sometimes contentious. And your roles—who is in charge, who is the parent—have been irrevocably altered.

Thrown into this partnership with little warning and few options, both caregiver and care recipient are likely to have moments of feeling resentful, uncertain, and, sometimes for no discernible reason, just plain crabby.

You can't change your parent, especially not at her age, but you can define the scope of your duties so that you protect your own sanity while also helping her. You can also try to see things through her eyes and adjust your expectations and reactions, which should ease daily tensions. Together this should help you form not an entirely different relationship with your parent, but a more peaceful one.

A Changing Relationship

When a parent grows frail, roles shift, sometimes uncomfortably. Who is in charge? How much should you intervene? Are you the parent now?

It's completely natural to have a get-it-done approach to this, to want to check things off your list and move onward. But sometimes a parent gets lost in the process.

> " No matter how difficult she is or how much we disagree, I can't shut her out. Never. It would be like shutting something in myself out. She needs me now tremendously.
>
> There must be something so deep in the relationship between mothers and daughters, more than we can ever realize. We're so connected, even when we're so different."
>
> —Betty H.

As you consider this task and your relationship with your parent, it's useful to examine your role, his role, and his best interests.

Are You Parenting Your Parent?

It is a common thought and one that is hard to avoid, especially if you are changing diapers, tying shoelaces, or dealing with irrational outbursts. But regardless of the circumstances, the answer is a flat-out no. You are not parenting your parent.

If your mother is no longer able to care for herself, you will have new responsibilities, ones that often resemble those of parenting. But you have not simply switched places. Your parent may have grown sick—she may be extremely frail and dependent—but she has not become a child.

That's not to say that you shouldn't use the same tricks that help in parenting—diversions to get her onto a new subject, a baby monitor so you can hear trouble, waterproof pads for incontinence. You should. But allowing yourself to think that the roles have reversed, that you are now the parent and your parent is a child, is a potentially disastrous way to look at this situation—for both of you.

For your parent, it is dehumanizing to be treated as a child, to be nagged, scolded, or bossed around, even if it's done in subtle ways. No matter how disease and age might have altered your parent's body or mind, no matter how much you are doing for her, she is an adult and deserves to be treated as one. She has a lifetime of experience and a wealth of time-tested opinions. She has earned her autonomy, respect, and pride. She might have reverted to childish ways, but that does not make her a child.

For you, reversing the roles will lead only to dead ends and frustration. After all, children grow and learn and, for the most part, do what their parents tell them to do. If you try to parent your parent as you would a child, without

perceiving the vast differences in the two situations, you will beat yourself up wondering why you are having such trouble with the task and be angry with your parent for not behaving as you want her to. *Why doesn't she listen to me?*

If you behave as an adult and treat your parent as an adult—an aged and frail adult who needs your respect, as well as your care—both of you will fare better.

> " Now that my mother's dementia is worse, she's given up and wants me to take over. I have to help her dress and get her to day care and feed her. It's gotten to the point now that if someone asks her a question, she'll answer but look to me to make sure it's right.
>
> Sometimes I get so frustrated and tired that I yell at her. I tell her what to do and then get mad when she doesn't do it right. And then I feel awful and I think, 'What in the world is happening here?'
>
> I have to keep reminding myself over and over that she's my mother and I love her dearly and I respect her. But it's hard."
> —Linda K.

REMEMBER THE GOOD OLD DAYS

If your parent is quite ill, if he has gotten crotchety in his old age, or if dementia has distorted his personality, find a photo from when he was younger—a photo of him at his best, a photo of him holding you when you were a child, a photo of him strong and well. Or put together a collage of photos. Then put it on your refrigerator or your desk, where you will see it often.

It should help you remember better times, when he was stronger. It should help you recall the father who hugged you, laughed with you, and taught you things. It should help you remember why you are doing so much for him now.

Foster Independence

You should not only avoid parenting your parent, but if possible go a step further and reinforce any independence that remains. Rather than cleaning his room, making his lunch, and getting him dressed, find a way for your parent to do things for himself. Rather than completely taking over his finances and legal affairs, keep him at the helm as much as possible, or at least make him feel that he still has some control.

Your job is not to control your parent's life, but to help him maintain as much control as possible.

Of course you want to say, *Stay there; I'll get it for you.* But movement, any movement at all, is good for his body. Mental stimulation, even if it's simple, can keep his mind running more smoothly and ward off depression.

More than anything else, a sense of autonomy is good for his soul. Your parent might welcome your help, but when elderly people are constantly catered to, when they no longer make their own decisions, when they are treated as needy and helpless, they only grow more needy and helpless, and often lose their spirit and drive.

Help your parent hang on to whatever abilities and independence he still has. Help him to help himself, whenever possible. Of course, this might mean more work for you—you may have to wait while he struggles to put on his pants or clean up after he spills the juice—but if he's able to give it a go, it is a great gift to him to get him to try.

Offer Respect

It's so easy when a parent becomes dependent to slip into a certain level of disrespect. She can't do simple things, she can't think clearly, and you might be taking on some pretty awful assignments; whatever respect you had for her is fading fast.

Don't beat yourself up. It's natural to be curt right now. But step back occasionally and rethink your approach.

Try not to boss your parent around or talk to her as if she were three. And never talk about her as if she were not in the room. Instead, make an effort to be civil and treat her with respect. Whatever her ability, give her choices and listen to her views. Protect her privacy and her dignity.

It will make her feel better, and oddly, it might make you feel better too.

So rather than snapping, *I told you to drink that Ensure! What's the matter with you? We have to go!* try, *Mom, we need to leave for the doctor's office. Do you want to bring that drink with you or have it later?*

Ask that others treat your parent with respect as well. If you witness behaviors on the part of a caregiver that you think are demeaning, talk with the caregiver. Give him or her specific suggestions for protecting your parent's dignity.

For example, caregivers might call your parent by a formal name if that is what he or she is used to—Mr. Hughes, Dr. Johnston, Mrs. Weber—not "Hon" or "Sweetie" (unless, of course, your parent likes that). They should place towels strategically when helping with a bath or caring for a wound. They should explain things at all times, telling your parent what they are doing even if your parent doesn't seem to hear or understand. (*I'm going to comb your hair now. I'm going to wipe your face and neck with a warm washcloth, okay?*)

" My mother was very sick, so I brought her to the hospital, and the doctor ordered some X-rays. They had taken her clothes off, and she was so weak that I had to hold her up. Her body, which used to be so strong and lean, was thin, her skin was loose, and I could feel her bones. I was holding her little body in my arms, and there was a great poignancy, a closeness, which I was so happy about. She was finally trusting me to care for her. She wasn't fighting me.

On that day, I felt what I had always wanted to feel with her. It was like a pouring out of tenderness."

—Betty H.

LOVE AND AGGRAVATION

You are doing so much for your parent. Why isn't he more appreciative? Why does he argue and criticize rather than thank you?

The truth is, he probably does appreciate what you're doing, more than you know and certainly more than he lets on. But here's the problem:

He's lost his freedom and autonomy. His life has been altered in ways he's not happy about. And although it isn't completely logical, those losses are connected to you.

So even though he might appreciate that you have opened your home to him, he's also angry that he had to leave his home and has to live with you. He might appreciate that you are helping him with his bath, but also feel angry that you have to help.

As hard as it is, know that he is grateful—even though he might not say it—and know that most complaints are not really about you at all.

Put Yourself in His Shoes

We know what it is to be children, teenagers, adults. Heck, most of us know what it's like to be middle aged. When we deal with rebellious teenagers, we might get annoyed, but we also understand because we have faint memories of what it was to be them.

But we do not have any idea what it is like to be our parents.

We have no idea what it feels like to be 85, to have diabetes, limited hearing, and a walker. We have no idea how it feels to look in the mirror and see not simply wrinkles, but a wisp of our former selves. We don't know how it feels to lose a spouse, friends, colleagues. Or how it feels to not simply stop working, but to lose our ability to work, to take care of ourselves, to tend to our homes, to take care of our own finances—to lose, perhaps, the ability to get ourselves dressed, or fed, or to the toilet. We haven't been there. We have no idea.

We can pretend for a moment. We can put on scratched glasses and glue toilet paper tubes to each lens so that we see, faintly, only what is directly in front of us. We can plug our ears with cotton so conversations are lost, and wrap our knees so tightly with bandages that walking is difficult and stairs are impossible. We can breathe through a straw so each breath requires effort. We can plug our noses so our favorite foods taste bland.

But we still don't know what it is, because our parents, even at their age, have hurts and hopes that we can't begin to understand. They have an acceptance that we haven't tasted, challenges we haven't faced, and joys that we haven't experienced.

And they come from a different time, when people didn't tweet, go to therapy, or rely on 15-minute meals. Many have lived through a world war, a depression, and segregation.

Your father might not understand your wish that he emote openly because he was brought up to believe that strong men don't do that. He might close the door on conversations about money because when he grew up, it was in bad taste to discuss such things.

So when you can't bear it another minute, when you lose your patience, when you want your parent to behave a certain way or do what you say, take a moment to remember that you don't know what it feels like to walk in his shoes.

Be Nice; You're Next

Hard to imagine, but true. How will you feel when your children tell you what to do, when those you raised think they know what's best for you and take control? How would you want your children and others to treat you if you were at this point in life?

Be nice because, in fact, you are next.

When They Won't Listen

Your father won't move out of his home, even though it is clearly unsafe for him to stay. Your mother is blind as Mr. Magoo, but refuses to stop driving. Your parent won't sign a power of attorney, let aides into the house, or relinquish the gardening chores.

It's enough to make a person scream.

Unfortunately, the need to protect your parent's autonomy can collide with the need to look out for his safety and welfare. So what do you do?

Taking Charge

Regardless of your mother's wishes, you have to take the helm if she is severely confused or compromised, or if she can

no longer understand options, make a rational decision, or communicate her views. (See page 378 for information on competency and guardianship.)

You also have to step in aggressively if your parent is being exploited, neglected, harmed, or mistreated. Contact the local office of Adult Protective Services, which you can find through the National Center on Elder Abuse (ncea.aoa.gov).

And finally, you have to act if someone else's safety or health is threatened. Specifically, if your parent is driving recklessly, you have to get her out of the car. You also have to act if your father's sudden rages or your mother's drinking threaten a caregiver or household member.

WEIGHING COMPETENCE

The question of when to intervene can get tricky when a person lingers in the gray area between competence and incompetence.

Say your mother is handing out chunks of cash to "that nice aide" or your father suddenly decides to change his will. What if your parent says one thing to you and something entirely different to your brother, or is lucid in the morning but becomes muddled in the afternoon?

If you face a troubling situation and don't know if your parent is competent or how much to intervene, talk with her doctor or get an assessment. (See page 378 for more on competency.)

Compromising

If your parent is largely competent and no one else's safety is at stake, your role is less obvious. Your duty to protect your parent might be superseded by his right to make his own decisions.

ASSESS YOUR CONCERNS. Why do you think your parent should do things your way? Why shouldn't she, for example, stay in her own home, shovel her own driveway, or save her money under her mattress? What are the risks? How serious are they? Can they be reduced?

When you think about the problem, focus on your parent's needs, not yours. Do you want your parent to move for her sake or because it will be easier for you? When it comes to her money, are you concerned about her financial security or worried about your own inheritance? Refocus your thoughts on what is best for your parent and what she needs and wants.

LISTEN TO HER VIEWS. Don't just assume you know better or that she's not playing with a full deck of cards. Why doesn't she want to move? What

does she like about her current living arrangement? What does she fear? How does she envision her future? Listen to her thoughts and reasoning. Try to understand how she sees the situation.

Maybe your parent is willing to take certain risks. Maybe cleaning the gutters is the only way your father feels valuable. Maybe your mother has reasons for not trusting that lawyer. Maybe she doesn't take the pills because of side effects that you don't know about.

DISCUSS THE PROS AND CONS. Perhaps your mother simply doesn't know that if she trips on the stairs and breaks a hip, it could land her in a nursing home or even kill her. Maybe she hasn't thought about how a move might provide her with companionship and activity. Maybe she doesn't understand how much money she needs for her future care or that the sweepstakes is a scam.

Be sure your parent fully understands the risks involved.

EXPLORE THE OPTIONS. Let your parent know that you heard her, and then explore some options and compromises.

If she can't manage the stairs and doesn't want to move, perhaps her bedroom can be moved to the first floor. If she can't shop and cook for herself, maybe she can have meals delivered. If she wants to drive, maybe she can limit it to local, daytime driving, and only in good weather.

BE CLEAR ABOUT YOUR LIMITS. If your parent's actions or inactions affect your life, be clear about what you can and can't do for him. In other words, if your father refuses to let strangers in the house or to attend day care, be clear about how much help you can offer and what you cannot do for him.

Don't be bullied into taking on more than you can handle simply because your parent refuses to use local services.

REQUEST A TRIAL PERIOD. If you want your parent to move and she won't, see if she will try it for a brief time. If your father flat out refuses to have an aide in the house, ask him to try it for, say, two weeks. *Dad, please try this for me, and if it fails, I'll drop it.*

GET OTHERS INVOLVED. If you hit a wall, get others in the family involved, as well as your parent's doctor, lawyer, or anyone else whom your parent respects. Sometimes a suggestion sounds different coming from a new voice.

It's maddening, of course, to suggest something a dozen times to no avail and then have your mother quickly agree (*What a good idea!*) when your brother makes the exact same suggestion. Oh well. Let it go. At least it worked.

HIRE AN INTERMEDIARY. A trained professional who is familiar with the issues and local landscape can listen to all the views, offer new suggestions, and ideally, facilitate a compromise. To find a mediator, contact the National Association of Professional Geriatric Care Managers (caremanager.org), the area agency on aging (eldercare.gov), or the Association for Conflict Resolution (acrnet.org).

Backing Off

After all of this, if your parent is competent and her actions are not endangering others, the final decision is hers. Not what you want to hear, but true.

All of us make decisions about personal health, finances, and safety every day, and some of these decisions are bad ones. Perfectly competent people

----

" My mother had a stroke about a year ago that left her very unsteady. She needed a cane to get around, and climbing stairs was almost impossible for her. Nonetheless, she started going back to her old routines almost immediately. She lives in the city and loves the theater, the opera, going out with her friends. I was worried sick. It was winter and the sidewalks were slippery, and I was afraid she was going to fall or have another stroke.

She got around pretty well with the help of friends. I began to realize that for her to stay in her apartment, to sit alone and watch television, would be a fate worse than death. My mother is going to get out and do things as long as she is alive. That's her nature. I worry, but I respect her immensely for it. I hope I have her gusto when I'm her age."

—Fran M.

text while they drive, smoke cigarettes, go bungee jumping, and make silly investments.

Your parent, even at her advanced age, retains the right to take risks—even ones that are foolhardy. When you are her age you will have the same rights, and you will be allowed to make your own decisions, despite the better judgment of your children.

Keep in mind that your parent is basing her decisions on different criteria than you are. Your only concern might be her health and safety, but at this point in her life she may place greater value on familiar routines, companionship, and independence.

You might worry because your mother insists on taking a morning walk and refuses to use her cane, even though she's tripped a couple of times, but for her, that walk, on her own, without a cane, is what makes life worth living.

> " Very late one night, I saw an elderly man I knew getting off the train. He was very frail, and I was astonished to see that he was not only traveling alone, but that no one was there to meet him at the station. I took him home in a taxi, and he seemed very grateful.
>
> I was furious at his kids, affluent people whom I knew slightly, for letting him travel on his own at that hour. I hated to think what might have happened to him, alone in the city.
>
> A few years later, when my own father became old and frail, he insisted on traveling on his own. He wouldn't put up with our telling him that it wasn't safe, and we finally realized that we couldn't cover his activities in a way that made us feel secure. I understood the man's kids for the first time and felt foolish that I'd been so self-righteous and critical. What can you do? You have to contain your anxiety. You have no choice."
>
> —Sara B.

WHOSE LIFE IS THIS, ANYWAY?

Early on, when a parent is newly ill or suddenly widowed, adult children often jump in with both feet to help. They discuss their parent's care and make a plan.

But when they present this grand plan, Dad is angry. He feels betrayed that discussions were held without his input, as if he were simply a problem that needed a solution.

His children are hurt that he is not happy about a plan they have worked

so hard to develop, and annoyed that he refuses to do what is clearly best.

Always keep in mind that your parent is still an adult and, unless he is severely incompetent, still in control of his own life. He doesn't need anyone making decisions for him—and certainly not without him.

If you are concerned about an aspect of your parent's life, express your concerns, but don't instruct him. Keep him at the center of all discussions about his future. It is his life, after all.

Likewise, your father might be willing to accept enormous risks in order to stay in his own home. Or he might be unwilling to give up cigarettes. Or he may not tell the doctor about a serious issue because he has no interest in the surgery that would be required. Or he might be more interested in living fully than in living longer.

Understanding your parent's point of view will help you let go of futile battles.

The fact is, you are wasting your energy and probably not helping your parent by pushing and pushing. For your own sake, as much as your parent's, let it go. At least for now.

Make other arrangements whenever possible. Do what you can to reduce any risk. Find other options. And then, as difficult as it may be, live with her decision.

In time, raise the issue again. See if her thoughts have changed.

Defusing Old Struggles

Parent-child relationships are loaded, even when the parent is well into her 90s and the "child" is in her 70s. The issues don't fade, and at times like this, they can be magnified.

Even close relationships come with buttons and nagging questions. *Why does she irritate me so much? Why does he set me off like this? Why does he say things like that?*

Although family therapy can be great, this might not be the time to try to sort through a deep bin of emotions with your parent. He needs help. You're a wreck. And time is running out. It's all you can do to get from one day to the next.

But a little insight and a couple of coping tips might help you find a little peace, patience, and forgiveness.

PINPOINT THE PROBLEM. What is it that troubles you about your parent and the way you relate to him? What is it

that you want and are not getting? What exasperates you, and why does it affect you so much?

Think carefully about this. Try to be precise. Does your parent's personality bother you because it is grating, because it has stood in the way of your being close, or because you see the same trait in yourself? Do you withdraw from your

> " My mother is very dependent, and always has been, but she never says thank you or shows any appreciation or cares that she is putting you out. I once said to her, 'Mom, don't you realize what you are putting us through? Don't you realize the anxiety and worry that you cause?' And she said, 'That's your problem.'
>
> I had to laugh at that. I mean, she's your mother. What are you going to do?"
> —Rhoda B.

mother's helplessness because it places too much of a burden on you or because it has caused you to become painfully self-sufficient? Do you cringe because of the way your father behaves now or because you still feel wounded by something he did in the past? Do you resent your parent for needing your help, or is the root of your anguish your parent's continuing power over you?

TACKLE SOME ISSUES. If your parent is relatively healthy and able to take part, and there is a specific issue you want to deal with—a recurring argument or an unresolved conflict—go ahead and try. You might get somewhere, but even if you don't, you will find some peace of mind in knowing that you tried, that you spoke your mind.

Keep your expectations low. If the subject is taboo or deeply painful, you might want to do this with a therapist who specializes in family relationships. However you choose to handle it, here are a few thoughts that might help:

- Bring up the topic at a time when you are calm. Instead of jumping into a heated discussion just when your mother has said the one thing that exasperates you, wait until the emotional climate is more temperate.

- Be composed. If you are confrontational or accusatory, you will put your parent on the defensive. Stay calm.

- Use statements that begin with *I* rather than those that begin with *you.* So instead of saying, *You are never satisfied. No matter what I do, you're not happy with it. All you do is complain,* try, *I feel unappreciated. I work so hard and yet I feel that nothing I do is enough.*

> 66 She's been a wonderful grandmother to my children. That's why I can forgive her and why I can do this."
> —Carla M.

- Ask her if she ever felt this way around anyone, and if so, how she handled it. What was her mother like? What sort of relationship did they have?

- Avoid old arguments. Steer the conversation away from familiar eddies with a history of going nowhere. As soon as you sense things slipping into old patterns, change the topic.

LET GO OF UNREALISTIC HOPES. There will be issues, especially those having to do with your parent's personality, current needs, or past events, that you can't change.

Personality traits tend to become more fixed later in life. For some reason this seems to be particularly true of less desirable traits. Someone who is gentle, giving, and selfless might become more saintly as the years pass, but more often someone who is trying will become very difficult indeed.

Unfortunately, a parent who has never asked you about your life or your feelings is not apt to get to know you now. A parent who endlessly criticizes and instructs is unlikely to stop now. A parent who has been needy may become more helpless. And a parent who has avoided a specific topic for a lifetime will be hard-pressed to venture into painful territory at this stage of life.

Of course, somewhere in your logical mind, you know all this, but accepting it can be wrenching. All of us want to have a loving bond with our parents

> " After my father died, I found his old letters and journals, and as I read them, I realized that there was this whole other side of him that I never knew, a sensitive and caring and emotional side that he never, even once, revealed to me. It makes me sad because I keep thinking, if only I had known this part of him, we might have had a very different relationship."
>
> —Alicia B.

that is based on mutual respect and trust. Accepting that such a person or such a tie will never exist, at least not in the way you believe it should, is almost like accepting the death of your parent—the parent you had hoped for and the parent you can never have.

Recognizing this might leave you feeling intensely alone, and perhaps betrayed. But accepting, and then mourning, this loss allows you to move on. Once you let go of unrealistic goals and accept what really is, you can stop struggling to make this relationship into something it isn't. And once you stop looking to your parent for approval and validation, you are free to get these things from yourself.

Ironically, when you no longer have high expectations, you might find that your relationship with your parent develops new strengths. You may notice qualities in your parent that you never saw before. Without that old tension, your parent may be able to appreciate certain qualities

in you. You may find that you actually enjoy what is, rather than constantly feeling cheated by what isn't.

LEARN ABOUT HIM. Sometimes we expect our parents to understand and respect us for who we are, but fail to give them the same courtesy. While there is still time—if there is still time—get to know your parent.

Ask your father about his life—his parents, his childhood, his schooling, his friends, and his loves. Ask him about his dreams, travels, successes, failures, challenges, hardships, and role models.

Get him to tell you stories he's never told you or to add new details to the old stories. Next time he begins a story that you've heard many times before, rather than rolling your eyes in exasperation, nudge him to tell a different angle of the story, or ask why that moment in time was so important to him.

SOMETHING UNEXPECTED

Every now and then, jump off the treadmill and do something unexpected with your parent.

When you're leaving the doctor's office and heading back to the nursing home, veer off to the park, find a spot in the sun, and have a banana split. When you should be making dinner and starting her bath, forget it. Call it a night, make some popcorn, and turn on a movie. Forget the physical therapy for a day; take him down to watch the fishermen at the dock.

Do something that has nothing to do with medicine, doctors, or paperwork. Spend time with your parent doing something you both enjoy. Break the rules. Have fun.

While you are at it, get him to talk about his current situation. Perhaps he is grieving or afraid of the future. Is growing old what he thought it would be? What makes him happy now?

Hearing about your parent's past, getting to know what makes him who he is, understanding something about how he feels now—all this should help you to see your parent as an individual.

It won't change what has happened, but it might help you let go of some anger and be more forgiving. It might give you a little more patience and tolerance.

Learning about him like this will likely also take conversations in directions that you never expected.

If your parent is able and willing to open up, these talks should be enjoyable for him too. Not only does he get to talk about himself, which is glorious, but he also gets to pass his stories on to future generations.

STOP BLAMING. Okay, easier said than done. But the fact is, whatever your father did in the past is done. He probably intended to be a good parent, just as you want to be a good parent to your own children. If you need an apology, or if it would make you feel better if you told him what you are feeling, then discuss the subject, but do it carefully.

Not only is the past over, but you both have a lot of other issues to deal with now. Once you've said what you needed to say, do what you can to move forward—to take that hurt, package it, seal it, and put it away. It won't be forgotten, but it won't be part of your daily life either.

IMPROVE THYSELF. Even though your parent may not be able or willing to change, you still can. Work on your own personality and relationships. Learn from his mistakes and be more open, honest, loving, or tolerant yourself.

Coping Day to Day

Moving from the big picture to the small, if your parent has a trait or habit that makes your chest tighten and your shoulders tense, there are steps you can take, day to day, to ease the stress and lower your blood pressure.

Be sure to read Chapter 3, "Caring for the Caregiver," as your own stress and resentment will trigger conflict.

PAUSE BEFORE RESPONDING. When your parent does or says something that's

abrasive, count to 10 before responding. Take a deep breath, and then exhale slowly as you count. That brief pause will help you stay calm and give you a moment to consider your response. If she demands that you say something, simply answer that you're thinking about what she's said. It might just make her think about what she said, too.

PASS BY THE HOOKS. Sometimes it isn't the big stuff, but the little stuff—a passing comment or look—that triggers a flood of emotion. Then you wonder what is wrong with you that you are so angry. Feeling bad about your reaction, you become even angrier.

For example, "That roast needs another 30 minutes" doesn't seem like the most awful thing for someone to say. However, when your mother has been instructing you on how to live your life for 60 years and now, at the end of a very long day, she is telling you how to cook a roast when you've cooked dozens of roasts just fine, well, that small comment can make you want to thump someone with the nearest frying pan.

Of course, getting angry, yelling at her, or just stewing for the rest of the evening doesn't help at all.

Find ways to ignore those comments that make you so hopping mad. Pretend you are a fish swimming along a mountain stream on a beautiful day and you spot a fat, scrumptious worm. It lures you, but you are no dummy. You know that there's a big, sharp hook behind it. You have two choices: Bite at the hook and get hurt, or swim on by and enjoy your day.

Next time your parent says something that makes your blood pressure rise, say to yourself, *Aha, I know what that is. That is a hook, and as much as I am drawn to it, I will not bite.* Swim on by.

Count how many hooks you pass by when you are with her (one is awfully good) and then try to do better the next time. It will be your own inner victory.

FINDING THE REWARDS

Caring for an aging parent is trying, without a doubt. However, there are rewards. This is, after all, your parent, and no matter how he might infuriate you, no matter how he might have erred in his role as parent, and no matter how much you must do for him now, no one will ever love you in quite the same way, and in truth, you will never love anyone else in this way.

Helping him now is an opportunity to reciprocate some of that love and attention. It is a chance to say, during quiet moments, things that you might not have said otherwise, and to care for him in tender ways that you never have before. Caring for your parent allows you to reaffirm family bonds and, in some cases, to strengthen those bonds.

Of course, these rewards may be hard to see or even imagine when you are in the thick of it. But when they come, cherish them. If you get a word of thanks, remember it. When there is some closeness, make a note of it. These are the moments that will get you through.

With each hook you pass, unfazed and unaffected, you win.

FORGET VICTORY. Instead of trying to win a fight with your parent, make it your goal simply to end the discussion peacefully. That will be a true triumph. Rather than saying, once again, *Why do you always bring up that same story? Why can't you just let it go?* ignore it. If you don't react at all, she might just stop telling the story or making that annoying comment.

RECOGNIZE YOUR HABITS. How do you typically react to problems in this relationship? Do you become angry and combative? Do you withdraw? Do you throw yourself into your work? Or take it out on other people? Or head straight for the nearest quart of ice cream?

Once you're aware of your reaction, you will be better prepared to alter it. If you typically snap at your children or shut out your friends after a visit with your parent, make a concerted effort to avoid those habits.

HEAD FOR NEW GROUND. If you find yourself falling into the same uncomfortable or annoying ruts with your parent, change the pattern. Play cards, go for a walk, talk about something new, or plan your visits for a different place and time. If you always visit in the evening when your parent is tired or has had a drink, stop by in the morning instead. If you always visit in her bedroom, take her into the living room or go out for lunch. A change of scene might do both of you some good.

REWARD YOURSELF. Ignoring the hooks, staying calm, avoiding old fights, and generally being more tolerant are no small feats. They require enormous patience and personal strength. Reward yourself for a job well done. Buy yourself a little present, treat yourself to a bubble bath, take a drive in the country, immerse yourself in some activity that has nothing to do with your parent and her illness.

INTRODUCE YOUR PARENT TO YOU, the adult. If you constantly fall into the childhood role you played in the family, pull your parent into your adulthood. If she is mobile, take her with you to your office or bring her to a local meeting in which you are involved. It's easier to be you, and not a child, on your own turf.

If she is less mobile, introduce her to your friends, show her your latest business report or artwork. Let her see you as an adult, be firm in your resolve to act

WHAT DOES SHE WANT FROM ME?

You have just spent the entire day racing around your parent's house, doing her laundry, changing the sheets, preparing her pillbox, and fixing her dinner. Two days later she laments that you never visit. What's a daughter to do?

It might be that your parent doesn't want more of your time, just more of you. That is, your company and affection might be more important to her than clean socks and hot meals. So while you are busy as a bee, she is feeling ignored. Later, she wonders why she never sees you because the truth is, she hasn't seen you.

The dilemma is that these tasks have to be done, and truth be told, it might be easier to be in the kitchen cooking than in the living room sitting with your mother.

Find a compromise—a little time in the laundry room, a little time with her. Or talk with her while you fold the laundry. You might let her know how much time you have and ask how she would like you to spend it.

By addressing her most fundamental needs for companionship and affection, you will be giving her an important gift, and you might head off some of the I-never-see-you laments.

> *Mom never has been lovable, and she never will be. She says things that are hurtful. She does it to all of us, but it's worse with me. She feels comfortable with me so she just lets it rip.*
>
> *I yell in my car. I call my girlfriends and unload.*
>
> *I love her, but I don't always like her."*
> —Suzanne W.

as an adult, and she might start to think of you as one and treat you accordingly.

ADJUST YOUR EXPECTATIONS. Not just your grand expectations about this relationship, but your hopes about each visit, holiday gatherings, and family togetherness. Lower your expectations to as close to zero as possible. If you envision your family as a Norman Rockwell painting, you are doomed to disappointment.

Likewise, if you approach your parent's door poised for a fight, it will probably happen. Family arguments can be ignited simply because you are primed for them. When there's the slightest trigger, you explode.

When you visit, keep your mind open and let things go as they will. Enjoy what's good and try not to make too much of the bad.

GET SUPPORT. Talk with friends, join a support group, find an online chat room. Unload. Getting feedback and support and knowing that others cope with similar issues will certainly ease the pain.

RESORT TO HUMOR. Humor is the great defuser. When things head into a familiar impasse, tell him a funny story. Watch a good comedy together. Read humorous books aloud. Laughing together will break a few prickly barriers.

MAKE NOTE OF THE GOOD TIMES. When you have a wonderful visit or a moment of closeness, share a warm hug, or receive a rare word of praise or thanks, don't sell it short. Believe it. Remember it.

MEDITATE. Take 10 minutes each day to sit quietly, soothe your soul, and find your strength. Feel the tension drain out of you with each slow breath. Find your inner calm.

Exceptionally Difficult Parents

There is no scale for rating difficulty when it comes to eldercare. Who has the most challenging parent? What situation is most taxing? Everyone's struggle is different.

Nevertheless, some parents are doozies. They refuse to accept any help, or demand constant attention. No matter what you do, they criticize and complain constantly. The aides stink. The food stinks. Life stinks. And they want you to know it, over and over again.

Sometimes they are awash in contradictions. A parent might lament that he doesn't want to be a burden, but then insist that you do everything for him. Or your mother is endlessly wishing that she would die, but is scrupulous about taking her medications and making doctor's appointments. You father cries because of loneliness, but then turns down dinner invitations.

Then there is the parent who was neglectful, abusive, alcoholic, and/or estranged. How do you care for someone who never cared for you, who was, and might still be, callous or cruel?

Many of the tips already offered in this chapter should be of use, but following are a few additional thoughts. Dealing with parents who suffer from depression, paranoia, anxiety disorders, and other mental illnesses is discussed in Chapter 13.

Complaints and Criticism

As suggested, try your best to stay calm, avoid the hooks, and take a moment to breathe before responding. A tall order, for sure, but you do not want to become a bickering, bitter person. Rise above it. Your calm, deliberate response might catch your parent off guard; she was looking for a fight, and you've taken the wind out of her disgruntled sails.

DISCERN THE REASONS. Think about what might be behind your parent's grievances.

Your mother says she hates your clothes, but it might be because they remind her that you used to go shopping together, and now she can't do that, or because she can no longer wear clothes that have small buttons. Your father says

you don't visit enough, but it might be because he is lonely and afraid of being abandoned.

REFRAME THE CONVERSATION. If you are constantly arguing or repeatedly reassuring her—*It's okay, Mom, you're not a burden*—find a new approach.

When she moans about being a burden, rather than reassuring her again that she isn't a burden, ask her why she feels like a burden. Or talk to her about what is most difficult for you and ways to ease the load.

When she says for the 28th time that she wants to die, don't say, *Mom, don't say that*. Instead, ask her (in your calmest voice) why she wants to die and what the worst part of living is. Let her know that although you can't make death come sooner, you are happy to talk with her and her doctor about protecting her from a drawn out death.

If you have some sense of the reasons behind your parent's comments, address the underlying issue.

Your mother says she hates the dinner you made, but perhaps it's because she misses cooking for herself. When she makes a face at the stew you've just laid before her, rather than tossing the spatula and huffing off, ask her if she misses cooking. What would be her perfect dinner? How would she make it, and where would she have it?

➕ MEDICAL ALERT

Incessant orneriness, social withdrawal, refusal to eat or see friends, unrelenting needs, accusations, and criticisms can all signal depression or dementia. Talk with your parent's doctor.

66 The difficult thing for me is the nonstop talking. I've had the same conversation over and over, heard the same exact stories. My mother is a compulsive talker, and those are long hours.

What I do now when I'm visiting is ration myself. After I've been with her for a while, I'll either go out and take a long walk by myself, which is great, or I'll try to get her out of the house. This is a new thing, and it works quite well.

It was so important to break that pattern of sitting in the living room, with her in her chair and me on the couch. It opened things up a little."

—Anne C.

Your father constantly says that he's just a useless old man. Rather than giving your usual retort, ask him when he felt most useful in his life, when he felt most productive, and what that was like.

Or simply say something clear and matter-of-fact that ends the conversation, like, *Dad, I'm so sorry you feel this way. I'm afraid that although I can help you with day-to-day issues, I cannot make you happy. That has got to come from you.*

AVOID MANIPULATION. Complaining, calling constantly, or becoming sick at just the wrong moment can be an effective way to control other people. Your parent gripes, and you come running or cancel your vacation. He got what he wanted. And so he grumbles some more, or needs you more, or ruins your next vacation as well.

He controls so little in his life these days, and this behavior works to his advantage. He might not be doing it consciously or maliciously. It just happens.

Don't fall victim to it. Set firm, clear limits on what you will do for your parent, and stick to them. Don't cancel your vacation or leave work for the eighth time this week.

If you are walking out the door and your father accuses you of neglecting him, rather than arguing with him or changing your plans, be clear and reassuring. *I know it feels that way. It must be very hard living here alone. But I will be back on Tuesday, and you need to know that I am never going to abandon you.* And then depart as planned.

Abuse, Neglect, and Addiction

If your parent was abusive, addicted, or otherwise failed in her role as parent, then your first decision is how much, if at all, to be involved in her care. It's an extremely personal decision and one that only you can make.

If you opt out completely, then talk with the area agency on aging (eldercare .gov) to see what options are available, and what community services and housing facilities exist. Or, if money allows it, hire a geriatric care manager to oversee her care. But be careful, though, when handing power over to a stranger. Best to maintain some control and decision-making power.

If you want to help in some way but would rather not provide personal care, then find things you can do from a distance. You can still be an overseer, organizing care and managing finances and legal issues, without actually spending much time with your parent.

If you choose to be more involved in your parent's care, then do so knowing that it's a choice and that you can change your mind at any time.

❝ My mother was was cruel to us. Emotionally abusive. Purposefully torturing us to see how much we would beg, how hard we would cry. Humiliating us in front of other people to get a laugh.

My siblings feel like she's getting what she deserves. They don't want to do this, to care for her.

I had a terrible relationship with her growing up. But now, I'm all she's got. I want to say, 'Why were you so cruel to me?' But I figure, what's the point? She has her own issues to deal with now. She's lonesome. Her husband's gone. Do I want to heap this on her?"

—Carla M.

CREATE BOUNDARIES. Decide exactly what you will do, what you will not do, and what situations you will not tolerate. Let your parent know your limits. *I will help you in the following ways and under these circumstances. If you say this or do that, we will have to find someone else to care for you.* Let her know that this is not up for debate.

DON'T LET OTHERS DICTATE HOW YOU HANDLE THIS. Only you know the depth of your pain, how this parent has affected your life, what you can manage, and what you cannot handle.

KEEP EXPECTATIONS REASONABLE. Don't go into this hoping for an apology or reconciliation. An aged parent, especially one who is ill, isn't likely to delve into the past, see the error of her ways, and suddenly apologize.

Remember, you did not deserve whatever your parent dished out. It is not your fault. And working hard now will not change your parent or the past.

TAKE CARE OF YOURSELF. This reconnection will likely stir up all sorts of old hurts, memories, and anger. Be extraordinarily gentle with yourself. See a therapist. Spend time with friends. Eat well, make time for exercise, and get enough rest.

A NOTE ON HEALING. None of this is to say that all is lost. Sometimes—*sometimes*—caring for an abusive parent can be healing. But that healing will have to come from within yourself, not from your parent. And it will take time. A lot of time.

Understanding that your parent probably had a difficult childhood, and that he might have been genetically predisposed for addiction or anger, will help some.

You might be able to forgive, or you might simply learn to detach, which is also healthy. With time, you might be able to stop owning it and reliving it and letting it shape your life.

Either way, your goal is to let go of the anger and move forward.

AND OF COURSE, SIBLINGS. You need to make your own, very personal decisions about your involvement in your parent's care. Your siblings need to make their own decisions too, and these are just as valid. You might decide to care for a father who abused you, but a sibling might not want to come near him. That's okay.

If your siblings refuse to be involved in the daily care, perhaps they can pitch in financially or help with paperwork or provide you with an occasional break. (See page 61 for more on working with siblings.)

Chapter 3

Caring for the Caregiver

Setting Limits • Emotional Minefields • 12 More Steps to a
Healthy Mind-Set • The Male Caregiver

Although it might not make sense immediately, caring for
yourself during this time is one of the most important things
you can do, both for yourself and for your parent.

Don't flip past this chapter, thinking that you simply don't have
time for such things. *My mother needs me. I can't worry about myself
right now. I'll be fine.*

Your parent's care can consume an ever-expanding piece of your
life and suck you into a swamp of anxiety, guilt, and resentment.
Before you know it, you are too busy for friends, snapping at your
spouse, distracted at work, hugging a bottle of wine, and constantly
trying to shake a cold.

Handling six things and worrying about another four while, on
some visceral level, feeling angry at the world isn't healthy. It leads
to irritability, isolation, depression, and, more often than one would
imagine, physical illness.

You cannot take good care of your parent if you do not take care of yourself. It's that simple. As any flight attendant will tell you, you have to put your oxygen mask on before you assist the person seated next to you.

So no matter what the demands on your time right now, take a step back. Breathe deeply and slowly. Get some perspective. And tend to yourself. Oddly enough, it will help you be a calmer, gentler, and more efficient caregiver.

Setting Limits

If there were such a thing as Caregivers Anonymous, the first step in the program would be to get rid of that little voice inside you that says, *I can do it all. I am responsible for everything. Whatever I do, it's never enough.*

Of course you want to make your parent well, make her happy, make her safe. In fact, if it were possible for you to be with her every minute of the day, perhaps you would be. This is your parent, after all. She needs you.

But the truth is, you can't be with her 24/7, and trying to do so will only exhaust and frustrate you without really helping her.

So how do you use your energies most effectively? If your mother has a sudden and severe illness, of course you'll want to be there. But when her needs are more chronic, when you find yourself taking on more and more responsibility, you have to step back, take a realistic look at the situation, and establish some boundaries for yourself.

This might require a seismic shift in thinking, a great realization that you are not responsible for everything, that you cannot fix everything, that you need help, and that you have a life (or some semblance of a life) of your own.

As hard as this is, you might be surprised to discover that setting some limits relieves your guilt, eases the tension, and gives you more patience and energy for those things that only you can give.

> ❝ Like the waves of the ocean, it sometimes overwhelms me. I think I'm this incredibly strong person, but I've been spending all my time taking care of stuff for my parents and I'm the one who's falling apart. It's way too much. They are doing much better than I am."
> —Lou Ann W.

EXAMINE YOUR MOTIVATION. Why are you helping your parent? It sounds like an odd question, but it's a healthy one to mull over. Do you feel that you have a cultural or religious duty to care for her? Do you view your parent's care as an unfair burden that was dumped on you? Or are you helping because, given your parent's situation and your priorities in life, this is what you gladly choose to do?

Your motivation might be complicated, but take a moment to think about it. Then consider your options, and make a conscious choice about

> For a long time, I visited my mother three times a week, but I was always running and always tired. I started to dread each visit, and I was angry with her because I felt it was all her fault. She was ruining my life.
>
> Then a friend said to me, 'This isn't her fault. It's your fault.' And, you know, she was right."
>
> —Fran M.

your involvement in your parent's care. If you can accept this as your choice, something you decided to do—not as

ACKNOWLEDGING THE JOB

Quite often, people tending to an elderly parent don't identify themselves as caregivers. They think they are just doing what needs to be done, what anyone would do. *She's my mother, for Pete's sake. She took care of me; I can take care of her. This is what families do.* Convinced that this is somehow normal, they don't understand why the task is so hard or why they are falling apart.

Although it's true that people have cared for their parents throughout history, across cultures, and around the globe, much has changed. In fact, the sort of eldercare we face today is a relatively new phenomenon.

Just a couple of generations ago, people grew old, became ill, needed some care, and died. Today, people live for years and years with complex medical issues. They don't simply need a loving touch and some hot food; they need catheters, oxygen, and eight different medications.

They need someone to put a spoon in their mouths, get them on the toilet, pull on their socks, and remind them what day and month it is.

The caregiver side of this coin has changed as well. Families often live far apart, and women, the traditional caregivers, are working and having children later.

For all these reasons, the job has become far more demanding, complex, and prolonged. It is not *just what families do.* Caregivers jeopardize their health, careers, finances, and relationships. They have a higher rate of depression, insomnia, illness, and even mortality. This task is literally killing them.

Caregiving is hard work. The first step in taking care of yourself, and thus taking better care of your parent, is to acknowledge that this is a big job, and that you cannot do it yourself. You need lots of help and support.

something your parent, your siblings, or a judgmental or unjust world has dumped on you—the work you do for your parent will still be difficult, but it will feel more like an interruption and less like an imposition. It will be a conscious decision that is more about love and family and less about old debts and unmet needs.

IDENTIFY THE NEED. You might know what needs to be done, but be specific. Write it down.

What does your parent need, and what is a luxury or perceived need? Does she need someone at her house every afternoon? Does she need help with bathing and dressing? Help with medications? Rides to the doctor? Make a checklist of her essential needs—the musts—and then a second list of what would be nice—the extras. Star anything on the list that only you can do (and be very selective here).

Writing it all down, preferably with her input, will help you see what is crucial, what can be skipped, and what can be done by others.

Now what about you? What are the "musts" in your life? What has to be done? What can be pushed off your to-do list? And what do you need in your life so you can stay sane? A night out each week with a friend? An hour each morning for exercise? Time with your kids?

CREATE A PLAN. Now that you have your lists, determine what you can reasonably do and, more important, what you have to stop trying to do.

Day to day, your parent's care may seem more pressing than other matters in your life—everything you do for your parent at this point might seem essential—but think about it. Visiting your mother every day may be ideal, but would she be okay with fewer visits?

As you decide what's truly necessary, consider what you may be ignoring or giving up because of your parent's care. Are you willing to jeopardize your own health? Neglect your children? Damage your career?

You might decide you will handle her finances, confer with her doctors, and visit twice a week, but not more than that. Or, if you live with your parent, you might create some parameters, some specific times of day when you can help her and other times when your family has some privacy.

Be conservative in your plan; it's always easier to increase your commitment than to decrease it. Don't promise to make three regular visits if that puts you over the edge; keep it at two.

GET COMPENSATED

If you are logging a lot of caregiver hours and your siblings simply can't (or won't) help much, then consider getting some compensation for all you are doing, especially if you have scaled back hours at your real job. Seriously. Don't be a martyr. A long-term caregiving job can wreak financial havoc in your life and create a lot of resentment. Some sort of compensation can ease the strain and mollify family relations. See page 66 on how to create a caregiver contract and calculate compensation.

> " I was so run down, going to work and then going to the hospital. If someone had a cold, I got it.
>
> I got *C. difficile*. It's an infection elderly people in hospitals get. I was in the ER with diarrhea, dry heaving, headaches. I was sick for 10 days.
>
> Then I realized, I am sacrificing my health for hers. I said to a friend, 'I'm 60. My mom is 91. I still have some good years ahead of me, if I'm lucky. She doesn't. I can't sacrifice my health for her anymore.'"
>
> —Maggie B.

DOLE OUT THE CHORES. In the beginning, caring for a parent can be like carrying around a backpack. It's not so heavy. And it feels kind of good, doing this for your parent. Anyway, he needs you to carry it.

With time, however, the backpack grows heavier. You trudge on because you must, but your step has slowed considerably, and your shoulders are sagging under the pressure.

You might think that (a) you don't need help, (b) no help is available, and (c) no one else will do it as well as you will. The truth is (a) you do need help, (b) you haven't looked hard enough, and (c) you're right, no one else will do it quite the way you do it, *but that's okay*.

Dole out any jobs you can. You do not need to take this all on by yourself, nor should you try to. Get other family members involved, use community services, hire help, and when necessary, consider other housing options.

Siblings, in particular, should be called on right away. They might have different ideas about your father's care or different ways of doing things, but they should be involved. If you begin this as a family effort when the tasks are smaller, you will have each other further down the road when the needs and responsibilities tend to be more monumental. (See page 61 for more on dealing with siblings.)

Get your parent hooked up with local services early so he has time to get used to them before his health declines further, and so he becomes less dependent upon a sole caregiver—you.

Let other people give you a hand as well. Someone might pick up your dog at the veterinarian, bring over a casserole, water your plants, or stay with your parent for an afternoon.

However you do it, get help!

LET GO OF FUTILE EFFORTS. Don't waste precious energy trying to get your parent to change her ways if it's clear that she won't. Talk with your parent about your concerns, get others to help in the effort, and show her other options. If she still won't budge, and she is mentally competent, you might have to give up.

For example, if you are spending a lot of time researching group homes for the elderly, and your mother has absolutely no intention of moving, at some point you need to stop the hunt and get on with more productive tasks, such as safeguarding her house and finding community and in-home services.

You might feel that you have failed, but you haven't. Your mother might be in a somewhat risky situation. She might fall or run out of money. But you have done what you can, and you cannot do

CAREGIVERS AS FROGS

It turns out that the old frog metaphor is not scientifically valid, but it's a good illustration anyway. Just don't try this at home.

The story goes like this: If you put a frog in boiling water (sorry, disgusting, but read on), it will thrash around trying desperately to escape the pot. However, if you put a frog in cool water and ever so gradually, degree by degree, turn up the heat, the frog doesn't thrash at all. Even when the water is boiling, the frog barely moves. Why? Because it doesn't sense any change; it learns to tolerate the heat. Before our little frog knows what has happened, it is cooked.

Scientifically inaccurate (frogs do try to get out), and yet strangely familiar.

If your parent suddenly, out of the blue, needed an enormous amount of assistance and services, you would frantically get help. But when this task starts with a few calls and visits and ever so slowly, degree by degree, requires more and more time and energy, you might not register exactly how desperate or unusual the situation is. You might simply, well, cook.

The point is, as much as you want to help—and you will help—don't ignore the fact that you might be in a pot that is simply too hot.

any more. You can't blame yourself if your parent's decisions are, in your mind, poor ones.

Likewise, if your siblings simply won't help, push and prod, but at some point learn to live with it. Urge them. Have a family meeting. But eventually, let it go. Don't waste valuable steam.

Letting go of hopeless crusades is an enormous accomplishment. Then you can accept life as it is and work within existing parameters.

LEARN TO SAY NO. Caregivers are often as bad at saying no to requests for help as they are at saying yes to offers of help. Women, in particular, often have trouble saying no, but such martyrdom is neither helpful nor good.

Convince yourself that saying no to certain things is not only okay, but necessary. Practice. Try it out on the dog.

Say no to the mirror. Just get the word out.

Confronted with a parent's escalating needs, you may learn, perhaps for the first time in your life, how to act on your own behalf.

> " When I retired, I didn't tell my mother. I didn't want her to think I was more available, that I had more time for her. I had been taking care of her for several years, and when I retired, I realized there was a lot that I wanted to do for myself, a lot that I had neglected because of her.
>
> I told her that I was working from home more, in case she called and found me there, but I didn't tell her that I had retired. And I have never regretted it."
>
> —Barbara F.

STICK TO YOUR GUNS. Sure, you can decide to cut back on some visits, even put a plan in writing, but how do you stick to it?

Say you decide that your marriage needs more attention, but just as you and your spouse settle in for a quiet evening together, the first in weeks, you find yourself feeling guilty for not being with Dad. You're short with your husband and end up calling your father in the midst of dinner, just to check in.

Be firm in your resolve. If you decide that you are not going to concern yourself with your father's financial affairs anymore because you have handed that job over to another family member, don't spend an evening researching reverse mortgages. If you've told your mother you cannot be interrupted during work, and she continues to call hourly, remind her gently that this is not the time to talk and that you'll call her when you get home. Then hang up. (Be aware, however, that a constant need for reassurance may be an early sign of dementia.)

NO COMPARISONS. Whatever you decide to do, and not to do, don't be influenced by what someone else is doing. Just because a friend visits her father every

> " I used to spend hours trying to convince my parents to move out of their big house and to organize their finances. But they didn't do anything. They would ask me questions and listen and act like they were going to do something about it. But they never did.
>
> And then I realized, they are not going to change. They are not going to move until something forces them to. And there is nothing I can do about it. It was terribly difficult to back off. You want so much to help, and you know things are only going to get worse. It took me three years to give up and let go, and I still struggle with it sometimes. I just have to go along and see what happens next."
>
> —Diane P.

afternoon doesn't mean that you should change your schedule. Just because a guy in your support group cared for his mother in his own home for 12 years, don't feel that you aren't doing enough.

Every situation is different. Every relationship is different. Each person faces different demands and has different supports. Only you can create the right balance for yourself. Find it and accept it.

Emotional Minefields

Simply surviving parentcare requires that you deal with some potent emotions. Believe it or not, the reactions you are experiencing now, even the ones that seem disturbingly illogical, cruel, childish, or out of character, are completely normal and common. Most of them can be tempered.

66 When I was taking care of my dad,
     I was so exhausted and I lost a lot
of weight. I went down to 103 and looked
gaunt. When you feel like throwing up all
the time, you don't eat."
                                          —Maggie B.

Guilt

Ah, guilt, the constant companion of caregivers. Women are particularly good at guilt. *I'm not doing enough, I'm not doing it right, I should have done something else.* And isn't it interesting that we can feel so guilty for not doing enough, and in the very same breath be resentful that we have to do so much?

Guilt is not a particularly useful emotion, especially in this case. So get rid of it. Summon it up, vomit it out into a trash bag, tie it up, and toss it out. And then do it again and again, because guilt has a sneaky habit of reappearing.

Stop focusing on what you are *not* doing, or what you imagine you *should* be doing, and focus instead on what you *are* doing for your parent (and for others in your life). Make a list of these things and be sure to include everything that you provide—emotional support, phone calls, visits, talks with doctors, help with financial matters, and so on. What would your parent's life be like without you?

Recognize and be proud of what you are giving, and give it generously. But please, dump the guilt.

Helplessness and Worry

Given all the medical issues, the costs, the paperwork, and the various players and services involved, it's no wonder caregivers often feel stymied and helpless.

The fact is, a lot is out of our control. No matter what we do, our parents become frailer. Death looms.

It's a downward trajectory that sometimes feels like a free fall. The sense of powerlessness and the worry that goes with it can be paralyzing.

TAKE ACTION. Don't stew—do.

Don't just complain to your friends about a chronically late home care worker, a rude orderly, or a poorly run meal service. Talk to the person involved, and if he's not responsive, speak to a supervisor. Be pleasant but persistent. Take action.

Ask questions when dealing with professionals. Be an educated advocate for yourself and your parent, and don't be afraid to speak up when necessary.

Getting answers and taking action is far better than letting problems fester. It will give you some sense of control. Most important, it often leads to solutions.

SET ASIDE A WORRY TIME. Rather than stewing during a meeting at work or lying awake at three in the morning, set aside a specific time, 15 minutes or half an hour each day, maybe during a walk or a commute to work just for worrying. It sounds ridiculous, but it works.

When you can't stop fretting, jot down whatever it is you are thinking about and know that you will contemplate it during your "worry time." Then, go back to sleep! It's been scheduled. In the light of day, you'll probably discover that it wasn't all that critical after all.

Resentment and Anger

Your parent's care is consuming your life. Your siblings aren't helping. Your spouse isn't supportive. The world isn't fair. And now, your heart is racing and your head aches. Resentment can be toxic.

It can also be self-perpetuating. You resent your parent for being a burden, then feel guilty for resenting him, then resent him because he's making you feel bad about yourself.

Anger is more difficult to deal with because it is so hot and blinding. Be careful. Anger can lead to rash acts, regrettable words, broken relationships, and abuse.

WALK AWAY. When you are angry, don't take any action. Get away from the situation and simmer down. Breathe deeply.

GET HELP. Right away. Contact the area agency on aging (eldercare.gov) and learn about adult day services, respite care, in-home care, and other local services. Then use them.

GET SUPPORT. A support group is great for defusing anger and resentment. These emotions are common; sometimes simply realizing that you're not alone can help. Or talk with a therapist individually.

ASK WHY. Once you're calm, address the reason for your feelings. You don't want to explode, but you also don't want to implode. What makes you so stomping mad? Is it really your parent's care, or is it your brother's criticism, your fears about your own old age, or a sense that somebody, somewhere, should be thanking you? What is causing this reaction?

REFRAME IT. That is, rather than simply being angry or wishing that a person or situation were different, think about what you can do to change the situation.

If you resent your parent because you are doing too much and missing out on

THOSE UNTHINKABLE THOUGHTS

Most people caring for an aged parent wish, at some point along the way, that their parents would die. It might be a fleeting thought or a constant presence. Either way, it can be very disturbing.

If you are hoping that your father will die soon because he is terminally ill and his existence is pretty miserable, you are not being unkind; you are being merciful.

But you might be wishing that your parent would die because he is a burden or a curmudgeon, or because you want an inheritance or your privacy, or because you are simply tired of waiting

and wondering. In other words, you want him to die not for his sake, but for yours. When this thought process starts parading around your brain, it can make you feel like an awful person.

Forget it. You're not. Caring for a frail parent, even if you are not providing hands-on care, is draining on many levels. Since there is really no other possible outcome, it is natural to want the struggle to end, for everybody's sake. You are not a bad person for feeling this way. You are only human. Get support and be sure your wishes don't translate into abusive actions.

> " What's difficult for me is the guilt that I'm not doing enough. After all the logistics of working stuff out and doing payroll every weekend, I end up not seeing my mother as much as I would like. It feels like I'm being pulled in a million directions. I don't see my friends, I don't see my grandchildren as much, and my children don't want to hear my 'laundry list' of reasons why I'm not available for them."
>
> —Diana R.

your own life, then back off. Do less. If your siblings aren't helping, talk to them about how they might help and/or arrange to be compensated for your work (see page 66). If you simply need a thank-you and some validation, let them know.

If you resent your spouse for not sympathizing or helping out more, talk with him (or her) about specific ways in which he can help and exactly what it

WHEN YOU'RE AT THE EDGE

The stress of caregiving can drive people to do things they never imagined possible. If you find yourself lashing out at your parent, neglecting him, threatening him, yelling at him, striking him (even lightly), or exploiting him financially or otherwise, get away from him immediately. Call a friend or neighbor to take over. You need help, and you need it now. Contact the area agency on aging (eldercare.gov or 800-677-1116) for support and respite services.

is you need from him. (You might also need to lower your expectations.)

Don't expect others to simply *know* that they should help out or thank you or do something different. Let them know (calmly, of course).

BEWARE THE PITY PIT. Don't be a martyr. It seems unthinkable, but it's easy to fall into a pit of self-pity and become so comfortable in that pit that you start to wallow in it. From this vantage point, the world is cleanly divided into black and white. I'm good; they are bad.

Of course, this will only hurt you in the long run.

WRITE. If you have trouble thinking clearly about this, write about it. Don't worry about grammar or style, just vent all over the page. Writing can help blow off a little steam without burning anyone in the process. It can also, with time, clarify some issues and, as a result, lead to solutions.

FORGIVE YOURSELF. If you snap at your parent, argue with your spouse, or devour a box of doughnuts, let it go. You've got a lot on your plate (besides doughnuts). It's natural and normal. Move on.

Disgust

This emotion might not be discussed openly, but most caregivers know about it, and it is no small matter.

Obviously, changing a diaper or cleaning up an "accident" will rattle anyone's nerves. Incontinence is one of the

> ❝ My mother has always been my best friend, and after my father died, we only became closer. She has always been there for me, always understood me. When she is gone, no one will do that for me. The idea of losing her is too painful for me to bear.
>
> Sometimes after I hang up the phone when she sounds down or weak, I feel helpless and sad. I cry so hard that I can't breathe. I guess I'm lucky to have a mother who I love this deeply, but sometimes I think that if I didn't, it wouldn't hurt so much. ❞
>
> —Carol P.

biggest reasons people get outside help or move a parent.

But more mundane things—a parent's eating habits, bodily noises, or odors—can also repulse. Even if you love your parent dearly, the scents and sounds that come with aging can bring on powerful waves of disgust. Your reactions will be compounded by your stress and exhaustion. Your reserve tank is on empty.

The fact is, some of this you simply have to get over. Your mother can't change the fact that she has difficulty chewing, and making her feel bad about it will only, well, make her feel bad about it. Try to understand that this is a byproduct of age, illness, and medications.

Some things can be improved with cologne (for her, not you), air freshener, mouthwash, and a box of tissues. Also, check out any relevant sections in this book for ways to improve the situation.

Your best defense is a good sense of humor. Talking with others (friends, a support group, an online chat room)

might also strengthen your resolve and, at least for a moment, help you laugh about it.

When you simply can't take it, get help. Maybe someone can come in the morning and help her with toileting and hygiene. Or maybe she can go to adult day care several days a week.

Get help, because although some discomfort is normal, disgust can lead to poor care and harsh words.

Grief

Parentcare is, at its core, about loss and grief. But it's not the normal sort of grief. It is a perverse grief, a good-bye that can't yet be said, although it hangs darkly overhead.

When a parent grows frail or forgetful, the losses come in small, unexpected doses—a fall, a missed name, a fender bender, a shaky hand, another nap. The loss drags on, always with us, weighing on us, and yet difficult to define or resolve.

And so, tears come in strange spurts. Grief explodes in anger and confusion. It's not clear what it is, this chronic, simmering grief, and it can be agonizing and unbearably lonely.

Whatever else is happening, whatever sort of relationship you have with your parent, try to acknowledge your grief. You might be grieving the impending loss of a parent you adore or grieving a relationship you never had. You might be mourning the loss of your childhood or feeling sad about your own aging process.

It's a complex mix, but whatever the cause of grief, it's important to recognize and allow it.

All of us grieve in our own way, at our own pace. The sadness can be constant,

BE ALERT TO DEPRESSION

Take care of yourself, get some exercise, see friends, set realistic goals, and make time for things you enjoy—ideally, *before* you're in trouble. Be alert to signs of depression:

- feelings of sadness, hopelessness, worthlessness, or anxiety
- fatigue, exhaustion
- changes in eating or sleeping habits
- loss of interest in activities you once enjoyed
- social isolation (not calling or seeing people who used to be in your life)
- difficulty concentrating
- irritability
- bouts of tears
- vague physical symptoms (stomachaches, headaches, general pain)
- thoughts of death

Depression can be treated effectively with counseling and/or medication. Call your doctor, or for immediate help, call the local crisis intervention, suicide, or depression hotline, or 911.

For information about depression, online support, or a referral to a local specialist, contact the International Foundation for Research and Education on Depression (ifred.org) or Mental Health America (mentalhealthamerica.net or 800-969-6642).

or it may crash over you in waves at odd times. Or it might show itself in other ways—anger, bitterness, and depression.

Allow yourself time to grieve. Have a good cry. Spend time alone, or share your thoughts with others.

If you love your parent and will miss her, don't allow this opportunity to let her know go by.

12 More Steps to a Healthy Mind-Set

Here are some additional ways to take care of yourself:

1. TAKE FIVE

If you are caring for your parent on a regular basis, especially if you are living with her, remove yourself completely from the situation once in a while. You need to refuel, and you can't do it without some distance. Get some respite before you are too distraught to plan or enjoy such a break.

You might take a vacation or you might simply take an afternoon off to sit in the park, see a friend, or have a pedicure. Set aside time in your regular schedule a few times a week to do as you please. If necessary, make arrangements for fill-in help or get your parent into a respite program.

Then, while you are away, be completely away. Think about something else. Talk about anything else. Clear your head.

2. A FRIEND, INDEED

When you are caring for an aging parent, quite often the first thing that goes is your social life. Invitations are turned down and friendships are put on hold because you simply do not have the time or the energy for them. If you are living with your parent, social isolation can become a serious problem.

Friends are more important now than ever. They can provide a sympathetic ear, make you laugh, get you thinking about other things, and remind you that you are not alone.

Studies show that caregivers who have social supports experience less depression and illness and are less overwhelmed by their responsibilities than those who don't.

Rather than cutting yourself off, reach out to your friends. Find a way. Make it a priority. Go out for lunch, go for a walk, or make a phone date. Just as you would be there for them, your friends want to be there for you.

3. GET SUPPORT

You might think that you are not the type to join a support group, that you wouldn't want to share with strangers, but try it. You can get practical tips, but mostly you'll see that others face the same difficult issues and turbulent feelings, and this in itself can be an enormous relief.

Support groups—whether in person or online—offer a safe arena in which to air intimate problems, vent anger, or talk about painful emotions. Because you face similar situations, you can understand each other in a way that others, even best friends, cannot.

Support groups vary widely in terms of purpose and membership, and you may need to try two or three before finding one that meets your needs. Some groups are designed for anyone caring for a sick parent, whereas others zero in on specific issues—family relationships, Alzheimer's, cancer, grief, or advocacy. Some are set up so people can share practical information and resources, and others function purely as emotional outlets. Some have leaders, others are unstructured. Although support groups are usually for the caregiver, some encourage parents to attend as well.

More and more venues for support and sharing are offered online,

> " Sometimes in the evening I reach a point when I think, 'I'd just rather not go out tonight.' But I always come home from the support group feeling better. Because everyone in the group is dealing with someone with dementia, it helps me see that what my mom is doing is perfectly normal for this disease. I also see that what I'm feeling isn't cruel or selfish or crazy. Even if I never see these people again when this is over, I'll never forget them."
>
> —Barbara F.

" The last time I went to my support
group, a woman was talking about
her father, who has dementia. She was
taking care of him 24 hours a day, and she
was so warm and had such a nice sense
of humor about it all that I thought, 'This
woman is a saint.' It made me feel terrible.

Eventually I had to come to grips with
it. That is her life; this is mine. I do the
best I can."

—Linda K.

which isn't as intimate but is a whole
lot easier—available when you want it
and completely anonymous. However,
be aware of advice given online; keep in
mind the source.

To find local a support group, contact your area agency on aging (eldercare
.gov or 800-677-1116). Caregiver Action

Network (caregiveraction.com) has an
online forum.

Most nursing homes, adult day-care
centers, senior centers, and mental health
clinics should also be able to refer you
to nearby groups. If you are interested
in a specific topic, contact the appropriate association, many of which either run
support groups themselves or can refer
you to one (for example, the Alzheimer's
Association, the American Cancer
Society, or Alcoholics Anonymous).

4. AVOID THE COULDA-SHOULDA-WOULDA'S

Also known as the If-Only or the More-
Better-Different Syndrome, this is a
dangerous mind-set. *I could have been
better about that . . . I should do more . . . If
only life were different. . . .*

Wishing for things that can't be,
regretting what is, or daydreaming about

MAINTAINING A SOCIAL LIFE

If you and your parent live together, or
simply spend a lot of time together, you
can still have a social life. You just have
to be a little more creative, flexible, and
determined.

If your parent wants to be included in
a social event (and you want her to be
included), have the guests come to your
house rather than going out. Home is a
more familiar and comfortable setting for
your parent. It also means she can leave
the room when she needs to rest, without
breaking up the party.

Of course you might not want the extra
work of cooking for a crowd, and there's

no reason for you to try to be Martha
Stewart. Have a potluck supper or just
order a pizza. People want to be together;
what's served is really secondary. (Friends
can help cook and clean up, too.)

If your parent would rather not go out,
or if you would rather not include her,
don't stay home just because it's easier.
Go out. Get a sibling or companion to
stay with her. Even though it may seem
like an extravagance, make yourself do
it. It's a worthwhile investment in your
well-being.

See page 486 for tips on socializing
when your parent has dementia.

what might have been is futile and potentially destructive if it keeps you from more productive tasks. It's human nature to think this way, but try to focus on what is and what can be.

5. SHIFT GEARS

Whenever you are feeling Type A, think Type B. Researchers have actually timed people who run through red lights and blast their horns at pedestrians, and have found that these racers don't save themselves any time at all. In fact, hurrying often slows things down because in the rush you are apt to spill food or misplace your car keys.

It seems contradictory, but sometimes when life is hectic, it helps to slow down. Stay calm. Breathe. Unhunch your shoulders.

If you are driving somewhere, and it takes 20 minutes to get there, don't try to make it in 19. Leave extra time and then relax. Use that time to listen to your favorite music or book. Or simply relish the silence. Stay in the slow lane, wait until the light turns green, and leave the honking to the geese.

6. EATING WELL

When a parent needs care, any thought of a decent diet vanishes. Stressed and overwrought, people either fail to eat or find that a bag of Doritos is a just reward for a taxing day.

And of course, racing from a doctor's appointment to a work meeting to the bank leaves little time for fresh food. It's 6:30 and people are hungry. What's fast?

Take-out food, chocolate fudge

HEALTHY BODY, HEALTHY MIND

The mind-body connection works in two directions. You can boost your physical health with a positive outlook, and you can improve your outlook by tending to your physical health.

Now, when your energy and optimism are taking a beating, it is more important than ever that you eat well, exercise, and get plenty of rest. Yes, you've heard it all before, but give it a real try. Make a concerted effort to take care of your body, and see if you don't notice a difference in your energy and mood.

---

brownies, and an endless stream of caffeine might seem, in the moment, like the only option (and you do deserve a reward), but rethink this approach.

Eating well will make a huge difference to your health, energy, and spirits. Furthermore, taking even half an hour to sit down with your family and have a real meal, rather than everyone eating out of a box on the fly, will have a surprising effect on everyone's day and relationships.

7. A LITTLE SWEAT

There is nothing like a workout to shed pent-up emotions, clear a muddled head, and revive a tired body. Exercise protects people from the harmful effects of stress, elevates mood, lowers anxiety, and promotes self-esteem.

MAKE IT DOABLE. Weight training and rigorous workouts are great, but if you hate that sort of thing, find something else. It's better to walk one mile five times a week and stick to it than to run three miles daily and give up after a week. An exercise regimen should last at least 20 minutes and be varied.

MAKE IT SOCIAL. Find an exercise partner. You will be less apt to excuse yourself from the routine, and you get to socialize while you sweat.

MAKE IT USEFUL. If you simply don't have time for the gym, rake the yard, sweep the floor, or walk to work. Read the newspaper on a stationary bike or talk to a coworker while you walk.

MAKE IT FUN. Exercise doesn't have to be boring. Play tennis, swim, skate, or dance.

MAKE IT CHALLENGING. Every now and then, push yourself. Challenging yourself physically seems to have a beneficial effect on stress and resiliency.

8. ZZZZZS

In studies of laboratory rats, scientists have found that severe sleep deprivation is always fatal. It is more harmful than starvation. For humans, life without sleep certainly feels deadly, causing irritability, poor concentration, lack of coordination, and forgetfulness. Make sleep a priority.

REGULAR CHECKUPS

Are you urging your parent to see a doctor but neglecting your own health? Stop postponing that physical checkup, mammogram, or dentist appointment. Your parent might provide a handy excuse for you to cancel (or fail to make) appointments, but don't.

> " During my father's illness I got very depressed and closed in. I realized that I needed some outlet, a way of dealing with the constant anxiety. So I started drawing.
>
> I hadn't done any sketches for years, but I bought a pad and pencils and dug in. I find I can express my rage and fear in drawings better than I can with words. I sketch each night. It's my sanity. I've actually gotten pretty good at it."
>
> —Eleanor R.

If you are having trouble sleeping, see the tips about dealing with insomnia on page 216.

9. PURSUE YOUR HOBBY

Hobbies, sports, crafts, and other such pursuits are not frivolous pastimes. They help clear your mind of your worries—perhaps just for a brief interlude—which allows you to regain some balance and energy.

If your parent's care is a prolonged commitment, don't forgo your pottery, gardening, painting, tennis, knitting, or javelin throwing—whatever it is that calms you.

Make it a point to find time for it. Take pleasure in it.

10. SPIRITUAL SUPPORT

Whether you are religious or not, spiritual issues often arise when a parent is sick. *How do I ease my anguish or grief? How do I face my own mortality? Why would a loving God do this?*

A little prayer can strengthen your will and focus your life. Nearly 75 percent of caregivers say they use prayer as a way of coping.

If going to religious services doesn't interest you, or if you simply want a more personal discussion, most clergy are happy to meet with people individually. Just call. (You can send a donation if you want to repay the favor.)

Devotee or atheist, sometimes it helps to simply sit quietly in a peaceful place, listen to your soul, and remember your priorities.

II. RELAX

You don't know how much stress you are carrying around until you sit in a relaxation or meditation class and let go of it. The techniques you learn there can be used anywhere, anytime, to ease the pressure. Classes in tai chi, meditation, and yoga, as well as in general relaxation, all relieve stress.

In fact, you can permanently change your response to stress and become a calmer, more relaxed person. So this is an opportunity not only for immediate relief, but also for personal growth.

12. LOVE TO LAUGH

Laughter is a forgotten healer. It makes the world sane (or at least it makes the insanity more fun), and the body healthier. A good dose of humor bolsters the spirit, and hysterical laughter strengthens the immune system, improves circulation, and relieves stress.

Of course, howling with laughter when someone you love is ill or dying can feel like a sacrilege. You might think

AVOIDING PITFALLS

A cup of coffee each morning can gradually turn into three. A glass of wine with dinner can become a scotch before dinner and half a bottle of wine during the meal. An occasional sleeping pill becomes monthly prescriptions. And food? Well, there's nothing like a pint of ice cream to soothe a frazzled soul.

But in the long run, these things will only sap your energy and make you feel worse. When drink, pills, or food call your name, pause, then find another way to cope with exhaustion and stress. Before embracing Sara Lee or Jack Daniels, do a few stretches, call a friend, grab some knitting, take a walk.

that you have to be solemn to reflect the seriousness of the situation and to show respect for your parent. But you don't. You really don't. It's okay to laugh, no matter how sick or incompetent your parent may be.

Find something funny about the situation. (Dentures are funny, especially

" My mother had a mastectomy, and sometimes forgets to put her prosthesis in. She'll come downstairs with her shirt all askew and sagging, and after standing there for a minute or two, she'll say, 'Something is not right.'

I look at her and have to laugh. 'Mom,' I say, 'you forgot your boob.' And we'll both giggle. She thinks it's funny, too. It could happen to anyone. If we didn't laugh, we would cry. It's that sort of thing."

—Greg C.

when your parent isn't wearing them. Certain sourpuss nurses are funny. The Jell-O served in hospitals is funny. Sagging, loose skin under the arm is mildly amusing when it's not your own.) See a slapstick movie, visit a goofy friend, scan the comics, play a joke on someone, clown around with your siblings.

Whenever you feel that you just can't take it anymore (and ideally long before that point), find some way to laugh—a long, side-splitting, teary, wet-your-pants kind of laugh. It's good medicine.

The Male Caregiver

E ldercare has traditionally been the province of women—leaving them to care not only for their own parents, but their husbands' parents as well—and they are still bearing the brunt of this job. However, men are becoming increasingly involved. Studies suggest that between 30 and 40 percent of caregivers are men (up from about 20 percent in 1996).

Although generalizations fail in so many ways (if you've seen one caregiver, you've seen one caregiver), there are some differences in how men and women typically approach this task. Both have strengths and weaknesses; the sexes might just learn a thing or two from each other.

Men are more apt to help with "hands-off" care, such as finances, legal matters, transportation, home maintenance, and hiring. Women, on the other hand, are more apt to handle the "hands-on" care, like dressing, bathing, feeding, toileting, and just plain being present.

Because most men grew up in an environment where women played the role of primary caregiver, they tend to be a little slow to get involved and, once there, question their competence as caregivers. They often feel helpless and uncertain. They don't know what to do or how to begin. Personal tasks are particularly awkward, especially when it's time to give Mom a bath.

Men are often reluctant to let others know that they are caring for a parent. They are particularly silent at work, fearful that revealing the situation will hurt their careers.

They are also less willing to get emotional support when they feel overwhelmed. They don't talk with their friends about the stresses of parentcare or join support groups as readily as women do. Likewise, they are less likely to talk with a doctor or other professional about depression or anxiety, or to take medication for it. Instead, they turn to alcohol (bad), work longer hours (bad), or release their stress on a playing field (good).

However, there are aspects of parentcare that men do better than their female

WHEN ONE PARENT IS WELL

When one parent is ill and the other is still able, everyone's attention naturally turns to the patient, but don't ignore your healthier parent—the caregiver. Your job is to help her so that she can do her job well.

Remember, her life has taken a dramatic turn. She has taken on enormous responsibilities. She stands to lose her mate and has already lost vital aspects of their relationship together.

You might not be able to extricate her completely, but you can lighten the load, be sure she gets a break, and offer emotional support.

Talk about the situation. Make a list of what jobs need to be done, which ones your parent feels that only she can do, and which ones others in the family or outsiders can do. Listen to her fears and needs, and help her understand the importance of taking care of herself and the ramifications if she were to become ill.

You might have to inch your way into this, taking over one small task and then another, or nudging her gradually toward community services and in-home help. Offer to take care of your father for certain shifts or to take over peripheral duties, such as home maintenance and bill paying.

Respect her desire to care for her spouse, but also be sure she gets away from the job occasionally.

Monitor her health, because she may be neglecting it now. Get her to eat well, sleep (which might mean moving to another bedroom), exercise, and see the doctor when necessary.

Helping your parent now will not only allow her to give her best to her spouse, but should also head off disaster. You do not want to find yourself with two ailing parents instead of one.

The Well Spouse Foundation (800-838-0879 or wellspouse.org) can help. It hooks members up with online and local support groups, and issues a newsletter.

---

counterparts. Women tend to get more emotionally overwrought, while men (yes, a huge generalization) tend to be more task oriented. They want to fix a problem and check it off the list. *What is going on here? What do I need to do to solve it?*

Although both sons and daughters suffer silently and wait way too long to get help, sons seem to be better at using community services, hiring outsiders, and delegating responsibilities. Daughters often feel they should do it all themselves.

Obviously, women should try to foresee problems, delegate, plan, make a checklist, and get help with daily tasks (and they might even benefit from a good game of hoops now and then), and men need to learn to talk and find emotional support when the going gets tough.

Some support groups are tailored just for men, and they can be very useful. If a support group is too touchy-feely, online support groups provide anonymity and don't require you to leave the house or office.

Chapter 4

The Inner Circle

Working with Siblings • Compensating the Caregiver •
A Family Meeting • Significant Others • Time for Kids •
Multilayer Sandwiches • Careers and Caregiving

C aring for an aged parent can strengthen relationships—
you might find a new appreciation for your husband or develop a
closer bond with your sister—but it can also revive old hurts and
create new divisions.

The issues are loaded, emotions are volatile, and old patterns are
hard to bear. Just when we need more from each other, we have less
to give.

Siblings who were at the fringe of your life are now in the center. A marriage that had a certain harmony is now strained. Children
want time that you simply don't have. At work, bosses and colleagues
offer a valuable diversion from your parent's care, but they create yet
another layer of stress as you struggle to balance all the competing
demands in your life.

When a parent's care becomes a long-term enterprise, don't let
it destroy the other parts of your life. Acknowledge your limits and
establish some boundaries. Keep the lines of communication open
and your priorities intact.

Working with Siblings

When a parent becomes ill, sibling relationships are tested, and even friendly alliances can become volatile. Old rivalries thought to be dormant reemerge, and new conflicts arise.

Reunited after many years, siblings are often haunted by childhood roles: the control freak, the black sheep, the martyr, the princess, the rebel. One is closer to Mom; another claims to be Dad's favorite. All are quietly competing for affection or praise.

While old issues might not be discussed, they are there, hovering silently at the edge of every conversation. The stolen diary, the broken promise, the lost boyfriend.

With this as a backdrop, siblings face the enormous matters at hand—a parent's safety, money, and eventual demise—and an inevitable inequality of duties.

It's the makings of a disaster.

Handle it tenderly, with as much love, forgiveness, and acceptance as you can muster, because you actually need your siblings now. And when your parent is long gone, these are the relations that will remain.

Together, Yet Different

Although you grew up in the same household, you and your siblings had different childhoods. And although you now sit in the same living room, each one of you views the current situation through his or her own lens.

Your father might have doted on you and criticized your brother. Or maybe your mother drank in the earlier years, but stopped around the time you were born.

Whatever the reasons, what you feel about your parent is not what your sibling feels. It might seem that your sibling is harsh to your mother or emotionally distant from your father, but this is their relationship, based on a long history. It is what it is for reasons you may never understand. You are not going to change it, nor should you try.

Likewise, each sibling has his own way of coping with stress—organize intently, go running, hide. Again, it's something to accept, not to judge or mock.

Finally, each person has different supports, resources (time, money, patience), and priorities. Be careful when determining what someone else should be doing.

One sibling might not have children, but this doesn't immediately make her responsible for Mom's care; perhaps she made a conscious decision not to have children so that she could have time for her artwork. Another sibling might seem to have the resources to support Dad financially, but your definition of wealth might not be his.

Because we grow up together and now sit together, we tend to feel we

> " My brother once said to me, 'How can I help you?'
> I said, 'I just need to know that I'm not alone in this.'"
>
> —Diana R.

AN ONLY CHILD

An only child does not have siblings to argue with, which is wonderful, but she also has no siblings with whom to share the worries, decisions, and responsibilities. If you are caring for a parent on your own, talk with a counselor or join a support group. Make time for close friends. Find others who understand your situation. You need a safe haven where you can express your concerns and get support and insights from others.

should all be on the same page, and yet our differences are vast. Try, as best you can, to accept them, even when you don't understand them.

The Primary Caregiver

Typically, when a parent grows frail, one sibling gravitates toward the role of primary caregiver and takes on the majority of the work. This person might be closest to a parent geographically or the closest emotionally. She might be the one with the most time to give or the one who typically takes care of others. (And yes, she is often a she.)

However this title is established and for whatever reasons, it can make everyone testy. The primary caregiver is resentful that she is doing more than her share, and others feel shut out or don't realize how much work is involved (or both).

If you are the primary caregiver, consider the following:

SHARE THE LOAD. Although you might believe that you can—or should—do

this alone, it's a mighty and exceptionally lonely undertaking. Get your siblings involved from the start.

It's better for you, it's better for them, and believe it or not, it's better for your parent.

It might seem that you are the only one who can do this because you live the closest or have the most time or are the most competent, but find ways for your siblings to help. Perhaps Mom can stay with your brother for a few weeks or your sister can come once a month to relieve you. A sibling from afar might handle taxes and other paperwork, contribute financially, or research an ailment or treatment or device.

You'll have plenty of reasons why only you can do this, and they'll have plenty of reasons why they can't help, but be careful. This can come back to haunt you later, when you are inexplicably furious at them all.

❝ My father moved in with me five years ago. He goes to adult day care. He pays rent. He's a pretty easy person.

But my sister doesn't understand the burden of day-in and day-out care, of not getting any personal time or time off. Why doesn't she see it? She's my sister.

I ask her to help. I say, 'We have a wedding to go to.' But she has reasons she can't take him. I can't hire help because she doesn't want me to spend his money.

It hurts."

—Patricia N.

> " Sometimes it's a gift to be the one caring for them. But sometimes I am resentful that so much falls on me when I do have other siblings.
>
> My sister goes to Arizona for three months. How nice that she can take off for three months.
>
> They say, 'How do you do all this?' They say, 'Thanks so much for all you do for Mom.' They say that.
>
> But if they were really thankful, they would help more."
>
> —Carla M.

COMMUNICATE. Talk with your siblings. Keep them posted about what's happening with your parent, what you are doing, what you need, and how they can help. And of course, listen to their concerns and opinions.

BE SPECIFIC. It might seem obvious that you need support, but your siblings are not psychics. They may not know that you need help or how to help. And honestly, if you have taken this on and are doing an excellent job of it, why would they butt in?

Ask for help. Be direct, but not accusatory when you approach them. (Use *I* instead of *you* sentences, as in *I am overwhelmed* rather than *You never help.*) Then be precise about what you need.

Just saying, *I need help* doesn't give anyone a clue about what to do. Tell them what you need. *I need someone to fill in every other weekend. I need someone to handle Mom's medical bills. I need financial help.*

COMPROMISE. Your siblings aren't psychics; they also aren't drones. If you want your siblings to help—and you *do* want

FOR VISITORS ONLY: THE BEST DAYS

Picture this: One sibling is front and center, handling the day-to-day issues and care. Her energy is focused on doctor's appointments, medications, hygiene, symptoms, and insurance bills. She has no free time and little privacy.

In comes a sibling who is visiting for the weekend. Mom has planned for this visit. She is showered, her apartment is tidy, the calendar is clear. The two of them have lunch together, talk about the grandchildren, look at old photos, and visit a neighbor. Afterward, Mom gushes about how wonderful the visit was and how much she appreciates the effort that was made.

Not only is Mom enamored of her other child, but this sibling thinks that things are pretty easy here, caring for Mom. What's all the complaining about?

If you are the one on the ground, do not clean up for a sibling's visit. Do not clear the calendar. Save tasks for your sibling to do. Use this time to take a break.

If you are the visiting sibling, know that you are getting the best of the best. Let your sibling know that you realize that. Get down to work, and offer praise and support.

your siblings to help—you have to let them do things their way.

Yes, you are in the trenches and they should defer to you on most matters. But you have to let go of some things. They won't do things exactly how you would, and they might mess up a few things, but that's okay. Really.

If you constantly criticize their efforts or correct them, they will stop helping—with good reason. So let it go.

Secondary Caregivers

If you are not the primary caregiver, of course you'll want to help your parent in

....

" My brother refused to believe that my mother had dementia. I would tell him specific things that she did and how impossible things were becoming, but he always came up with an excuse for her. And then he would tell me that I was the one with the problem, that I was being overprotective.

I brought Mom to his house one Saturday. I knew that the only way he would realize what was happening was if he saw it for himself, if he spent some real time with her. When we arrived, I told him that I had to go out of town and left Mom with him for the night. I didn't give him an out.

When I came back for her the next day, he took one look at me, and for the first time in my life, I saw my brother cry. It was very sad, and I felt sorry for him. I understood—he really hadn't wanted to see it. But I had to do it. I needed his help and his support. I couldn't handle it alone any longer."

—Terry B.

....

whatever way you can and stay in touch regularly.

But the best way to help your parent now is to support the sibling who is bearing the brunt of this. Jump in and help. Call. Ask how she's holding up. Let her vent. Tell her how much you appreciate what she's doing. Send her a gift certificate. Fill in so she can get away from it.

Try to understand that there's more to this than meets the eye. The primary caregiver is not simply handling reportable tasks—*I took Mom to the doctor this afternoon*—she is dealing with constant worry, huge responsibility, lack of privacy, and all the buttons and stresses that come with being with a parent regularly (even a nice one). She is on call 24/7, expected to jump at the hint of a problem. Even when the hours aren't enormous, the load can be unbearable.

Support her, practically and emotionally.

If you feel shut out or ignored or don't like the way your sibling is handling things, talk to her, but be tactful. Start by giving her credit for all she is doing, but then explain, gently, your concerns.

If the primary caregiver is not your favorite sibling right now, remember that she is under a lot of stress, living and breathing this job. It's hard for her to worry about you or see beyond the day's urgent problems. And wrong or right, she probably feels a bit resentful (or more than a bit).

Know that although you might see things differently from a distance, the primary caregiver knows quite a lot about your parent's care. Unless you think things have really run amok, you'll have to defer to her judgment.

> " I wish I was there with my father. Absolutely. I saw him a lot over the summer, and that really made me happy. I loved being there for him. But I guess that's easy for me to say from a distance. While I feel a bit at a loss, the grind of being there on a daily basis is very hard on my brother. Because I'm far away, I appreciate each visit, each minute. I am always afraid when I leave that it might be the last time."
>
> —Jane C.

If you have no interest in helping your parent for whatever reasons, or simply can't, then you might offer to help the primary caregiver—do her taxes this year if you're a financial whiz, pick up groceries for her, watch her kids, treat her to a massage.

When Siblings Won't Help

If your siblings are not helping with your parent's care, try the steps outlined earlier. Be clear that you need help, specific about how they can help, and willing to step aside and let them do it.

If none of that works, hold a family meeting to discuss your parent's care (see page 69). If necessary, get a geriatric care manager, family mediator, counselor, or social worker involved.

Be leery of excuses. *I live too far away. I'm too busy with the children. I'm not good at this.* There's no reason for you to nod and mope your way back into the job. Everyone can do

something. Siblings who live far away can handle finances, research local services, and offer the primary caregiver regular respite. Those with young children can cook meals for your parent, get prescriptions filled, pick up groceries, and fill in from time to time.

If you've tried all of the above and then some, and nothing works, stop wasting your breath. If a sibling absolutely will not help no matter how you plead, this is his or her decision.

Your sister might not be able to accept that your parent is sick or dying. Your brother might have such a complex relationship with your father that he can't begin to deal with any of this.

Drop it. Try to understand that their relationship, perspective, and supports are different from yours. Your sibling has his reasons—ones that you may never

THE SIBLING FROM AFAR

Be forewarned of a common occurrence that some in the field call the Brother from California Syndrome (or from Massachusetts, if you live on the West Coast).

It goes something like this: One or more children are dealing with an aged parent regularly. In sweeps a sibling from far away for a brief visit. Sizing up the situation quickly, he lets his siblings know what they are doing wrong and tells them what should be happening instead.

This does not go over well. If you are the sibling from afar, avoid this. If you are the one with Mom, prepare for it. Do your best to remain detached (worth a try); explain how it feels from your end, perhaps in an email; and be sure he gets to the airport on time.

COORDINATING CARE ON THE WEB

S everal websites help caregivers manage tasks, schedules, medications, appointments, and communications. Check out Lotsa Helping Hands (lotsahelpinghands.com), Caring Bridge (caringbridge.org), CareZone (carezone.com), Saturing (saturing.com), and Tyze (tyze.com).

It's understandable. You've been in charge for some time. You know her doctors and her medications and her symptoms and preferences. You have a system. Someone else might not do it right. Someone else might need so much instruction that it's easier to do it yourself. Getting help might suggest you are inadequate or unloving or weak. Getting others involved might be complicated.

Think about what it is that is keeping you from sharing this load. What are you afraid might happen if others do this job? What are you trying to achieve by doing it all yourself?

understand—and in the end, he will have to live with this decision. Let go of it; move on to more productive tasks.

Do not be a martyr, amassing resentment as though it were some prize, because it is a very destructive prize indeed. Far better to find a way to share the work.

Learning to Share

Sometimes—surprisingly often, actually—primary caregivers complain that no one helps but then don't really let others help.

Compensating the Caregiver

W hen one sibling is doing the bulk of the work, families should consider some way of compensating that caregiver. Yes, this work is done out of love and duty, but it is also a job, and it can be quite an enormous commitment. People often have to stop working or cut back on their hours, and then struggle financially. They forgo sleep, meals, and their own health care, and jeopardize their marriages and their sanity.

Compensating the principal caregiver can mean better care for your parent, and should also ease any resentment, guilt, and tension.

It might seem distasteful at first, but don't reject this notion too quickly. It has saved many families from estrangement. Everything is aboveboard, and (hopefully) no one feels cheated.

Some families take an informal approach to this. The primary caregiver might keep Mom's car or live in Mom's home rent-free, or Mom might send the caregiver's family on a vacation each year. Sometimes a parent includes a gift to this child in her will.

However, more and more families are drafting formal agreements and paying family caregivers an hourly or weekly rate, or reimbursing them when a house is sold or an estate is settled. Obviously, this needs to be discussed fully among all involved, and any agreement should be put in writing.

CONSIDER THE IMPLICATIONS. It's sometimes useful to have an elder law attorney involved in this, as these agreements can affect estate taxes, the caregiver's taxes (payments are income and taxed accordingly), and Medicaid eligibility (payments have to be seen as legitimate expenses and not gifts).

Indeed, if your parent is nearing Medicaid eligibility, paying a family caregiver makes perfect sense because it will make your parent eligible sooner. But the agreement has to be done properly.

DEFINE THE NEEDS. Make a list of your parent's needs. If this contract will affect Medicaid eligibility or taxes, get your parent's doctor, a home care agency, or a geriatric care manager to document the need.

Be specific: scheduling, bill paying, conferring with doctors, rides to appointments, making meals, supervision, help with baths, laundry, and so on.

The services and hours involved will change and need to be updated regularly.

ESTIMATE THE HOURS. Given the work involved, how many hours a week will it take? A caregiver will not be paid for every minute of his or her time. (No, you cannot include the time you spend fretting at 3 a.m.) Some of this *is* done out of love and duty. But siblings also need to realize that there is a lot of time spent organizing and handling the unexpected that is hard to quantify.

Once a contract is in place, the caregiver should keep a log of the hours worked and what was done. This will help family unity and it is critical if your parent applies for Medicaid.

AGREE ON THE PAY. Find out what people are paid for comparable work in the area by calling local home care agencies.

If your parent pays you hourly, then he becomes an employer and you an employee. Tax forms and insurance come into play; you might want a bookkeeper or payroll company to handle this.

If this is not showing up as wages, the annual gift limit to an individual is roughly $13,000 (it changes each year, so be sure to check).

If your parent has a home but no money, a caregiver might keep track of all hours and get paid when the home is sold. Or, your parent might be able to transfer the house to the caregiver's name in return for a promise of lifetime care.

Most states, when considering Medicaid eligibility, allow a lump sum payment that is based on a monthly rate multiplied by the parent's life expectancy. (Sometimes money is held in escrow to prevent caregivers from getting paid and hightailing it.)

Also, if your parent is on Medicaid, see if the state allows for payments to family caregivers. Some states, in an effort to keep people out of costly nursing homes, will compensate family caregivers as if they were hired privately.

DISCUSS OTHER REIMBURSEMENT. If the primary caregiver has expenses related to your parent's care—if he is buying groceries, paying for gas, or installing ramps—then those expenses obviously need to be reimbursed as well. He should keep careful records and share them with siblings regularly.

Often a parent who lives with a child pays rent as well. This might or might not factor into the compensation scheme, depending upon the rent and her needs.

ADDRESS THE DETAILS. The best-laid plans can derail when the details are ignored. For example, let's say Dad lives with one child and makes a monthly payment that covers a share of household expenses as well as caregiver compensation. But that caregiver still needs a break, so twice a year Dad visits another sibling's house for two weeks.

Should that other sibling get the rent plus hourly wages during those days? If not (for surely a little respite is to be expected), should the original sibling continue to get the rent (yes, as the mortgage is still due) or the caregiving compensation (maybe not, unless paid vacation was part of the contract)? How does this equation change if the other sibling takes Dad more often? Figure out the answers to these sorts of questions in advance.

WRITE A CONTRACT. Write a precise job description, detailing services, hours, and pay. Again, if this will affect Medicaid eligibility, get an elder law attorney involved. You also need a doctor, home care agency, or care manager to confirm the need and spell out the services required, and you need documentation of the going rates for such care. All involved should sign it. (See page 649 for a sample contract.)

LIVE WITH IT. Once everyone has had a say and agreed to a contract, they need to believe in it. No hard feelings. No secret resentment.

It's worth noting that just because a sibling is being paid for his or her duties, it does not mean others get to

> ❝ My mother lives with me, and my two sisters got very resentful because I was telling them when they could visit her. I didn't want them just dropping in whenever it was convenient. It's invasive, and besides, I hoped they would plan their visits when I couldn't be home so Mom wouldn't be alone.
>
> I would say, 'I have a class on Tuesday and Thursday, and it would be helpful if you could visit then.' But they got indignant and accused me of trying to keep them away from her. It got so that we were hardly speaking.
>
> When Mom needed more help, I talked to a social worker at the hospital, and she asked everyone to meet with her. When we explained how we were feeling without yelling at each other, everything seemed so simple and sort of childish.
>
> I think we were all worried about Mom and taking it out on each other. We have a lot more understanding now. There are still sparks, but we've really pulled together as a family."
>
> —Carol G.

disappear. Everyone still needs to pitch in and be involved. The primary caregiver should be paid for the daily grind, but she is handling more than that, and others need to offer support and give her a break from time to time.

More important, this is everyone's parent, so everyone needs to spend some time with her, check in, and be sure all is going well.

A caregiver's agreement can lead to improved care and better sibling relationships. But you need to communicate, reexamine it regularly, and keep your options open. Listen to everyone's views, and try to be friends when it's over.

A Family Meeting

Whether you face a family conflict or just want to plan ahead, it's helpful to get your family together, either informally or for a structured meeting with an agenda and a mediator.

Such a gathering will enable all of you to take a hard look at your parent's situation, hear your parent's views (when possible), make plans for the future, and dole out responsibilities. If caregiving duties are lopsided, this is an opportunity to bring things into balance.

Such a meeting also provides a forum where each person can air his or her views, learn what others are feeling, share much-needed emotional support, and devise a way to work as a team—if not in harmony, then at least under some sort of temporary truce.

The first meeting may be a little rough if you and your siblings don't get along. Siblings will have their own agendas, viewpoints, fears, and needs.

Don't give up. This is the beginning of a process. Just getting together and acknowledging that your parent needs attention and that you need to work together is in itself an accomplishment.

If a gathering is geographically impossible, organize a telephone conference

MEDIATION

When sibling relationships, financial issues, or any caregiving situation becomes too complex, heated, or entangled, consider mediation. Mediators are often successful at finding a resolution and are far less expensive and time consuming than, say, going to court.

To find a mediator, contact the National Association of Professional Geriatric Care Managers (caremanager.org), the area agency on aging (eldercare.gov), or the Association for Conflict Resolution (acrnet.org).

FAMILY MEETING TOPICS

- What are your parent's current health problems and physical and cognitive limitations? (It sounds obvious, but siblings can disagree even on this.)

- Is her current living situation working out? Can you make it safer and more manageable?

- Is it time for a move? What options are available should a move become necessary? Should you get on any waiting lists?

- What is her financial situation? Does she need help managing her money or paying bills? Can she afford the services she needs? Is she eligible for, or nearing eligibility for, Medicaid? Are there other benefits she might be eligible for?

- Given all of the above, what exactly needs to be done at this point? Is there research or planning that needs to happen?

- What must be done by family? What tasks can each person take on?

- What community programs or home care services are available to meet her needs?

- Beyond her pressing needs, what would be enjoyable for your parent? (Your parent might *need* someone to deliver meals, but she might *enjoy* visits from grandchildren, daily walks, and audiobooks.) Who can do some of this?

- How will each person help and support the primary caregiver?

- What services, housing, and financial assistance might your parent need in the future? How can you prepare for that now?

- What are your parent's wishes concerning aggressive medical care? Is everyone in agreement on how to follow her wishes?

- Is anyone in the family feeling unfairly treated, unheard, or unsupported?

- When will you meet or communicate next?

---

call or a video chat. Or, you might organize a Facebook or iChat group message, which is not ideal but can be helpful when siblings have particularly bitter relationships.

WHO COMES? It's important to keep your parent centrally involved in any discussion about his care and future, if at all possible. It is his life, after all, and no one likes to be instructed on how to live.

Beyond your parent, limit participants to siblings and anyone who is integrally involved in your parent's care. You might also have a geriatric care manager, or some other professional present. But try to keep the number small and manageable.

A MODERATOR. If emotions are fraught and the issues complex, find an outsider who can guide the discussion, make sure everyone has a chance to talk, and encourage people to listen to each other.

A moderator should be a neutral party, someone who is not related to the family and who is good at mediating disputes—a member of the clergy, a hospice counselor, a social worker, or a geriatric care manager.

AN AGENDA. Although it might seem oddly formal, having an agenda will help keep the conversation on course. Your parent's daily needs, finances, housing, medical care, and future are obvious topics, but ask siblings about other topics they want to discuss. A moderator or a sibling who's been chosen in advance to organize the meeting should incorporate these suggestions into a manageable agenda.

Don't try to get through a mountain of issues in one sitting. Prioritize issues and set a time limit on the meeting.

ADVANCE RESEARCH. If necessary, get family members to research certain issues before your meeting. For example, one sibling might look into financial and legal matters while another checks out community resources and housing options. Then, when you get together, you'll know some of the options and have a better idea of what needs to be done.

SOME GUIDELINES. To make sure that everyone is heard and the meeting accomplishes what you want it to, agree upon some guidelines in advance. Ask others for suggestions or adapt the following to suit your needs:

1. No one is allowed to dominate the meeting. If you don't have a moderator to direct and focus the discussion, agree that each person will talk for no more than, say, five minutes at a time—and use a timer, if necessary.

2. When someone is speaking, others must listen without interrupting. Listening, and really digesting what others have to say, is an essential goal of these meetings. If you get nothing else accomplished, be sure that you all hear each other's views. If people have trouble absorbing what others are saying, ask each person to briefly repeat the last speaker's message before taking his turn.

3. Each person should use sentences that begin with *I*—speaking only about his own opinions, feelings, and actions—and avoid finger-pointing statements that begin with *you*.

4. All discussions should relate directly to your parent's care. Steer away from old arguments and debates that are not relevant or helpful. If there are particularly touchy issues floating about that are simply unresolvable, then state on your agenda a list of issues that are *not* to be discussed.

> I live with my mother and needed help. At our first family meeting everyone agreed to pitch in, but it didn't work. So finally, when I couldn't deal with it anymore, I left home.
>
> It's hard to admit that I did that, but it got results. I told them, 'I'm not going back home until there's a written schedule and it's adhered to.' Of course, then they all had to pitch in.
>
> Once they realized exactly what was going on, once they lived it and saw what I was dealing with, they were willing to help. We made out a schedule, and most of the time it works."
>
> —Linda K.

5. Once you have all agreed on a plan, put it in writing, detailing schedules and assignments. Make a copy of the plan for each person.

6. Give your plan a trial run. In a few months, reconvene to discuss how things are working, to reassess your parent's needs, and to make any necessary adjustments to your plan.

Significant Others

If you have a strong and supportive relationship with a spouse, it will be an enormous help to you now. A spouse who listens, empathizes, and takes on some additional household responsibilities is a godsend and deserves your gratitude.

If you don't have that, whatever problems exist in the relationship may be magnified now. A parent's care often causes marital rifts, some of them deep.

If your parent needs you for the short term, your spouse will have to make do without you for a time. Your parent's care is a priority, and you both have to make compromises.

However, if your parent's care becomes a long-term undertaking, if you are consumed by her needs for more than a few months, do not let it destroy your marriage. Your parent will have to do with less of you because your spouse, even if he (or she) doesn't say so, needs a little more of you. Here are some approaches that should help during this time:

CLARIFY WHO'S RESPONSIBLE. Is each of you solely responsible for your own parents, and not at all responsible for

each other's parents? Is the woman responsible for both sets of parents? (Of course not, but this assumption is made with frightening regularity.) Should a spouse be expected to give up his weekends, vacations, or evenings to join you when you visit your parent? Should a spouse be expected to live with an in-law? Should a spouse who has developed a strong relationship with an in-law have a say in her care?

The answers will vary enormously from couple to couple. But talk about them. Don't make assumptions or hang on to unspoken expectations.

COMMUNICATE. Set aside time to talk (preferably when you are both calm and won't be interrupted; put the phones away). As always, use sentences that begin with *I* instead of those blaming *you* sentences. Small misunderstandings can expand into large ones if not attended to. Talk.

BE CLEAR. Don't assume that your spouse knows that you need help or knows how to help. Tell him, in concrete terms, what you need from him, whether it is emotional support or tangible

> **❝** Last time I visited my mother, my husband came with me. I got a sinus infection and spent a lot of time in bed, so he was in charge. Each day, when he went off to read the paper, Mom would come down and say, 'Now don't let me disturb you, dear. Keep on reading.' But then she would talk and talk and talk at him for hours.
>
> I wouldn't have wished this on him, but in retrospect I'm relieved that he had that experience. Now he can understand why I come home from these visits feeling so exhausted."
>
> —Carla P.

assistance. *I need to stop by Mom's house two nights a week. Could you please shop and make dinner on those days?* (Of course, if you leave dinner in his hands, you have to accept what he considers to be dinner, for better or worse.)

RECOGNIZE THE DIFFER-ENCES. Men and women really do come from different planets. Although there are plenty of exceptions, men are often uncomfortable with all the emotional hubbub and seek a little distance, which makes a wife feel abandoned just when she needs support most.

Sometimes men want to help but truly do not know how. (Yes, he stepped right over the laundry basket.) What seems obvious to you (a pile of dishes in the sink) might truly be invisible to him.

Finally, men often want to solve a problem, so they offer advice, thinking they are being helpful, only to find that they've ignited a fuse. *I want understanding, not answers!* Unable to fix things, or even have a discussion that isn't explosive, they feel inadequate and withdraw.

Be clear. Don't assume he should intuit your needs and feelings. Tell him. And then calmly remind him a week later. (If only "calm" could be bottled and purchased.)

CONSIDER HIS FEELINGS. You are not the only one affected by this. Your spouse will certainly feel the impact of your stress and the changes in the house-hold. Not only is he getting less of your attention, but he also has to cope with other fallout: bad moods, burned dinners, and crying jags.

He might feel shut out when he can't share or understand your anxiety and grief. Or he might be afraid that if he voices his own needs or opinions, he will appear selfish or unsympathetic.

KEEPING SANE AT HOME

In addition to the sibling meeting described in this chapter, you may want to call a meeting of your spouse and children. A planned discussion, rather than talking about your parent's care here and there over the laundry or TV, will be more productive.

Follow the guidelines outlined earlier. Let each person talk about what he or she feels, and then discuss how everyone can work together and support each other, assigning specific chores and duties if necessary. When the issues are knotty, a family counselor, found through a mental health center, can be helpful.

Also, no matter what is happening with you, or what sort of relationship your spouse has with your parents, he may have his own grief to deal with. He might be reminded of the loss of his parent or haunted by his own aging process.

With all that you are dealing with, it's hard to think about someone else's

sadness or anxiety—or the reasons someone might not be as helpful or supportive as you'd like—but try. Don't let this be *all* about you. Encourage your spouse to talk about his feelings, and give him the time and the space to vent.

MAKE THE EFFORT. Yes, your time is limited, but sometimes even small efforts, the ones that don't take much time, can make a big difference.

A weekend getaway would be amazing. Dinner and a movie, terrific. But having a sandwich together on a bench or a 10-minute walk in the evening can recharge a marriage. Next time you're sitting in the doctor's waiting room, text him. Let him know that you're thinking of him.

(It's understandable that you might not want to have sex right now, but your spouse might take that as a personal rejection. Talk about this too, if possible.)

SAY THANKS. Even if the help you receive is minimal, thank your spouse for it. He (or she) might not be doing anything more than putting up with your stress and busier hours. Express gratitude. He'll be more likely to help in the future. Positive reinforcement is not just psycho-speak; it works.

LAUGH. Did you, along the way, forget how to laugh together? It takes no time, burns calories, improves circulation, and strengthens bonds, and it's free. What's not to love about that?

> " When my mother-in-law became sick, I started visiting her, fixing her meals, making sure that she was all right. I guess it's my nature to take care of people.
>
> But then I became resentful. I don't really like her—she is very critical—and I had my own parents to take care of. I couldn't hide my resentment, and it caused regular spats between Steve and me.
>
> Finally, I told him that I was glad to help, but that I would not be responsible for her care. I was firm about it. I explained what I would and would not do. Honestly, it was very unlike me to be so assertive.
>
> He was incredibly understanding. He didn't realize that I had been feeling any of this. He began to realize that he'd been denying the whole thing about his mother and dumping it on my shoulders.
>
> I still visit her, but not nearly as much, and usually with support from him, which is all I really wanted in the first place."
>
> —Rose M.

Time for Kids

Your parents are old, your children are young, and you are caught in the middle, pulled by both ends of the age spectrum and feeling a bit like Plastic Man (without so much elasticity). Each day you face a dilemma: Do you take Dad to his doctor's appointment or get your son to school on time? Do you visit your mother or watch your daughter's soccer game? Do you give her a bath or make dinner for your family?

When the day is done, there is practically no "you" left, just the echoes of all the people who need you.

The dual demand of child and aging parent is so common that it has its own names—"the sandwich generation," "women caught in the middle," "the caregiver crunch." For working moms, the dilemma would more appropriately be called "mission impossible."

Having children around when a parent grows frail actually has some benefits—a child can pitch in and help, a grandparent might enjoy a child's company, and children learn from watching us care for those we love. But it can also leave you feeling torn, guilt-ridden, and irritable. (What else is new?)

Don't let your child get lost in the commotion, slipping down your ladder of priorities until he is hardly on it anymore. Address his needs and concerns, and be sure that your parent's care does not unhinge your number one job: being a parent.

STOP, BREATHE, ORGANIZE. If you are running in circles and never catching up, stop. Consider the demands on your time, prioritize. Make a plan. Accept that you cannot do it all (and be okay with that because, truly, you cannot do it all).

With all that you are juggling, it is vital that you be organized—very, very organized. Take a moment to think ahead. Learn about community services and housing options early. And always, always have a Plan B. Keep a list of available sitters and senior companions up to date.

BE HONEST. Children, even very young children, can understand much more than we give them credit for. Certainly, a child of any age feels the stress in the household and your anxiety.

Talk to them, but keep it simple and at a level that is appropriate. Tell them that Grandma is sick, how that is hard for everyone, that it makes you sad and tired, and that you don't have as much time for them as you'd like.

> " It's pretty well known that my mom was not a nice mother, that she was cruel to us. But my kids have watched me. They see how I treat my mom.
>
> My son said to me, 'You know, Mom, the way you turned out and the way you take care of your mom when she wasn't a good mom to you . . . I'm really proud of you.'
>
> That's part of the gift. They have never resented me for it, for all the time I spent caring for my mom and dad. I think, maybe when it's my time, they'll be there for me."
> —Carla M.

Then, encourage them to ask questions, and answer their questions directly. If a parent is dying, talk about that as openly as you can, too. (For more on children and grief, see page 579.)

TAKE TIME TO LISTEN. Don't assume that you understand a child's concerns. Let her tell you about them. Children respond to illness in unexpected ways and worry about issues that adults might not even consider. For example, a child might be wondering if she is going to have to give up her bedroom if Grandpa moves in, or she might be concerned that Grandma's ailment is contagious.

Your child won't open up on your schedule, so be ready and attuned. When you sense that a child wants to talk, stop what you are doing. Get off the phone; put dinner on hold. A child might not "save" his emotions for later, when you are free.

When he does open up, no matter what he says, be careful not to make him feel that his emotions are wrong, trivial, or silly. Let him know you've really heard him and that you take his concerns seriously.

SET ASIDE TIME FOR THEM. With everything going on, it may seem impossible, but carve out some time for just the two of you (or five of you), and do something, anything, unrelated to Grandma. If you can't set aside an afternoon for an excursion, take a short detour on the way to the grocery store and go to the park, even briefly. Or make a lunch or dinner date, perhaps going out with just one child.

LET HIM HELP. If a child shows any interest in helping with your parent's care (or even if he doesn't), give him a job to do.

Keep your requests reasonable. Even a toddler can carry Grandma's blanket to her, or draw a picture for her. Children want to be included in family life and will be proud that they helped.

LET HER REFUSE TO HELP, TOO. Younger children might be willing to be involved, but older children, especially adolescents, might want to keep a distance. They may be uncomfortable with their grief or sadness, or feel "grossed out" by aspects of your parent's care. Or they may be preoccupied with what they consider more important aspects of life—friends, parties, dates, music, or sports.

Although these priorities might seem skewed to you, they are a normal and necessary part of teenage development. Urge teenagers to understand the importance of family and responsibility, and get them involved in some way, but allow them to be teenagers, too, even if it means distancing themselves somewhat from you and your parent's situation.

GET AT THE CAUSE OF BAD BEHAVIOR. Children have an uncanny ability to pick up on stress. Your stress makes them stressed, which makes them whine and run in circles (if they are young) or slam doors (if they are older).

They can also feel jealous of a grandparent who is getting your love and attention. Or they might wish that a grandparent would leave or die. They feel awful for feeling this way and they feel bad for being bad, which only makes them more cranky and out of control.

A child's behavior might be his way of expressing his pain, jealousy, and confusion, or a way to get your attention—his way of saying, *Help me. Notice me.*

Remember that you are the adult here. Your child is far less able than you are to deal with all these emotions. Spending time with him and talking openly should fend off some problems.

Let him know that it's normal to feel jealous and confused, and that his feelings are understandable.

When there are outbursts, remain calm and try to understand the root of the problem. Don't condone his behavior, but do allow some of it. Everyone needs a little forgiveness right now. If things become unmanageable or worrisome, talk with a school counselor or a child psychologist.

SHOW YOUR CHILDREN YOUR YOUNGER PARENT. If your parent is very sick, confused, or grumpy, pull out some old photos or home movies. Show your children what Grandpa used to be like in his younger and stronger days. You might tell them stories of things you used to do together. Help them understand who this man used to be.

> " My father has been quite frail for three years, and sometimes I feel angry that my children aren't seeing the man I knew. I tell them what he used to be like, but they just see this very weak person who needs a lot of peace and quiet.
>
> Last time we were there, the kids were playing in the garden, and he said, 'When the hell are you going to leave? This noise is too much.'
>
> I don't know whether to bring them next time I go. It's hard on him and hard on them."
>
> —Jane C.

Multilayer Sandwiches

" The sandwich generation" might be squeezed between parents and children, but many of us are facing a far more complicated sandwich than that.

When you are caring for children and aged parents, and aging in-laws, aunts, uncles, or grandparents are added to the mix, a simple sandwich becomes a triple-decker. Or, better yet, sticking with the sandwich analogy, a hero.

Just as you get Mom settled in a nursing home and Dad set up at adult day care, your husband announces that his father needs help. The pileup is beyond anyone's dreams (or worst nightmare), and an overwhelming task suddenly takes on colossal dimensions.

It's time for some serious restructuring and a lot of help. You are no longer a daughter, niece, or in-law. You are a general. And this is war.

Gather the troops. Call in the reserves. Enlist volunteers. Assign duties. Use every community service available. There's no room for emotion now. (Guilt? Are you kidding?) This has to be handled quickly and effectively. Do what you can to get the most pressing jobs done.

Take each person's situation, one at a time, and formulate a quick plan of action. What are the most pressing needs? What services are available? Who can help and how? Unload *all* extra duties.

If possible, find a geriatric care manager or case manager who can help you identify community services and draw on all the benefits to which your parent/aunt/in-law/grandparent is entitled. This is especially important for those relatives who live far away.

Careers and Caregiving

You're at work when your phone rings. It's your father. His speech is garbled and he seems confused. You're worried, but you have an important meeting with your boss in 10 minutes. What do you do?

Your mother goes to adult day care until 4 p.m. each day, but today you can't leave work until 7. What do you do?

The hospital just called. Your parent broke her hip. She's in intensive care. Even if you leave work now, you wouldn't be at the hospital for several hours. What do you do?

Caregivers often quit, change jobs, accept a demotion, or cut back on their hours. Others continue on, but jeopardize their careers by leaving work early, coming in late, making calls at work, and generally being exhausted and distracted.

Before you veer off your career track or quit your job, think long and hard about your options. There might be a way to care for your parent and keep your day job.

PLAN, PLAN, PLAN. Regardless of the situation, plan ahead. When you work, it is vital that you are always prepared, always one step ahead. Learn about housing options and local services, even if you don't need them yet. Make provisions to get your job done or to get someone to cover for you if you are suddenly called away.

HAVE A PLAN B. Always, always, always have more than one plan in place, more than one name and number to call. If your parent is dependent on a companion who comes each day, have the name of a second one or an agency that can send someone over on a moment's notice. If you rely on your parent's neighbor to keep an eye on things, get the name of someone else who can run over when there's a crisis and the first neighbor isn't answering her phone.

SET PRIORITIES. Write a list of everything that you need to do, and then scratch some items from it. Prioritize. What has to be done, what can be put off, what can be forgotten?

ENLIST HELP. This is no time to be the martyr. Get help! Talk to relatives, friends, and neighbors about how they might pitch in. Find volunteers who can check on your parent regularly or when a crisis strikes. Use community services.

CONTACT THE HUMAN RESOURCES DEPARTMENT. Many large companies and some smaller ones have personnel who can provide information about eldercare and community services. Others are hooked to a national service that provides referrals and counseling. Some companies offer flexible hours and job sharing. Others sponsor support groups, seminars, and information fairs on eldercare.

ORGANIZE YOUR TIME. Make a schedule of your day, and look for ways to be more efficient. Are there errands that can be skipped, or done in the morning or during breaks at work? Can you shop for a week's worth of food in one hit? Can you do some research while sitting in the dentist's office?

COMPARTMENTALIZE. Sometimes it can't be helped, but making phone calls or searching the Internet on company time is a risky habit if you want to keep your job. Make phone calls during a lunch break or in the evening whenever possible. When at work, be at work.

YES, ONCE AGAIN, TAKE CARE OF YOURSELF. The boss is yelling at you, your spouse is tired of all this, your children are whining, and then, well, there's your parent. You are on the right path for a nervous breakdown or at least a good case of the flu.

Take 10 minutes out each day for stretches, deep breathing, meditation, or even just a quiet moment alone. Find a local support group, or join an online group. Remember your own needs.

SET LIMITS. When you are working, this is critical. Set realistic expectations for yourself. You cannot do everything for your parent, so define what you can and will do, and what you can't and won't do.

LET GO OF SOME THINGS. Your house is a mess, the garden's all weeds, and you haven't organized family photos for more than three years. Forget it. The cobwebs can wait.

ESTABLISH RULES. If your parent or a health aide calls you at work regularly, set down firm rules about when you can be interrupted and under what circumstances. It sounds cold, but it's better to be clear than to be annoyed with your parent and reprimanded by your supervisor. *Mom, I love you and I want to help you, but I can't do anything until I get home from work. I will talk to you about it then, not now.*

DISCRETION AROUND THE WATER COOLER

At work, be careful what you say to whom. It's fine to use eldercare services offered by the human resources department. It's fine to talk to your boss about changing your schedule. But you don't want to stand around the water cooler griping about your parent's needs and all the time you spend at work dealing with her care.

THE FAMILY AND MEDICAL LEAVE ACT

Under the 1993 Family and Medical Leave Act, employees must be offered at least 12 weeks of unpaid leave to care for a new child or an ill family member—a parent, spouse, or child (but not a grandparent or in-law). The act applies only to businesses with 50 or more employees. An employee must have been with the company for at least one year and must have logged at least 1,250 hours in the previous 12 months (about 24 hours a week) to be eligible for leave.

The act mandates the following:

- If possible, employees must give 30 days' notice that they are taking a leave.

- Employees (except for those in the 10 percent of highest-paid positions) are entitled to get their old job back, or a post with equivalent duties, benefits, and pay.

- Employees are entitled to their full health benefits while on leave. However, an employer can demand to be paid back for the cost of premiums if the employee quits the job at the end of the leave.

- Leave can be taken in bits and pieces—a few days or even a few hours at a time—if the employer and employee both agree on the arrangement.

- An employer can require that vacation or sick days be used at the beginning of the leave.

GET YOUR PARENT TO USE THE INTERNET. If your mother calls you at work 10 times a day, teach her how to use email. She can contact you to her heart's content, and you can read it when you get a chance.

Negotiating with Your Boss

Most people are hesitant to speak with a boss about family responsibilities, and rightfully so. You'll have to use your own judgment here. It will depend on your boss and your relationship with him or her. In most cases, bosses would rather know what's going on and work out a plan than have you sneaking out early and coming in late with no explanation.

A boss's number one concern is getting the job done. So when you talk to a boss about changing hours, taking time off, or other work arrangements, couch it in terms a boss can appreciate.

Rather than telling a sob story and asking your boss to help you, come up with a plan and explain how you will ultimately get your work done. (*I'll leave at 3 p.m. but come in at 7 a.m. when it's quiet and I can get more done.*) Work out all the details in advance and show why your plan will be at least as good as the current way of operating and perhaps even better.

As you pitch your idea, be sure to keep the focus on your professional goals and the goals of the company rather than on your personal needs. And let the boss know that you are committed to this job.

Propose a trial period, which gives both you and your boss a chance to test this arrangement before accepting it.

The
Golden Years

Chapter 5

A Healthier Body

**In the Gym • The ABCs of Diet • The Liquor Cabinet •
Up in Smoke**

Y**our parent is old, frail,** and has a medical file as thick as a New York City phone book. She has real problems, and you have serious concerns. She can't hear well, she can barely walk, money's a problem, and she's got a life-threatening illness. You are sleepless from worry and more than a bit overwhelmed. *Healthy aging* is really not a concern right now; your parent is beyond needing a few vitamins and is certainly not about to go to the gym.

Well, hold on just a minute.

Eating well, exercising, dealing with stress, and otherwise taking care of oneself are no less important at 85 than they are at 50. The old adage is true: Use it or lose it. And if your parent has already lost most of it, she might get some of it back, or at least enjoy what remains.

The truth is that some of the decline that we attribute to aging—frailty, poor balance, immobility, confusion, anxiety, depression, and forgetfulness—is the result of inactivity, poor diet, and isolation as much as passing years.

By tending to her body and—just as important—to her heart, mind, and soul (see the following chapter), your parent will increase her mobility, independence, and stamina. It won't cure disease, but it will help her make the most of what she still has.

Do not assume that she can't do it, or that she won't do it. She can improve her life by simply eating a little better, stretching a bit, and getting out from time to time. Small lifestyle changes can reap big rewards.

In the Gym

E ven if your parent can't hobble across the hallway or push herself out of a wheelchair, she can still benefit from some gentle exercises. Don't be overprotective here—*But my parent is really too feeble for this.* And don't let her fear stand in the way, either. If she can't or won't go to a gym or pool, maybe she can walk to the mailbox, sway to her favorite music, sweep her own front step, or do some easy stretches.

If your parent uses a wheelchair or is bedridden most of the time, she might be able to do neck rotations, arm stretches, and foot flexes each day. Pretty much everyone can do something, and every little bit helps.

Why Bother?

The benefits of exercise for very elderly people (or anyone, for that matter) are enormous. Numerous studies have shown that even the frailest people in nursing homes become more mobile and people with dementia become calmer when they exercise. Your parent might groan at the thought, but exercise is more effective than many of the medications he takes. Here are just a few specific benefits of exercise for even extremely frail and/or confused people:

- Increased mobility, stamina, and energy

- More independence and a higher level of functioning

- Less depression

- Less anxiety

- Enhanced self-esteem and optimism

- Reduced risk of heart disease, diabetes, osteoporosis, and some types of cancer

> ## ✚ BEFORE HE BEGINS
>
> Before your parent embarks on any exercise regimen, he should first talk with his doctor, a physical therapist, or a sports medicine specialist.

- Improvement of existing vascular or heart disease, osteoarthritis, and diabetes

- Better balance and coordination (which reduces the risk of falls)

- Stronger bones, muscles, and joints

- Loss of extra weight

- Relief of pain

- Deeper, more restful sleep

- Improved bowel function

- Boosted immunity

- Improved memory and less confusion

- Less agitation

- Better interactions with caregivers

Did you notice that last one? Yes, it's true. Elderly people who get some exercise get on better with their caregivers. Do you need any other reasons to pull out the Jane Fonda DVDs?

IN THE POOL

If your parent has access to a pool, swimming and water exercises are great for muscle mass, cardiovascular function, and overall health. As with other exercise, your parent might start with just 5 or 10 minutes and work up to 20 minutes three times a week.

Many pools offer senior exercise classes—such as water Pilates, water aerobics, and aqua therapy—but if not, just walking back and forth in the shallow end holding on to the edge and bringing the arms up and down in the water are two terrific exercises.

If your parent is reluctant or downright refuses to move a muscle, find out his reasons. Some elderly people are afraid they will get hurt; some worry that they will have to join an expensive gym or buy special equipment, still others think exercising is only for young people; and many are just used to their sedentary way of life. All of these issues and concerns can be addressed.

Finding the Right Exercise Program

Your parent's exercise regimen should suit her specific needs and be something she will stay with. Some people will enjoy a short walk, some like yoga, and others are drawn to the pool. Your parent might spend 10 minutes in the morning stretching and doing resistance exercises in bed while watching the news.

Sometimes exercising is simply a matter of doing more for oneself—getting up and about, taking care of the house or garden, walking to the grocery store. Your instincts might tell you that your parent should sit down, but don't listen to them. Let him sweep the walkway or rake the leaves or hobble to the kitchen to get himself a sandwich. It's good for him.

If your parent is bedridden or uses a wheelchair, she obviously needs to keep it simple. A physical therapist can help. Some exercise videos are made especially for older people with physical disabilities.

If your parent is willing, a good regimen has four

TAI CHI

Tai chi (short for tai chi chuan) is a Chinese martial art that is known for its health benefits. It involves slow, synchronized, almost dancelike movements, and measured breathing, that help both body and mind. It is sometimes referred to as "moving meditation."

According to ancient Chinese thinking, focusing one's concentration and breathing, and moving deliberately through the various postures, improves the flow of Qi (pronounced "chee"), which is the vital life force.

Whatever the reasons, tai chi helps coordination and balance, significantly reducing the risk of falls among the elderly. It also reduces stress, alleviates depression, lowers blood pressure, eases arthritis pain, treats insomnia, improves immune function, and increases independence.

The moves are easy to learn, easy to do, and can be done anywhere, at any time, in any clothing, and by anyone who can stand up. They are gentle, graceful, and soothing, with names like "white crane spreads its wings" and "waving hand in the cloud." (Very frail people might want to avoid the Chen style of tai chi, which is a faster version.)

It is best learned with an instructor. Classes are available through local Arthritis Foundation chapters, YMCAs, recreation centers, senior centers, some churches and synagogues, community centers, and gyms.

---

components: aerobic, strength, flexibility, and balance exercises. Ideally, he should alternate, doing aerobic exercise one day and strength exercises the next, for example.

AEROBIC. Aerobic exercises give the heart and lungs a workout and improve endurance. Walking, riding a stationary bicycle, swimming, or other water exercises (which are especially good for people with arthritis, osteoporosis, or back, knee, or hip problems) are all good choices, but so are raking, dancing, and mopping.

STRENGTH. Lifting weights is not simply for those seeking rippling abs and bulging biceps. In fact, after lifting weights, your parent might not notice any visible increase in muscle, but the effect will still be there—more strength, better metabolism, less risk of osteoporosis.

Strength exercises can be done with small weights, a large band of rubber for resistance (found at sports stores), or jugs, bottles, or socks filled with sand, beans, or water (but don't put water in the socks!). Your parent can also stand in a doorway and push against the doorjambs, squeeze his palms together, let someone else act as an immovable barrier, or work against the weight of his own body by doing push-ups or sit-ups.

If your parent is particularly frail, he might lift his shoulders slowly and lower them, make a fist and release it, and so on.

FLEXIBILITY. Bending and stretching improve range of motion, alleviate arthritis, and relieve tension. With the

> **"** My mom is 80 and has a list of med-
> ical problems. She uses a walker
> and needs oxygen at night. But somehow
> she just keeps on going. She swims in the
> pool at the senior home she's at and rides
> a stationary bike. She's always seeing
> friends, going out to dinner, going to lec-
> tures. I call her and she's like, 'Oh, I can't
> talk right now. So-and-so's coming for
> lunch.' It's as though she decided that she
> is not going to get old, and so she doesn't.
> I think, Please, please let me be like her!"
> —Anne C.

lack of use that comes with age, muscles
and bones shrink, and tendons and lig-
aments fail to extend. As a result, older
people often stoop over, have trouble
with their balance, and experience back
pain.

Your parent should take it easy,
stretching gently until he feels a slight
pull, then hold it for anywhere from 8
to 30 counts, depending on how it feels.

BALANCE. This is critical for the elderly,
as it helps prevent falls (which in the
elderly are extremely serious and often
fatal). Balance exercises are often part of
strength exercises, but they also include
things such as holding the back of a chair
and going slowly onto tiptoes or bending one leg up and back.

Rules of the Game

Your parent should be sure to observe
the following guidelines:

- Start slowly and work up gradually,
  doing a little more each week. Your
  parent might get winded after only a
  few minutes of walking, for example.
  That's okay. Go slowly. It may take
  several weeks for her to build up more
  stamina.

- Rest whenever necessary. Your parent
  should stop exercising immediately
  if he has palpitations, chest pains, or
  cramps, or if he becomes nauseated,
  dizzy, faint, light-headed, breathless,
  or exhausted.

- Drink plenty of fluids, especially if
  it's a warm day (but avoid ice-cold
  fluids, which can cause cramping).
  Elderly people tend to lose their sense
  of thirst, so drinking water might not
  come naturally to your parent. She
  might need a reminder from
  you.

- Stay balanced. Stand with
  legs planted slightly apart,
  back straight, body aligned,
  and eyes focused ahead. Your
  parent should have something nearby that he can grab
  if he feels off balance.

- Begin and end with simple,
  easy stretches, warming up
  beforehand and then cooling
  down slowly at the end.

VIDEO EXERCISE

There are dozens of exercise videos
especially for older people and those with
disabilities. Look for them at your local library
or search online. The Arthritis Foundation has
several DVDs that are good for most elderly
people (afstore.org). The National Institute
on Aging has a DVD as part of its Go4Life
campaign (go4life.nia.nih.gov).

WALKING FOR LIFE

Walking is a great form of exercise for an elderly person (actually, for all of us). It's easy on the joints, it's entertaining, it's cheap, and it can be social. It requires no special skills and can be done virtually anywhere.

Your parent might just walk to the end of the driveway and back. For more serious walkers, schools often have outdoor tracks, and some malls are open early for walkers.

Get your parent to start with a short walk—which may be a few paces or a few blocks, depending upon his abilities—three times a week, and then add a little more each week.

As he walks, he should stand straight, with his head erect and arms swinging loosely at his sides. Tell him to lift his feet rather than shuffle, so he doesn't trip on cracks and bumps.

Make sure your parent has comfortable sneakers with arch supports and thick rubber soles. Find sneakers made of nylon, mesh, canvas, or other material that lets the air circulate. If he needs to carry things with him, like a cell phone, get him a fanny pack. If he doesn't have a cane or walker, consider a good walking stick for support.

Someone should always know where he is headed. Remind him to drink before he's thirsty, because once he's thirsty, his body is already seriously low on fluids (remember, the elderly often fail to register that they are thirsty).

- Vary exercises. He might do strength exercises one day and aerobic the next, or work on one muscle group one day and a different group the next.

- Avoid getting dizzy. Your parent shouldn't get up too fast or change directions too rapidly.

- Keep breathing! People tend to hold their breath when exercising. Your parent should breathe regularly with each repetition.

- Exercises should not be painful.

- Watch the temperature. Choose a comfortable time of day, when it's not too hot or cold.

- Wear loose, comfortable clothing that doesn't impede movement. Opt for

" When I was pregnant, I did stretching exercises from a video. My mother, who is in a wheelchair, would watch me. She enjoyed the music and energy of it. And it was something for her to do. I encouraged her to join in, and with some reluctance, she finally did. She did simple versions of what I was doing, or she would swing her arm out to the side when I was swinging my leg, that sort of thing. But she had fun with it.

After the baby was born and I wasn't using the tape anymore, I gave it to her. She says she still uses it most days. I know it helps her keep moving, and it's entertaining."

—Jane D.

YOGA AND PILATES FOR ALL

Yoga, a mind-body exercise that originated in India and involves doing asanas, or poses, seems to be effective at reducing pain and depression and improving health, flexibility, and balance in seniors. It also seems to alleviate lower back pain. Look for classes aimed at the elderly or beginners, which will be easier and more instructive.

Pilates focuses on developing a strong spine and torso, or core, which improves balance and coordination (and helps with lower back pain). Again, try to find classes targeted to seniors.

layers that can be shed as the body warms up.

• If your parent is exercising in his house, he should clear plenty of space to allow for safety and freedom of movement.

• Make exercising part of each day's routine. It might be helpful to keep a daily record—how many minutes, what movements, how many repetitions, and so on.

Where Do We Sign Up?

Exercising with others can be fun and inspire your parent to stick with it. If he is interested in a group activity, find an exercise program for elders that is oriented toward his particular needs and abilities.

Inquire at the local senior center, community center, department of recreation, Jewish center, or YMCA. Ask at local gyms and health clubs about exercise classes for the elderly.

For more information and exercise ideas, check out the National Institute on Aging's Go4Life program (go4life .nia.nih.gov).

The ABCs of Diet

Does your parent skip breakfast, dine on half of yesterday's saved sandwich, or return meal trays that have barely been touched? Or is your father obese and filling up on pound cake despite repeated warnings from his doctor?

Whereas most of the country is talking about obesity and buying diet books by the boatload, the elderly have very different weight and nutrition issues. Perhaps the most important difference is that when it comes to the elderly, extra weight is not the biggest concern; malnutrition and weight loss are.

Studies suggest that nearly a quarter of the elderly in this country are

WHEN EATING SLOWS

If your parent is not eating, talk to his doctor, as it can be a sign of illness or a side effect of medications. But also try to figure out the source of the problem yourself, because there could be an easy solution.

With age, the sense of smell diminishes, and with it goes taste, making food less appetizing. Loneliness and depression can also make eating less enjoyable and interesting.

Your dad might say he's not hungry, but in truth he might have trouble getting to the grocery store, affording food (for real or perceived reasons), preparing food, and using utensils. If he is acutely ill or has oral problems, he may be having difficulty chewing and swallowing. If your parent has dementia, he might simply forget to eat. Certain medications can also hinder appetite.

A more sedentary lifestyle also leaves a person less hungry—you burn fewer calories, so you need fewer calories. And let's remember, institutional food—like that served in a nursing home—can be pretty dreadful.

You can make shopping, cooking, and eating more manageable for your parent, or you can have meals delivered. Or maybe see if someone could sit with him at mealtime and help him eat. For more tips on making shopping, cooking, and eating more manageable, see page 133.

---

malnourished. That doesn't mean they are bone-thin and starving; it simply means that for various reasons, they are failing to get the vitamins, minerals, and other nutrients that their bodies need.

The problem is often overlooked by doctors, who are focused on heart function and brain waves, not lunch plates. It is even overlooked in hospitals, where, according to at least two studies, nearly half of elderly patients do not get proper nutrition. So take a look at your parent's eating habits and any weight changes, and ask the doctor about any concerns you have.

Not Too Fat for Me
One good thing about old age is that, finally, a little pudge is not a bad thing. The body stores calories in fat, and that extra reserve can be useful in times of illness or surgery. It also makes nice padding, possibly protecting frail bones and vital organs from falls.

Whatever the reasons, the evidence suggests that elderly people who are a little overweight fare better than those who are underweight. So unless there are compelling reasons for your parent to lose weight, don't bug her, and tell her not to worry about it.

When the Weight Should Go
If your parent has arthritis, osteoporosis, heart disease, diabetes, or another condition that requires weight control, and he is more than a little plump—20 to 30 percent over one's desirable weight is considered obese—then it's time for a change.

DIETARY ADVICE

If you are worried about your parent's eating habits and the doctor isn't much help, your parent, or you, may want to consult a nutritionist. Since anyone can hang up a shingle, be sure to look for a "registered dietitian," a certification that means the person has, at the very least, received a bachelor's degree in nutrition or a related field and has passed a special exam.

To find a registered dietitian, call the state dietetic association, ask at the doctor's office, or contact the American Dietetic Association (eatright.org), which can refer you to a registered dietitian in your parent's hometown.

Your parent doesn't need to lose it all. Getting rid of even a few pounds (maybe 5 percent of his weight) should help lower his blood pressure, reduce his cholesterol level, improve his diabetes, and relieve the pressure on his joints. A modest goal will be more attainable, and who wants to start a painful diet at 89?

Forget the fad diets, which tend to fail and usually aren't healthful. Have a doctor or registered dietitian work out a meal plan for your parent, or use common sense. Basically, he needs to skim some fat and calories from his daily diet while being sure he gets the nutrients he needs.

If your parent has put weight on suddenly, he should see his doctor. There are various conditions and medications that might be behind sudden weight gain.

Sudden Weight Loss

Unintentional weight loss is a warning sign of a number of serious illnesses, including depression, cancer, heart failure, and dementia. If you notice weight loss, talk with your parent's doctor.

After a lifetime of lectures about low-fat, low-calorie diets, it's time to forget all that. If your parent has become frighteningly thin, he should eat any food he likes—peanut butter, cheese, ice cream, doughnuts, whatever. At some point, it's just about getting calories in (unless he has diabetes, in which case he needs to confer with his doctor or a nutritionist).

When weight loss is an issue, it is often better to offer five or six small meals or a series of snacks, as a large plate of food can be overwhelming. Keep a bowl of high-calorie treats on the table. Or try a shake of ice cream or yogurt and fruit with some protein or high-calorie powder thrown in.

Nutritional drinks, such as Boost and Ensure, are useful as supplements, but they should not replace real food and should, preferably, be given between meals and not in place of meals.

Healthy Eating

In general, if your parent has a reasonably good diet and the doctor says he's fine, let him be. As we've noted, a few extra pounds are not a concern. Some Fritos in the afternoon or a slice of cake after dinner is nothing to worry about. The truth is, you've got enough on your plate (no pun intended) and don't need another issue to fret about.

That said, the fact remains that most elderly people do not eat well, and their bodies often do not absorb the vitamins and other nutrients they need. Many have health problems that would be alleviated by better nutrition. Eating well reduces the risk of disease, improves recovery from illness or surgery, and generally makes people feel more robust. So, if you have the time and energy for it, and he's willing, see if you can't improve his diet.

Your parent should stick to the same basic principles the rest of us should follow (along with any special medical orders)—plenty of fruits, vegetables, fiber, fluids, and whole grains, and not so much fat, sugar, and salt.

Fluids and fiber have to be emphasized. Elderly people often lose their sense of thirst (and the desire or ability to get up and get a drink), so be sure your parent has a glass of water nearby at all times. Don't let him skip it in an effort to avoid going to the toilet, as this can actually make incontinence worse.

And because constipation is so common and can be so serious, be sure your parent is getting plenty of fiber (prunes, apricots, lentils, carrots, certain cereals). Of course, he needs water so the fiber can do its job.

Beyond that, a few key words: *variation, moderation,* and *real.* That is, a good diet includes a variety of vegetables, fruits, rice, grains, nuts, and so on, but there's no need to be extreme. An occasional doughnut is fine; a mound of kale each day is not necessary. And obviously,

NUTRITIONAL SUPPLEMENTS

While the experts are still hemming, hawing, and disagreeing about the virtues and dangers of dietary supplements, the business of dietary supplements is exploding. It's not just vitamins and minerals anymore, but amino acids, hormones, herbs, antioxidants, and a whole assortment of unpronounceable and unrecognizable items. And they are not just found in pills sold at the pharmacy, but in chocolate bars and vitamin drinks sold at every market in the country.

The best way to get nutrients is through healthful food. However, many elderly people have health and other problems that make it impossible for them to get the nutrients they need through diet alone.

A daily multivitamin—and some are specifically designed for the elderly—or a hit of B vitamins might help, but before taking any kind of supplement, your parent should talk to her doctor or a registered dietitian.

As for the medley of supplements claiming to cure illness, reverse aging, and boost memory, energy, happiness, and well-being, forget it. Very few dietary supplements have been scientifically shown to do anything beneficial. Most are a waste of money, and some are dangerous. According to the National Institute on Aging, supplements can cause high blood pressure, nausea, diarrhea, constipation, fainting, headaches, seizures, heart attacks, or strokes. They can also interfere with the action of certain medications. Talk to your parent's doctor.

food should actually be just that—food. Stuff that came out of the earth or was fed by the earth. It should not contain 48 ingredients, half of which you can't pronounce. It should not be a reconstituted, processed, fortified, food-type product.

For more information on diet and nutrition, check out these two websites: the federal government's nutrition site, nutrition.gov, and the American Dietetic Association's eatright.org.

The Liquor Cabinet

Although it might seem that sipping a couple of scotches every evening is one of your father's last little pleasures in life, beware. Alcohol, even seemingly reasonable amounts of it, can cause serious health problems in the elderly and exacerbate some of the more routine troubles that come with old age. In other words, those highballs might be making your dad's day-to-day life more miserable than you—or he—imagine.

Alcohol is a drug, and like other drugs, it has a more pronounced effect in older bodies. So even if your father has always had an evening cocktail without any trouble, it might simply be too much for him now. Studies show that when a 60-year-old and a 20-year-old drink the same amount of alcohol, the older person's blood-alcohol level is 20 percent higher than the younger person's. A 90-year-old is apt to have a blood-alcohol level that is 50 percent higher.

Although one drink with dinner may not be cause for alarm (and, yes, wine in moderation might reduce cardiovascular risk), even small amounts of alcohol can intensify problems that your parent might already be struggling with (confusion, incontinence, insomnia, poor appetite, poor balance, and depression). It also

SIGNS OF TROUBLE

Your parent may have a problem with alcohol if he:

- Gulps his drinks

- Has a heightened reaction to alcohol (appears flushed, confused, or unstable after drinking moderately)

- Hides or lies about his drinking

- Has little interest in food

- Is irritable or unreasonable

- Withdraws socially

- Neglects his personal hygiene

❝ My mother used to love to have a couple of old-fashioneds every night. Then we decided that her drinking might be contributing to the dizziness and the falls, so Elizabeth, Mom's companion, got her down to one small glass of sherry. I was amazed, but Elizabeth can get Mom to do almost anything—things that I could never convince her to do.

One evening when I was visiting, Mom said, 'Oh, I think I'll have a real drink tonight.' And I said, 'No, Mom, please don't do that.' I was a little nervous about what her reaction would be, but she didn't say a word, and she didn't have the drink. I was truly shocked. And very relieved."

—Greta N.

hinders coordination and slows a person's reactions, increasing the chances of a serious fall. In addition, alcohol can make a person more susceptible to infections, colds, and other illness.

Perhaps most disconcerting, alcohol and medications, including over-the-counter (nonprescription) medications, can be a dangerous mix—and most elderly people take between two and seven medications a day.

Because of all this, the National Institute on Alcohol Abuse and Alcoholism recommends that people over 65 have no more than one drink per day. One drink, by the way, is not served in a mug. It is defined as one 12-ounce beer, 5 ounces of wine, or 1.5 ounces of distilled spirits—gin, vodka, scotch, and so on.

Unfortunately, boredom, pain, and insomnia can make alcohol a welcome analgesic. Those who have routinely had one drink every evening begin to have two or three; former teetotalers decide that a little nip each evening might help them sleep.

As for heavy drinking, there is no question that it is very serious. In addition to all the risks mentioned above, your parent now faces a higher risk of liver disease, stroke, immune disorders, hypertension, vitamin deficiency, certain types of cancer, and permanent brain damage.

If you are worried about your parent's drinking, talk with him about your concerns or ask his doctor to talk with him.

If the problem is dire, have a family meeting and confront the issue with your parent. Talk about the effect his drinking is having on the family. Point out the medical risks he is taking and what he is doing to his body. Talk about the benefits of quitting, particularly how it will affect his life and his relationships. Let your parent know that if he decides to quit, you will all support and encourage him. You can also seek help from one of the groups listed on the next page.

➕ MEDICAL ALERT

If your parent routinely drinks alcohol and is placed in a situation in which it is not available, such as a nursing home or hospital, he is likely to go through withdrawal. The symptoms include shakiness, sweating, rapid breathing, agitation, and sometimes delirium, hallucinations, and seizures.

Alert the personnel about his drinking habits, and be sure the information is entered in his record. Withdrawal is a medical emergency that requires immediate treatment.

ⓘ FOR MORE HELP

Alcoholics Anonymous
aa.org or 212-870-3400

....

Al-Anon Family Groups
al-anon.org or 800-356-9996

....

**National Institute on Alcohol
Abuse and Alcoholism**
rethinkingdrinking.niaaa.nih.gov

....

**National Council on Alcoholism and
Drug Dependence Hope Line**
ncadd.org or 800-622-2255

Your parent might be able to cut back or abstain on his own (although it's unlikely). Counseling from a doctor is often helpful. (Sometimes seeing the results of a liver function test or some other clear indication of the consequences of his drinking is useful.)

Structured programs or more intensive counseling is just as effective among the elderly as it is among younger people; however, those who started drinking recently will be helped more easily than those who have an entrenched drinking problem. Some research suggests that treatment is more effective when it is done in a setting with other elderly people, where they can talk about pertinent issues (life in retirement, physical ailments, family life, and so on).

Because withdrawal can lead to medical complications in the elderly, such as delirium, hospitalization is sometimes recommended.

Up in Smoke

Everyone knows the perils of cigarette smoking, but what's the point of stopping late in life? After all, your mother has smoked for more than 50 years. Isn't the damage done? Is there any real benefit to stopping at her age?

Surely you know the answer: Absolutely. The rewards are enormous at any age, and they start immediately. As soon as that last cigarette is put out, the body begins to repair and restore itself.

Within minutes, blood flow improves and blood pressure drops, reducing the risk of heart attack, stroke, and other circulatory disease. Within hours, carbon monoxide levels in the blood return to normal. Within a few weeks, a person's sense of taste and smell return, and breathing becomes easier. Within months, coughing and shortness of breath improve. According to the American Lung Association, smokers who quit at age 65 added 1.4 to 3.4 years onto their lives.

Okay, if your father is lying in a bed, months away from death, let him be. It's agonizing to see people with acute emphysema lighting up a cigarette, but it might be too late to make a fuss about it.

But if your parent can quit, he will not only be healthier, but he will also be more energetic, have a better appetite, sleep better, and goodness knows, smell a whole lot better (in both senses of the word).

And just think of the money he'll save. (It's not a bad idea to do the math with him so he can see how much he'll be saving each year.) By quitting, he will also safeguard other family members, particularly grandchildren, from diseases caused by his smoking.

Kicking It

Although some people can quit on their own, most people need help. Nicotine replacement therapy (patches, inhalers, lozenges, nasal sprays, and gums) can be effective. Some medications can also help. Your parent should confer with her doctor.

To be successful, most people also need some sort of cessation class, counseling, and/or support group. At the very least, it helps to have a smoking buddy who is quitting at the same time or who knows what your parent is going through. Some people also find techniques such as acupuncture and hypnosis helpful.

If your parent decides to quit, he will need enormous support and encouragement from you and other loved ones. Nicotine is very addictive. Until his body adjusts, the craving will be powerful.

The first few weeks will be the hardest, for everyone. Your parent is likely to be cranky, angry, and tired. He might swear and yell or just retreat into his smoke-free hell. Some people have headaches. Some have trouble breathing in the beginning, although this will vastly improve with time. He may have trouble sleeping and concentrating, and may feel anxious and depressed. He might gain some weight, but not enough to worry about; the pounds are a whole lot healthier than the tar and nicotine.

Put up with his moods. Tell him you're proud of him. Keep him busy and distracted. Support him. Set goals or milestones (one week without cigarettes, for example) and then celebrate when he reaches them. Remind him of all the good things he is doing for his body (and yours). Avoid situations that he associates with smoking. Find substitutes for that hand-to-mouth habit, like popcorn, carrot sticks, and sunflower seeds. If he's willing, exercise will help distract him and relieve some of the stress he's under.

And finally, cigars, snuff, chewing tobacco, and pipes are *not* safe alternatives to cigarettes. These habits are also addictive and can cause cancer and heart disease.

ⓘ FOR MORE HELP

Smokefree.gov
(Run by the National Cancer Institute)
smokefree.gov or 800-QUIT-NOW
(800-784-8669)

···

Quit for Life
(Run by the American Cancer Society)
quitnow.net

···

Freedom from Smoking
(Run by the American Lung Association)
lung.org or 800-586-4872

Chapter 6

A Happier Soul

The Quest • Family and Friends • Spiritual Fulfillment • Reminiscing • Volunteering and Working • Involved and Active • Dating, Sex, and Marriage

It's terrific if your parent lifts weights, eats spinach, and throws out his cigarettes. Scientific research shows that this will all contribute to a healthier and more independent life.

But the anecdotal evidence suggests that tickling a grandchild, laughing with an old friend, hearing an inspiring sermon, planting a garden, or stirring an intoxicating beef stew might be the strongest medicine of all.

Those who have close family ties, social contacts, a hobby or intellectual pursuit, optimism and humor, and a spiritual base—or at least one or two of these ingredients—get sick less often, recover faster, live longer, and are less apt to suffer from memory loss.

Most important of all: They enjoy life.

We caregivers get so focused on the immediate crisis—the medical, financial, and safety problems, the aides and the doctor's appointments—that we sometimes forget there is a person here, and that for this person, longevity is not the only goal. Your parent might rather sip a cup of tea with friends or take a drive in the country than undergo one more blood test.

Oh, but she needs the test. Maybe. But at this point in her life, which does she need more? Which should take priority in these waning years, medicine or meaning? As Frederick Nietzsche once said, "He who has a *why* to live can bear almost any *how*."

Our parents face tremendous physical obstacles, but often what is most problematic for them—intolerable, really—is the boredom, loneliness, and lack of purpose. And sometimes, what they need most is not more scans and prescriptions, but more time with loved ones, more opportunities to share, learn, enjoy, create, or reminisce.

The Quest

We're not talking about anything major here. You don't need to arrange for your parent to visit the Galapagos Islands (although if he likes that kind of thing, there are trips for the disabled, as well as terrific videos). The simplest activities or events can have a major impact.

Talk with your parent about what she enjoys now and what she used to enjoy in her younger days. What made life interesting? What gave it meaning? What made her happy?

If it was raising her children, maybe she can become a foster grandparent or dictate letters to her grandchildren or review family photos. If she loves her church, arrange for her to get there, or record the services, or see if a member of the clergy will visit. If she was always involved in politics, see if she can't volunteer in some small way, perhaps by stuffing envelopes. If she loves nature,

get her out to a park or preserve, watch nature videos, or buy her a bird feeder.

If your parent is in a nursing home, she might receive visits from a grandchild, listen to her favorite music, arrange flowers, or if she can get around at all, volunteer by delivering books or visiting other residents.

If she is largely out of it, just playing her favorite music or audiobook might give her comfort and make her feel less alone. Sometimes just stroking a cat or dog is immensely soothing.

Look through the newspaper, read bulletin boards, and scan community calendars for activities that might interest her. Ask her friends or other elderly people in her community what they do with their days. Don't give up. You may have to try a couple of ideas before something strikes your parent's fancy. But eventually you will find something or someone to warm her heart.

Family and Friends

While you are racing around remembering medications and talking to doctors and nursing homes—all essential tasks—it's easy to forget your parent's most basic need: you. At the end of the day, humans need social bonds. They need friends and family.

....

> **When my mother moved up here to live with me, she sat in the house watching TV most of the day. Back in Texas, she had been very active, so this felt like a disaster. I thought I'd made a huge mistake moving her here.**
>
> **I suggested she go to the senior center and see what other people were doing, or sign up for a class or something at the library. She didn't budge. Just sat there. Said she was fine.**
>
> **I work, so I didn't have a lot of time to entertain her or find activities for her, and honestly, I was annoyed that she didn't make more effort. Every day I'd come home and she'd be sitting there, doing nothing.**
>
> **I think, looking back on it, she was in shock, what with all the change in her life. She needed time to adjust. And I think that she needed an activity that made her feel useful, something that gave her value. She didn't want to take classes or sit in a senior center.**
>
> **It took her a few weeks, but eventually she got involved in our local food pantry. It was perfect because it didn't require a lot of physical work, but she felt really needed. "**
>
> **—Emily P.**

They need to love and be loved. This need is written deeply into our genetic codes, and it is basic to our survival. And although it is with us throughout life, it seems to be most acute at both the beginning of life and the end, when the body is weak, life is uncluttered, and one's needs are primal.

So slow down for a moment. Sit with your parent. If you can't visit often, call, Skype, or email. It can be brief. Any sort of contact is better than none. Even a parent who is very ill and can't actually take part in a conversation will enjoy hearing the voices of people he loves.

Include your parent, whenever possible, in family activities. Even if he can't actually participate, he should be there. Or, if he can't be there, set up a video chat.

Friends, Old and New

Many of your parent's old friends might be just that, *old*. They are deceased, or too disabled to get out, or perhaps they live elsewhere now. Digging up friendships and a social life is difficult at any age, but it is hardest just when you need it most. Your parent might need a little push from you.

Urge her to call an old friend or new acquaintance for lunch, supper, or a movie. If she can't get out, maybe someone could come visit her.

If she doesn't know many people nearby, get her to join some club, class, or activity—the League of Women Voters, a painting class, a bridge club. If she's in a nursing home or other senior facility, check out the activity schedule and encourage her to participate. Even if she doesn't like crafts or sing-alongs, urge her to try some of the activities.

Many communities have programs in which volunteers will visit homebound elderly. If there isn't one, you might find a volunteer through a service club, high school, senior organization, or religious organization.

Once she makes a friend or two, or if you've found a friendly volunteer, set up standing dates—a card game every Tuesday night, lunch every Thursday— so she doesn't have to think about creating new social events each week.

Cyber Connections

Although it doesn't replace real friendship and face-to-face social contacts, the Internet is a powerful tool that can give your parent access to an abundance of information and activities, and most important, link her to family, friends, and new acquaintances.

Grandparents can suddenly communicate with children, grandchildren, and friends all over the world through video chats and email. If your parent can't get out, it's a wonderful way to bring the world in. If you're far away or at work, it also offers you another way to check in and see how your parent is doing.

With the Internet, your parent can pursue lifelong interests or delve into new topics. She can look up her family tree, track down relatives or friends, and read her hometown newspaper. She can learn about foreign places, go back in history, read about a favorite movie star, pursue a hobby, or play games. It will give her a sense of independence and involvement, and keep both her brain and fingers active.

Your parent can also visit chat rooms or join online support groups and talk anonymously with others who share her interests or concerns.

She doesn't have a computer? Most libraries, senior centers, assisted living facilities, and nursing homes have computers for public use.

If she's buying a computer, search for laptops or tablets especially made for seniors. Although a tablet, like the iPad, is easier to operate (you can buy a stand and keyboard if touchscreen typing is difficult), the screen might be a little small for dim eyes. Take your parent to a computer store where she can try various options and talk to an expert about her specific needs and disabilities.

> " My father is 83 and has Alzheimer's. Last year, old family friends invited us to a Christmas party. My immediate reaction was to leave him home. He is often oblivious. He's not terribly mobile. But my sister urged me to take him, so I dressed him up, put on his old holly tie that he always used to wear at Christmas, and got him out the door.
>
> I felt like I was making a mistake, that people would stare, that he would embarrass himself, that he wouldn't know what was happening.
>
> It turned out that, of course, all these old friends were in their 80s too. One was crumpled over in a wheelchair with Parkinson's. Several had walkers. Half of them couldn't hear.
>
> They were so kind and patient with him. He came to life. He didn't remember anyone's name, but he had so much fun. I hadn't seen that spark in his eye in ages."
> —Sally R.

Many senior centers, libraries, computer stores, and nursing homes offer Internet classes specifically for the elderly. Although some websites offer tutorials, most are too complicated. (Try seniornet.org and aarp.org/technology.) You can also download Eldy (eldy.eu), free software that makes any PC easy, easy, easy.

Remember, a computer can be adjusted so that text size is larger, contrast is greater, and colors are brighter. The mouse pointer can also be enlarged. Tools such as Microsoft's Magnifier work like a magnifying glass. Speech recognition software is great for those who have trouble typing, and you can also find software that converts text into speech. Similarly, most computers have applications that help shaky hands by ignoring repeated or very brief keystrokes.

If all else fails, get any teenager in the family to teach her how. They are the computer experts.

Spiritual Fulfillment

Unlike other age groups, most elderly people consider themselves to be at least somewhat religious. This may be because of their upbringing, but it might also be because questions about mortality, the purpose of life, and spirituality often take on greater importance at this time.

As it turns out, this is a very good thing. A number of studies have shown that people who are religious get sick less often, recover faster, and have a greater ability to cope with illness, disability, and loss. They view ailments and disabilities as less painful and less cumbersome than those who are not religious. They clearly have less depression and anxiety, and they have more motivation, hope, and optimism.

Religion gives people a sense of meaning and hope. These feelings help them do more, take care of themselves, and reach out to others. Hopelessness and worry, on the other hand, contribute to heart disease, high blood pressure, stroke, and other disorders.

For many people, the church, synagogue, or other place of worship is the most important source of social support outside the family. If your parent attends services, he is getting out, making friends, and seeing people, and they are seeing him (which is important, since someone is likely to notice if something is amiss).

Whether or not your parent practiced a religion in his younger days, he might like to go to church or synagogue, attend a religious discussion group, speak to a member of the clergy, or simply have someone read to him from a religious text.

Encourage your parent to pursue his religious beliefs and explore his faith. Even without strong spiritual views, weekly services can be a good thing.

Reminiscing

The next time your father drifts back several decades and tells you stories you've heard a dozen times before, rather than shaking your head in despair, encourage him to tell you more—more details, more stories, more memories.

He's doing something that's enormously healing. Reminiscing allows him to review his life, think through important issues, see his accomplishments, let go of his regrets, and pass on experiences to the next generation. It also returns him, temporarily, to a time when he was younger, stronger, more confident, and more capable.

If you can get your parent to tell new stories or flesh out the old ones, reminiscing can be a wonderful experience for you, too. Or your children might like to share this activity with their grandparent. Exploring these details gives you insight into your parent's life and background, and it may be one of the last chances you have to learn about your heritage.

Record your father's tales because you are sure to forget important details or a tone of voice that made the story his. Ask about his life and about historical events he witnessed. What was his childhood house like? What about the school he attended? What were his parents like? How did he travel or dress as a young boy? Why did he choose his career? Who did he date? What political events or inventions were most exciting to him and why?

If your parent is up to it, get him to talk about your ancestors. Draw a family tree together, gathering additional information from other relatives. This is wonderful information that you can pass down to your children and grandchildren.

As your parent talks, let him ramble about the subjects he most enjoys. Don't correct him or force him to stay within some chronological order. Just listen, encourage him, and enjoy it.

If your parent can't speak or grows tired easily, he might enjoy hearing you reminisce about his life and things you all did together. You can flip through a photo album with him to spark conversation about various events in the past.

> " Dad and I always had what I call a business relationship. We talked about finances and health and practical matters, but never emotions.
>
> Then one day I was visiting him in the hospital and running out of conversation, and for some reason, I asked him about a girl he dated in college. His eyes got misty and he started telling me all about being in love for the first time and and how hurt he was when she left him. He got lost in his past, lying in that bed, with tubes all over the place. He told me about other women he dated, his friends, funny things that happened, and how he met my mother.
>
> He was like a kid, remembering all this stuff. And for the first time I saw this very human, vulnerable, and youthful side of my father."
>
> —Alicia B.

Volunteering and Working

If your parent is able, volunteering is a wonderful way to regain a sense of purpose. It will also help her meet new people of different ages, take her mind off problems, and be involved in the community, politics, the arts, children, medical care, women's issues—whatever interests her. She might help at a food pantry, school, or hospital, or help out at a fund-raising event.

Even if your parent can't leave the house or her bed, she might be able to make phone calls or edit letters. If she is in a nursing home, she may be able to give tours, answer visitors' questions, deliver meals or flowers, or visit patients in the infirmary.

If your parent would like to help other older people in the community—delivering meals, reading to people with poor vision, visiting homebound elderly, escorting people to medical appointments—contact the area agency on aging (eldercare.gov) and ask about volunteer programs.

Senior Corps, a federal program, runs several large senior volunteer programs, including the Retired and Senior Volunteer Program (RSVP), Foster Grandparents, and the Senior Companion Program (seniorcorps.org or 800-942-2677).

If your parent is a retired business executive or small-business owner, he or she might like to get involved with the Service Corps of Retired Executives (SCORE), which provides free counseling to small-business owners (score.org or 800-634-0245).

To find out about other possibilities, call local churches, synagogues, community centers, hospitals, libraries, schools, day care centers, fund-raising groups, political campaigns, museums, theaters, nature centers, the United Way, the Red Cross, or the local chapter of

REFUSING TO BUDGE

Your parent's most serious obstacle to social, mental, and spiritual involvement may not be disability or illness, but her own attitude. She might believe that she's too old to do, learn, give, or care.

Of course, this negativity is self-fulfilling. Inactive, she becomes lonely, bored, and weak, which leads to more feelings of worthlessness and, in turn, more inertia.

See if you can spark her enthusiasm and get her engaged. Start small, and focus on her particular interests and needs. If your parent continues to reject your efforts, if she is lethargic and withdrawn and has no interest in the things she used to enjoy, it might be a sign of depression or early dementia. Talk with her doctor.

A RIDE IN THE COUNTRY

If your parent is very frail and doesn't get out much, he will benefit from a change of scene and some fresh air. Even if it takes some logistics to get him into the car, try it. Driving down a country road, by the sea, or along a busy city street may cheer him up considerably. If you don't have time for pleasure trips, take him with you when you run your errands, just to get him out of the house.

AARP. You should also contact the local volunteer center in your parent's area, which you can find through the Points of Light Foundation (pointsoflight.org) or Volunteers of America (voa.org or 800-899-0089).

Working for Pay

If your parent doesn't want to work for free and she is relatively fit, she may be able to find a job that pays. Owners of shops and restaurants are finding that older people can be more reliable than teenagers, and some senior organizations specifically look to hire older people. The area agency on aging should know of local employment programs for seniors. Also, look through the want ads or call businesses that interest your parent—a museum gift shop, a hospital, a clothing store, a movie theater. You might also contact local senior centers to see if they know of any such jobs.

Lending a Hand

If your parent is bored, give her a project, something that might also help you. Ask her to sort through old photos, write addresses on holiday greeting cards, look something up in the library or on the Internet for you, snap beans, repot some plants, or otherwise give you a hand. You get a task done, and she feels useful. Or, you don't get a task done (and actually have to redo the job) and she feels useful, which is also good.

" I was doing everything for my mother. I was miserable and she was miserable. She'd say things like, 'Don't trouble yourself,' 'I really wish you wouldn't do this.' She felt I was ruining my life for her, which I was in a way, and that made her unhappy.

I found a note pinned to a bulletin board in town that a teenager was looking for after-school work. I called her and set her up visiting my mom.

It's been amazing, like the daughter she never had. They bake cookies. Well, my mother sits in her wheelchair giving instructions while Sarah bakes, I should say. They talk about their lives. My mother gives Sarah constant advice about friends and boys and schoolwork.

I arranged for Sarah to come by twice a week, but she stops in almost every day because I think she loves this almost as much as my mother does. She's a godsend."

—Jerry B.

Crossing the Generation Gap

If your parent has always been good with children, he can still have them in his life. Even if he never liked them much, he might enjoy them now that he has more time on his hands.

A connection between the young and the old enriches the young, and certainly makes the old feel younger.

Call local schools, day care centers, Boy Scout and Girl Scout troops, religious organizations, and other groups to find out about ways your parent might either help or be helped.

The Foster Grandparent Program, run by Senior Corps, puts elderly citizens to work (for a small compensation) in hospitals, schools, and day care programs. Participants can help children who have been abused or neglected, care for premature infants or young children with disabilities, or mentor young mothers and troubled teens (seniorcorps.org or 800-942-2677).

AARP's Experience Corps works with older volunteers, hooking them up with urban schools where they serve as advocates and role models for children, teaching them to read, helping with homework, and supporting school programs (aarp.org/experience-corps or 202-434-6400).

_____

" My father lives in a nursing home, and he gets very bored and lonely. When anyone visits him, it's as though he won the lottery, he gets so excited. The rest of the time he basically sleeps and roams the hallways and talks to the nurses. He's not interested in any of the games or activities at the home and says all the other residents are 'too old' or half crazy.

I've tried a lot of things, and I think my most successful effort was signing him up as a foster grandparent. This little boy, Tyler, not only visits, but also sends him games and calls when he has homework questions. They've developed a really nice relationship."

—Eleanor R.

_____

Involved and Active

Exercising the Mind

It's never too late to learn. Call local colleges, community centers, high school extension programs, museums, and senior centers and ask about classes and lectures. If your parent is able, he might paint, cook Italian food, or play an instrument. Perhaps he wants to study music or learn about architecture.

Find out about tours of museums and art galleries, many of which have special courses and prices for the elderly.

Chronic illness and bed rest can muddle your parent's mind and make him listless. If your father is unable to get out of the house, get him books, audiobooks, or lectures on DVD from the local library or the Internet.

He doesn't have to take it all in—there are no exams. He doesn't even have to take much of it in. But learning gives a person energy, optimism, and pride. And it will take him briefly away from his pain and troubles.

Creative Outlets

Even people who have never shown much interest in art, dance, or music during their younger days sometimes find a passion for it once they have time on their hands. Don't predetermine what your parent likes to do or can't do.

See if she might be interested in taking an art class or picking up some charcoal pencils and a pad, or give her a ball of clay to mold.

Drawing, painting, and sculpting help people release tension, sort through conflicts, and grieve losses. Creativity also taps into an important part of the brain, and the soul, that might not get much use.

Music also soothes. Did your parent ever play an instrument? Would she like to try again? Would she like to listen to a new song or an old favorite, and dance or just sway to the beat?

Research shows that music triggers the release of opiates and endorphins in the body, which help lower blood pressure, improve breathing, alleviate pain, and generally make a person feel good. Dance, even in some limited way, does

SO MANY GADGETS AND GIZMOS

Don't assume that just because your parent is severely arthritic, deaf, shaky from Parkinson's, or blind that he can't do things he enjoys. In this era of accessibility and technology, a vast array of gadgets, gizmos, and other products can make gardening, sewing, fishing, reading, bowling, hunting, swimming, and other hobbies, sports, interests, and adventures possible. Search the Internet for your parent's favorite activity and add the word *disabled* or *accessibility* or *elderly* to the search window.

all this and adds an element of exercise to the activity.

If your mother doesn't want to "do," maybe she would like to watch or listen. You might take her to a play, a gallery opening, or a concert. If she can't get out, rent or buy a DVD. Or she might just like to lie in bed and listen to old show tunes, songs from her youth, or pieces by a favorite composer.

Travel and Exploration

Even if he uses a wheelchair, your parent can go on a tour—to foreign countries or nearby cities, colleges, botanical gardens, and historic sites and monuments.

Most senior centers offer discounted trips, from day excursions to weekend foliage tours to full vacations. Colleges, museums, environmental groups, and history clubs often offer tours for seniors.

Numerous travel agencies specialize in travel for people who are elderly and/ or have disabilities. Look on the Internet under "disability travel," "wheelchair travel," or "senior travel," or call a local travel agent and ask for suggestions.

Road Scholar (formerly known as Elderhostel; roadscholar.org or 877-454-5768) offers an enormous array of trips, tours, and courses for older people. Their staff can suggest trips that might be right for your parent. (One of their repeat participants was 100 years old, legally blind, and in a wheelchair.)

Some older people find that cruises are the easiest form of travel.

The key is to keep plans simple, with lots of breaks and rest periods.

Movies and Books

If your parent is laid up or just tends to stay in, get her some books and movies. She may not have the initiative to do this for herself, but once she is involved in a good story, she may get lost in it. How about some of her favorite old films? Was she a Jimmy Stewart fan? Did your father have a crush on Audrey Hepburn?

If she is active, suggest that your mother join a book club, gathering with

> " The thing my mother loved most was music. The home where she lived had concerts and even a music therapy class, but she couldn't go because she was afraid of riding in the elevator by herself, and the nurse said there wasn't enough staff to escort her. One day in the hallway I ran into the woman who directed the program. I told her about my mother, and she said she would be happy to bring Mom to and from the class each day. It was such a relief. Her spirits seemed to pick up right away."
>
> —Barbara F.

friends once a month to discuss a book they have all read (or listened to); or she might get some friends together to see a weekly movie at home or in the community room at her residence.

You can get her a small laptop, mini DVD player, or tablet so that she can download films. She can use earphones if she needs the volume particularly loud.

If your parent has trouble seeing, there are large-print books and devices that enlarge the words in a book onto a screen. Or get audiobooks. Contact your local library or bookstore, both of which should have numerous audiobooks and large-print books. You can also contact the Library of Congress (loc.gov /nls or 888-657-7323) or go to largeprintbooks.com or any online bookseller. Sometimes local volunteers will read to older people.

For people with hearing loss, the Described and Captioned

SIMPLE PLEASURES

If your parent is severely ill, heavily medicated, or suffering from dementia, it may take very little to entertain him. Children's games, such as checkers or Go Fish, an otherwise monotonous task like sticking labels on envelopes, stroking a pet, or listening to the jingle-jangle of children's songs may give his day a boost. What might seem silly to you might engage or even delight him.

Media Program (dcmp.org) lends videos with captioning free of charge.

Projects and Hobbies

Maybe your parent isn't into making birdhouses, but what about other hobbies and projects, like gardening, bird-watching, fishing, collecting, model building, or painting?

Think small-scale. If she doesn't want to take care of a full garden, she can have a few small planters in a window.

Ask what she used to do in her younger days; she might enjoy reviving an old hobby. If she doesn't want to do things on her own, ask at senior centers about hobbies, crafts, and classes.

Sports and Games

Sports and games are a terrific way to exercise, meet people, and build some confidence. It might be bingo, bridge, or shuffleboard, or it could be walking, playing golf, or swimming. Your father may have to take it easy, but that doesn't mean he can't participate. Some other activities to consider include fishing, horseshoes, darts, bowling, croquet, badminton, archery, miniature golf, or pool. Local gyms, YMCAs, and senior centers may arrange or know of such offerings, or you can call the local department of recreation or community center.

Nintendo's Wii allows your parent to play tennis or bowl from a chair at home. Wii has taken hold in nursing homes and is often referred to as Wii-habilitation.

Senior Center Activities

Senior centers and adult day care centers offer elders a place to socialize, talk about the events of the day, attend lectures, go on trips, learn new skills, and in some cases, find out about practical matters such as estate planning and budgeting. If there is more than one center in the area, your parent is welcome to sign up for classes at any or all of them.

Creature Comforts

What has come to be known in medical lingo as pet-facilitated therapy, or PFT—basically, having a dog or cat—clearly boosts people's emotional states as well as their physical health. Animals make people feel loved and less alone, they ease depression, and they give elderly people a sense of responsibility. And, since Rascal needs a daily walk, a dog can provide a little exercise as well. For someone who is anxious or agitated, just stroking a pet is calming.

The findings about pet-facilitated therapy have been so conclusive that federal law now mandates that elderly

> " After her stroke, my mother was confined to bed. As the winter dragged on, she became bored and depressed. I could only get over to see her about twice a week, so she was there, watching TV.
>
> We had a huge storm and her aide went out and built a snowman right outside Mom's window. She wrapped a scarf around his neck and put a hat and mittens on him. Mom loved him so.
>
> She put a block of suet on his head and the birds came, right outside Mom's window, and she could watch them all day. She was sure she knew one bird from another. She was so delighted, so happy, with her snowman and the birds that ate his hat."
>
> —Marjorie C.

people living in subsidized housing be allowed to keep pets, so don't let the landlord shoo Patches out the door.

Although a dog or cat provides the most companionship, a bird, hamster, tank of fish, or other animal can also ease loneliness and provide entertainment. These smaller, simpler pets are particularly useful if your parent is very frail or confused. Even a bird feeder can be entertaining.

Dating, Sex, and Marriage

Your parent may be old, but he's not dead. Just because his hair has turned white, his joints have grown stiff, and his hearing is weak does not mean that he is immune to the arrows of love or, yes, the draw of a physically intimate relationship. Arthritis, diabetes, hypertension, and hearing loss have not made your parent any less of a person. All people, until their last breaths, need love and intimacy almost as much as they need food and water.

Dating

It can be unsettling for a child, even a fully grown child, to discover that Mom has fallen in love, or that Dad is acting like a teenager around a certain someone. *He's 92 years old, for Pete's sake. He can hardly see, much less walk. Someone has to cut up his meat and lay out his pills and help him get his pants on. So what is this about? Is he some kind of pervert? Is she after his money?*

Late in life, even very late in life, flirting and dating, touching, and gazing into someone's eyes is heavenly. It provides companionship and feelings of youthfulness, of being alive. Really alive. It boosts self-esteem and gets the old ticker beating. Hooray, hooray! Love and sex are not stripped away at the nursing home door, nor are residents deprived of their rights to engage in such activities.

If your parent is interested in meeting someone new, the popular online dating sites (Match.com and eHarmony, for

> ❝ Two years after my dad died, my mother met a man and they began to go out for lunch occasionally. She was so nervous about it, like a schoolgirl. I kept saying, 'It's okay. Just enjoy it. He's nice.' I could see her, right before my eyes, becoming young again.
>
> They've been together now for several years. She's bent over with arthritis and he can barely hear or see, but they are so happy together. It's like a whole new life has opened up for her. It makes me feel like there's so much promise, that life doesn't end at 80."
>
> —Jenny R.

example) have plenty of older men and women looking for matches. Other sites cater specifically to seniors (although many consider people over 50 "seniors"). "Speed dating" is also being offered in some communities and senior centers.

Sex

The whole idea of love at a late age may seem sort of "cute" until you wake up to the obvious: Your parent is staying in the heartthrob's apartment. At night. All night. *What are they doing in there?*

Ageism hits its lowest point with the assumption that people in their 80s are beyond dating and could not possibly be having S-E-X.

Sex very late in life, if your parent is fortunate enough to have it, is sometimes more about intimacy and companionship than about physical pleasure. Sure, there's a physical need and sometimes a response, but at this stage of life, sex tends to be more about caring, closeness, understanding, sharing, and loyalty.

The emotional and psychological aspect takes on greater importance.

Not that you want to hear it, but sex is not a bad form of exercise, it reduces anxiety, and it reassures a person that, yes, this old body still functions.

Forgetting your reaction for a moment, the idea of dating, much less having sex, might be frightening and daunting for your parent. She might think she's too old for such behavior and worry that her body might not respond the way it once did. And gee, will she remember what to do?

All of these worries can get in the way of meeting people, becoming intimate, and finally, sharing a bed. Your father might not function, simply because he is so afraid of not functioning.

Sex at an old age usually takes longer, men require more time to become erect, women require lubrication, and the two might have to find an imaginative position because of sore knees and replaced hips.

SWEETHEART SCAMMERS

Not all attachments are innocent and loving. There are heartless fiends out there who prey on elderly hearts. A younger woman meets your father, and the next thing you know they are getting married.

Age, isolation, and boredom are volatile ingredients. If you suspect that your parent's new love has bad intentions, act immediately. The sooner you do something, the easier it will be to break this off.

Most important, be involved in your parent's life. Visit unannounced. Call often. Ask questions. This alone can scare a scammer away. If that doesn't do it, call the area agency on aging (eldercare.gov) or Adult Protective Services (napsa-now.org). Ask a lawyer how to protect your parent and his assets.

Of course, his assets are not the only thing at risk. Financial exploitation often leads to neglect and other forms of abuse. Trust your instincts. Don't delay. See page 330 for more on financial exploitation.

DATING, SEX, AND DEMENTIA

People with dementia can also fall in love and, yes, have sex. In the early stages, that might be perfectly fine—wonderful, in fact. If your parent is still somewhat competent and seems to know, at least to some extent, what he is doing; if this is consistent with other things he has done in his life; and if there is no abuse or exploitation involved, then it's probably nothing to worry about. Indeed, it's something to celebrate.

But later in the disease, when your parent's ability to reason is largely gone, dating raises a number of issues. If you are concerned, talk with his doctor, a psychiatrist who knows about such things, or others involved in his care.

If your parent is living among others who have dementia, and someone is making unwanted sexual gestures or advances, talk to the staff of the facility. Urge your parent to keep a distance, and talk to her about how she should respond if this person were to undress, make rude remarks, or make some other sexual advance. Remember, this lack of inhibition is part of a disease, not part of the person.

If your parent is inappropriately sexual, see page 516 for ways to curb it.

One of the major causes of sexual dysfunction, aside from all the psychological ones, is medications. Antidepressants, tranquilizers, and a host of other medications, as well as alcohol, can douse desire or otherwise interfere with normal sexual functioning.

Finally, your parent might worry that medical problems, such as arthritis, heart disease, incontinence, or surgery, make it impossible or dangerous for her to have sex. But this simply isn't true. Most obstacles are surmountable. And the benefits certainly outweigh any risks.

(The good news: no interruptions from children, lots of free time, and slower male responses. Also, no worries about pregnancy, unless Dad has found someone much, much younger; men can still make babies late in life.)

Support and encourage your parent. Okay, it's not a subject you're eager to bring up with her. But try to be accepting of any hint of interest on her part. Encourage it. Ease any tension and remind your parent, if possible, that romance and passion are good for the soul.

" My mother was widowed after 60 years of marriage, and two years later she met someone and is about to remarry. She's 85 and he's 80. I think it's wonderful. I am delighted for her.

My sister is concerned that he has memory problems. She worries that Mom will have to take care of him. Actually, because my sister lives closest to them, she worries that she will have to care for both of them. I don't think we have any say in the matter. This is what Mom wants. It makes her happy."

—Dianne D.

If this "date" is kind and responsible, wouldn't it be nice if your parent were no longer alone? If she had a companion? No, you won't have the control over her that you once had. Yes, there is a chance she will remarry, which might muddle some issues for the family. But what a joy for her if she finds someone to do things with, to share life with, to love.

And Marriage

Your mother is getting married. You might like this fellow; you might not. Either way, all sorts of questions arise. Will he take good care of her? Will he now be making decisions about her care? Or is she going to end up taking care of him? Maybe you will end up taking care of both of them!

It's time to talk.

Romance and wedding planning are exciting, but when marriage is in the air, be realistic and get some practical advice. Marriage will drastically affect your parent's living situation, daily habits, other relationships, finances, and estate.

Talk with your parent, and get her to talk with an attorney. She needs to protect herself.

Who is going to make medical decisions on her behalf? Who will decide if she needs nursing home care at some point? Who will handle her assets should she become incapacitated or incompetent? Has she assigned power of attorney to someone? Does she have a health care proxy? In other words, will this new spouse make all decisions about living, medical care, and finances, or does that authority reside with

you or some other trusted person?

How will all of this change your role and responsibility? How will it change family dynamics and traditions?

And critically important, how will it change her financial situation? How can she protect her finances and be sure that she has enough to cover her own care? And if passing something on to her children has always been important to her, how can she be sure this marriage doesn't interfere with that goal?

Ideally, the couple should sort everything out in advance. What are each person's assets, income, expected future income, debts, and other financial obligations? What insurance policies exist, and who are the beneficiaries? How will this merger affect Medicaid eligibility? Will assets be held individually, as "joint tenants," as "tenants in common," or in a trust for someone else?

Because these issues get particularly messy late in life, when people have various accounts, assets, and financial needs, and might also have some cognitive

STDS AND HIV

One is never too old to have sex, but also never too old to contract sexually transmitted diseases, such as genital warts, herpes, chlamydia, or hepatitis B. And certainly everyone who is sexually active is at risk of becoming infected with HIV.

Your parent should talk with a doctor about how to protect himself, or he should use a latex condom. For more information about HIV and the elderly, contact the Association on HIV over Fifty (hivoverfifty.org).

impairment, your parent should sign a prenuptial agreement detailing everything. Any agreement should be updated from time to time, as assets, needs, and relationships change.

Once again, the focus is your parent's happiness and choices. Unless real trouble is brewing, it is not about whether or not you approve of or like the situation. Your parent is an adult. You are not her parent. If she is competent and not under any undue influence (someone taking advantage of her age and loneliness), you have no say in this decision. This is her money, her life, and her choice. If she is happy, try to be happy for her.

Homosexuality

Homosexuality was not widely accepted in your parent's generation, but it is far more so now. As a result, many elderly homosexuals who have never revealed their sexual orientation before are suddenly becoming open about it. In fact, they might have been in a heterosexual relationship for years, perhaps unhappily, perhaps happily (sort of), because they did not want to admit their sexual orientation.

Elderly homosexuals (as well as transgender and bisexual seniors) endure all the same stresses and worries as elderly heterosexuals, plus the added hardship of discrimination. If your parent is in a nursing home or other group facility, the isolation may be compounded.

Support your parent. He or she needs your love and compassion now more than ever.

You can search the Internet for information and support groups in the area. Also contact Senior Action in a Gay Environment, or SAGE (sageusa.org or 212-741-2247).

Life at Home

Chapter 7

Tips for Daily Living

Safety First • Monitors and Alert Systems • Preventing
Falls • Room-by-Room Modifications • Bathing and
Grooming • Dressing • What's for Dinner? • In the Driver's
Seat • Gadgets and Gizmos

W ho can help but worry about an elderly parent
getting through the day, or even part of the day, alone? *What
if Dad falls? Should Mom still be driving? Is he eating anything?
Is she remembering her medications?* And yet, in this country, more than two
million people over the age of 85 live alone, and millions more spend at
least part of the day on their own.

If your father has arthritis, diabetes, and fuzzy vision, it doesn't
mean that it's time for a nursing home or that you have to follow him
around tending to his every need. You don't want to, and he probably
doesn't want you to, either.

Whether your parent lives alone, with you, or in some sort of group
facility, you can do minor renovations and rearranging, buy some useful gadgets, plug into local services, and take advantage of a few tips
so that he can live as independently as possible, for as long as possible.

Ask your parent about the details of his day or hang out with him and observe how he goes about his basic tasks. Does he have trouble holding his razor, operating his phone, walking down stairs, heating up spaghetti, or locking the front door? Does he have a way to get groceries or visit a friend?

Once you know the day's snags, brainstorm solutions. There are all sorts of ways to make cooking more manageable, dressing more doable, exercise more feasible, and free time more entertaining.

If the biggest problem is your worry meter—he's managing, but you're holding your breath waiting for a disaster—you can address that as well with various monitors and alerts (and a few relaxation skills).

If you need help with a specific problem and don't find a solution here, contact an occupational therapist, visiting nurse, carpenter, or electrician, depending upon the situation. For tips on making day-to-day life easier if your parent has dementia, also see Chapter 24.

Safety First

You won't think that you need an emergency plan until, of course, there's an emergency. Think preventively. With any luck, you'll never need any of it, but why take that chance?

Vial of Life
A vial of life is a simple plastic container that saves lives. It's so low-tech, it's ingenious, and so easy that there's no excuse not to have one for your parent.

In an emergency, rescue crews and hospital personnel need information that a person in a crisis often can't relate.

The vial, which can be a large plastic vial or a plastic bag, holds just that information.

The vial or bag can be taped inside the front door, where it's clearly visible, or on the refrigerator door, or stored inside the fridge (where it won't be damaged by smoke or fire). Red decals are then placed on the front door and/or on the outside of the refrigerator and/or over your parent's bed, notifying crews of the vial's existence (although many emergency crews know to check the fridge).

The vial should include the following:

- Name, address, phone number, date of birth

- Primary language spoken

- Emergency contact telephone numbers (including yours)

- Doctors' names and numbers and preferred hospital

- List of medications (including over-the-counter drugs and dietary supplements)

- Medical conditions or injuries (including cognitive decline)

- Allergies

- Past surgeries and hospitalizations

- Height and weight

- Blood type

- Hearing or vision difficulties, oxygen, cane/walker

- Health insurance information

- Do Not Resuscitate orders, health care proxy, living wills, or other special instructions

- Identifying information, such as a photo or description (so they know they are dealing with the right person)

Vials of life ("life" is sometimes written as LIFE, and stands for Lifesaving Information For Emergencies) are available at most pharmacies, some senior centers and doctors' offices, and online.

But honestly, you can very easily make your own. See page 639 for a form. Or just write out the above information

(legibly) and put it in a clear plastic bag, along with any medical orders or proxy forms. Write "emergency medical information" in large red letters on a piece of paper and place that in the bag, facing out, so the words are clearly visible, and tape the bag to the door of the fridge. Then place notices, in red, on the inside of the front door and by your parent's bed, explaining where the information is.

Make a copy of this information and place it in your parent's purse, wallet, glove compartment, or anywhere else it might be helpful, and keep a copy for yourself (we all get muddled in an emergency). And be sure to update it regularly (old medical information won't be terribly helpful).

Medical Emergency Identification

Your parent also needs any crucial information with him when he's away from home. So today (seriously, do this today) get your parent some sort of identification so emergency crews will know his name and address, whom to contact, and if any medical conditions require special attention.

The simplest thing to do is to put a medical identification card in the front of your parent's wallet. (We've provided one on page 637.) Although emergency crews might not check a wallet immediately, it's certainly better than nothing.

If there is information that an emergency crew absolutely must know—if, say, your parent is allergic to some medication—buy a medical alert bracelet, necklace, or dog tag.

Beyond that, a few other options exist for giving emergency crews access to medical and contact information when your parent is away from home. For example, you can get a medical ID number to put on the aforementioned tag or bracelet. A responder contacts an emergency call center and, using this ID number, receives all necessary contact and medical information.

Or you can put your parent's pertinent medical information on a flash drive and attach that to a medical alert necklace, wristband, or key chain. Just be sure it is clearly marked "Medical Alert."

Most pharmacies sell a variety of medical alert options, and numerous companies sell them online.

ICE (In Case of Emergency)

ICE stands for In Case of Emergency, and although not all medical crews are aware of it, enough are that it's worth the small amount of effort involved. Your parent (and you, while you're at it) identifies someone in a cell-phone contact list as "ICE" so crews know whom to contact in case of emergency.

You can go a step further and download an ICE app on a smartphone and then put it on the first page of apps, in the upper left-hand corner. Ideally, you should also put a sticker on the phone announcing that ICE information is available. The app provides more information—emergency contacts and home address, as well as medical information, medical history, wishes, doctor, and preferred hospitals.

Safety Checklist

Bad eyesight, arthritis, poor hearing, imbalance, multiple medications,

---

ID YOURSELF AS WELL

If your parent is dependent upon you, get yourself a medical alert bracelet or wallet-size card identifying yourself as a primary caregiver, in case something happens to you. The bracelet might say something like, "My father has dementia and will need help. Please call 123-456-7891." Provide the phone number of a family member or other caregiver.

---

confusion, and other health problems all put your parent at risk for accidents. Look through her house for hazards and use some preventive strategies.

❑ Put a 911 reminder near the phone or, better yet, designate one speed-dial button for 911. Don't assume your parent will remember your number, 911, or anything else if she's injured, burglarized, or in some other trouble. Even the keenest minds go blank in moments of panic.

❑ Put her street address (and the nearest cross street) in clear letters by the phone in case she becomes muddled when talking to emergency crews.

❑ Keep a clearly written, large-print list of other emergency phone numbers by every phone, or program them into the telephone's memory. The list should include police, fire, ambulance, your home and work numbers, and the phone number of another nearby relative or a neighbor. Some phones let you put photos on the speed-dial buttons.

❑ As mentioned, put medical information in a vial of life and get your parent a bracelet or wallet-size card with emergency info on it.

❑ Because of their thinner skin and slower reactions, elderly people are at risk for scalding. Set the hot water heater to 120°F.

❑ Clearly label chemicals, harsh cleaners, insecticides, medications, paints, and so forth. Or put them out of reach completely.

❑ Check that smoke detectors and carbon monoxide detectors work. Your parent's waning sense of smell makes a smoke detector that much more important, but smoke detectors can have dead or missing batteries. Change the batteries every year. You might want to set off the alarm so that your parent knows the sound and what to do when she hears it. (It obviously does no good if it simply scares her out of her wits and she suddenly can't think to get out of the house.)

❑ Check for manageable escape routes. Your parent probably won't be able to climb out a window, so look for escapes she could use. Is the back door wide enough for your mother's wheelchair? Is there a back stairway that your father can manage? If your parent might not be able to escape because of a disability, call the local fire department and ask for safety instructions.

❑ Buy a small fire extinguisher that is easy to handle and put it in a clearly visible place, preferably in the kitchen, where fires often start. Show any aide or companion (and your parent) how to use it.

❑ In case of a blackout, be sure your parent has a backup generator ready to kick in.

❑ Have at least two flashlights (with working batteries) ready to use (and easy to find) in case of a power outage (even if you have the generator).

❑ Make sure all bathroom and kitchen outlets contain working circuit interrupters to prevent shocks. Be sure that outlets are not overloaded.

❑ In the kitchen, check that all burners and the oven work properly. Is your mother apt to reach for equipment located above the hot stove, in which case a sleeve or apron string might catch fire? If so, rearrange things.

❑ If your parent gets cold easily, buy him some good long underwear and turn up the heat. Be careful with space heaters and electric blankets, as they can cause burns and fires.

❑ If your parent has even mild dementia or confusion, register him with the Alzheimer's Association's Safe Return program. Your parent will be given an identification card and become part of a national photo database. Learn more about it through the association (800-272-3900 or alz.org).

❑ This should go without saying: Lock up any firearms.

❑ Inform the police and fire departments that your parent is elderly and lives alone. Don't rely on window decals to alert them to her presence (although these are useful, too, and available through the local fire department). Ask if there are any special precautions you should take.

AVOIDING COMMON SCAMS

One of the most common crimes against the elderly is financial exploitation. It may be a sweepstakes or credit card scam. It could be a repairman who finds a bounty of expensive problems that need fixing. But usually it is a family member, adviser, or new "friend" making off with the cash.

The best way to protect your parent is to warn him of common scams and be sure he isn't too isolated. For more on fraud and exploitation, see page 326.

Crime Precautions

The elderly are easy prey, but there's no need for your parent to lock herself in the house. Even if she is physically frail, knowledge and common sense can protect her from most dangerous situations.

Talk to your parent about the precautions she should take and what she should do in specific situations. Most of it is obvious stuff—streets to avoid at night, times when it's best to have a buddy, what to do if a stranger comes to the door. You might also do the following:

❏ Let the local police department know that your parent is elderly and living alone, especially if she lives in a small town where the police might pay special attention to her.

❏ Make sure your parent can properly operate all his home door locks and that he uses them. If he has trouble using a key, he might switch to a coded lock.

❏ Install a peephole in the front door. Remind your parent that she should not open the door for anyone unfamiliar—a salesperson or repair person—unless she has asked that person to the house. She might also invest in an intercom for the front door.

❏ If your parent doesn't already have one, install a security alarm system in his house. Then, make sure he actually uses it. You can also install "panic buttons" by his bed or favorite chair, or get an emergency response system.

❏ Look into installing outdoor lights that are triggered by motion; they will go on as soon as your parent nears the property—or if someone else does. You can also install exterior floodlights that can be operated from the bedroom.

❏ Several companies sell systems that operate house lights, as well as thermostats, home appliances, and a radio or television, from afar. When your parent is heading home, he can light up the house and even make it noisy several minutes before entering, allowing burglars time to escape (and the house time to warm up).

❏ Suggest that your parent leave jewelry or expensive watches at home when traveling or if he goes into the hospital or rehab center.

Monitors and Alert Systems

"I 've fallen and I can't get up" was part of an ad campaign that led to a lot of jokes (one placed the quip on each bra cup). But the ad's message was deadly serious.

When elderly people live alone, the fear is that something will happen—a fall, heart attack, or some other crisis—and they won't be able to get to a phone to call for help. Getting help immediately not only saves lives, but also significantly reduces the odds of being hospitalized or laid up for a long time.

Of course, having a cell phone in her pocket will serve in many emergencies, but what if she's fallen in the shower, or she's too injured to call, or she simply can't think clearly enough in that crucial moment to pull out her phone and talk to emergency crews?

Traditional Systems

A traditional personal emergency response system (PERS) works within your parent's home and an area just outside her home, and requires that your parent push a button in an emergency. The help button can be worn as a pendant or on a wristband, like a watch.

When your parent pushes the button, a call goes into a response center, where your parent is identified by a code. Someone at the center will then talk to your parent through an intercom on her phone and then contact the appropriate people. If your parent does not answer the intercom, the responder sends emergency crews immediately.

Dozens of companies sell emergency response systems. You can find them in the Yellow Pages or on the Internet or check with a medical supply store.

Prices and contracts vary, so know what you're getting into. Some sell the system (usually for $200 to $2,000) and then charge a monthly service fee ($10 to $40). Others rent systems (usually about $30 a month, but it can vary from $15 to $60).

When possible, renting is preferable because you don't have a big initial expense and don't have to worry about repairs or a company going defunct or moving. Also, the technology is changing rapidly and in a year you might want a different machine. Some companies charge an installation fee (no, thank you). Others require a one-year contract (no, thank you).

Although most insurance companies do not cover the cost of such a system, some hospitals and social service organizations offer the systems for free or at a discount to people with low incomes.

When comparing systems, ask about the staff receiving emergency calls. Are they available 24/7? How are they trained? Do they speak your parent's native language? Find out the company's average response time (if they are not checking their response time periodically, they should be). How often do they test the system to be sure it's working? Is the equipment guaranteed? Will the system function even if the phone is off the hook or in use?

Be sure your parent can test the system for a trial period or get a 30-day, money-back guarantee. During this time, check that your parent can operate the buttons. Also, see how well it works within his house and how far one can venture into the backyard before the system fails.

Once your parent has an emergency response system, check the batteries regularly. It's no good to have it if it's not working.

Most important, be sure she will actually push the button in an emergency. People often don't push the button, even after a serious accident, either because they can't or—more often—because they "don't want to be a bother." Tell your mother that she'll be much more of a "bother" if she fails to call for help. When in doubt, she should push.

Mobile Systems

If your parent is out and about on her own, you might want to invest in a system that links to her mobile phone. Known as a mobile PERS, or MPERS, this system will allow her to have an emergency call button wherever she goes. A GPS lets the call center know exactly where she is when the call comes in (assuming she's not completely out of range). A base unit is usually a couple hundred dollars, and then there is a monthly fee of around $30 to $60.

Fall Sensors

Because seniors often fail to push their emergency call buttons, you might want to purchase a sensor that detects when someone has fallen. The gadget

A (SIMPLE) PHONE CALL AWAY

Wouldn't it be great if your parent could use her mobile phone to text, video chat, log her appointments, and keep track of her medications? If only.

Alas, many older people have trouble operating smartphones, what with all the apps and tiny buttons. Eventually, in frustration, they leave the darn thing on the bureau and you're left calling into voicemail all day.

You can buy phones for the elderly that are larger and have big fonts and simple steps for taking pictures and sending emails. In the meantime, if you go to "settings" on a regular smartphone, there is often an "accessibility" option that allows you to adjust settings for imperfect vision, hearing, and motor skills.

You can also get an extremely pared-down cell phone that is easy to use. No Internet. No camera. Just a phone. So no texting or calendars, but at least your parent will have a phone at all times.

These phones (Just5, Jitterbug, and Doro, to name a few) have giant, easy-to-see buttons, simple speed dialing, and amplified sound. Some lock when they aren't in use (so no pocket calls). Some have bright flashlights. Some have a single, large speed-dial button that initiates a string of calls to a preprogrammed list of emergency numbers (for example, 911, you, your sister, your mother's neighbor).

WATCHFUL EYES

If your parent lives alone and doesn't have regular visitors, ask a neighbor to alert you if anything seems out of whack (the lights don't go on in the evening or the newspaper isn't picked up). You might also ask someone who sees your parent on a regular basis—the apartment superintendent, a barber, or rabbi—to contact you if anything seems wrong. (Of course, you should approach only those individuals you trust completely; you don't want questionable strangers to know that your parent is frail and alone.) People who work for meal delivery programs, like Meals on Wheels, are usually taught to recognize signs of trouble as well.

recognizes a fall automatically; there's no need to push a button.

Some of these go beyond detecting falls; they also let you know if there is any significant change in your parent's daily routine—your parent doesn't get up from her nap, for instance, or hasn't moved out of her chair to eat lunch.

These sensors are like small pagers, which clip onto a belt, attach to a band that's wrapped around the chest, or are worn like a pendant. They don't simply detect when someone has become horizontal (possibly a nap and not a fall); they measure motion and changes in acceleration. Some also use pattern recognition to distinguish your parent's normal movements from falls. By most reports, they are pretty accurate.

If a fall is detected, and your parent doesn't get up immediately or hit the "reset" button, the unit alerts a call center. Then, like the PERS systems, the call center tries to speak with your parent via phone, and if there is no response, responders call 911. You can set it up so that you are also alerted, by either text or phone call.

In most cases, if your parent fails to wear the monitor for any length of time, a message is sent to a designated caregiver, alerting that person (you) that the device is not being used. You can also check a web page to see how active or inactive your parent has been. Unlike a webcam, which comes with all sorts of privacy issues, an activity monitor simply tells you whether your parent is on the move—or not.

You can opt for a system that works in the house or buy a mobile unit, a version of the MPERS, that works with your parent's cell phone.

Home Sensors

Home sensors let you know if your parent is up, getting meals, or straying from her usual routine.

The systems vary greatly, but the basic idea is that motion detectors are placed in key areas of the house—the bathroom, bedroom, kitchen, front door, and so on. Sensors can also be placed on a walker or cane, refrigerator door, coffeemaker, or other appliances. If you know that Dad gets up and has coffee every day at 8 and today you notice that it's 9:30 and the coffee hasn't been made, you can call him and see if anything's wrong.

Granny Cams

It is possible to install tiny video cameras in your parent's house. For many people, this is an unimaginable invasion of privacy, but for others it is the difference between living at home and moving to a nursing home. Let's say your mom is frail and a bit confused. You could install motion and fall detectors, but would you know if she left the stove on or fell asleep in the tub?

Although this raises both legal and ethical questions, people also use hidden cameras to keep an eye on aides. Are they kind? Abusive? Honest?

The cameras are legal in all states, but many states do not allow audio recording without a person's prior consent. You'll also need permission from your parent if you want to place them in her home, of course.

With cameras streaming constant video to your laptop, you can get on with your life (sort of) and glance over from time to time to be sure Mom is okay.

But would she really want this? And do you really want to be aware of her every move? Would she allow the cameras in her bathroom? If they aren't covering every corner of the house, are you really getting the oversight you hoped for? Will you watch the video stream often enough to make it useful? Also, think about how you would handle it if you see a problem—you need a plan in place if she falls or doesn't get up from bed or wanders aimlessly out the door.

If it helps, go for it. Just think through the various, and important, privacy and trust issues.

Preventing Falls

Everyone catches a toe or trips on a step occasionally, but at your parent's age, even a minor tumble can have major repercussions. Older bodies break more easily than younger ones, and they don't heal as quickly or as completely. Then, while they are trying to heal, enforced bed rest exacerbates existing medical ills and causes new ones—pneumonia, infections, bedsores, and constipation.

Each year, one out of three Americans 65 years or older and living in the community (and 60 percent of those in a nursing home) has a serious fall. About 10 percent of these falls result in fractures of the hip, spine, pelvis, hand, and wrist, as well as spinal cord and brain injuries.

Half of all older people who fracture a hip never fully recover—they end up needing canes, walkers, or wheelchairs for the rest of their lives. Twenty-five percent of them die within six months of the injury. Furthermore, 40 percent of elderly people entering nursing homes cite falls as a reason for the move; 25 percent say it is the primary reason.

❝ My mother was always active. At 96, she volunteered, traveled, read. But when she fell and broke her ankle, she was immobile for a couple of months, and that really killed her spirit. She could never get around well after that, and so her mood, her body, everything just went. She died a year later."

—Mel T.

Any fall, even a minor tumble, can create fear and uncertainty, leading to less exercise, fewer social interactions, and reduced independence.

To put it simply, falling is one of the most serious health risks facing older people. Preventing falls should be a primary concern for you and your parent.

The problem is that most people do exactly the opposite of what they should do. Afraid of falling, elderly people become extremely cautious and are reluctant to move around. We caregivers encourage this guarded approach by urging our elderly parents to remain stationary—*Don't move, Dad. I'll get it for you. It's not a problem.*

Ironically, this is a surefire way to increase the risk of falls (not to mention making life dull and miserable). Sedentary, your parent will have less strength, balance, and flexibility, and will be more apt to, yes, fall.

Furthermore, an inactive lifestyle will make your parent dependent, isolated, and depressed, and it can cause health problems.

It's a downward spiral, so try to avoid it. Your parent needs to get up and out, but safely.

There are several ways to reduce the risk of falls:

REVIEW MEDICATIONS. Many drugs cause dizziness, confusion, and fatigue or affect blood pressure. Your parent should ask her doctor if she can reduce, quit, or change certain medications, especially sleeping pills, antidepressants, antianxiety drugs, and blood pressure medications.

URGE YOUR PARENT TO GET UP AND MOVE. Exercise and physical therapy that improve balance, coordination, flexibility, and strength will all help considerably. Tai chi, which involves slow and controlled movements, is also an excellent way for elderly people to improve their balance.

MAKE HER HOUSE FALL-SAFE. Be on the lookout for household hazards, such as meandering electrical wires, loose rugs, piles in pathways, and dishes or hanging plants that must be reached with a footstool. Be sure the house is well lighted. Add handrails and grab bars. Read "Room-by-Room Modifications" on the next page for more on preventing

---

➕ MEDICAL ALERT

If your parent has a serious fall and is in pain, stay calm. Call an emergency crew. Don't move her unless you need to restore her breathing or get her away from fire, out of water, or clear of some other danger. If you must move her, don't pull on an arm or leg; wrap your arms around her chest and then pull up using your legs, not your back.

Otherwise, let her be. Cover her with a blanket if it's cool and assure her that medical help is coming and she is going to be just fine. Continue to talk to her in a slow, calm voice until help has arrived.

PRACTICE MAKES PERFECT SENSE

Your parent should practice getting up slowly from a chair and, if necessary, practice using handrails and other supports as he moves about a room. It's not what he's done for the past eight decades, so it will take some time to get used to it.

Also, show your parent what to do in case he falls. (First, use that emergency button.) If he's not hurt, he should roll onto his belly and push himself up onto his hands and knees, and then crawl to a piece of furniture that he can use for support while he pulls himself up.

If possible, have him try doing this. Such a drill may sound silly, but when people fall, they often become confused and disoriented. If they have practiced what to do, it should come to them more easily when they actually need it.

Any time your parent falls, his doctor should be notified.

---

falls, and if you still have concerns, get an occupational therapist to assess the house.

GET HER VISION AND HEARING CHECKED. If necessary, your parent should have cataract surgery or consider a hearing aid.

OPT FOR STURDY, NONSLIP SHOES. Sneakers or other rubber-soled shoes provide a solid base. Avoid shoes with open heels or toes. Slippers or socks should also have rubber bottoms.

BE ALERT TO DRINKING. Alcohol has a pronounced effect on the elderly and will skew balance and reflexes.

CONSIDER VITAMIN D SUPPLEMENTS. Although they can increase the risk of kidney stones, research suggests that elderly people who are at risk of falls can benefit from taking 800 I.U. (international units) a day. Vitamin D helps prevent bone loss and appears to improve muscle strength and balance in this population.

Room-by-Room Modifications

There are all sorts of ways to make a house safer and life easier.

A visiting nurse or an occupational or physical therapist can examine your parent's home for hazards and show you how to make it more accessible. If the inspection is done as part of a hospital discharge, Medicare or other insurance policies might cover the cost. The local agency on aging should also be able to help. Many of these agencies cover some or all of the costs of home inspections and modifications for eligible seniors.

Or, you can simply tour your parent's house yourself and look for places where she has to bend, reach, stoop, or step over something. Look for anything that might trip her up or get in her way.

Be sure knobs, faucets, and switches are easy to use; pathways are clear; and lighting is adequate. A variety of things will make life easier: ramps, lever faucet handles, lights that go on when someone enters the room, handrails and grab bars, doors that open automatically, and large-print phones and thermostats.

If she spends a lot of time at your house or elsewhere, check out those places as well.

Entranceways

• Be sure there's a sturdy handrail on each side of any entrance steps. If necessary, add a ramp.

ON ICE AND SNOW

Obviously, walking on ice and snow is not a great idea, but sometimes these things can't be avoided. In such cases, your parent should walk slowly, with his weight centered and his knees slightly bent, and look for small patches of grass, sidewalk, or loose snow where he can plant a foot with more traction. (And remember, he should always wear shoes with rubber soles!)

You might want to get him some simple, light snow chains, cleats, or coils that slip over any shoe. Check out Yaktrax, Snow Trax, and Stabilicers. A walking stick should also help in snowy regions.

• Install a bench or chest near the front door, where groceries and other bags can be placed while your parent manages the lock.

• Likewise, put a shelf inside the door for packages, keys, and other items.

• Depending on the climate, keep a bag of salt or sand by the door for when it's icy out. If money is no object, a contractor can put a heater in the stoop (and even in the driveway) so ice melts.

• Entranceways throughout the house should, ideally, be extra wide to accommodate a walker or wheelchair.

Floors and Pathways

• Check carpets for worn areas and rips. Tack down any flaps or curled edges.

• Use low-pile, wall-to-wall carpeting wherever possible.

• Get rid of throw rugs or make sure they have a rubber, non-skid backing on them. (You can buy an inexpensive thin rubber mat to lay under a rug.)

• Make sure floors are even and level. Repair loose floorboards and remove thresholds at doorways.

• Clear hallways and other pathways of wastepaper baskets, footstools, magazine racks, electrical wires, and other small objects.

• Install handrails in hallways.

" My father has this little, three-legged pine table in his living room, right by his favorite chair. Every time he got up or sat down, he would lean on the table, using it for balance. I told him a hundred times that the table was wobbly, and that one day he was going to lean on it, fall over, and kill himself. I even bought him a new table, but he didn't use it. He's pretty stubborn. He said, 'I've had this table here for 45 years and I haven't fallen yet. Why would I fall now?'

But I think my warning sank in a little, even though he would never admit it. I've noticed that he doesn't really lean on that table anymore. He puts more weight on the chair. He listens if I bother him enough about something. I just have to be a little more stubborn than he is."

—Skip K.

Stairs

- Avoid stairs completely, if possible. This might mean turning a downstairs den into a bedroom or building ramps onto short stairways.

- Sturdy handrails that extend the full length of the stairs should be placed on both sides of the stairwell. Don't forget the stairs leading to a basement and those by the front and back doors.

- If your parent is particularly wobbly, urge her to go down stairs backward, holding on to the handrails, as if she were climbing down a ladder. It's easier for most people, and if she falls, it's better to fall forward onto the next step than straight down all the stairs.

- Mark the edges of steps—or any place the floor changes elevation even slightly—with brightly colored, glow-in-the-dark adhesive tape.

- Use nonslip treads. Consider getting rid of carpeting on stairways, as it rounds off the edges of steps and shortens the depth of each step, making footing more precarious. Use rubber mats instead.

Furniture

- Chairs should be tall enough to get into and out of easily, and have strong armrests and high backs that can be used for support. If necessary, keep a walker or cane by the chair or look into electric-powered pneumatic chairs that lift a person up and lower him down. You can also buy wedged cushions that provide a little help in getting out of a chair.

- Likewise, make sure the bed is not too high or too low, so your parent can get in and out easily.

- Get rid of beds and other furniture with nonlocking wheels.

- Furniture legs that curve outward create a tripping hazard. Move such furniture out of any pathway or get rid of it.

- Avoid three-legged tables, which are not sturdy.

- Repair broken or wobbly furniture immediately.

- If your parent is largely bedbound, consider bringing a hospital bed into the house. A hospital bed can be raised and lowered (higher while you help her dress or eat, and lower while she gets into and out of bed).

Bathrooms

- Install grab bars near toilets, in showers, and around tubs (before you think it's necessary). Your parent should not rely on towel bars for support.

- Lever faucets, rather than knobs, are easier for arthritic hands.

- A raised toilet seat or convertible commode (which has arms and is positioned over the existing toilet) will make sitting and getting up easier.

- A shower stool allows your parent to sit while showering.

- Attach a wall-mounted liquid soap dispenser in the shower so your parent is not fumbling around picking up bars of soap.

- Install nonslip strips or rubber mats on the floor of the tub or shower, and on the bathroom floor.

- Avoid bath oils, which make feet and hands slippery.

- A showerhead that can be raised and lowered is ideal, as your parent will want it lower if she's seated. A handheld showerhead can be placed in a holder at the right height and makes it easier for a second person to help out.

- If your parent has trouble getting to the bathroom, consider putting a commode next to her bed, at least at night.

Kitchen

- If you're renovating, install low cabinets or cabinets that are adjustable (so that someone in a wheelchair can reach them).

- Pull-out shelves make it easier to reach things.

HOME RENOVATIONS

Your parent's home can be renovated to accommodate almost any disability. In addition to the suggestions listed throughout this chapter, you can make a house even more accessible with ramps, lower sinks, wheelchair-accessible bathrooms, automatic door openers, and so on.

A website funded by Weill Cornell Medical College (thiscaringhome.org) provides simple instructions and guidance on how to make a home safer and more accessible for an elderly person and has a section focused on dementia.

AARP (aarp.org or 888-687-2277) also has information on how to make a home user-friendly for seniors.

Homemods.org, a service of the Fall Prevention Center of Excellence, (homemods.org) has information about home modification as well as a database of local programs and contractors who specialize in such work and will do other maintenance work for seniors at a discount.

The National Rehabilitation Information Center (naric.com or 800-346-2742) has information on disabilities, rehabilitation, home modification, rehabilitation equipment, and local organizations.

- A pull-out counter provides a work space if your parent is in a wheelchair.

- If your parent has poor eyesight, use contrasting colors: a light countertop and dark backsplash, for example, or a light countertop with a contrasting edge.

- You can install a sink that can be raised and lowered to suit someone standing or in a wheelchair.

- Replace faucet knobs with levers, and replace small button knobs on cupboards with large horseshoe-shaped knobs. Levers are great not only because they don't require grasping, but because they're easy to use when one's hands are full or slippery. If that's not possible, buy soft foam covers for knobs to make them easier for arthritic fingers to grasp.

- If your parent uses a gas range, make sure the dials are easy to read. If she has poor vision or suffers from mild confusion, mark the "off" position clearly with a strip of colored tape. (If she's more severely confused, you might have to shut a gas range off.)

- Several manufacturers make wheelchair-accessible stoves.

- Countertops with rounded edges can reduce injuries.

Lighting

- Older eyes need more light and don't adjust quickly to changes in lighting, so lighting should be bright and evenly distributed. Avoid having dark hallways that lead into brightly lighted stairways, for example.

- Reduce glare by aiming lights at a wall or the ceiling, and use low-glare bulbs and lampshades. If there is a sunny window facing your parent as he uses the stairs, hang curtains or shades to block the glare.

- Make sure light switches are easy to use and easy to reach. They should be placed at the entrance of each room and at both the top and the bottom of any stairs, so your parent isn't walking through a dark room to get to a light switch. Better yet, get motion-activated light controls.

- Use night-lights in the hallway, the bathroom, the kitchen, the stairway, or anywhere else your parent might venture at night.

Other Measures

- Put outlets high, so that your parent doesn't have to bend over to plug something in. If you'd rather not hire an electrician, use duct tape to run an extension cord up a wall.

- Check the temperature. Both low and high body temperature can make a person dizzy and thus susceptible to accidents. In general, the thermostat probably needs to be higher than it used to be, even at night, when it should be around 65 degrees. When temperatures rise, be sure your parent's home is air-conditioned or at least well fanned. (If she doesn't have air-conditioning, she might need to install a room air conditioner or move to an air-conditioned facility during the hottest part of the day.)

- Organize things so that frequently used items are within easy reach.

HEAVY LIFTING

When helping your parent move, you don't want to hurt him, and you certainly don't want to put your back out or otherwise injure yourself.

- Support him along his larger muscles and bones. Rather than holding a hand, hold a shoulder. Rather than turning him over by pulling an arm and leg, pull the shoulder and thigh.

- Bend your knees and push up using your leg muscles, not your back. You don't want to pull your back out in this process.

- If you can't lift or maneuver your parent, don't. Call for help from a neighbor, friend, or, if necessary, the police.

- You can buy a "transfer belt" (at a medical supply store or on the Internet) that helps in lifting people to a standing position. You might also consider buying chair lifts, straps for cars, and other devices aimed at lifting and maneuvering people.

- Teach your parent how to rise from chairs and beds gradually to avoid light-headedness. She should get up in stages, with two hands planted firmly on strong armrests or other supports.

- Install grab bars by the bed and the closet, so that when your parent is getting out of bed or dressing, he has something to grab and steady himself.

- If necessary, encourage your parent to use a cane or walker. A doctor should fit it, and your parent should be taught how to use it correctly.

- If your father uses a cane, attach a loose wrist strap to one end. Then, if he drops it, it won't fall to the ground and leave him in the precarious position of having to stoop to pick it up.

- If your parent has any hanging plants, be sure she doesn't have to duck to get past them or reach up on tiptoes to water them.

Bathing and Grooming

Life with an aged parent becomes a whirl of compromises. In this case, you'll have to strike some balance between ease and vanity. Your mother might like to shower daily and have her hair done regularly, but is this practical or even doable?

Good hygiene and personal care is

> " When my mother's hair started to fall out after the chemotherapy, I didn't think much about it. We all knew it would happen, and she's never been terribly concerned about her appearance.
>
> A friend of hers suggested that she buy a wig. I thought, 'Mom? In a wig? Never!' But sure enough, she bought one and she wears it all the time. She looks pretty good in it, and it's made a big difference in how she feels. She has a lot more confidence."
>
> —Diane M.

important, not only because it prevents infections but also because it lifts a person's spirits (and of course, smelling vaguely off will keep other people at a distance). But for most people, a couple of baths a week are enough; sponge baths in between are fine.

If you or someone else is helping your parent bathe and brush her hair, these tips should help:

- Buy a chair made for the shower or use a small stool, as long as it's stable and won't slip (and is waterproof). You can also buy a rubber device that deflates to lower a person gently into a tub and then inflates to get him out again.

- As mentioned, grab bars and a raised toilet seat can make everyone's life easier and safer. And lever handles are easier to use than knobs.

- If your parent is immobile, a sponge bath is as good as a regular bath. (It's not easy, but be sure to get into all cracks and under every fold of skin, and then dry thoroughly.)

- You can buy a rubber basin for washing your parent's hair while she is in bed or in a chair.

- An electric toothbrush is easier to use. If your parent is quite sick, gently use a wet, soft toothbrush or dental swab (available in medical supply stores) to wipe the teeth, gums, and tongue.

- A new, short (chic) hairdo might be just the thing for a woman who can't get to the beauty parlor or shower regularly.

- Finally, medical supply stores, mail-order catalogs, and online stores sell a mind-boggling array of bathroom gizmos, such as a razor holder that attaches to the hand (so arthritic fingers don't have to grasp a thin handle), sponges with long handles, toothbrushes with thick handles, and nail clippers, toothpaste dispensers, mirrors, showerhead attachments, and urinals that are made for arthritic fingers.

> " In my mother's era, you took baths. She never used the shower. Ever. But I couldn't get her into the tub. And if I did, she couldn't get up once she got down. I said to her, 'A shower is so wonderful. You don't know what you're missing.' But she absolutely would not do it.
>
> Finally, she did try it not long ago. She had her first shower at 90-some years old. I said, 'Isn't this wonderful?' You know, I'm standing outside and she's in there, but I'm holding her and I'm getting all wet. She wouldn't say that she liked it. But she accepted it."
>
> —Margaret F.

Dressing

If your parent has trouble reaching the zipper on the back of her dress, managing the tiny buttons on her sweater, or getting her shoes tied, explore the latest line of "easy clothing" for both men and women—pants with Velcro closures, shirts with snaps, dresses with large zipper handles or ones that pull on from the front and then are sealed with a Velcro closure down the back, large jerseys that pull over the head, shoes that slip on, and skirts that pull on.

Or check the racks of a shop your parent already likes. Jersey dresses with wide necks slide over the head, and wraparound dresses pull on like a coat. Sweatpants and tops are the easiest (and most comfortable) outfits to wear, and many stores sell attractive elastic-waist pants. Do your best to find clothing that suits your parent's style and that you think she'll like.

But before you purchase a new wardrobe, think about ways to make the clothes she already owns easier to use. Buttons can be replaced with Velcro, and elastic laces turn tie-up shoes into slip-ons.

> " After her stroke, my mother had a terrible time getting dressed. I bought her several pairs of elastic-waist pants and a pair of slip-on Keds, and I lent her several of my larger pullover shirts. But there was still one problem. I couldn't seem to find a bra. I was looking for something that closed in the front with Velcro or wrapped around. In the meantime, I told her she'd just have to go without.
>
> Now, my mother is large-chested. No bra meant—well, it was obvious she didn't have one on.
>
> I told her I was still looking and she said, 'You know, I kind of like it like this.' She was all guilty smiles. 'I don't think I want one after all,' she said.
>
> It was the 1960s all over again. She was liberated. She was never going back.
>
> So I bagged the bra and bought her a fleece vest, just to make it all a little less obvious. She never wore a bra again."
> —Marjorie C.

A Few Other Tips

- When buying new clothes for someone who has trouble maneuvering, consider going a size larger, which will make it easier to get clothes on and allow room for movement.

- For sensitive skin, find silky materials or soft knits.

- A variety of gadgets can make dressing easier, such as metallic arms or "grippers" that help pull socks and pants on, devices that pull buttons through their holes, and extra-long shoehorns.

- Dozens of online stores sell clothing designed for people with disabilities, including people who use wheelchairs, people with diabetes (who often need special shoes), and those who suffer from incontinence. Search "adaptive clothing."

- Buck fashion. Style may have to give way to ease.

MORE THAN CLEAN—BEAUTIFUL

People feel better when they look good. A new hairdo and some makeup may seem unnecessary, but it might improve your mother's outlook. Your father will feel more dapper with a clean shave and combed hair.

Make sure your parent has the proper tools not only for basic hygiene, but also for a bit of primping. Your father may be able to use the toilet safely, but can he open his aftershave? Can your mother manage her lipstick? Easy-to-open lids and other handy devices should help.

Also, find out about local barbers and beauticians who make house calls. Some offer discounts to senior citizens.

Don't forget the little touches that make your parent feel attractive. If your father likes to wear a tie but can no longer tie it, buy him a clip-on. Give your mother a colorful silk scarf, which hides humped shoulders, surrounds the face with color, and makes her feel special. (You can tie it permanently so all she has to do is slip it over her head.)

What's for Dinner?

Getting healthy meals on the table can be a struggle for the most able among us—it may be even more difficult for your parent. And as discussed in Chapter 6, it's very important that he eat regularly and well, and that he maintains his weight. A poor diet can lead to all sorts of medical problems and worsen existing illness, not to mention make your parent feel tired and apathetic.

Are logistical issues getting in the way? Can he get to the grocery store? Can he open a can? Is he used to his wife cooking for him and now she is gone?

Here are a few thoughts on making healthful eating easier for your parent (for tips on dining when someone has dementia, see page 501):

Getting to the Store

- If your parent can't get to the grocery store, contact local transportation services or a senior center to see if a senior van or volunteer can give her a ride.

- If transportation is not the issue—if she simply is not mobile—see if there's a grocery store that delivers, or talk to a volunteer service, her religious organization, or perhaps even a neighbor or friend to see if someone might do the shopping for her.

In the Grocery Aisles

- Once a month—perhaps on a shopping trip with you or with someone else who can help with heavy bags—

WHEN APPETITE GOES

It's terrifying to watch a parent lose her appetite. Whatever you offer—her favorite chocolate pastries or the grilled cheese sandwiches she used to love—she's just not interested.

Sudden, unintentional weight loss is a sign of serious trouble. It may be the result of depression, cancer, heart disease, alcoholism, confusion, loss of smell or taste, or swallowing problems, to name a few. Loneliness is a contributing factor (who likes to eat alone?). Multiple medications can also dampen an appetite. Whatever the reasons, weight loss can weaken the immune system, lead to depression, and cause muscles to waste away.

Don't ignore a sharp change in appetite or weight. Talk to your parent's doctor and try to determine the root of the problem. Whatever the underlying cause, a little exercise can boost an appetite. Treating depression will certainly help. Some medications promote weight gain.

At this point, don't worry about what your parent is eating; any calories are good calories, even if they are from a milk shake or candy or doughnuts.

If things get serious, think long and hard before agreeing to a feeding tube. An NG, or naso-gastric, tube is inserted in the nose and down into the stomach, and allows for liquid nutrition. A G tube, or gastric tube, is inserted through an incision directly into the stomach, and allows for all nutrition. While feeding tubes can keep people alive, they can also cause aspiration and pneumonia.

If your parent is severely ill and nearing death, know that loss of appetite is normal. It's hard to accept, but the body is simply shutting down and can't process food. A feeding tube can cause complications.

your parent should stock up on frozen and canned foods, pasta, rice, beans, cereal, and other staples that keep well. (Bread, butter, and meats can all be frozen and used at a later date.) Interim shopping trips can be used for getting light loads of fresh fruits, vegetables, and dairy products.

- When purchasing perishables he should buy only as much as he can use. If your father is shopping for one, he can ask the grocer to break open large containers and give him just a few potatoes or a half dozen eggs. Most will do this readily. He can buy small portions of cheese, cooked meat, a pint of milk, and a half pound of hamburger so unused food doesn't spoil, or he can get regular portions of some things and freeze small amounts for later use.

- "Long-life," or UHT, milk (heated at ultra-high temperatures) costs a little more but can be stored on the shelf at room temperature for up to six months. (Once it is opened, it must be refrigerated, and lasts about 10 days.) It is perfectly safe, quite tasty if chilled, and as nutritious as regular milk.

- Dietary supplement drinks, like Ensure or Boost, and powdered breakfast drinks are useful now and then as just that—a supplement—but they should not replace regular meals.

- If your mother walks to the corner grocery or has to transport her bags from the bus stop, get her a handcart.

- Prepared foods have come a long way, and a few now are nutritious and delicious. Just look for ingredients you've heard of.

- If money is a concern, rice, dried beans, pasta, and frozen vegetables tend to be cheaper. See if there is a food pantry in town. Learn about meal programs and whether your parent is eligible for food stamps.

In the Kitchen

In addition to the suggestions listed on page 128, consider these:

- If your parent has stiff joints or weak muscles, dozens of aids—jar openers, spoon holders, lightweight cookware, and so on—can make cooking easier.

- Small toast-and-broil ovens, microwaves, and woks are convenient for single-serving meals. Food processors are helpful for chopping.

❝ My mother-in-law seemed to be shrinking away—getting tinier and skinnier. She just wasn't interested in food. But then one of her aides starting cooking for her and she transformed. She put on weight and has a real cushion on her now.❞

—Daisy S.

❝ In the months after my father died, my mother didn't eat much. She couldn't be bothered to make a real meal just for herself. She said she hated eating alone. So she lost a lot of weight, which was bad because she was thin to start with.

I taught her how to sauté vegetables in a wok and showed her a few easy pasta and rice recipes—all things she can do in one pot with very little work. Whenever I visit, I load up her shelves and refrigerator with food. She protests a lot, but she eats it. Maybe only because she can't stand to see things go to waste.❞

—Jennifer S.

- Put lazy Susans in cabinets that are full of small items so your parent has easy access to them.

- Move utensils, plates, food, pans, and other frequently used items to mid-range shelves or onto the countertop so your parent doesn't have to reach high shelves or stoop to get things from low places.

- Buy your parent a cookbook (large-print, if necessary) with easy recipes that serve just one or two people. Some cookbooks cater to special diets, with low-salt or fat-free dishes. Or show your parent how to make a few easy dishes, and then write down the directions for him. He can add vegetables, beans, tofu, or rice to a can of broth or other soup; toss some tomatoes, cheese, vegetables, or leftover meat into a helping of pasta; fold all sorts of food into a small omelet; or sauté an assortment of favorite foods in a wok.

- If you leave food for your parent, make sure that he can easily open and heat whatever you bring. He may just toss it out, not wanting to admit that he couldn't undo the twist-tie or unwrap the foil.

At the Table

- Make dining social. Elderly people often fail to eat well purely because they don't like to eat alone. When you can't be there, urge your parent to get together with friends, or see if a volunteer program might send someone over at mealtime.

- If your parent has trouble with fine-motor skills, buy him forks and knives with longer, heavier, thicker, or bent handles; glasses with built-in straws; and plates with rims.

- Food that doesn't have to be cut up is easier for less dexterous hands, and finger food is often easier for people with dementia, who can be confused by utensils.

- When one's sense of smell and taste recede, food becomes less appetizing. To perk up food, rather than adding more salt, throw in some herbs, spices, extracts, lemon, or garlic, and heat food whenever possible, so it gives off more aroma. A variety of textures on the plate—crunchy vegetables, creamy sauces, crispy crusts—also makes a meal more appetizing.

- If your parent's appetite is diminished, keep portions small. A large volume of food can be overwhelming. Several small meals or snacks over the course of the day may be preferable.

- A few ideas for easy, healthful snacks: fresh fruit, cheese cubes, vegetables with dip or hummus, raisins and other dried fruit, popcorn, yogurt, chicken nuggets, tea sandwiches, egg rolls, meat slices, and peanut butter and crackers.

MAKE IT SPECIAL

Eating is not a chore. It is, or should be, an enjoyable part of the day. It should fill the senses and please the soul. There should be rich aromas and interesting textures. And it should be social and relaxing. Not every day, perhaps, but at least some of the time.

Of course, life isn't perfect, and right now, your life and your parent's life are far from perfect. But do whatever you can to make meals special, and remember, even small things count.

When your mother dines alone, encourage her to put her dinner on a plate, rather than eating it out of the pan, and to sit down at the table to eat. You might even arrange to eat at the same time and set up a video chat on your respective tables.

If she's in a nursing home, eating propped up in bed off an institutional tray, bring a pretty linen cloth and a small vase of flowers (fake ones will do) to make dining seem a bit more special.

WHEN COOKING ISN'T POSSIBLE

There are all sorts of programs to ensure that the elderly have access to nutritional food. Congregate meals offered at local community centers, churches, and senior centers are nutritious, social, and inexpensive or free. Some senior centers provide transportation to meals.

If your parent can't go out, find out about meal-delivery services, which can also be free or inexpensive. (See page 152 for more on meal programs.) If your parent can afford it, she might hire someone to drop off a meal each day or to pack her freezer with a week's worth of homemade food, which should be fresher and more interesting than a delivery service.

- Be sure his dentures fit properly and that he has no other dental problems that are hindering his eating.

- When your family dines together, let your parent eat at her own pace. Have her start before the others sit down, or let the children leave the table while she finishes. If she feels that others are waiting for her, she may quit mid-meal, or worse, hurry and choke on something.

- If your parent lives with you, don't enforce "normal" mealtimes. Sometimes, as people grow older, the established routines don't work anymore.

When Swallowing Is Difficult

If your parent has trouble chewing and swallowing, or is unable to feed herself, you or some other caregiver will need to be more involved.

People who have had a stroke or have dementia, pulmonary disease, Parkinson's disease, head or neck cancer, or injuries to the head, neck, or chest sometimes suffer from dysphagia, a condition in which swallowing is painful, difficult, or impossible.

This puts them at risk of malnutrition, dehydration, or choking. They can also inhale liquid or food into their lungs and develop pneumonia.

Signs of dysphagia include wheezing, drooling, or gagging; congestion; or simply taking a long time to swallow foods. Your parent should talk with a doctor. A speech therapist can teach him exercises and ways to make swallowing easier.

If swallowing is difficult, try the following:

- Offer your parent small meals several times a day rather than a few large meals.

- Get her to eat sitting up. She should eat slowly, pausing between bites. She should take small bites or sips, and absolutely not try to talk while eating.

- Semisolid foods, such as mashed potatoes and thick soups (without chunks), are best. Pretty much anything can be pulverized into a thick, smooth consistency. A food processor or blender will grind meat, mash potatoes, and puree vegetables and fruit. Also try scrambled eggs, oatmeal, egg salad, creamed sweet potatoes, bread pudding, custard, applesauce, flavored gelatin, and milk shakes. Honestly, baby food straight from the jar is soft, nutritious, tasty, and perfectly good for adults. If you must mash foods into an unappetizing-looking lump, garnish it with lemon or herbs.

- Often, thick liquids are easier to swallow than thin ones. Add powdered milk, ice cream, honey, powdered eggs, pudding, gelatin, or a commercial thickening agent to liquids.

- Serve foods that are either warm or cool, as this might help trigger a swallow reflex.

- If you are feeding your parent, never hurry her or thrust oversize bites at her. If you don't have the time (and one meal can take an hour or two), see if a home health aide or a local volunteer can help.

Food Safety

Although younger people can tolerate most germs without any ill effects, the elderly, who have weaker immune systems, are vulnerable to the bacteria, parasites, and chemical contaminants in food. They also don't recover easily once they become sick. As a result, you and your parent need to take some extra precautions.

The problem is, this is a time of life when people tend to be particularly bad about food safety. Your parent might forget to put food back in the refrigerator, or forget how long the meat has been cooking, or be certain that he just bought that month-old milk. Sometimes they don't want to spend money on a new carton of milk, or they might not realize the milk has spoiled because their sense of smell isn't what it used to be.

Although much of this is obvious, be aware of food safety and be sure your parent is food savvy:

- Elderly people should avoid raw or undercooked fish, meat, poultry, and eggs; raw or unpasteurized milk or cheese; unpasteurized or untreated fruit or vegetable juice; and (yes, it's true) raw alfalfa sprouts.

- When shopping, put raw meat, fish, and poultry in separate bags so they don't drip and contaminate other foods.

- Don't buy food in cans that are dented or bulging, or jars that are cracked or have loose-fitting lids.

- Check the dates on food and buy those with the longest shelf life remaining.

ⓘ FOOD SAFETY INFORMATION

For more information about food storage and safety, contact the following:

Government Food Safety Information
foodsafety.gov

USDA Meat and Poultry Hotline
www.fsis.usda.gov
888-674-6854

- Prepare raw meat on a separate work surface. Bacteria from the raw chicken, for example, can easily travel to the salad if the two are chopped on the same surface or if unwashed hands handle both.

- Meat and eggs should be cooked thoroughly. Cook roasts and steaks to 145°F and poultry to 180°F. Ground beef should be cooked through (sorry, no rare for your parent), egg whites and yolks should be firm, and fish should be opaque.

- Remind your parent to throw out food that is past the expiration date, moldy, or smelly. He (or you) might mark food clearly with the date when it should be tossed.

- Thoroughly rinse all raw produce in cool water.

- Thaw frozen foods in the refrigerator, under cold running water, or in the microwave, but not on the counter. When thawing food in a microwave, cook the food immediately afterward.

- When microwaving, turn the food during the cooking time to be sure there are no undercooked spots.

- Perishable food, leftovers, and take-out food should not be left out for more than two hours (and that's pushing it; in warm weather, stick to a one-hour limit).

- Don't forget the water. As with food, your parent will be more susceptible to contaminants in water. Buy her a water filter.

- Wash the kitchen sponge in the dishwasher or wet it and throw it in the microwave (on high for at least one minute) every other day to kill bacteria.

In the Driver's Seat

So, your parent is still driving. Every time he shuffles to his car, maneuvers his arthritic knees under the steering wheel, squints over the dashboard, and pulls into oncoming traffic, you worry. Or maybe he's already had a few fender benders and gotten a couple of tickets. But how do you stop him? You try to bring it up tactfully, but he won't listen to a word of it.

Anyone who has followed a snail-paced car or one that darts past stop signs (*What stop sign?*) knows that plenty of people in their 80s and 90s shouldn't be behind the wheel. The most danger-ous people on the roads are males under 20 and all people over 75.

The skills needed for driving tend to fade in these last decades. It starts with sensory input—noticing what's going on in all directions. Older people typically have a narrower field of vision, are more sensitive to glare, need more light to see, and can't follow moving objects well. So they might not notice immediately that a woman with a stroller is entering the crosswalk up ahead.

Also, they process information more slowly, so even if they see the woman, it takes an extra second to connect the dots: *I am headed for her. I need to put my foot on the brake.*

And finally, reflexes slow, coordina-tion declines, and bodies are less flexible, so the actual process of lifting a foot off the accelerator and slamming on

> " I took my father, at the age of 91, to the eye doctor. The doctor said that Dad couldn't see out of one eye. So I said in a loud voice, loud enough for my dad to hear, because he's also pretty deaf, 'Do you think it's a good idea for him to be driving, what with him being blind in one eye and all?'
>
> The doctor said, 'Yeah, it's fine.'
>
> So that was it. I didn't raise it again.
>
> My brother refuses to get in the car with him, and that hurts his feelings. But none of us will say, 'You have to stop.' He couldn't live without his car.
>
> He has started using a van service more, and we tell him how happy that makes us. But he hasn't stopped. I guess we should do more."
>
> —Sam B.

the brake—or looking in the rearview mirror, or turning the wheel—takes a moment longer than it should.

Illnesses such as dementia, arthri-tis, insomnia, diabetes, depression, and Parkinson's disease compound the haz-ards. Medications also make driving more dangerous, especially sleep aids, antihistamines, painkillers, antidepres-sants, and diabetes drugs.

In other words, don't wait for a stroke or diagnosis of Alzheimer's to address this. Your parent may be capa-ble in other parts of her life but unsafe behind the wheel. The changes can happen slowly—sometimes impercepti-bly—and yet be severe enough to cause a deadly accident.

Of course, driving is a way of life. Who can forget the exhilaration of get-ting a driver's license? It was a ticket to freedom and a sign of maturity. Throughout life, driving gives us inde-pendence and autonomy. To give up this mobility, and the independence, can be devastating. Your parent might suddenly be left with no way to get out, to do things and see people. Even if she has no place to go or if ample public trans-portation is available, her driver's license and the car keys are a vital part of her identity.

Talk About It

Conversations about driving will be touchy, no doubt, but it's critical to *start them early*. It will be much easier to dis-cuss driving and slowly wean your parent off his car than to suddenly demand that he stop.

Think carefully about who should raise the subject. It's probably best not to pick the loudest, most authoritarian person because this topic needs to be handled with kid gloves. Save that sibling for later, when someone needs to take a firm stand.

When it comes to this issue, people are more apt to listen to a spouse or a doctor than a child. A physical or occupational therapist might be the best one to broach the subject, as a therapist sees your parent's limitations objectively.

If you are raising this subject, start by asking him what he thinks. Does he believe he is a safe driver? Are there any issues about driving that concern him (driving at night or in the rain, for example, or seeing over his achy left shoulder)? Would it be helpful if other people drove sometimes? Does he worry about accidents? Has he ever gotten lost while driving? How much longer does he think he will be able to drive?

Mostly likely, he'll say all is fine. Stay calm. Don't disagree or roll your eyes. Show true interest and pause before responding.

Once you've listened, let him know that you heard him, and that you understand how important this is to him. Tell him that you want to be sure that he can drive for as long as possible.

But also let him know that even very capable, independent people often lose some visual acuity and hearing, and that reflexes and reaction times often slow a bit, so it's important to see what he can do so that he can hang on to his license. (It doesn't matter if you are certain it's time for him to give it up; you are inching your way to that place and, with any luck, letting him arrive there on his own.)

Suggest that he try some of the things described here to evaluate his driving and refresh his driving skills while you continue to wean him from his car. If he needs to stop driving immediately, skip ahead to page 143!

Safety Behind the Wheel

Go for a drive with your parent and see whether there actually is a problem and what it is. Is your parent having trouble turning his neck to see behind him? Is he getting caught in intersections while trying to turn left? Is he squinting to see the road in the evening? Once you see what is happening, address specific issues.

- If your parent hasn't had his eyesight and hearing tested recently, he should make the necessary appointments at once. One of the simplest and most effective ways of improving driving skills is cataract surgery. Sometimes people aren't aware that their vision has declined, or they put off the surgery.

- Exercise will improve his reaction time, his range of motion, and his attentiveness. Simply stretching his neck each day by rotating his head side to side and up and down, and circling his shoulders may help him twist around to parallel park or check oncoming traffic with greater agility and safety.

- If your parent suffers from dizziness, fatigue, confusion, or blurred eyesight, all of which affect driving, ask the doctor about ways to reduce these symptoms. They may be caused by an untreated illness or, more likely, by inappropriate medications.

- Safety courses for "mature" drivers have been shown to help, if your

EVALUATIONS AND REFRESHER COURSES

Many organizations provide information and driving tests on their websites. The AAA Foundation for Traffic Safety (seniordriving.aaa.com) has exercises, driving tips, and a self-exam for older drivers. AARP (aarp.org) also has an assessment, as well as a variety of guides, for older drivers.

A driving evaluator can test your parent's driving and determine if she is safe on the roads. Many occupational therapists are trained to evaluate driving skills, or you can contact the local AAA (seniordriving.aaa.com). You can also find referrals on the website of the American Occupational Therapy Association (aota.org) or the Association for Driver Rehabilitation Specialists (www.driver-ed.org).

Before giving up the keys, your parent can take a refresher course, which will not only help her be a safer driver and keep her license, but as a bonus will qualify her for a lower insurance premium in most states.

AARP offers a Driver Safety course, which can be taken in a classroom or online, and many local AAAs offer classes. Senior centers, driving schools, and the Department of Motor Vehicles might have information about other senior driving courses in your parent's area.

parent has the motivation. They can be taken in a classroom or online (see box above).

- Although there's still debate about whether mental games, or "cognitive training," improve driving, there's nothing to lose if your parent is willing. The exercises, which you can buy online, are essentially video games that require one to think fast, react quickly, and use a broad field of vision.

- Be sure your parent wears her seat belt, both at the shoulder and at the waist. (Airbags are not a replacement for seat belts.) Be sure that she can fasten and unfasten the belt easily, as elderly people often skip the seat belt because it's difficult to clasp. Automotive shops can adjust the shoulder strap so that it is comfortable or reset the belt so it can be easily hooked and unhooked.

- Obvious, but often forgotten: Make sure that your parent's car is in good working order, including brakes, defroster, defogger (for front and rear window), battery, wipers, dashboard light, exterior lights, and turn signals. Headlights should be clean and wipers should be replaced periodically.

- Install large mirrors and add extra mirrors if your parent is having trouble turning his head to see what's behind him.

- A number of devices are available to solve specific problems. Automotive stores sell seat cushions (if your parent has shrunk with age), gadgets to raise the pedals, and spinner knobs that make a steering wheel more responsive. Large knobs for climate control will be easier to see and use. A program called CarFit helps improve your parent's car to fit his specific needs (car-fit.org).

- If your parent is buying a new car, opt for power everything—brakes, seats, steering, locks, and so on.

- Be sure that your parent plans trips ahead of time and knows exactly where he is going without looking at a map or GPS.

- Even if it means that the drive takes a little longer, he should take a route that avoids complex intersections or difficult left turns.

- Avoid distractions, like the radio, cell phone, and chatty passengers. All attention should be focused on the road.

- If he feels at all sleepy while driving, he should pull off the road and have a short nap, get out and stretch, or stop for coffee.

Steering Away from the Car

Even if your parent is still pretty adept behind the wheel, you'll want to begin to wean him from his car, because chances are, eventually he will not be able to drive. It's easier to do this when he has some time to make the transition.

For starters, your parent might avoid driving:

- at night, dawn, or dusk

- during rush hour

- on unfamiliar routes

- in city centers or on busy streets

- long distances

- in bad weather

- when he's feeling sick, stressed, or tired

As he adjusts his driving habits, introduce him to car pools, senior vans, and public transportation, and try to get him used to letting other people drive. Find friends, relatives, neighbors, or volunteers who are willing to give him a ride occasionally.

If he complains that public transportation is inadequate and using a taxi is ridiculously expensive, let him know that the average cost of owning and operating a car is $8,000 a year. That's a lot of money to put toward taxis!

Many communities have programs for helping seniors find transportation. Find out what options exist in your parent's community by contacting the area agency on aging (eldercare.gov) and local senior centers.

Also, although it's important to get out of the house, most things, including groceries, medicines, meals, and clothing, can be delivered.

When It's Time to Quit

The question of quitting is a hot potato that no one wants to touch. Family members often know that an elderly person is a danger on the road, but they don't dare do anything about it. They might not want Grandpa driving their children around, but then look the other way when he's by himself. Taking action is simply too difficult.

But when it's time to stop, do not cross your fingers and look the other way. Get him out of the driver's seat. This isn't just about his life; it's about the lives of others.

Unfortunately, you can't rely on the state to monitor his driving. Most states, reluctant to alienate a large population of elderly voters, refuse to retest or otherwise restrict older drivers.

As noted earlier, an occupational or physical therapist can often determine if your parent should get off the road and will turn this into an unofficial medical order. Or talk to your parent's doctor and see if he or she will talk to your parent about stopping.

When you confront your parent, brace yourself, because he is bound to be hurt, if not furious. Be sensitive to the gravity of what you are suggesting, and to the implications, both practical and emotional, but remain firm in your resolve. And be ready with solutions to his travel problems. If your parent uses his driver's license for identification, call the Department of Motor Vehicles to request a photo ID card.

If all else fails, you can report an unsafe driver to the DMV or your state-licensing agency. It's a difficult step, but it may be your only choice. Of course, be sure to find out in advance what happens when someone is reported, as states have varying procedures. And ask that your name be kept confidential.

In the meantime you can disable the car and then say it's beyond repair.

Gadgets and Gizmos

There are literally hundreds of gadgets you can order from catalogs, find in medical supply stores, or purchase on the Internet, all to make health care, dressing, dining, shopping, reading, walking, gardening, and everything else easier for your parent. From talking thermometers for aged eyes to special fishing gear for stiff fingers, if your parent needs it, someone sells it.

You can buy emergency alert buttons and fall sensors; pill reminders and dispensers; various sound amplifiers and visual alerts (like a blinking light for the doorbell or phone) for people with poor hearing; easy-to-use phones and computers; and a host of products that make flipping switches and turning knobs easier for people with arthritic fingers. For people who have poor vision, there are audiobooks, e-readers, talking alarm clocks, and large-print everything, as well as devices that send an enlarged image from a book to a TV screen.

Telehealth devices, or remote patient monitoring (RPM) devices, as they are also known, monitor oxygen, pulse, heart rate, glucose, weight, and the like. Information is sent wirelessly to a modem on the phone, and a health care provider or family member is alerted if the readings fall out of a certain range.

You can buy lifts that carry a person up stairs, supports and pulleys for people

WHERE TO FIND THAT DOOHICKEY

To find helpful devices, start by contacting AbleData, a federally funded database of assistive products and manufacturers, which also has specialists on hand to help you (abledata.com or 800-227-0216).

Each state also has a federally funded "assistive technology project," which is dedicated to helping residents get the assistive devices they need. To find the program in your state, contact AbleData or go to the website of the Association of Tech Act Projects (ataporg.org).

Beyond that, there are literally hundreds of companies that sell low-vision aids, hearing devices, gadgets for arthritic fingers, and more. You can find some in a phone book, but better to look online. Search under "disability products" or "assistive devices" or something more specific, such as "vision aids" or "canes."

who have trouble getting out of bed or out of a chair, automatic door openers, lights that respond to verbal commands, and ramps for vans. There are keypad locks and fingerprint readers for people who can't manage a key, big-button TV remotes, and remote-controlled thermostats.

For cooking, there are all sorts of teakettles and jug tippers, crumb trays, large bibs, weighted utensils, large-print cookbooks, jar and can openers, automatic stove shut-off devices, and special cutting boards, knives, and electric choppers for easy slicing, dicing, and baking.

For bathing, you can buy a variety of stools, chairs, and benches, as well as basins for washing someone's hair in bed. For dressing, there are grabbers that help pull on socks and pull down zippers, special easy-to-wear clothing, and hooks that help with buttons. Long-handled brushes and combs are easy for those who can't reach around easily.

You can buy phones that allow you to put pictures of friends and family on large speed-dial buttons, and phones with voice-activated dialers. For people who always lose essential items (you might want to buy one of these for yourself), you can get a base unit with buttons that trigger a beeper on corresponding items: keys, eyeglasses, cell phones, purses, wallets, and so on.

And there are dozens of grabbers, turners, levers, and openers to help people reach high items, turn taps or knobs or keys, open jars, or pick up sewing needles.

For the enthusiast, you can buy card-holders and card shufflers, reels that bring in the big fish, magnifiers for sewing, or cradles from which to launch a bowling ball.

You can also find a number of canes, walkers, and electric scooters for a parent who is weak, stiff, or otherwise finds movement painful or impossible.

Medicare and other insurance plans generally don't cover these items, and the truth is, a lot of it is junk. But some of it can change your parent's day, or even save her life. It's worth browsing the Internet to get a sense of what's available.

If you see something that's potentially useful, with a little ingenuity, you might be able to duplicate it. For example, you can make utensils heavier or give them thicker handles by simply taping padding to the handle; you can lengthen an unreachable zipper or a light cord with a piece of ribbon; or you can make a dress easier to wear by replacing buttons with Velcro.

Finally, just remember, technology can assist you, but it is not a replacement for human interaction, and it is useful only if someone uses it properly. An emergency button won't help if your parent is unable or unwilling to push the button. An electronic pill dispenser might alert you if your parent fails to remove her medication, but what if she takes it from the dispenser, but then, on her way to get some water, forgets to actually swallow it? In other words, use the gadgets, but don't depend upon them blindly.

Chapter 8

Getting Help

Assessing the Need • Family and Friends •
Community Services • Geriatric Care Managers

Your father needs someone to come over for a few hours each week to do some light housekeeping and buy groceries. Or perhaps your mother has dementia and needs intermittent nursing care, as well as a full-time person who can bathe and dress her, feed her, and guide her through the day. Whatever the needs, you can't possibly do it all, which means that you have to find some help. And the sooner, the better.

Learn what's out there, even if you don't think you need help yet, because you will probably need it sooner than you think. By starting early, you will know where to turn as the situation changes, and you can get your parent on any waiting lists for popular programs.

You might think you can do this yourself, but honestly, the most successful caregivers get plenty of help. You want to give your parent your best, but you can't do that if you have five to-do lists piled on top of your didn't-do lists. Share the load so you can spend less time running errands and more time giving what others can't: your love and attention.

This chapter looks at community services and programs, and the next looks at hiring help in the home.

Assessing the Need

Before you sign your mother up for extensive and expensive care, consider modifications to her home that would allow her to do more for herself. Sometimes renovations to the bathroom, kitchen, and/or stairwell can make life a whole lot more manageable. See Chapter 7 for tips on how to make the tasks of daily life simpler and safer for her.

Then, think about exactly what it is she needs. Does she need help first thing in the morning getting showered and dressed? Does she need a ride to the grocery store, or someone to shop and cook for her, or would a meal delivery program be just the ticket? Does she need someone to take her to the doctor's office now and then? To keep her company?

In the end, you might discover that she doesn't require round-the-clock home health aides after all. Maybe she'll be fine with some help each morning getting dressed and making breakfast, going to a day care center during the day, and having her dinner delivered in the evening.

If you are not sure what sort of help she needs, or there is some disagreement in the family about what to do, an area agency on aging might have a caseworker who can do a formal assessment and guide you in finding help. You can also hire a geriatric care manager to create a game plan.

SIGNS THAT YOUR PARENT NEEDS HELP

- She's losing weight unintentionally.
- Her personal hygiene isn't up to par.
- She's missed appointments or forgotten events.
- She's not getting out.
- She's not doing things she once enjoyed.
- The mail is piling up.
- Bills aren't being paid, or finances are otherwise in disarray.
- There's no food in the fridge or what's

there is moldy or expired.
- She stumbles, limps, or shuffles when she walks.
- She has fallen.
- She has trouble getting up from or into a chair.
- Her clothes aren't laundered.
- She forgets to take her medications.
- She's had a car accident.
- She's gotten lost in a familiar place.

Family and Friends

This cannot be stressed enough: When your parent needs help, don't take it all on yourself. Get other family members involved from the start (see Chapter 4). Close friends might also be willing to pitch in with small tasks or keep her company from time to time.

You may be reluctant to ask for help, but keep in mind that even though people may not readily volunteer their services, they are often more than happy to help out once they are asked. Keep favors small. Perhaps a friend will pick up a few extra groceries for your parent while doing her own shopping, or get books or videos at the library once a month. A neighbor might be willing to take your parent's garbage out once a week when he's hauling out his own bags. A local teenager might get credit for community service if he comes by one afternoon a week to keep your parent company and help around the house.

Don't forget your own friends and acquaintances. If someone is in the same situation, she (or he) might share some of the workload—you check out local day care and home care options while your friend investigates Medicaid eligibility and rules.

Those who aren't in the same situation might be willing to exchange duties with you in the name of mutual relief and a refreshing change of pace—a friend sits with your parent while you take her children to the park. Or maybe you make dinner for both families on Tuesday nights while your friend does dinner duty on Thursdays, giving each of you one night off.

Several websites help you organize chores and communicate between a group of family members, neighbors, and friends. (Check out lotsahelpinghands.com, caringbridge.org, carezone.com, saturing.com, and tyze.com.) Most let you post tasks that need to be done on a calendar and then the members of your community can check the calendar and attach their names to whatever tasks they will take on. They can also post messages and keep the group updated on your parent's health and activities.

Community Services

Communities establish services for the elderly in response to the demographics and specific needs of the local population. As a result, most communities offer a handful of basic services to elderly residents, but the scope and

COMMUNITY SERVICES AT A GLANCE

TYPE OF HELP	SERVICES PROVIDED	AVERAGE COSTS*
Telephone reassurance and friendly visitors	Phone calls or brief visits to check on your parent's well-being	Free or minimal charge
Chore services	Minor repairs and handyman chores	Free or based on a sliding scale, plus materials
Meal programs	Group dining at a community center, or meals delivered to the house	Free or minimal charge, but sometimes available only to disabled and/or low-income seniors
Transportation services	Rides to day care, senior centers, shopping malls, or appointments	Free or minimal charge
Senior centers	Clubs that provide social activities, lectures, meals, and information	Usually free
Adult day care (or adult day services)	Supervision, recreation, meals, and some health care and counseling. Transportation often provided	$70 on average, but range from $30 to more than $150 a day; some are subsidized; covered by Medicaid in some states
Case managers and geriatric care managers	Assessment, guidance, advice, and more	Community agencies may provide some consultation for free or on a sliding scale; if hired privately, between $50 and $250 an hour

*Prices vary widely depending upon the area and whether you hire workers through an agency.

details of those programs are as different as the communities themselves.

The funding sources, costs, and sponsors are equally diverse, with services being offered by public agencies, private businesses, churches and synagogues, civic groups, and charities. Some services are free and some are subsidized. Obviously, some free services are available only to seniors living on a marginal income.

Telephone Calls and Visitors

Many organizations provide a telephone reassurance program in which someone calls once a day or once every few days to see how your parent is doing. The callers are typically volunteers, often other senior citizens. Whatever the specifics, someone will speak with your parent briefly, and if anything seems askew, the volunteer will alert you or another designated contact.

Some of these programs actually have a person stop by. It's just a quick visit, to make sure everything is okay.

The programs are usually run by senior centers, religious organizations, and other public or nonprofit agencies; if they are offered by home care agencies, there will mostly likely be a fee. Contact the area agency on aging (eldercare.gov) or search online for "telephone reassurance" in your parent's town.

You can also contract with a private company for automated calls. Your parent gets a recorded message. If she doesn't answer the phone or if she says that, no, she is not okay, a responder is notified.

Although they're not terribly personal, using such a service should ease your mind that your parent is okay on the days when you can't check in yourself.

Companions and Homemakers

Companions and homemakers are discussed in the next chapter, "More Help at Home," but they are mentioned here because some organizations provide visitors who do more than just visit.

Volunteer companions, some of whom are other seniors, will check in with your parent and have a chat and a cup of tea. Although some will do an odd job or take your parent to the store or library, in general these volunteers are offering friendship and are not there to do the heavy lifting.

Volunteer homemakers are less common, but they do exist. They will do some laundry, tidy the kitchen, and vacuum. Some will help with grooming or transportation.

Some communities have free or low-cost companion programs run by a public agency or a private group. Churches or other religious organizations also sponsor companions. Local senior centers often know of companion programs in the area.

Volunteer programs are wonderful if your parent simply needs company. But if she needs reliable and consistent help, you need to hire a paid companion.

Chore Services

Chore-service programs enlist workers, often volunteers, to do minor repairs and odd jobs for elderly residents. Most won't tackle major renovations, but they will usually build ramps, weather-strip

A REMINDER

Be organized, even if you're facing a crisis, or before you know it, you'll have crumpled brochures tucked in kitchen drawers and illegible notes scribbled on napkins and scraps of paper. As you learn about community services, keep a master list of all relevant agencies and representatives, with their phone numbers and extensions.

windows, put up storm windows, or install grab bars. Some will shovel a sidewalk or rake leaves.

Chore services, like visitor and telephone services, are sometimes offered by local nonprofit groups such as senior centers or churches. Your parent pays for the materials that are needed, but the labor is often free or charged based on need. (Your parent may have to meet some minimum income guidelines to be eligible.)

Try the area agency on aging and senior centers first. Homemods.org, a service of the Fall Prevention Center of Excellence (homemods.org), also has a list of carpenters and handymen who will do home renovations for the elderly at a discount.

> " My father has a person who comes by every other day for an hour and tidies up. But he's a hoarder. There is stuff everywhere, piled up the walls, covering the floors. Boxes, chairs, old books, broken appliances, newspapers. He can't throw anything out.
>
> She was aghast at first, but she's learned his ways. She knows what she can do, and mostly what she can't touch. He doesn't let her touch much.
>
> It's more about the friendship. He likes her a lot. She talks to him, worries when he's sad, and hugs him. He likes the company.
>
> He says to me, 'She is like my family. I see more of her than I see of you.' That's my dad. He always says the wrong thing."
>
> —Sandy B.

Meal Programs

If your parent can't cook for himself or isn't eating well for some other reason, or if he simply needs companionship, look into congregate dining and meal delivery programs.

Congregate meals are typically hot lunches served in schools, community centers, religious centers, apartment buildings, senior centers, adult day care centers, or other community sites. Most programs are open to all elderly people, and they often provide transportation to and from the site. The meals meet federal nutrition guidelines, and some programs have kosher, vegetarian, low-salt, diabetic, and other special meals.

Congregate meals are usually free. Some programs request a voluntary contribution based on income, but the average donation is less than a dollar a meal, and many programs accept federal food stamps.

The best part is that these meals are social. If your parent doesn't know people in the group, the first few visits may seem a little awkward, but eventually he will meet people and become accustomed to the routine. And a social routine is a good routine.

If your parent can't leave the house, meal delivery programs will bring a hot lunch and sometimes a frozen or cold bagged dinner to his door.

These programs, which are called by a variety of names but are widely known as "meals-on-wheels," are operated by senior centers, religious organizations, and community groups. Most are free (they have to be free if they receive federal monies), although they will solicit a donation (and they need it badly, so give if you can). Some private groups charge a nominal fee.

To be eligible, your parent must be unable to prepare meals alone, but there is no income limit. As a bonus, the volunteers who deliver the food are usually trained to look for signs of trouble.

To find out about meal delivery programs in your parent's area, contact the area agency on aging (eldercare.gov) or local senior center, or go to the Meals on Wheels Association of America's website (mowaa.org).

Transportation Services

If your parent needs a ride to a doctor's appointment, the grocery store, day care, or elsewhere, a number of public and private groups provide door-to-door transportation specifically for elderly or disabled people. These community vans are usually free, but some groups ask for a donation or charge a minimal fee.

Some services pick up groups of people on a set day and take them to a shopping center, for example. Some take elderly people door-to-door for appointments and errands on an on-call basis. Most of the vans are equipped to take people in wheelchairs.

The area agency on aging (eldercare.gov) should know about vans, buses, and volunteer and private drivers who serve elderly residents. In addition, the local department of public transportation should be able to tell you about bus routes, discounts to seniors, and other accessible transportation services.

Senior Centers

Senior centers were established as social clubs for relatively healthy elderly people, and most of them still serve that function; they are geared for people who are independent and active, offering recreation, lectures, and social events.

BENEFITS, DISCOUNTS, AND SPECIAL SERVICES

If you put on your sleuthing cap, you may find that your parent is eligible for a number of free and discounted community services. The National Council on Aging has a website (benefitscheckup.org) that helps people find services and benefits for which they are eligible. The area agency on aging (eldercare.gov) and, if appropriate, the Veterans Administration (va.gov) should also be helpful.

Also contact local senior centers, community groups, and organizations aligned with specific diseases and issues (such as the Alzheimer's Association).

Beyond government and community programs, businesses often offer special services and discounts to the elderly. See if the library might deliver books, a grocery store might deliver groceries, or a hairstylist might make house calls. Some doctors even make house calls. Whatever the need, it's worth a few calls to see what is available.

WHEN YOUR PARENT BLOCKS THE PATH

After numerous phone calls, you've found a reliable homemaker as well as a good adult day care center, but your mother says, flat-out, no. She insists that she doesn't need help (she forgets that she has set off the smoke alarm three times in the past month), and she doesn't want strangers in her home, thank you very much. When you persist and send the homemaker over anyway, she makes unbecoming remarks and fires her on the spot.

Before you blow your top, take a deep breath. You have every reason to be angry, but try to see this from her point of view. Having lost so much already, she might be unwilling to let go of anything else (her independence, her privacy).

Telling her that her fears are silly won't erase them. Instead, encourage your mother to express her concerns, and then let her know you hear her. Tell her that you care and that you will not abandon her. Assure her that getting help will allow you to spend more "quality" time with her.

Finally, be candid about the risks and opportunities the situation presents. Ask her how she sees this playing out if she doesn't let people help her. What risks is she taking? Does she understand what she stands to gain if she does allow them in—hot meals, a caring companion, and help with all sorts of daily tasks? (If your parent is confused because of dementia, see page 491 for tips on using services and hiring help.)

If the situation is not dire, proceed slowly as you introduce new services. For example, you might introduce a worker in some neutral location, like a restaurant over coffee. Or, start by getting someone to do her shopping or drop off a meal a few times a week. No one need cross her sacred doorstep immediately. Once she trusts one person to enter her home, she may be open to more help, more hours, and other workers. Or, start with a trial run, perhaps a few hours a week.

If this doesn't work, or if the situation doesn't allow for such small steps, be gentle, but stay firm. Once you've heard her and reassured her, let her know that there is no other way, that you simply cannot do this alone. If it isn't dangerous, you might leave your parent for a period of time without your help so that she understands the severity of the situation. A day without you may help her understand how much assistance she needs.

If the situation is dangerous, talk to her doctor. Perhaps your parent will listen to him or her. Or, find a geriatric care manager or a social worker from a family service agency who can help resolve the matter.

However, the focus is changing. As the population grows older and more frail, senior centers are serving a more diverse group. Some are still small social clubs that operate out of a church basement, but others are large, publicly funded organizations, housed in freestanding buildings and offering an array of services, including help with chores, volunteer visitors, homemakers, recreational programs, meals, health screenings, counseling, exercise and computer classes, lectures, and field trips.

....

" We visited the adult day care center, and on the way home, my mom cried. She thought she was too young, that the other people were much older than she was. Really, she is no younger than they are. But somehow seeing them all together, she just didn't think she belonged.

She finally agreed to try it, three days a week for three weeks, and if she still hated it, we'd do something else. It was a pact we made. I was like, please, please, please let this work.

The center had a children's day care program attached to it, and at some point during the day, the kids would come in and spend time with the old folks. There was a baby, Maria, and because Mom was pretty capable, physically, they let her hold her, rock her.

The second week she was there, I came in and Mom was holding the baby, rocking her, and she looked so serene, so happy. Now it was my turn to cry."
—Janet S.

....

Find out what your parent's senior center offers, because it probably does a lot more than run bingo games. In addition, it should be a good source of information and referrals to other local services. Senior centers are usually free and open to all elderly residents of any age, income, or health status.

Adult Day Services

Your mother uses a walker and her memory is starting to fade. She can't get her own meals, she needs help getting to the toilet, and she cannot remember why she called you. She's pretty well covered on the weekends when you are home, but what do you do the other five days of the week?

One answer is adult day care (also called adult day services), which provides care and supervision outside the home to elderly people who might otherwise be in an assisted living facility or nursing home.

Generally, what happens is something like this: Your mother is picked up by a van in the morning, taken to a center where she is cared for by trained staff, and then dropped off at home in the evening. While at the center, she sees friends, listens to music, has breakfast and a hot lunch, does some gentle exercises and crafts, and receives occupational therapy and routine medical attention.

Just as important as what she gets, however, is what you get—a break from the work and stress of her daily care.

Most centers provide door-to-door transportation, meals, exercise, social activities, counseling, and help with grooming, toileting, and eating. Many offer more intensive medical care and rehabilitative therapy. And still others provide care specifically for people with Alzheimer's and other forms of dementia.

Some offer periodic home care, pharmacy and laboratory services, and transportation to appointments and errands. Most centers have a nurse or nurse's aide and a social worker and/or case manager on staff. And many provide support and counseling to caregivers.

All adult day programs provide care during normal business hours, but some are open in the evening and on weekends, as well. A few provide overnight respite care.

The best ones will have waiting lists, so get on this early.

A typical center costs about $60 a day, although prices range from a few dollars up to $150 a day. Medicare might cover the cost of any physical, speech, or occupational therapy your parent receives at the center. Medicaid, which is governed by states, will often cover adult day services, especially if your parent would otherwise be in a facility of some sort.

Some centers are subsidized or publicly owned and charge a lower rate or assess fees on a sliding scale, and some communities have programs to help with such costs.

Larger communities often have more than one center, and some cities have dozens of them. Unfortunately, rural areas often have nothing. If your parent has choices, see which center offers the level of care that she needs and then, if there is still some choice, tour the centers.

Obviously, a center should be clean, attractive, well ventilated, and safe. It should be arranged to meet the needs of clients—no open door if someone with dementia might roam out, a bathroom wide enough for people using

wheelchairs, and so on. It should allow for some time spent outdoors. Activities should actually be interesting (they shouldn't rely on television and bingo games) and manageable for your parent. And meals should be nutritious and appetizing (of course).

Staffing is vital. A program should have a nurse or social worker on staff, and at least one "care provider" for every six clients (or one for every four if the clients are severely impaired and need a lot of assistance), and it should provide training for the staff. Perhaps even more important, staff members should enjoy older people, be upbeat and involved, and interact easily with the clients.

If you're uncertain, visit a couple of times. Is the staff harried and flustered? Annoyed by client requests? Standing to the side chatting among themselves? Talk to the staff about how they might handle particular issues involving your parent, such as incontinence, aggressive behavior, confusion, diabetes, immobility, and so forth.

Go when the program is letting out and talk to other clients and caregivers as they leave the facility.

People are often surprised by how much they enjoy adult day services once they get used to it. But it can take several tries before your parent reaches the point of acceptance.

To find adult day services, contact the local area agency on aging (eldercare .gov or 800-677-1116) or the National Adult Day Services Association (nadsa .org). Also, go online to the National PACE Association website (npaonline .org) to see if one of their Programs of All-Inclusive Care for the Elderly is available in your parent's community.

" My mother would stay in bed almost all day. I could not get her up to do anything. She would eat and that was it. Day care was the answer to my prayers.

I still have a hard time getting her to go each morning, but once she's there, she's fine. She does things and meets people. She's really started coming out of her shell. We've even started playing cards together in the evenings."

—Linda K.

WHERE TO FIND HELP

To learn about the services in your parent's community, contact the following:

THE AREA AGENCY ON AGING. Begin your search with the local agency on aging, which can direct you to services and discuss your parent's specific needs. Some also offer legal, financial, and family counseling free of charge. You can find it by contacting the Eldercare Locator (eldercare.gov or 800-677-1116).

LOCAL SENIOR CENTERS. Some centers provide services directly, and some sponsor senior advocates who counsel residents about community services.

EMPLOYERS. See if your workplace has an employee assistance program that provides information, referrals, and counseling to people who are caring for an elderly person. A few companies offer referrals nationwide (very helpful if you live in Tulsa and your parent is in Tucson).

RELIGIOUS ORGANIZATIONS. Even if your parent is not affiliated with any faith, such groups often provide direct help to people of all faiths or can refer you to programs and services in the area.

NATIONAL ORGANIZATIONS. For virtually every ailment or interest— from asthma to veterans—there is an organization that can guide you to services, refer you to professionals, and provide information (for a partial listing, see page 610). Many, such as the Alzheimer's Association and the Arthritis Foundation, have local chapters that provide services directly.

211. Many communities have information and referral lines, which are contacted by visiting 211.org or dialing 211.

Geriatric Care Managers

If you are far away, busy with other things, facing a crisis, arguing with family members, and/or just need some guidance and support, a geriatric care manager can be your salvation. He or she can assess your parent's situation, counsel your family, connect her to appropriate services, and oversee some or all of her care on an ongoing basis.

Care managers (also known as eldercare consultants and case managers, although these terms often refer to people who offer less extensive help) are usually social workers, nurses, or psychologists with training in geriatrics or gerontology. They can handle almost any facet of your parent's care, either short or long term.

You can hire a manager to simply assess the situation and create a plan. Or you might hire one to oversee a particular challenge, say, finding a good nursing home or mediating a family dispute.

A care manager can also take over the whole kit and caboodle—hire, coordinate, and monitor home care workers, work with financial advisers and lawyers, get your parent to appointments, and so on. In most cases, you can take it a day at a time and expand, reduce, or cancel the service at any point.

Sometimes the area agency on aging or a local family service organization has case managers who will, for free or on a sliding scale, advise families on various issues, and they might even do an at-home assessment.

Private geriatric care managers, on the other hand, sometimes charge a flat rate for a particular service, which might range from $200 to $2,000, depending upon the task. Others charge an hourly rate, at anywhere from $80 to $250 an hour. An initial assessment will cost $200 and up, depending upon the region and what's involved.

You can minimize costs by helping with some of this. (You can ask the manager to give you a list of jobs, such as getting information from the doctor or calling a nursing home about a particular issue.)

Keep in mind that a care manager's fee does not include the cost of services themselves—home health aides, nurses, medical supplies, and so on. Plus, geriatric care managers will often charge their hourly rate for travel time, not just time with your parent.

Most states don't regulate care managers. Anyone can hang a shingle. So it's best to hire someone through the National Association of Professional Geriatric Care Managers (520-881-8008 or caremanager.org), which sets standards and vets their members.

When hiring, check the person's training and experience. He or she should have formal education in social work, nursing, gerontology, or a related field, and ideally should have been doing this in your parent's area for several years.

If you are hiring someone for extensive help (and not just an initial consult), ask how many clients the person is currently serving and what the maximum number is. The fewer clients, the more time and attention the care manager can give to your parent. Someone with more than 30 clients might spend, on average, only an hour a week considering and monitoring your parent's situation.

Be sure there is backup in place—another care manager or a family member. As with other employees, get a written agreement regarding the job description and fees.

Chapter 9

Paid Help at Home

In-Home Care • The Hiring Process • From Day One • Managing the Troops • When There Is Trouble • Respite Care

Although it's expensive, private in-home care can be a godsend. Once it's set up, you'll be shaking your weary head, wondering why in the world you didn't do this sooner.

Even a few hours of help a day so you can get a break will be money well spent. And starting this early, even in a small way, will get your parent used to the idea of strangers caring for her. So once again, don't delay. Find out about local home care services and use them.

You can hire individuals on your own or contract with a home care agency. The former is much cheaper and works fine in most cases, but the latter means that workers have been screened, that backup help is available, and usually that they are insured.

Medicare does not cover most long-term care. It covers nurses and therapists under specific, and very limited, circumstances, but it does not pick up the cost of the humdrum help with daily tasks that most people need. Medicaid covers these services, but one has to be impoverished to qualify for it. Your parent may have to pay out of pocket, and unfortunately, the costs add up. (See Chapter 17 for more on Medicare and Medicaid coverage.)

Hired help won't be perfect. Others won't care for your parent exactly as you want them to. You might not be crazy about Dad's caregivers. But if the care is adequate, take advantage of this break. Turn down the worry meter. It's time to attend to your own life and recharge.

In-Home Care

I n-home care comes in two basic flavors, "skilled" and "custodial."

Skilled care refers to medically necessary care: nursing; physical, occupational, and speech therapy; and some related services.

Custodial care is help with the stuff of daily life—bathing, dressing, cooking, shopping, and other routine tasks—and is typically provided by aides or companions.

In-home care is usually a blessing, an enormous relief. But you need to hire people carefully and then keep an eye on what's going on. If you sense trouble—someone is drinking or stealing, or otherwise abusing, exploiting, or neglecting your parent—don't wait a moment to find someone else. If, on the other hand, you find a reliable, trustworthy, and caring home health aide, treat her (or him) like gold.

Companions and Aides

People use these words interchangeably—caregiver, companion, aide, personal care assistant. It's largely a matter of semantics.

That said, usually companions keep your parent company, help him with minor tasks, and generally watch over him, but the focus is on companionship.

An aide will prepare meals, tidy up, change your parent's bed linens, help your parent get dressed, remind her to take her medications, drive her to appointments, and pick up occasional groceries and supplies. Most will also help with bathing and eating.

Most companions and aides do not do heavy housework or chores (sadly, you are not going to get those windows washed), nor do they work for anyone but the patient (your linens won't be changed).

If your parent simply needs company, and not hands-on care or heavy supervision, check with a local senior center or community center first. Sometimes volunteers are available. If your parent lives in a senior housing complex, there may be another elderly person who is perhaps more capable than your parent who would visit regularly.

You can find more formal companions or aides through an agency, or you can look on your own, in much the same way you would hire a babysitter. Ask friends who have an elderly parent in the area, as well as those who might know about good nannies and sitters. Many of these people care for young and old alike.

If referrals don't get you anywhere, post a sign in a senior center, church, synagogue, or community center. Be sure to leave your telephone number, not your parent's; you don't want to publicize her vulnerability.

Companions and aides cost anywhere from $5 to $30 an hour, depending upon the area, the services provided, and whether you use an agency. Live-in caregivers should not charge by the hour, but rather, by the day or week (which should be significantly lower than an hourly rate, as they are presumably sleeping during some of this time). Live-in fees vary wildly. Of course, someone who lives in will need a bedroom, meals, television, and possibly use of a car.

BRAINSTORMING ALTERNATIVES

Before you spend a fortune on private caregivers, think about more creative options.

For example, if your parent simply needs a little help and companionship and he has a spare bedroom, find a college student, a writer, or a young couple who would like a place to live in exchange for some help around the house. You can supplement daytime care with a boarder who gets free or reduced rent for making dinner and being on call at night. Your parent speaks Italian? What about a foreign-exchange student from Italy?

This type of arrangement might provide less constant or reliable care than a paid caregiver, but if your parent doesn't need extensive help, it is essentially free, and it can work out wonderfully for all involved. It will also make your parent feel less like an invalid (because he'll have a roommate, not a caregiver).

Call a college housing office, put an ad in the newspaper, or contact the local shared-housing program. Obviously, you'll need to thoroughly vet the person before he or she moves in. You can also find organizations that arrange such housing through the National Shared Housing Resource Center (nationalsharedhousing.org).

Another possibility is for your parent to share an aide or homemaker with another elderly person who lives nearby. The rate might be reduced because you are giving an employee more hours and less travel time between jobs.

Also, most paid workers require at least four hours of work per shift. By sharing, you have a bit more flexibility. For example, a caregiver could get your mother up, bathed, and dressed and do some tidying, then go to the neighbor's house for two hours to help out there, and return to your parent later.

Or maybe your parent can share a house with an elderly friend or a couple of friends. They can share an aide and each other's company.

Sometimes all it takes is a little ingenuity and flexibility.

> ❝ After his wife died, my father-in-law went into hibernation, staying at home watching television. My husband said he was fine, but I was worried. He aged so quickly and was so lonely. I had him for dinner once a week, but we both work and we have two young boys, so we couldn't do much.
>
> I learned about a companion program and convinced Dad to try it. It's really been great for him. Scott, the companion, is in much the same situation as Dad. He's alone and can't get around all that well. But he visits two or three times a week, and they play rummy and have lunch. Last week they went to a hockey game together, which is something Dad always loved but hadn't done in years.
>
> What's been really interesting, and totally unexpected, is that his health has improved so much. He literally looks 10 years younger."
>
> —Lucy A.

Homemakers

Homemakers generally do more physical work and less socializing than companions, but the distinction is faint and largely depends upon the individual. Homemakers do laundry and light housecleaning, prepare meals, and might do some shopping. Most will also help your parent bathe and dress, although some stick to household work.

Many homemakers, especially those hired through home care agencies, are trained specifically in caring for elderly people. But again, the quality and extent of the service depends upon the individual worker.

In most cases, your parent has to foot the bill, but in some areas, homemakers are available at no charge or on a sliding scale and are paid for by public monies. However, there can be long waiting lists for such services.

In many states, under certain circumstances (if, for example, your parent is considered eligible for nursing-home care), Medicaid will cover the cost of homemakers.

As with companions, if homemakers are not offered through community programs, you can hire one through most home care agencies or find one by putting an ad in the local newspaper or on a community bulletin board.

Home Health Aides and Nurse's Aides

Home health aides and nurse's aides bring some medical training to the task and generally care for people who are pretty severely ill, cognitively impaired, or disabled.

They help with bathing, dressing, getting to the toilet, and other personal tasks. Some will prepare meals and do light housekeeping (but only that which pertains to your parent, such as changing

> ❝ I used to stay in the house the whole time the aide was there. It was a control thing for me. I felt that I had to oversee everything and that I couldn't trust anyone with my father. I was afraid that if I left, something would happen.
>
> I've gotten over that. Now I leave the minute the aide arrives. I go shopping, run errands, or visit friends. A couple of times I took my bills and mail to the library just to be out of the house. It's really an important break in the day for me."
>
> —Grace D.

OMG, SO MANY INITIALS

Health care and home care providers often talk about ADLs, IADLs, and the like when evaluating function and need. Here are some of the initials you might come across while finding services for your parent:

ADL. Activities of Daily Living refer to personal tasks, such as bathing, grooming, dressing, using the toilet, eating, walking, and moving from, say, the bed to a chair.

IADL. Instrumental Activities of Daily Living are those tasks that allow a person to remain independent, such as shopping, doing laundry, and taking medications.

LTSS. Long-Term Services and Supports refers to any housing or services that someone needs when he or she cannot perform ADLs.

HCBS. Home and Community Based Services include transportation, adult day care, meal programs, and chore and personal care services.

and laundering his sheets and tidying his room). They can also do simple medical procedures, such as changing bandages, checking catheters and intravenous lines, taking temperatures, or administering medications.

Certified home health aides usually work for an agency, under the supervision of a nurse. Fees range from $13 to $35 an hour, depending upon the experience and training of the aide and the cost of living in the area. Medicare and other insurance will cover the cost of home health aides only when their services are needed as part of a package of "skilled" nursing care.

Social Workers and Nutritionists

Social workers often work as part of the home care team, counseling clients and their families about social and emotional issues, reviewing the living situation and needs of the elderly person, and referring families to appropriate community services.

Nutritionists will get your parent on a diet that is healthful, manageable, and compatible with his medications and any illness that might be affecting him.

These individuals all make house calls, often through a hospital or home care agency. Medicare or other insurance often covers the cost if it is medically necessary and part of a hospital discharge plan of care.

Therapists

As part of your parent's home care, a doctor might recommend that he see some sort of therapist on a regular basis.

Physical therapists work the muscles and joints to improve mobility, flexibility, and strength, usually after an injury, surgery, or an illness (such as a stroke). They use various exercises, heat,

BROADER USE OF MEDICAID FUNDS

Every state has some sort of "waiver" program that allows Medicaid recipients (and veterans) to get home and community care, rather than going into a nursing home. Some allow clients to design their own care—to decide how they want to spend funds, rather than getting prescribed services from certified agencies. Some even allow recipients to hire relatives and friends as caregivers. So before you set out to hire a stranger from an agency, see what Medicaid allows in your parent's state.

To find out about these programs, contact the area agency on aging (eldercare.gov), the local Medicaid office, and the National Resource Center for Participant-Directed Services (participantdirection.org).

massage, and other techniques to restore mobility.

Occupational therapists train people with rigid fingers, stiff hips, dim vision, or other disabilities to perform daily tasks by working on muscular control and coordination, teaching them new ways to do things, setting them up with special equipment, and making adjustments to the home.

Speech therapists help people who have trouble speaking or understanding speech (because of a stroke or other illness or injury) to communicate again. They can also help people who have trouble swallowing or breathing.

Nurses

Doctors stopped making house calls some time ago, but nurses make house calls routinely these days, and they do much of the work that doctors used to do. They can monitor your parent's health, change dressings, insert catheters and intravenous lines, administer medications, give injections, and perform other medical tasks. They can teach your

> When my father left the hospital, I took a leave from work to help my mother care for him. It was grueling. We had to be with him, or within earshot of him, every minute.
>
> We were lifting him, turning him, feeding him, cleaning him, and helping him go to the bathroom. Mom stayed with him night and day, and wasn't getting much sleep.
>
> Two weeks into it, we realized we needed help. We hired a home health aide who came for three hours every morning to get him up, cleaned, and fed. But even with that, we were still both exhausted. So after three more weeks, we hired a companion who came five afternoons and stayed overnight three nights a week.
>
> That changed everything.
>
> I'm not sure why it took us so long to get help. I don't know why we were so resistant. We should have had all that in place the day he came home from the hospital."
>
> —Gloria J.

IN-HOME CARE AT A GLANCE

TYPE OF HELP	SERVICES PROVIDED	AVERAGE COSTS*
Companions and home care aides	Companionship, supervision, light housekeeping, and help with meals and daily tasks	$5 to $30 an hour. Some are subsidized through state programs. A live-in companion can cost from $200 to more than $1,000 a week, depending upon how much care someone needs.
Homemakers	Light housekeeping, laundry, cooking, errands, sometimes help with bathing and dressing	$20 or more an hour from an agency, but range from $8 to $30. Sometimes free or charged on a sliding scale through community programs.
Home health aides	Personal care (bathing, feeding, dressing, toileting, etc.), minor medical care, and light housekeeping	$7 to $35 an hour; might be covered by Medicare or Medicaid
Physical, occupational, and speech therapists	Training in physical movement, doing daily tasks, or communication	$20 to $90 an hour; might be covered by Medicare or Medicaid
Nurses	Medical care	$20 to $90 an hour; might be covered by Medicare or Medicaid
Respite programs	A break for caregivers, from a few hours to a few weeks	Cost varies widely, but in some instances, it may be free, subsidized, or provided by volunteers.

*Prices vary widely depending upon the area and whether you hire workers through an agency, which can add significantly to the price.

parent or family members how to perform some tasks, and they oversee other workers.

Registered nurses, or RNs, have at least two years of nursing school and are licensed by the state in which they practice. Licensed practical nurses, or LPNs, have at least one year of specialized education and must also be licensed. LPNs work under the supervision of an RN.

The Hiring Process

When a member of the congregation volunteers to call on your mother, or you find an aide through a friend, you can go on instinct alone. But if you are contracting with an agency or hiring a freelance worker to care for your parent on a daily basis, do your homework. Ask a lot of questions, get referrals, and get any agreement in writing.

You can hire home care workers either through an agency or directly. There are advantages to each route.

If you hire workers directly, you will pay less and you will have more control over whom you hire and the work that's done. An agency will have rules about what an employee can do. For example, an aide from an agency might not be allowed to give medications or offer a massage or join your parent for a meal. If you hire directly, you're the boss and you determine the rules. If you have some referrals and find someone good, this can be a perfect arrangement.

Agencies will cost more—sometimes quite a bit more—but they generally make life easier. Good ones will assess the situation, develop a plan, find workers, screen them, and oversee scheduling. Most important, they will (or should) send a replacement to fill in if a worker is sick or can't otherwise get to work.

If you find a reputable agency that offers a full range of services, the care tends to be better coordinated and more comprehensive than anything you can arrange on your own. A registered nurse and/or case manager will oversee the work and will typically know about other resources in the area. Also, agencies should have insurance in case of an accident, and they will handle all the paperwork, such as insurance forms, and Social Security and tax forms for employees.

Most important, if your parent expects Medicare to foot the bill, she has to receive care from a certified agency. Certification also means that the agency and workers meet health and safety standards set by the federal government. In some cases, Medicaid services must also be provided by a certified agency, although states are getting more lenient about this and most now allow you to hire independently.

Be aware that home care agencies are popping up all over and some are not terribly reputable. They hire staff off Internet sites, do minimal background checking, provide little training, and fail to supervise the work.

In some gray zone between agencies and hiring someone on your own are sort of "quasi" agencies—that is, a person loosely organizes a group of aides and companions, finding jobs for them and taking a cut. Rates should be slightly cheaper than those charged by certified agencies, but generally they won't screen workers as carefully, and they might not provide insurance coverage for workers.

If your parent is paying privately, she might get some financial relief if she works with an agency associated with the local health department or one that's operated by a religious organization or a Visiting Nurse Association.

> " I have two companions who come in shifts to watch Mother while I'm at work. One is excellent, and I love her dearly, but Mother is really awful to her. Frances is an articulate, intelligent, retired professional who is doing this work in order to keep active. She is very thoughtful, kind, and sympathetic. Mother was a nurse, and I think she feels resentful and threatened by having this capable person take care of her. She is rude, uncooperative, and mean to her.
>
> The other companion is young and sweet, but nobody's home. Every day is a new day for her. I have to tell her everything all over again. Mother gets along just fine with her—perhaps because she is so simple.
>
> I spend a lot of time apologizing to Frances and a lot of time explaining things to Susie. I guess there's no perfect solution. Anytime you have someone caring for your parent, there's bound to be some problem."
>
> —Barbara H.

These services are sometimes subsidized by public monies or donations, meaning that your parent will pay only what she can afford.

Contracting with a Home Care Agency

Which agency you use depends, in part, upon whether your parent needs skilled nursing care, and whether Medicare or Medicaid will cover her care.

If your parent is leaving the hospital or has recently left the hospital, talk with the hospital's discharge planner or social worker about setting up home care. These people are usually pretty savvy about what's available, what's covered, and what's reliable. They will also call and make arrangements for your parent, in most cases. (Keep in mind, however, that some hospitals have financial arrangements with certain health care agencies, so there might be some bias.)

Check out Medicare's Home Health Compare (800-633-4227 or medicare .gov), which lists agencies in the area and explains how they compare on various fronts with state and national averages (how often patients improved, how often the staff checked patients for pain or depression, and so on). You can also get referrals from your parent's doctor, contact the area agency on aging (eldercare.gov), or use the "agency locator" at the website of the National Association for Home Care & Hospice (nahcagencylocator.com).

If you don't need a certified agency (because Medicare is not footing the bill), the National Private Duty Association (privatedutyhomecare.org) has the names of many private-duty companies on their website.

Whatever arrangement you make, ask to have all agreements, including services to be provided and financial arrangements, put in writing.

QUESTIONS FOR AN AGENCY

- Exactly what services does the agency provide?

- Who is on the team—physicians, nurses, therapists, dietitians, social workers, home health aides, homemakers, companions?

- Can the staff meet the special needs of my parent (medical, physical, cultural)?

DAYS OF CARE OUTSIDE THE HOUSE

If you are patching together care at home, wondering how to afford it all, and starting to think about nursing homes, keep in mind that adult day care has taken a *giant* leap forward.

As explained in the last chapter, most centers now provide a full spectrum of services—transportation, exercise, activities, and meals, as well as medical care, therapy, rehabilitation, and care for people with dementia.

Not only is this cheaper than hiring in-home care (about $60 for eight hours of care versus $20 an hour for an aide), but it's far more social, it gets your parent out of the house, and it's generally more consistent. Also, it's good to have an elderly person under the watch of more than one set of eyes.

The centers will usually pick up your parent in the morning and deliver him home in the evening, although some programs have evening and weekend hours. Ah, this is sounding better by the minute!

Most of these programs are supported with public money, as well as charities and fund-raisers, which keeps the prices low. In most states, Medicaid will cover the cost if your parent would otherwise be in a nursing home.

To find a center, contact the National Adult Day Care Association (nadsa.org). Also check out the Programs of All-Inclusive Care for the Elderly (PACE) website (pace4you.org). PACE provides extensive care in the community and at home 24/7/365. Although few and far between, it's worth seeing if there's one in your parent's community.

- How does the agency determine what services my parent needs? Will a nurse evaluate him? Will he or she consult with my parent's doctor and my family?

- How often will his Plan of Care be updated?

- How will his care be coordinated? Who oversees workers? Will a supervisor visit regularly?

- How do I reach a supervisor if there is a problem?

- Is someone available 24/7 in case of emergency?

- Are backups provided when workers cancel or don't show up?

- Will the same person care for my parent consistently, or will the guards change regularly (which is certainly less desirable, but often unavoidable)?

- If my parent doesn't get along with a particular worker, can someone else be assigned to him? Can we interview two or three aides and select one?

- How do you recruit and screen staff? What training or experience is required? Do you do background checks on workers?

- What sorts of additional training does staff receive (care for patients with dementia, caring for a blind person, caring for someone who is incontinent, and so on)?

- How does one file complaints?

- What is the cost for these services? Is there a minimum number of hours per week or for each visit? (If your parent only needs help bathing and dressing, will you be charged for a four-hour minimum?) Is there any maximum to how much care will be provided?

- Is the home care agency certified to receive Medicare and Medicaid reimbursement?

- Can it subsidize care for people who cannot pay for themselves? (Government and voluntary agencies, such as a Visiting Nurse Association, often have public or private money to cover some care.)

- Is the agency licensed by the state and in compliance with all state regulations? (Agencies that provide nursing and therapeutic care must be licensed.)

- Is the agency accredited by a trade association, such as the National League for Nursing, which sets standards for the industry? (Accreditation means that an agency has met certain requirements with regard to staffing, training, and supervision, but not all agencies choose to take part even if they meet the requirements, so don't rule out an agency simply because it is not accredited.)

- Is the agency insured and bonded (which protects your parent in case of theft or accidents)? Does it provide worker's compensation (so you are not liable if an employee is injured while caring for your parent)?

- Under what conditions can the client or the agency terminate services?

- Can the agency provide references? Be specific when you ask for references (so you don't talk to two selected people who were happy with the service). For example, ask for the names of two clients who live within five miles of your parent, or two clients with dementia who received care within the past month.

Hiring Independently

To find a caregiver on your own, ask friends, neighbors, and your parent's doctor for referrals, and check with the agency on aging and local senior center. Look through the classified ads or take out an ad yourself.

You can find online registries that will provide you with names of freelance workers (they take a cut of the worker's fee). These are essentially employment services for health care workers. They are not the same as home care or private duty agencies; workers are not screened or supervised in any way, nor are such registries certified or regulated. Although they can be useful, you need to screen workers carefully yourself, and you will be responsible for any paperwork, filing state and federal payroll taxes, and supervision.

Interviewing Caregivers

Weed through candidates by phone first, asking a few broad questions, such as these:

- What credentials, qualifications, and prior experience do you have?

- Have you ever worked with a patient with [your parent's specific disease or disability]?

- What is your primary language and how fluent are you in [your parent's primary language]?

- What hours are you available, and how many months or years can you commit to this?

- Do you smoke?

- Do you have a valid driver's license and a car?

- Can you provide references?

When you meet someone face-to-face, don't make snap judgments. Of course, you want someone who is on time, respectful, kind, and well groomed. Beyond that, stay open-minded. Remember, what you want in a best friend is not necessarily what you want in a caregiver.

Watch how he interacts with your parent and moves about in his space. What sort of rapport do they have? Does he treat your parent with courtesy and kindness? Humor? Does this person seem to grasp what needs to be done? Is he well versed in the issues of elder-care, or at least eager to learn? Does he use touch in a way that would be comforting to your parent?

Some things to check on:

- Is the caregiver physically capable of meeting your parent's needs—can she support your parent so he can move from a bed to a chair or get out of bed?

- Exactly what chores and services will she perform? (And what *won't* she do?)

- Depending upon the nature of the work and the employee, find out if the worker or any coordinator is bonded (to cover any lawsuit that might arise).

- If you have any concerns, online companies will do a background check for about $25. Search "background check" or "crime check."

❝ Mum's caregivers adore her. They are on the front line, day in and day out. They spend much more time with her than we do. My sense of things—and perhaps my guilt at not being that front-and-center person—is that they believe the family doesn't do enough.

It's about projection, both ways. You walk into her home and there is the peachy smell from a plug-in that you know she never would have considered using. You drop by for a visit and she is being fed a hot dog with cheese. She says she doesn't feel like eating. Strike one against the caregivers.

Her caregiver wants the weekend off. You've worked all week long and have vague plans for yourself, and you don't want to give up the day to sit with Mum. Strike one against the family.

Both sides feel they are the ones who have her best interests at heart."

—Diana R.

From Day One

I t's tempting, in those first few days when everyone is a bit anxious, to just "see how it goes" and focus on everyone's happiness. But this is the time to be clear about what is expected, lay down any ground rules, and make any compromises. (Really. It only gets more awkward the longer you wait.)

Be kind and gentle, of course, but do it. Put the details of the job in writing, so there is no confusion later about what is expected. Of course, give the caregiver a chance to make revisions or add her own particulars to the "contract."

Be specific about the hours, responsibilities, pay, bonuses, vacation days and sick days, and the types of things that would lead to termination. (See page 646 for a sample contract.)

It can be useful to provide a detailed daily schedule or list of duties so there are no misunderstandings about exactly what's involved in the job.

Be clear about what should happen if, say, the worker can't come to work one day or if she has a complaint or problem.

Let her know how often you want to be updated, whether you prefer to be contacted by phone, email, or text, and whether there are times when you shouldn't be called (unless it's an emergency).

Outline how finances are to be handled—what day she'll be paid and who will pay her, and how she'll be reimbursed if she picks up groceries or other supplies.

HEADING OFF TROUBLE

E lderly people—even the competent ones—are easily exploited and mistreated. Make the rules crystal clear from the start. The best protection is prevention.

Be absolutely clear that no money or lavish gifts (aside from paychecks) are to exchange hands, regardless of the circumstances. You don't want your ever so appreciative mother to start writing extra checks or giving away her jewelry.

Likewise, let your grateful parent know that an aide is getting paid adequately

and that a letter to a supervisor or a bonus over the winter holidays is appropriate.

No matter how much you trust an employee, don't push your luck. Don't leave valuables or cash lying around; keep booze locked up; and don't let a worker have access to any bank accounts, passwords, or a Social Security number.

Once you have workers in place, stay involved. Be sure that your parent gets out and/or that family, friends, and neighbors come in. The more eyes on the situation, the better.

Relay any house rules—about smoking, noise levels, food, alcohol, phone or TV use, guests, the car, or anything else that concerns you or your parent. You certainly don't want a caregiver texting friends all day.

Depending upon the situation, you might want to include other specifics. For example, when and how medications are to be given, whether you want your parent massaged to avoid bedsores, what food preparation is expected. Will she have access to a car? Can she eat whatever is in the fridge? And so on.

Of course, your list should include provisions for the aide, too (for example, time for breaks, options for meals, a private space where she can go if your parent is napping). Ask if she has any specific requests or needs. And be ready to compromise.

> " We hired what was essentially a babysitter to stay with my father. Kim was about 17 at the time, trying to earn some money over her summer vacation.
>
> One afternoon I arrived when she was leaving—we had a sort of changing of the guards each day—and I realized that she had been crying. I followed her out on the porch, and we had a long talk about how my father reminded her of her grandfather, who had died a few years earlier.
>
> Apparently, she had been really close to her grandfather, and she was reliving his death every day. It was very sad, but also very sweet. I had thought of her as a sitter, but after we talked, I saw her as someone who was really sharing this pain with me, someone who really cared about my father."
>
> —Grace D.

Managing the Troops

Home care workers perform personal tasks in the most intimate surroundings, which can lead to close bonds, but it can also be a recipe for frustration, friction, and, keeping with the alliteration, fury.

Jealousies arise, and benign habits can make you want to thump your head against a wall. *Why does she click her tongue like that? Is she really going to tell me about her granddaughter again? I've told her repeatedly that Dad takes his coffee with skim milk, not cream.*

If your parent needs constant care, you have the added challenge of handling multiple workers, juggling schedules, filling in holes, and trying to create some sense of organization and continuity.

Even if you're used to managing people, this is a taxing job. Communication, compromise, and a Zen mind-set are key (*I am* not *going to let this bother me; I am at peace with the world . . . I am calm*). A few things to consider:

EMERGENCY INFORMATION

- Post emergency numbers—fire, police, ambulance, and poison control—in large clear writing near all phones or have them on speed dial. Include your parent's street address and the name of any cross street (to give to emergency call responders.)

- Have a list of other important numbers by the main phone or on the fridge, including your home, work, and cell phone numbers; numbers of other family members, friends, or neighbors; the doctor's office; and possibly a handyman.

- Any medical information that might be needed by an emergency crew should be on a medical bracelet or displayed prominently on the refrigerator or over your parent's bed. (See page 115.)

- Be sure any worker knows where to find medical supplies, secondary fire escape routes, breaker boxes, and water shut-off valves.

IT'S A TWO-WAY STREET. A worker who is treated with respect and kindness is more apt to treat your parent (and you) with respect and kindness. During these tough times, it may be hard for you to think about anyone else's needs, but do what you can.

Welcome any worker into your parent's life. Make sure she has a place for her belongings and decent food to eat. If she is living-in or working long shifts, she will need regular breaks and privacy. Be sensitive to her needs and the pressure she faces, both on the job and away from it.

Remember, little acts of kindness matter. When she walks in the door, even if you are completely frazzled, take a few moments to say hello and ask how she's doing.

When there is a problem, don't immediately assume it is her fault, or at least don't lambaste her the first time around. There might have been some miscommunication, or maybe she got busy with other things. Offer a gentle reminder. *You are sweet to bring doughnuts. What a generous gesture! With all that's going on I probably didn't make this clear, but Dad's got diabetes, so he can't have those. Would you mind terribly eating them before you come?*

FOSTER THIS RELATIONSHIP. It is important that your parent gets along with her home care worker. So encourage their budding friendship. Tell a caregiver about your parent—what makes her tick, what she used to be like, what will win her over, and what will upset her. Likewise, tell your parent a little something about the worker—where she comes from, if she's married or has children, if she has interests. Then, step back and let them get to know each other.

If your parent is thrilled that an aide has arrived and hardly notes your departure, or if she lets you know that you're doing something wrong and that Sarah or Kevin does it just right, gulp down the old pride. Sure, there will be a pang of jealousy, but hallelujah, they've hit it off!

COMPROMISE. No one is going to do things exactly as you would, which means that you have to accept change and ignore a few minor mishaps or irritating habits.

Try several people if necessary, but be ready to compromise, or you will be hiring and firing in rapid succession.

The aide might not make your mother's eggs as you would. She might put on music that you wouldn't choose. She might pile the pillows differently or spray the room with an air freshener you hate, but if your parent likes her and she is doing a reasonably good job, learn to live with it.

This means loosening your grip, turning down the old control meter. Repeat your new mantra: "I will be flexible and kind because she takes good care of Mom, and that allows me to have a life." Okay, it's not the shortest mantra, but you get the idea.

COMMUNICATE. If there is a problem, raise the subject sooner rather than later, because the longer you wait, the more difficult it will be to institute change. Likewise, ask that workers be candid with you about their problems or frustrations. Don't let things fester.

MONITOR THE WORK. If your parent is able and alert, then he can supervise his own care. But if he isn't, make unannounced visits occasionally.

If you can't drop in and your parent isn't alert enough to monitor things, ask a friend or neighbor to check in from time to time.

MAKE SMOOTH TRANSITIONS. Accidents frequently happen during the changing of the guard—one caregiver leaves and another shows up, unclear about what's been done and what needs to be done. Has your mother been given her medication? Has she had her lunch? Has she had fluids today?

Talk to workers about the critical importance of passing on information. Post a clear checklist—and get workers to use it—so everyone knows, for example, who gave what medication, at what time, and what is to happen on their shifts. (See page 648 for a sample checklist.)

MAKE IT EASY. Whatever tasks need to be done, make them as manageable as possible. Perhaps an alarm goes off when your parent needs to take medications, or you buy a raised toilet seat so there isn't so much lifting, or you play soft music to ease any agitation. The point is, don't just hand over a list of instructions

> " My mother is now on Medicaid, but I supplement the pay of the two women who take care of her. They earn so little and they work so hard. They are incredible with her.
>
> Vicky will wash Mom's hair, not because it needs it, but because Mom enjoys it so much. Kathy will stop at the store on her way to the house in the morning to pick up anything Mom needs. They really are wonderful. They are almost like family. And because of them I can stay in my own apartment and continue working. So I pay them extra and do anything else I can to keep them happy."
>
> —Jacqui L.

and walk out. Talk with the worker to find ways to make this job easier.

PROTECT THEM. If a family member is giving a worker trouble, protect her. Step in on her behalf. Or at the very least, acknowledge your uncle's ornery behavior, apologize, and thank her for putting up with it.

OFFER PRAISE AND THANKS. When things are done well, show your appreciation. A simple "thank you" will usually suffice, but if a worker is exceptional, write a note to her supervisor, give her a bonus, or buy a small gift. (People working for agencies don't get paid as much as you might think; the agency takes a hefty cut.)

When There Is Trouble

Serious problems are rare, but they happen. A worker mistreats your parent, steals from him, lies to you, or gets drunk on the job. Or, perhaps your parent is the problem. He yells at caregivers, fires them, or, in his confused state, makes sexual advances.

When the Caregiver Is the Problem

Be alert to signs of physical abuse, such as unexplained (or poorly explained) bruises, burns, or other injuries.

Emotional abuse (threats, insults, humiliation, isolation) will be harder to detect. If your parent can't communicate, he might develop irrational fears, nightmares, or new symptoms or behaviors, such as twitching, incontinence, or rocking. He might withdraw socially or become unusually quiet.

Unusual withdrawals from a bank account, any change to a trust or will, or the disappearance of valuables are clear indicators of financial exploitation, which is shockingly common.

And finally, there's neglect. Your parent is losing weight, but eats whenever you visit. He's got bedsores. His clothes are unwashed, his bed is unmade, his appointment is missed, and so on. Although neglect is usually the result of a misunderstanding, ignorance, inability, or laziness, it can be intentional (a caregiver withholds food or leaves your parent in soiled pants to "punish" him).

When you suspect serious trouble, don't ignore your intuition. If it's dire and urgent, call 911. Dismiss the worker immediately and call the local elder abuse hotline (ncea.aoa.gov). Notify the bank if the problem has to do with your parent's accounts.

If Medicare covers your parent's care, contact the Quality Improvement Organization in her state. Medicare contracts QIOs to be sure that patients receive quality care. You can find the local QIO through Medicare (800-633-4227 or medicare.gov).

If your parent is confused, she may make accusations that are false because she is paranoid or anxious about having a stranger in the house. Investigate her complaints, and if you are certain that she is inventing problems, reassure her that you understand her fears and remind her that she is safe. If her accusations continue, even if they are untrue, find another worker with whom she is more comfortable.

When Your Parent Can't Be Pleased

If your parent has lofty expectations for his care, if he is never pleased with any worker, if he resents the fact that he needs care and takes it out on workers, stay calm. Again.

Find out what's really going on. Is this worker no good, or is your parent just miserably unhappy and not letting any new caregiver into his life?

Let him air his hostility, fears, and hurts. Your calm reaction and willingness to listen will get you further than arguing. Once he's stated his case, let him know that you hear him, that you understand that this is all hard for him. And then explain—slowly and clearly, but firmly—that although this situation is not ideal, it is the best option. Remind him that you are not abandoning him,

> " When my parents were getting frail, we hired help through a home care agency. Both my parents were physically challenged, but mentally with it.
>
> One day, Dad called and said, 'Joe needs his family to come over from Tonga, and I'm going to loan him 3,500 bucks.'
>
> Joe was the aide sent over by the agency. I got off the phone with Dad and called the agency and said, 'Get Joe out of that house NOW!'
>
> He was gone within a few hours. I didn't want Dad to know why, or that he had anything to do with this. The agency simply told him that they had to shift workers and someone new was coming over."
>
> —Mark S.

and that you will continue to see him and care for him.

Talk with the worker as well. Help her understand your parent's situation and fears. Help her see that this is not personal, that it is not about her (although it seems that way). Encourage her to be flexible and have a sense of humor. And beg her to please put up with some occasional wrath. Tell her to call you if she needs to let off some steam, and be sympathetic when she does.

Respite Care

Anyone with hands-on responsibility for a frail parent needs a break occasionally, if not regularly. Start using respite care as soon as possible. You need it before you think you do. You also need to get your parent accustomed to other caregivers before he is deeply established in a routine that includes only you.

Respite is a broad term that may mean having someone come over one evening a week so you can go out for dinner, but it usually means moving your parent temporarily to a nursing home or other facility, or hiring ample help for a week or two while you go on vacation, deal with a family emergency, or simply escape the day-to-day rigors of caregiving.

You might believe that you are the only one who can oversee your parent's care. You may be afraid that if you leave, your mother will have a stroke or your father will hate you for "deserting" him. You may worry that if you move your parent temporarily or have someone replace you for a few days, everything will fall apart. You may worry,

----

❝ I have decided to take a week off by myself. I am going to a little cottage near a lake. I haven't told Mum yet, but I feel no guilt at all.

At first it felt like a ruthless decision. I thought I should keep being here for her. Or, if I took some time off, I thought I should visit friends or do something with my grandchildren. But the pressure has been intense. I feel so time-bound, so scheduled, as if my life is just about the needs of other people. I really want a week to myself, for me, not for anyone else. Just to look at the water and clear my head. That's my gift to myself."

—Ann S.

----

and he may not like it, but you need to do it.

Ask the area agency on aging (elder care.gov) about respite programs, or call nursing homes, which sometimes provide respite care. Veterans' hospitals may provide respite as part of your parent's regular medical care. Some adult day care programs also offer respite care.

Medicare covers respite when it is part of hospice care, but not in most other cases. If insurance won't cover it and the cost of respite is prohibitive, talk to family, friends, and neighbors and see if you can't patch something together. You have to get away from this.

When Using Respite

If you are an integral part of your parent's day, try a brief trial of leaving him with someone before heading off for an extended trip.

When you go, leave detailed, written instructions about your parent's medications, meals, and habits, even if you have discussed each item thoroughly with any staff or workers ahead of time.

Leave a list of all emergency phone numbers, and names and numbers of at least two backup contacts.

Show respite helpers where to find emergency medical supplies.

Have a backup plan. A home care agency should have backups, but privately hired companions and aides can cancel just when you are about to drive away. Talk to others who might step in if your parent is deserted.

Don't be talked out of this break, even if your parent complains.

The Halls
of Medicine

Chapter 10

Rx for the Elderly

The Age Difference • Finding a Doctor • A Wellness Visit •
A Geriatric Assessment • A Personal Health Record •
An Informed Advocate • Complementary and Alternative
Medicine

W hether your mother is having regular appointments
with several doctors or a series of tests and treatments for
an advanced disease, she needs one primary physician at the
helm. One doctor should keep track of all her ailments and medications,
refer her to specialists when necessary, and coordinate her care.

This sounds so basic that one wonders why it is even mentioned.
But when it comes to elderly patients, nothing is simple, and what's
obvious often doesn't happen.

Most elderly people see numerous doctors, have a calendar full of
medical appointments, and have such a large stack of prescriptions and
instructions that even a mindful caregiver can't keep track of them.
Doctors are issuing orders that don't jibe, and medications are given
that are just plain unsafe together.

At the risk of giving you more work than you already have,
the other thing that your parent needs is a strong advocate.
And because you are front and center, this hat probably goes to you.

It's important to ask questions. Lots of them. *Why is she getting this medication? Is it safe with her other drugs? Can we start with a lower dose? What is the goal of this treatment? When can we stop it?* This is no time to be shy.

Keep an ongoing record of her medical history, symptoms, treatments, and instructions. Be sure those involved in her care are aware of all instructions, especially if she moves from one location or caregiver to another. And, if something seems amiss, speak up.

The Age Difference

The medical wisdom that worked at 30 might be medical malpractice when a patient is 80. Old bodies digest, absorb, excrete, and metabolize differently than younger ones. And rather than having just one isolated illness, they often have any number of diseases and symptoms, which complicates things enormously.

The fragility and complexity of the system mean that an otherwise benign illness might be life threatening. A common disease can cause uncommon symptoms. A recommended dose can bring about dangerous side effects.

For example, withdrawal, sadness, and apathy might look like depression but could actually be signs of an infection, stroke, or heart disease. A drug that a young person can use without any problems can cause confusion, incontinence, or blurry vision in an older patient.

When heart disease, diabetes, arthritis, and dementia are all at play, even a stellar doctor will be hard-pressed to determine exactly what's causing what and which treatments are most appropriate.

A doctor treating your parent should look beyond any immediate symptoms or test results and consider your parent's age, medical history, and other ailments and treatments. Ideally, he or she will also consider your parent's housing arrangements, exercise regimen, diet, daily habits, social supports, and even her financial situation, because each of these plays a role in her health and medical care.

In other words, the doctor shouldn't simply mend a broken ankle; he or she needs to recognize that your mother has fallen because her vision is waning, and that the combination of her arthritis medication and her heart pills is making her dizzy. The doctor should also realize that your mom lives alone and will have no way of taking care of herself if she has a cast on her leg.

THAT CRITICAL OUNCE

Prevention is perhaps the most important aspect of medical care. The elderly cannot bounce back from an illness or an injury as easily as their younger counterparts, so prevention is essential.

Of course, prevention might not have been part of your parent's upbringing. He might come from the school of if-it-ain't-broke-don't-fix-it. You might have to do some gentle but forceful persuading.

Make sure your parent's living situation is safe, see that he is eating healthfully, urge him to get a little exercise, and encourage him to be mentally active. He should have regular physicals, eye exams, and dental checkups (as should you). He should also have a one-time pneumococcal vaccine to fight pneumonia, a one-time shingles vaccine, and a flu shot each fall.

Most important, the doctor should know your parent's priorities and goals, and should make every treatment decision with those goals in mind. Geriatric care is, for better or worse, a matter of trade-offs. Does she want whatever treatment will let her live as long as possible, at any cost? Or is her primary goal to be free of pain? To be lucid for as long as possible? To be mobile? To avoid the ICU? Or to attend some specific event? Her doctor and your family need to keep this in the forefront of all decision making.

Finding a Doctor

If your father has a primary doctor whom he trusts, he may not need to look any further. If he is hunting for a new primary doctor, or if he needs to find a specialist, the best bet is to get a referral from a trusted professional or friend.

If you are searching websites for a new doctor, proceed with caution. Most doctor-rating websites aren't terribly useful or accurate. Some are simply marketing tools. The Informed Patient Institute (informedpatientinstitute.org) grades various sites, so see what they recommend in your parent's state. It's also worth checking out the federal government's site, Physician Compare (at medicare.gov/physiciancompare), which provides basic information.

Every state has a licensing board, which has information on doctors who have been sanctioned or have been the target of malpractice cases. Although a single lawsuit isn't a big deal, disciplinary action or repeated suits raise a red flag. You can get much of this information at the Association of State Medical Board of Executive Directors' DocFinder (docboard.org).

Finally, some health insurance plans offer information about the doctors in their network.

While hunting, here are a number of issues worth considering:

> Mom has one general doctor, who is what I would call a social doctor. He's sweet, but he is not a help. He has missed so many things, it's amazing.
>
> When she was in the hospital after her hip operation, he was going to let her go home without night nurses even though she couldn't get out of bed. Last fall, he failed to realize that she had severe congestion in her lungs. He'd prescribed diuretics for her, but he never checked to see whether she was taking them. He just reassures her and says, 'You're doing splendidly.'
>
> She says, 'I know he isn't a good doctor, but I can't leave him. He's been Dad's doctor and my doctor for too long.'
>
> I can't push her to do anything once she's made up her mind. It just means that we have to keep closer tabs on her health and press him when we think something is wrong.
>
> Once I called to see when he would be on vacation and then made an appointment for her during that time just so another doctor in the practice would examine her."
>
> —Betty H.

WILL THIS DOCTOR TAKE ON YOUR PARENT? The biggest problem you are likely to run into is that doctors aren't thrilled to take on new Medicare patients, and even fewer will see people on Medicaid. So that should be the first question: Does this doctor accept your parent's insurance?

AN UNDERSTANDING OF ALL THINGS GERIATRIC. Although it is ideal to have a geriatrician either at the helm or consulting, it is by no means essential. Good general practitioners and internists are perfectly capable of caring for your parent, especially if they have a lot of experience with elderly patients.

Your parent needs a doctor who understands the complexities of geriatric care, someone who doesn't just diagnose and treat but considers all aspects of a patient's life, including her goals for her care.

A MATTER OF INSTINCTS. The healing process starts in the mind. Your parent will fare better in the hands of someone who instills confidence in her, someone she trusts and can talk to easily. (Of course, gut instinct is less important when you are looking for a specialist. Then, credentials and experience are essential.)

A SHARED PHILOSOPHY. Does your parent want aggressive medical care at all costs, feel strongly about avoiding extraordinary treatments, or have an interest in alternative medicine? Find a doctor who respects—and will uphold—your parent's wishes.

CREDENTIALS. Take a look at a prospective doctor's credentials—medical school, residency training, board certifications,

✚ WHAT TO BRING TO THE DOCTOR'S OFFICE

Before seeing a new doctor, you or your parent should gather insurance cards and make a list of relevant medical information, as well as any questions you have. The doctor will need to know about the following:

- Past illnesses or injuries, tests, hospitalizations, and surgeries.

- Any current symptoms—dizziness, confusion, swelling, weight loss or gain, and so on. Has there been any change in physical ability or cognitive function? When did any symptoms begin? Did they come on suddenly or gradually? Rank these concerns in order of their importance rather than mentioning them vaguely or with equal emphasis.

- Current medications and those taken in the past, including prescription and over-the-counter drugs and any diet supplements (also include any dietary aids, nicotine gum, vitamins, laxatives, decongestants, sedatives, eye or nose drops, medicated creams, patches, and so forth). You might have to search your parent's medicine cabinets and drawers to compile a complete list.

- Allergies or sensitivities to medications or other substances.

- Daily eating, sleeping, toileting, and exercise habits.

- Eyeglasses, hearing aids, dentures, or other such devices.

- Any obstacles faced in daily life— problems with bathing, getting dressed, balancing the checkbook, climbing stairs, communicating.

- Family history of physical or mental illness (including parents, siblings, grandparents, children, and blood-related aunts and uncles).

- Any tobacco, alcohol, or other substance use.

- Prior exposure to heavy metals or chemicals (usually in a workplace).

- Names and phone numbers of previous and current doctors.

and any other qualifications. To learn about these, ask the office secretary.

EXPERIENCE. More important than what college someone attended is a doctor's experience in treating elderly patients and in dealing with the problems that plague your parent. Find out what percentage of the practice is devoted to elderly patients and, in particular, what percentage is devoted to patients with your parent's ailments.

AFFILIATIONS AND ASSOCIATES. Check whether a doctor has admitting privileges at your parent's hospital of choice. If the doctor is in a group practice, find out whether your parent will see this particular doctor or an associate.

LOCATION. Is it relatively easy for your parent to get to the doctor's office? Is there ample parking? Is it on a bus route, or is there a van service that will take her there? Will your parent have to go someplace out of her way for tests and lab work? A smaller office might send her far away to have tests done, while a larger office or one that is within a medical center might just send her down the hall.

A Wellness Visit

I t's an annual rite. You wrap your naked body in a piece of paper towel and wait, shivering, for someone to come take your blood pressure, listen to your lungs, and check that you haven't gotten markedly shorter or fatter since last year. Blood and urine are offered up and, sore throat or not, you say, "Ahhh . . ."

Although physical exams have been the cornerstone of medicine for eons, Medicare does not cover them. What Medicare does cover is an annual "wellness visit," which looks nothing like the above. In a wellness visit, which typically lasts about 45 minutes, no one strips down. No paper gowns.

Instead, doctors check a few basics, such as height, weight, and blood pressure. Then most of the visit revolves around questions and a discussion about risk factors, family history, medical history, medical concerns, and ways to stay healthy. For example, a doctor and patient might discuss weight control, ways to avoid falls, concerns about memory problems, the risk of diabetes, or signs of depression.

Some doctors aren't happy about this setup, and some patients feel cheated when they think they are booked for a physical and don't even get to take their clothes off. However, there is a growing consensus that discussions about risk and prevention, and about gait and memory, are more useful than routine lab tests, at least in the case of elderly patients.

The bottom line: Know what your parent is booked for, and if no one has advised her to have a wellness visit, she should ask for one.

Medicare does cover other preventive services (mammograms, glaucoma tests, bone mass, colorectal screenings, diabetes screenings, and so on). And the fact is, most doctors have figured out ways to check lungs and test blood and urine in the course of other appointments, so despite Medicare's restrictions, most people are getting general physicals of some sort or another.

By any name, an exam should cover some basic territory:

THE BODY. A doctor should review your parent's medications regularly and check your parent for problems that are common in the elderly (arthritis, weight loss, thyroid problems, and heart disease, for example).

A doctor should examine your parent's gait or steadiness and his physical abilities. With a few quick tests, the doctor can

IN THE EXAMINING ROOM

I f you are with your parent during any segment of an exam, stay in the background. Relay any pertinent information, but be careful not to answer questions addressed to your parent. Quite often, the doctor is not looking for an answer, but is observing how your parent responds.

find out if your parent can reach, bend, walk, turn, sit down, and get up without difficulty; hear what's being said; pick up a spoon; or read his own pill bottles.

THE BRAIN. An exam might include a quick test of your parent's cognitive abilities and mental state. A doctor might, for example, ask her to name three items and then recall them a minute later, draw a figure, and have her count backward from 100 by sevens. If there is any question about her mental abilities, the doctor will conduct a more comprehensive exam or refer her to someone else for further evaluation.

THE MIND. The doctor should also ask about your parent's moods, fears, and anxiety. If there is any suggestion of depression, an anxiety disorder, or other mental illness, the doctor might refer your parent to a geriatric psychiatrist for further evaluation (although most will simply write a prescription).

THE PERSON. A doctor (or assistant) should ask about your parent's daily activities (eating, sleeping, exercising, dressing, hygiene, and so on), how she is functioning, and also about her housing situation and social supports. Such information will alert a doctor to possible ailments, such as depression, insomnia, or incontinence, and uncover practical problems and potential risks. If your mother isn't eating, does she need to be put in touch with a meal-delivery service? If she lives alone, is she at risk of falling or having other accidents?

A Geriatric Assessment

Because the medical care of the elderly can be so complex, many hospitals and clinics have established geriatric assessment centers (also called geriatric evaluation units). In these centers, a geriatrician heads a team of medical specialists (neurologists, psychiatrists, rheumatologists, and so on), nurses, social workers, physical and occupational therapists, case workers, and dietitians, who address all facets of your parent's health and life.

Although some of these centers provide primary medical care, replacing the family doctor, most act as consultants in cases where the patient has dementia, multiple ailments, difficult-to-diagnose symptoms, or serious problems managing at home.

Patients are typically referred to a geriatric center by their personal doctors, but you can make an appointment directly if you have nagging concerns that aren't being addressed.

A geriatric assessment can last several hours, or it might be broken up and done in pieces over several visits. It includes a detailed physical, neurological, and mental exam. It also includes evaluations by social workers and nurses who will talk with your parent, and perhaps with the family, about your parent's daily life and future. The team will provide counseling as well as practical help, hooking your family up with local services and housing options.

Geriatric centers are usually found in major medical centers or hospitals in large cities, although some have opened in smaller hospitals and cities. To find one, ask your parent's doctor or call hospitals in the area.

A Personal Health Record (PHR)

Every time your parent sees a new doctor, is raced to the emergency room, or goes into a rehab facility, the staff will ask about her medical history. If you are like most people, you will reel off a doctor's name, allergies, when she had her stroke, the names of a few drugs, and a few vague descriptions. *It's pink, and as I recall, it has a Z on it, or maybe it's an N. She started taking them last spring. Or maybe late winter.*

Or because of your excellent organizational skills, you have written down all her medications and treatments on a list, which is, oh, oops, at home.

That list is, in fact, a personal health record, or PHR, although maybe not a terrific one.

Electronic PHRs, which are stored on the Internet and available through any computer, tablet, or smartphone, make it easier to update information and are always accessible when you need them. Beyond keeping track of basic health information, some can also be used to refill prescriptions, make doctor appointments, and submit medical claims. Some also come with a medical

emergency card, which staff can scan to access information.

Not only is this handy when your parent shows up in the ER, but it also helps you stay on top of things. You'll be more apt to know if a medication is working (*She's been on it for two weeks and she's still coughing*), if a refill is needed, and the dates of various appointments.

Of course, a PHR is only as good as the information that's on it. In other words, you actually have to keep it up to date, or you might as well go back to Plan A—the scrap of paper stuffed in your purse. Also, a PHR needs to be on a secure, reputable website, requiring a password and ID.

And finally, you need access to your parent's PHR, which isn't always easy. Be sure that you have any authorization required so you're not shut out when you need that information most.

A PHR, whether it's paper or electronic, should include the following:

• doctors' names and phone numbers

• medical conditions and symptoms

• allergies

- medications, doses, and start and stop dates, including nonprescription medications and supplements

- dates of surgeries or treatments

- advance directives

- contact information for health care proxy

It might also include these items:

- dates of doctors' appointments

- vitals, such as height, weight, blood pressure, cholesterol

- names and numbers of pharmacies

- family medical history

- recent test results

- additional emergency contacts

Many companies, as well as some providers, insurance companies, and nonprofit groups, offer electronic PHRs. Some do it for free; sometimes there's a small fee. You can get free PHRs through Medicare (mymedicare.gov) or the American Health Information Management Association (myphr.com). The Veterans Administration offers veterans a PHR called My Health*e*Vet at www. myhealth.va.gov.

Note: An electronic PHR is not the same as an electronic health or medical record (EHR), which is something hospitals, doctors' offices, and insurance companies keep. However, if your parent wants to see her EHR for some reason (she can't recall when she started a medication or wants to see a test result, for example), or if you, as her proxy, need to see it, you can have access to these as well. Increasingly, providers are giving patients direct access to their health records online.

An Informed Advocate

A good doctor is only part of the medical care team; the patient and family play a critical role as well. As your parent grows more frail or more confused, you will become his advocate and possibly his sole spokesperson. The medical world can be confounding and intimidating, but be bold.

GET A MEDICAL POWER OF ATTORNEY.
A medical power of attorney, or health care proxy, is a legal form that gives you or some other person the authority to make medical decisions on your parent's behalf if she cannot make them for herself. This document is easily obtained from a lawyer, a local hospital, or online. Be sure to get one that is specific to your parent's state (or two states, if she spends time shuttling between places).

Be sure your parent's doctor has a copy of this and any other advance

IF HER DOCTOR KEEPS YOU IN THE DARK

The Health Insurance Portability and Accountability Act (HIPAA) was passed in 1996 to protect patient privacy because medical information was being stored electronically, and that made people understandably nervous.

The problem is that many health professionals misconstrue HIPAA (as well as privacy acts that followed) and refuse to share information with family members. This has led to no small number of angry outbursts in hospital hallways.

The fact is, doctors and other health care professionals are allowed to discuss your parent's medical care with you, and the rules are extremely lenient. But to avoid problems, get your parent to sign a medical power of attorney and to name you on any HIPAA or other privacy agreement that the doctor or hospital might require.

If you have questions, the U.S. Department of Health & Human Services website explains patient privacy and the various rules in some detail (hhs.gov).

---

directives (such as a living will). Your parent should talk with you or her chosen proxy about her priorities, preferences, and feelings about medical care, especially the kind of care she wants when death is near.

ASK QUESTIONS. If you are overseeing your parent's medical care, or even if you are on the sidelines, don't hesitate to ask questions. If your parent is handling her own care, remind her to ask questions and to write down the answers. Don't be embarrassed that you don't know what the liver is, where it is, or what it does. Don't pretend that you know what an abscess, an antigen, or a fistula is, nodding agreeably as the doctor races on. Ask, ask, and ask again. It's important that you (and ideally your parent) understand the issues.

Before an appointment, write down any questions you have and give them to the doctor so he or she can allot time for them and address the most critical ones first.

If you have questions or concerns that can't wait until the next visit—*Is she supposed to take the new medication with dinner or before going to bed? Is this dizziness serious?*—call.

TAKE NOTES. Your parent returns from seeing the doctor and gives you the lowdown. *He said I had some kind of bowel problem—oh, what did he call it? Irreversible? Irrational? I don't remember. Something to do with the bowel.*

Or maybe you go with her and return clutching her new prescriptions. *Oh dear. Was she supposed to start the antibiotics this afternoon or tomorrow morning? Take the nausea drugs before breakfast or after?*

Every time you talk with a doctor or nurse, take notes. It's so easy to forget specifics when you're in a medical office. If your parent is still in charge, encourage her to take notes, or ask the doctor to write down any information and instructions.

DO YOUR HOMEWORK. When the doctor hasn't explained the facts clearly or your parent gives you only partial information, do some research on your own. You don't have to look up every study done on Coumadin, but find out what blood clotting is about, what the drugs do to prevent it, and what side effects are possible.

Of course, the Internet is loaded with garbage. Don't trust sites set up by drug companies, articles in popular magazines, or advice from friends (and certainly not advice doled out by strangers!). Check out the sites listed in the box on page 191.

BE A KEEN OBSERVER. If you are involved in your parent's medical care and you see her regularly, be alert to changes in her moods, habits, and complaints. A minor fall, a dull pain, or changes in weight, sleep habits, or moods can all indicate a serious medical problem and should be brought to the doctor's attention.

KEEP RECORDS. Again, maintain an updated list of all your parent's medications (prescription medications as well as nonprescription ones), including the dose, the dates she started and stopped taking them, and any adverse side effects from them; any allergies; the names, addresses, and phone numbers of all doctors seen; special dietary needs; and the dates, places, and reasons for any hospitalizations or surgery.

This might seem like extra work you don't need, but honestly it will save you time later (searching through the trash for an old pill bottle) and is critical to her care.

USE ONE SPOKESPERSON. When it comes to your parent's medical care, one sibling should be the family spokesperson. Typically, this will be the person who lives nearby and goes to doctor appointments with your parent. This person, and this person only, should be in contact with the doctor's office; he or she can then relay information to others.

If multiple family members are calling the doctor, chances are there will be miscommunication, misunderstanding, and frustration—on all sides.

That said, if the doctor has offered to meet with the family to discuss a diagnosis or prognosis, then it's best if all are present, so everyone hears the same thing and it doesn't turn into a mangled game of Operator (although, oddly enough, even when all are present, siblings often leave having heard different things).

GET A SECOND OPINION. Even if your parent's doctor is terrific, get another opinion on any serious matter, particularly if surgery is recommended. Another doctor will either offer new options or reassure you that this is the best way to proceed.

USE CAUTION WHEN COMPARING. Don't give too much weight to the tales of other people who had a similar illness. A stroke is not a stroke is not a stroke, particularly when it happens in an elderly body. So don't second-guess the doctor just because Aunt Ashley was cured when she had these same symptoms.

BE A TEAM PLAYER. Although you should be a staunch and persistent advocate for your parent, you also need to work with the doctor and other health professionals. Be open about your concerns and questions, but also be patient and understanding. Doctors and nurses work under enormous pressures, and there are limitations to what they can do.

UNDERSTAND THE PROCESS. Medicine is as much an art as it is a science. Your parent's doctor doesn't know everything because everything isn't known

FINDING GOOD INFORMATION ON THE NET

The Internet is loaded with medical information. A little of it is useful, most of it is inaccurate, and a scary amount of it is simply a guise to get you to buy a product.

Be cautious. Many well-known and seemingly respectable sites are tightly linked to drug and insurance companies, and thus have biased information. Others are written by, well, just about anyone.

Use sites of reputable foundations, medical associations, government agencies, medical journals, or other established organizations. Beware of any site loaded with ads or trying to sell something, even remotely.

Some good starting points for medical information:

- For easy-to-read, basic health information aimed specifically at seniors, try the National Institutes of Health's NIH Senior Health website, nihseniorhealth.gov.

- For more detail about a wider range of issues, go to healthfinder.gov, another federal website, which will lead you to articles from a variety of respected institutes, universities, journals, and agencies.

- The American Geriatrics Society Foundation for Health in Aging has a consumer website with detailed and reliable information on a broad range of health topics for the elderly, healthinaging.org.

- The Mayo Clinic has a helpful and trustworthy site, mayoclinic.com. In addition to good information about specific diseases and symptoms, the site has a Symptom Checker, First Aid Guide, and Health Manager (for tracking health information).

- MedlinePlus (nlm.nih.gov/medlineplus) will lead you to an abundance of information from the National Institutes of Health and the National Library of Medicine.

- Most illnesses and disabilities have established associations and corresponding websites, such as the Alzheimer's Association, the Arthritis Foundation, the American Cancer Society, and so on. Healthfinder.gov can lead you to most of these organizations (simply click on "find services and information," and then "find a health organization"). For information about less common ailments, contact the National Organization for Rare Disorders (800-999-6673 or rarediseases.org).

and because each person is different. No one test or treatment is likely to provide "the cure" or "the answer"; it is all part of an ongoing process.

Your desire for clarity, answers, and action may push a doctor to act in ways that are not in your parent's best interests. A doctor might, for example, order an unnecessary test or prescribe a potent drug simply to appease anxious family members who want *something* done. A linear "cure" mentality is apt to lead to disappointment, and it might distract from your parent's true goals and day-to-day care and comfort.

Also, remember that the doctor's primary responsibility is to your parent, not you. While he or she will take family opinions into consideration, your parent's needs should be front and center.

Complementary and Alternative Medicine

Although it's not the stuff of your parent's generation, don't rule out nontraditional forms of therapy. Yes, much of it is ineffectual, and some is downright dangerous, but some therapies are safe and effective.

"Alternative medicine" is, as the name suggests, treatment that is used in place of conventional practices. "Complementary medicine" is that which is used at the same time as conventional treatment. "Integrative medicine" is the use of conventional medicine in conjunction with an unconventional treatment that is widely thought to be safe and effective.

Although many of these therapies have been used for thousands of years, there is scant scientific data on their value. The most up-to-date information is available from the National Center for Complementary and Alternative Medicine (nccam.nih.gov).

Broadly speaking, most complementary and alternative medicine (known as CAM) can be broken down into three categories—dietary, manipulative, and mind-body therapies. A few of the more common therapies are described briefly here.

Dietary Supplements

A *supplement* used to refer to a group of vitamins and minerals, usually provided in a once-daily tablet. But now the word refers to a broad array of amino acids, herbal products, animal tissues, and questionable ingredients usually given in pill or liquid form but increasingly loaded into drinks, "health" bars, and candy. (A daily vitamin is not considered alternative medicine.)

Dietary supplements, or "nutraceuticals," are virtually unregulated. Manufacturers can make all sorts of outlandish and unproven claims, as long as they don't claim to cure a specific illness. And who can resist a pill that promises to improve memory or treat arthritis or boost energy? Especially a pill that is "natural."

But most of this is a waste of time and money, and just because something is "herbal" or "natural" does not in any way mean that it's safe. Many are toxic, and others interact dangerously with conventional drugs.

For example, studies suggest that ginkgo increases the risk of bleeding and that raw ginkgo seeds can be toxic. St. John's wort can interfere with antidepressants and chemotherapy. Kava has been linked to liver disease.

Read up on any supplement from reputable sources, talk to your parent's doctor, and buy only from large, established companies.

Body Manipulation

Body-based, or manipulative, practices refer to those treatments where someone puts their hands on you to readjust, realign, rebalance, or relax muscles, bones, and various bodily systems. The most common of these are massage, acupuncture, and chiropractic therapy.

MASSAGE

Massage feels good and is therapeutic because it relieves tension, which helps to reduce stress and ease pain. However, for an elderly person who is not comfortable with physical contact, this obviously will not be relaxing.

If your parent is game, a massage makes a nice gift. Many massage therapists make house calls. As always, check with your parent's doctor first.

ACUPUNCTURE

Acupuncture, which originated more than two thousand years ago in Asia, is based on the notion that the human body has an energy called *Qi* (pronounced "chee"), which regulates spiritual, emotional, physical, and mental balance. Qi moves about the body on "meridians." By stimulating points along these meridians, the acupuncturist restores balance so a person's Qi flows smoothly.

In this country, the most common form of acupuncture involves inserting extremely fine needles into particular points in the body.

Although Western doctors have not discovered physical evidence of these meridians or concrete evidence that acupuncture is any more effective than a placebo, it does help many people, particularly when treating pain.

Most states now have standards in place for certification and licensing of acupuncturists. Many medical doctors are also now being trained in acupuncture.

CHIROPRACTIC

The theory behind chiropractic medicine is that misalignments (called "subluxations") in the skeleton, particularly in the spine, interfere with the work of the nervous system and the body's natural defenses. When the scaffolding is adjusted, the body can begin to heal itself. It is an ancient practice dating back at least two thousand years.

Chiropractic is particularly useful in treating ailments in the muscles, joints, and bones, such as neck pain, headaches, strains, and arthritis. Evidence suggests that it is as effective at treating low back pain as conventional medicine. (Some

A WORD OF CAUTION

Your parent should check with his doctor before adopting any integrative regimen, or even taking supplements—not necessarily to get the doctor's support of a particular therapy, but to make sure that it won't interfere with his ongoing medical care or cause troublesome or dangerous side effects. Also:

• Never rely on an alternative medicine practitioner for a diagnosis. Always check back with the primary doctor.

• Older bodies typically don't tolerate things as well as younger bodies do, and the confluence of medical ailments makes treatment complicated. In other words, your parent should use extra caution when trying an alternative therapy.

• Just because something works for your friend does not mean it is right for your parent.

• Learn the credentials, training, and fees of any practitioner. Ask your parent's primary doctor for a recommendation, or contact professional organizations. Some large medical centers have CAM (complementary and alternative medicine) clinics.

• Most nontraditional therapies must be paid for out-of-pocket. Insurance coverage is limited.

• Beware of quick fixes, grand promises, and medical breakthroughs. They don't exist.

studies suggest that doing nothing is also as effective; that is, the pain eventually goes away by itself.)

Chiropractors usually have four years of specialized training and get a D.C., or Doctor of Chiropractic, degree. Many insurance companies, as well as Medicare and, in some states, Medicaid, offer some coverage for chiropractic treatment.

Check with your parent's doctor first, though. It's important to rule out other ailments (such as compression fractures, tumors, and so on) and to be sure that such manipulation is safe for your parent.

THERAPEUTIC TOUCH
Therapeutic touch is based on the notion that the hands of these therapists have a healing force. Despite the name, the therapists don't actually touch the client, but rather slide their hands two to four inches above the skin (or clothes; a person does not have to undress for this). In doing so, the healer identifies energy imbalances and corrects them.

Whether or not energy is actually rebalanced, therapeutic touch has been known to to reduce anxiety, increase relaxation, and reduce pain.

Mind-Body Connections
Clearly, the state of the mind affects the state of the body. On the simplest level, placebo studies repeatedly show that people get better simply because they believe they are being treated. And there's no doubt that fear, pain, and anxiety become cyclical—anxiety increases

pain, fear of pain increases anxiety, and so on.

The simplest and most immediate approach is to get your parent to pause and take three slow, deep breaths (you should do this too!). Breathe in through the nose and out through the mouth, feeling all the muscles, one by one, relax. It takes almost no time and can immediately make a person feel calmer.

Many mind-body approaches stem from ancient practices that have been used for thousands of years in Asia. The Chinese therapy qigong, the Japanese therapy Reiki, and the Indian system of Ayurveda all emphasize the body's energy and balance. The ancient art of tai chi is effective in improving balance and preventing falls in the elderly (see page 85).

MEDITATION

One of the most common mind-body therapies is meditation. Your parent might pooh-pooh the idea of meditating, but research suggests that meditation is great for both body and soul.

....

" I wouldn't say that my mother is into alternative medicine—she doesn't try anything terribly radical. But when she was diagnosed with cancer, I bought her a couple of books on diet and nutrition. She started taking vitamins. She also started reading books about emotional states and healing—Bernie Siegel stuff. I think it has helped. She is stronger both physically and mentally. I can see the change in her. It makes her feel like she still has some control, like she can take charge and fight this thing herself."

—Diane S.

....

(Note: Meditation is beneficial for stressed caregivers, so read on.)

Meditation is conscious relaxation. It means paying attention to one's breathing, relaxing the muscles, and clearing the mind of all the rubbish. Once someone is successfully meditating, his breathing becomes deep and regular, and his mind is detached from the problems of daily life.

Meditation is useful for anyone, but it seems to be particularly effective in treating stress, pain, hypertension, and heart disease, and is thought to strengthen the immune system.

VISUALIZATION

Visualization, also known as guided imagery, can be very helpful for elderly people, particularly those who are in chronic pain, anxious, worried, or depressed.

In one form of imagery, the person imagines a relaxing scene or situation. For example, you might have your parent close her eyes while you speak slowly and softly, getting her to imagine herself, say, lying on the beach—the warmth of the sun on her skin, the steady sound of the waves, the weight of her body as it sinks heavily into the soft sand, and so on. Putting oneself into this other place, entering it completely with the mind, relaxes the body and relieves anxiety, tension, and pain.

In another type of visualization, a person imagines his body healing itself, imagines weak areas growing stronger, important nutrients entering the bloodstream, or strong immune cells fending off an enemy infection. This sort of thinking fosters a sense of control and power, which might help a person heal.

Chapter 11

The Body Imperfect
Part I

A Muddle of Medications • Vision • Hearing • Sleep •
Temperature Regulation • Dehydration • Skin Care •
Arms, Legs, and Feet • Teeth and Mouth

Your overriding concern right now may be stroke, cancer, dementia, heart disease, or some other life-threatening illness, and rightfully so. But don't lose sight of your parent's seemingly more mundane complaints, such as blurry eyesight, incontinence, and restless nights.

Doctors will attend to severe illness, but they often ignore these other ailments, which can be more bothersome day-to-day than any specific disease. Your parent's poor hearing will distance him from people he loves, his itchy skin will keep him awake at night, and his achy knees will prevent him from doing the things he most enjoys.

Moreover, these nagging problems can cause or exacerbate serious illness. Poor hearing can mimic or worsen dementia. Cataracts are a leading cause of falls. And sleeplessness, well, sleeplessness is something you might know all about. It, too, can look like dementia, cause falls, and lead to depression, among other things.

Be careful not to pass off these complaints as unavoidable aspects of old age. *That's what happens at 86. What do you expect?* Certainly, these ailments are common in old age, but that doesn't mean they are untreatable or unworthy of attention. In fact, many are preventable or treatable, and a few are curable. And life with almost any disability can be made more manageable.

The information supplied here is not meant to replace the advice of a doctor, but if you are aware of the problems, the symptoms, and some remedies, you can alert the doctor and brainstorm solutions. You can also make changes around your parent's house and in his daily life to keep him comfortable and independent for as long as possible.

ON THE LOOKOUT FOR SYMPTOMS

PROBLEM	SIGNS OF TROUBLE
Overmedication	A cabinet filled with prescriptions from multiple physicians, unexplained confusion, memory loss, disorientation, instability, drowsiness, agitation, weakness, dizziness, nausea, rash, and any symptom that arises soon after a new drug is added to the list
Vision loss	Squinting, pulling back to read small print, failing to notice stop signs, trouble following sporting events or driving at night, complaints of "halos," floaters, or glare
Hearing loss	Saying "What?" a lot, constantly turning the volume up, staring vacantly while others talk, not "remembering" what was said or asking that things be repeated
Insomnia	Complaints of fatigue, long periods in bed, frequent naps, wandering at night
Hyperthermia	Sweating, dizziness, nausea, or, in severe cases, hot and dry skin, rapid pulse, and confusion
Hypothermia	Lethargy, confusion, paleness, shallow breathing (even in normal temperatures)
Skin problems	Unusual-looking moles, itchy, cracked, red, or irritated skin
Mouth ailments	Pain, dry mouth, difficulty chewing

Understanding what your parent is up against—why he doesn't remember what you said (he didn't hear it), why he is so grumpy (he is in pain), or why he didn't eat that beautiful meal you made (he's having trouble swallowing)—should also give you more patience and compassion as you try to help him now.

A Muddle of Medications

The thought of your father as a druggie may seem absurd, but take another look in his medicine cabinet. A prescription for pain, a blood thinner, a little something to help him sleep, a pill to aid digestion, medication to lower his cholesterol, a pill for his memory, and something for his arthritis. Then, of course, he's got his vitamin D, a stool softener, and fish oil.

It's not uncommon for an older person to make weekly visits to the pharmacist and take half a dozen medications or more.

This would be dicey for anyone, but for your parent, it could be lethal. Remember that older bodies do not tolerate drugs in the same ways young bodies do. Changes in hormones, body fat, water content, metabolism, blood flow, stomach acids, and kidney function all affect the way bodies absorb, use, and discard drugs. So those pills that your mother took years ago might not be safe for her now.

Add to this the number of ailments and medications involved, and then factor in the odds that instructions won't

be followed exactly (*Oh, I thought I was supposed to take the ones in the tall bottle three times a day and the blue ones in the morning, and the big ones after lunch . . .*) and you're prime for a disaster: falls, seizures, confusion, dizziness, depression, delirium, hemorrhage, incontinence, rashes, heart failure. The list goes on.

Doctors sometimes overprescribe, fail to stop medications that are no longer needed, and fail to ask what other pills a patient is taking. Patients don't take medications as directed, forget pills, or skip doses to save money or avoid side effects.

If you are involved in your parent's medical care, ask plenty of questions when a new drug is prescribed, and keep careful records of the medications she takes—the names, doses, reason for them, dates they are started and stopped, side effects, and instructions. Include over-the-counter drugs, such as aspirin, or cold medication, vitamins, and alcohol or recreational drugs. (For a form you can use, see page 640.) Show this list to any doctor or health care professional she sees. If your parent has a new

GOOD MEDICINE

- Be sure your parent's primary doctor has a complete list of all medications and supplements your parent takes.

- Get a doctor's okay before making any change in a medication routine. Your parent should not take more of a drug to increase the effect or stop taking a drug because she feels better.

- Make sure doctors know about any allergies your parent has.

- Your parent may be taking medications, especially over-the-counter medications, such as antihistamines or sleeping pills, out of habit, unaware that these may be dangerous for him. Talk to the doctor.

- Keep pills intended for emergencies in a place where they can easily be found by your parent, you, or some other caregiver.

- Never let your parent take a friend's pills, even if he has the same symptoms.

- If your parent has missed a dose, call the doctor or pharmacist to find out what to do.

- Don't crush or break a pill without first asking the pharmacist. You might destroy a coating designed to protect the stomach or upset the action of a time-released medication.

- Don't leave pills where a child can get them. Children are often poisoned by a grandparent's pills.

- Throw out drugs that are old or no longer needed.

- Know both the trade and generic name of medications so your parent is not mistakenly duplicating doses, especially if prescriptions are obtained from different sources.

symptom or says she just doesn't feel like herself, alert the doctor.

Questions for the Doctor

When your parent's doctor prescribes a new medication, learn all about it. Here are some questions to ask.

- What is this drug supposed to do? Is it treating the cause of the problem or only the symptoms? If it's the latter, is there any way to treat the cause?

- Is there another way to treat this problem (change in diet, exercise, or lifestyle)?

- Is it safe for my parent to take this, given her other medications and supplements?

- What is the proper dose for someone her age? (The elderly should start at very low doses—often one-quarter to one-half of that given to a younger or larger person—and then the dose can be gradually increased as needed.)

- What time or times of day should she take it?

- How should she take it? Should she take it with food or drink?

DANGEROUS DRUGS

Certain drugs are extremely dangerous for elderly people. Of particular note are "anticholinergic" drugs, which affect the brain chemical acetylcholine and cause confusion and hallucinations. Anticholinergic drugs include some commonly used antihistamines, muscle relaxants, sleeping pills, antidepressants, pain relievers, Parkinson's medications, and cardiac medications. Even over-the-counter anti-inflammatory medications, such as ibuprofen and naproxen, can cause serious side effects if taken on a regular basis.

If your parent takes one of these drugs, ask his doctor about it. Sometimes the benefits outweigh the risks, but other approaches should be tried first, and the drugs need to be carefully managed. Of course, your parent should not stop taking a drug without checking with the doctor first.

The Beers Criteria, put out by the American Geriatrics Society (AGS), lists drugs that should not be given to elderly patients or should be used with great caution. You can find the list at the AGS website, americangeriatrics.org, as well as at the AGS's consumer site, healthinaging.org.

- Should she avoid any particular foods, drinks, dietary supplements, or activities while taking it?

- What side effects or reactions should we watch for? What should I do if my parent has a bad reaction? (There may be trade-offs—for example, your parent may need to take a drug that worsens her confusion in order to get rid of the far more troubling hallucinations. Weigh the pros and cons.)

- How long does it take for this drug to have an effect? How will she know if it's working?

- Is there a goal (a particular blood pressure, for example) that she is trying to achieve?

- Should she continue to take it even after she feels better? If not, when should she stop taking it? (Your parent or you should check regularly with the doctor to find out if the drug is still needed or if the dose can be lowered.)

- What should my parent do if she misses a dose?

- Is it habit-forming?

- Is there an alternative that requires fewer doses each day (which might then be an easier regimen for your parent to follow)?

- Are there remedies that might counter expected side effects (such as stool softeners for constipation or the active cultures in yogurt to fight yeast infections)?

- Is there a generic version that is just as good as the brand name but less expensive?

> " My mom, who's always been one of the most chipper, upbeat people I know, became very depressed last fall. She was lethargic and mopey and didn't want to go out with her friends. On one visit I brought up the subject of her grand-daughter's upcoming wedding, knowing she'd been looking forward to it for a long time. She sort of shrugged and said she'd go 'If I'm still around.' That was so uncharacteristic of her that I urged her to see a doctor.
>
> He took her off the blood pressure pills that she'd been taking since she was 65—that's about 18 years. He said that age had changed her body chemistry, so he changed the medication and greatly reduced the dosage. And sure enough, as soon as her medication was adjusted, her spirits returned to normal. Not only did she get to the wedding but, as usual, she was the life of the party!"
>
> —Lorenzo R.

Questions for the Pharmacist

- How should this medication be stored? (Away from light? In the refrigerator?)

- If your parent has trouble swallowing, is there a way to get it down more easily? Is the medication available in liquid form, can the pills be crushed, or can a capsule be opened and the powder mixed with food to make it easier to swallow?

- If your parent has trouble seeing, does the pharmacist have large-print labels?

- Can you get the medication in easy-to-open bottles (without those darn childproof caps)?

- What is the expiration date?

- Is it possible to fill just half the pre-scription, to be sure there are no adverse effects, before paying for the entire bottle?

Check that you receive the right medication. Read the label and make sure both the patient's name and the drug name are correct. Some medication names differ by just a letter, and busy pharmacists have been known to dole out the wrong drug.

Keeping Tabs on Compliance

Most of us have trouble remembering to take medication, especially if the pills have no immediate effect, the symptoms are already gone, or the drugs have unpleasant side effects.

For the elderly, who have so many pill bottles and a tendency toward for-getfulness anyway, noncompliance is a serious problem.

Impress upon your parent the impor-tance of following instructions to treat

DRUG MONEY

Talk about sticker shock. Your parent's pharmacy bill might make you wonder what's in those little caplets. Truffles? To learn about programs that provide free and discounted drugs, go to benefitscheckup.org or medicare.gov. For more information about ways to save on medications, see page 347.

MEDICATIONS IN A NURSING HOME

If your parent is in a nursing home, be particularly vigilant about her medications. Nursing home residents take enormous amounts of medications, and there is evidence that many of these drugs are unnecessary or inappropriate. Given a resident's frail status, this is extremely risky.

Be sure that your parent is not being sedated as a way to dull aggressive or difficult behavior (or at least be sure that nondrug approaches have been tried first). Antipsychotics may be dangerous and are usually not terribly effective in nonpsychotic people. But they are often used, particularly when a person suffers from dementia. They can cause sedation, dizziness, restlessness, and confusion, as well as a muscular disorder that causes tremors, called tardive dyskinesia, which is often irreversible.

the illness completely and avoid complications. Just because she feels better doesn't mean she should stop.

If your parent insists everything is fine, but you are unsure whether she is taking her medications properly, check her pill bottles. Look at the prescription date and see if the appropriate number of pills have been taken. If things don't match up, she may be less able to manage her medications than you thought.

PILL REMINDERS

A number of gadgets remind people to take pills, but before you spend, try a little old-fashioned ingenuity. Keep pill bottles where they will be remembered (pills to be taken at bedtime might be placed on the toothbrush stand, and those to be taken in the morning, on the breakfast table). Label each pill bottle in large, bold letters: "Take one with breakfast" or "Take two before bed." And post a checklist so she can cross it off each time she takes one. You can also program her smartphone with reminders.

If she's taking numerous pills—and odds are that she is—buy her a pillbox. That might be a simple plastic box with multiple compartments, or you can buy an electronic pillbox that flashes or beeps when it's time to take a pill—and voilà, the pill pops out. Some models will send a text message to you if your parent skips a dose. (Of course, if between grabbing the pill and getting a glass of water she forgets to actually swallow it, you won't know.)

You can contract with a company to place automated phone calls at pill time (about $15 a month)—your parent has to respond that yes, she did indeed take her meds. Also, some emergency response companies have pill-reminder systems as part of the package.

You can buy an array of pill reminders and related paraphernalia at pharmacies, medical supply stores, or online. Be sure to get a device she can actually operate, as some have tiny buttons and print that will frustrate her no end.

When a revolving group of caregivers is dispensing your parent's medications, make a large chart, running from a.m. to p.m., listing what pills to take when. (See

page 641 for a sample chart.) If necessary, color-code the chart, matching the
color of the bottle or pill with a similar
color on the chart (*blue pills at two, white
pills at six, pink liquid at ten*, etc.), so there
is no confusion.

If worse comes to worst, call your
parent at pill time and have him take
his medicine while you wait on the
phone. Of course, if he's on a number
of medications, this will not be a lot of
fun for you.

Vision

You may be wearing (and forever
losing) your own set of reading
glasses, never mind hunting for your
mother's.

With time, the lens of the eye
becomes more rigid, making it hard
to see small print. But this presbyopia,
which sets in around 45, is just the beginning of the eyes' aging process.

Older eyes get weepy because they
are more sensitive to wind, temperature,
and light. This tearing can also be caused
by dryness (common) or an infection
(not common; requires medical help).

Older eyes also get dry because of
aging, medications, and certain medical conditions. Lubricating eye drops,
sometimes called artificial tears (not
saline solution or eye drops for redness), can help, but if dry eyes persist,
your parent should see an ophthalmologist; chronic dryness can lead to more
serious problems.

Floaters, those tiny specks that drift
across your field of vision, are generally
just annoying. They cannot be wiped
away because they are inside the eyeball.
If they are severe, your parent should

talk to an eye doctor, as floaters can be a
sign of more serious problems, like reti-
nal detachment.

➕ MEDICAL ALERT

The American Academy of Ophthalmology
recommends that people over 65 have
their eyes examined every two years,
or more often if a person has an eye
disease, a family history of eye disease,
or another risk factor, such as diabetes.
Your parent should see an eye doctor
immediately if:

- her vision becomes blurred or
  distorted, or she complains of
  "seeing double."

- she sees flashes of light or halos.

- her eyes are sore, swollen, or have
  unusual amounts of discharge.

- she has wandering or crossed eyes.

- she loses her peripheral vision or
  vision in one eye.

- she becomes acutely sensitive to
  light and glare.

A number of more subtle changes in vision typically occur late in life, changes that your parent may not be aware of, but that will make life harder.

Older eyes can't see well in dim light, are more easily blinded by glare, and can't refocus quickly from near to far or from light to dark. They also don't discriminate easily between colors and contrasts, such as the edge of a step, and they have trouble following moving objects, such as cars on the highway.

Even if your parent insists that her vision hasn't changed, assume that it has. Get her to a vision specialist for an eye exam, and compensate wherever you can around the house—making things brighter, adding contrast to steps, and getting rid of glare.

Eye Diseases

In addition to the normal vision changes that happen with age, there are four eye diseases that frequently afflict older people:

CATARACTS. More than half of people over age 65 have cataracts, although the symptoms are often mild. With age, areas in the transparent lens of the eye become cloudy, hindering vision, especially if the cataract is in the center of the lens.

Having cataracts is a little like viewing the world through a pair of fogged-up goggles, but the change happens so gradually that your parent may not realize anything is wrong. He might have trouble doing things and become frustrated and embarrassed because he doesn't understand why simple tasks have become difficult for him.

Although your parent might get by just fine using magnifiers and stronger lighting, he should talk to an ophthalmologist and, if possible, get the problem repaired sooner rather than later.

Cataracts will increase your parent's risk of falling and will affect his ability to drive, as they dull night vision and make the eyes sensitive to glare. Untreated, they can lead to blindness.

If that's not enough to send your parent to the ophthalmologist, a few intriguing studies suggest that cataracts hinder far more than vision. As the eye ages and clouds, it lets in less sunlight, which interferes with the body's natural circadian rhythm. Normally, when the sun comes up, our bodies release the hormone cortisol, making us feel chipper and alert, and then, as daylight dims, we release melatonin, making us

> When my mother's vision began to fade, she became depressed. She always loved to read, but that became more and more difficult until finally she couldn't do it at all. She started listening to the radio and watching television up close. But she missed her reading terribly.
>
> It was a nurse at the home who set her up with audiobooks. She listens for hours, and the funny thing is that she has expanded her reading repertoire. She used to just read mysteries. Now it's political books, biographies, racy romances, classical books, everything. She listened to a book last month about World War II planes, and she was telling us all about them. She's like a kid again, learning all this stuff."
>
> —Mel T.

feel droopy and ready for bed. Research suggests that when sunlight (particularly the blue light at the end of the spectrum that is blocked by cataracts) doesn't get through, that natural rhythm gets out of whack and people become prone to insomnia, memory loss, and depression, and possibly heart disease, diabetes, and cancer.

When cataracts are repaired (especially when lenses are replaced with intraocular lenses that allow this critical blue light to enter), people tend to sleep better, nap less, and have better reaction times and fewer falls.

For most people, cataract surgery is a relatively simple and painless procedure. It takes less than an hour, and your parent can return home the same day.

The eye takes about a month to heal fully and several more weeks to adjust. In the meantime, your parent can resume his regular daily activities, including driving, reading, and working, although he may have to wear large (and unglamorous) dark glasses to protect his eyes.

GLAUCOMA. People usually don't experience symptoms of glaucoma until the damage is done. An eye doctor can detect the problem early and treat it. But untreated, glaucoma can lead to partial or total blindness that cannot be reversed. Another good reason to get your parent (and yourself) to the ophthalmologist regularly!

For a variety of reasons, fluid inside the eyeball fails to drain adequately. It builds up until it squeezes the optic nerve in the back of the eye. Over time, the nerve is damaged irreversibly, which leads to vision loss or blindness.

> " My mom had cataract surgery, and at a follow-up visit the doctor gave her a prescription for new glasses. Her nursing home fills her prescriptions.
>
> A few weeks ago my mother told me that she was seeing double. We went to see the doctor who did the surgery and he was testing her eyes and he says, 'These aren't your glasses. This isn't the prescription I gave you.'
>
> The nursing home had given her her old prescription. They had the new one; they just didn't fill it. They said, 'Oh yeah. She needs the new one. But that will take four to six weeks.'
>
> I said, 'She got that prescription two months ago. She's seeing double. I want to talk to the head of nursing.'
>
> Finally they said, 'We're doing it today.'"
>
> —Maggie B.

Glaucoma tends to run in families and is more common among African Americans, people with diabetes or previous eye injuries, and people who have used steroids over an extended period of time.

When the trouble is spotted early, medications (oral medications or eye drops) can stop or slow the damage. If your parent is given medications for glaucoma, it is critical that she continue to use them even if she doesn't notice any change in her symptoms.

When medications don't help, doctors often recommend surgery to repair the eye's drainage system. Laser surgery, which can be performed in less than 20 minutes and is painless, is usually tried before traditional surgery.

MAKING THE WORLD MORE VISIBLE

Improve lighting

- Up the wattage, especially in stairways and places where your parent reads. Older people need nearly three times as much light as younger people. A 75-watt bulb placed one or two feet away is usually fine for reading, but try different intensities to see what's most comfortable for your parent. (A reading light should be positioned behind the shoulder on the same side as your parent's better eye.)

- Make sure light switches are accessible at the entrance to all rooms, and/or install lights that are triggered by movement.

- Put night-lights in the bedroom, hallways, and bathroom.

- Distribute light evenly (old eyes have trouble refocusing when going from light to dark).

Reduce glare

- Cover shiny surfaces and avoid waxy floors (which you should do anyway to prevent falls).

- Aim lights at a wall or ceiling to create indirect light.

- Add blinds or curtains to windows that tend to be filled with bright sunlight.

- Get your parent sunglasses (preferably polaroid) to cut down on glare and to protect her eyes.

Create contrast

- Use reflector tape or colored tape on the edges of stairs to make steps easier to see.

- Use dark dishes on a white countertop, or put white plates on dark mats. Put dark wallpaper behind a white toilet.

- If your parent's vision has grown quite poor, wear bright colors when you visit.

A few more tips

- Write notes in big, clear letters.

- Always place keys, eyeglasses, TV remotes and such in the same place, so they're easy to find.

- Use bright nail polish to mark dials on the stove, washing machine, and other appliances so she can clearly see the OFF position.

- If your parent's vision is very faint, encourage her to touch things—hold your hand, feel your face, or explore a new object with her hands.

MACULAR DEGENERATION. Or, more precisely, age-related macular degeneration, or AMD. This is a disease affecting the retina, a thin layer of cells lining the back of the eye, which converts visual images into electrical impulses and sends them on to the brain.

AMD occurs when the macula, the part of the retina responsible for seeing fine details, deteriorates. This slowly creates a blind or fuzzy spot in the center of one's vision. Straight lines might seem curved, and printed words may look disjointed.

Macular degeneration usually affects both eyes (sometimes one at a time) and worsens steadily until the blurry area completely blocks out, say, several words on a page—the very words the person is trying to read.

Most people have what's known as the "dry" form of AMD, which comes on slowly and is caused by deposits in the macula. The "wet" form is less common and more severe. Small blood vessels leak into the eye, and eventually a person can lose all central vision.

Age-related macular degeneration is the leading cause of severe vision loss among people over 60.

Your parent should get medical help early. Although there is no way to reverse the damage, there are ways to slow the disease. Certain supplements (vitamins C and E, beta-carotene, zinc, and copper) can slow the loss of vision, but your parent should talk to his eye doctor and his primary doctor before taking any supplements. In some severe cases, laser surgery can be helpful. Luckily, for those with the wet type of macular degeneration, the process may be slowed or halted by injections into the eye (this is not as scary as it sounds).

DIABETIC RETINOPATHY. The longer someone has diabetes, the greater chance he has of developing retinopathy. Essentially, blood vessels in the retina of the eye leak, blurring vision and, if left untreated, cause blindness.

The best prevention is proper care of the diabetes and annual eye exams. Laser treatment can often improve vision and slow the decline, or at least prevent blindness.

Low-Vision Aids

These days, low vision isn't as much of a problem as it used to be because computers can zoom, reading tablets can enlarge type, and goodness knows televisions are enormous.

In addition, a vast assortment of low-vision products can make the world more visible—from magnifying glasses, big-button phones, and large-print books, to watches that vibrate and computers that talk.

These products can be found in some medical supply stores, through company catalogs, or online. Search under "low vision aids" and you'll find dozens of companies.

The National Federation of the Blind (nfb.org) and Lighthouse International (lighthouse.org) have online shops. An eye doctor or other low-vision specialist can also guide your parent to appropriate aids.

Many companies have special services for people who are totally or partially blind. For example, some telephone companies provide dialing aids, free operator assistance, and a list of special products to people with vision or hearing disabilities. Other companies may be willing to send bills in large-print format (although it might be easier to get bills online and just zoom in).

Large-print books, magazines, newspapers, cards, games, calendars, and so on that are printed in 18-point type like this, for example, are a godsend. The local library and all major bookstores should have books in large print, as well as audiobooks that you can download or get on CD. Of course, the font in e-books that are read on a tablet (Kindle, Nook, or iPad, for example) can be enlarged as needed.

If the local library doesn't have much, the National Library Service for the Blind and Physically Handicapped (800-424-8567 or loc.gov/nls), which is part of the Library of Congress, lends audiobooks and magazines, as well as the equipment needed to play them, all for free. Postage is also free when returning equipment, tapes, or disks. Anyone with poor eyesight or a physical handicap that prevents him from holding a book or turning a page is eligible for these services.

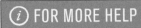

FOR MORE HELP

American Macular Degeneration Foundation
macular.org
888-622-8527

The Glaucoma Foundation
glaucomafoundation.org
212-285-0080

Lighthouse International
lighthouse.org
800-829-0500

National Eye Institute
nei.nih.gov
301-496-5248

National Federation of the Blind
nfb.org
410-659-9314

Hearing

Hearing loss among the elderly is a silent epidemic, so to speak. Statistics suggest that about half of people over 75 have trouble hearing. But very few—maybe 15 percent—of these people do anything about it. That means that millions of older people are walking around with little or no idea of what others are saying, even though help is available.

These people are not simply missing out on some interesting conversations; they can be shut out of life. Conversations become a chore and eventually, social gatherings, religious services, and movies are no longer fun. As a result, they begin to withdraw and often become isolated, irritable, and depressed.

Loss of hearing, and the social isolation and inactivity that accompanies it, can lead to physical decline, as well as delusions and other psychotic symptoms. Hearing loss also increases the risk of falling.

People with hearing loss can be misdiagnosed as having dementia. And

FEELING DIZZY

Up to 30 percent of elderly people feel dizzy frequently or regularly, making them even more prone to falls and more apt to avoid the sort of activity and exercise that might help them become more stable. Dizziness can also lead to social withdrawal, loss of independence, and depression.

Dizziness is an imprecise term, describing a number of sensations. Your parent might feel that the room is revolving or that she is tilting and unsteady, or she might feel light-headed and faint.

Whereas dizziness in a younger person is usually a symptom of a specific problem, in the elderly it can be the result of myriad diseases and impairments.

We feel balanced because numerous systems (cardiological, respiratory, psychological, auditory, visual, neurological, psychiatric, and chemical) are functioning properly. When any of these systems is out of whack, a person can end up feeling light-headed or dizzy.

Medications are a frequent cause of light-headedness or dizziness. This is especially true if the dizziness occurs within three minutes of getting up from a lying or sitting position. In addition, inner-ear disorders, infections, stroke, and head injuries can all contribute to dizziness.

Bring this to the doctor's attention. Even if one cause is treated, it should reduce the severity of the problem.

Consider getting your parent to use a cane. Get her to rise slowly from any chair or bed (as that can momentarily worsen the situation). Urge her to avoid caffeine, alcohol, and tobacco, which can all make things worse.

certainly, poor hearing will exacerbate any existing cognitive problems. If your parent is frequently saying, *But you never told me!* find out whether learing loss is the cause of the problem.

On the most basic level, it's dangerous. Your parent might not hear fire alarms, oncoming cars or honking horns, emergency sirens, or other alerts. He also might miss important information or misunderstand questions about medical problems or financial issues and then give answers that get him into trouble.

So, if your parent is saying *What?* a lot, insisting you never told him things, or nodding blankly, urge him to have his hearing checked by a doctor. Sometimes the problem can be treated—for example, if an infection, earwax, or another obstruction is found.

Even if the problem is not curable (which it typically isn't), all is not lost. Although it takes some effort, there are ways to communicate more clearly with your parent and a variety of devices that will help with hearing, phone calls, TV, and communication. An audiologist can measure your parent's hearing and suggest solutions.

You may not find an easy fix, but simply understanding the problem and finding small solutions—buying a phone amplifier, or learning to speak to your father only when he can see your face—should be an improvement for all involved.

MAKING THE WORLD MORE AUDIBLE

- Sit or stand within three feet of your parent when talking to him. (Don't yell to him from the kitchen.)

- Face your parent when you speak and be sure he is looking at you. (And make sure his good ear is aimed in your direction.)

- Sit in the spotlight. There should be ample lighting, and it should be aimed at you, the speaker.

- Don't put your hands over any part of your face while speaking.

- Turn off the television, the running water, or other background noise.

- Speak clearly. Don't try to talk to your parent while you are eating, chewing gum, or smoking. Enunciate clearly, but don't exaggerate the movement of your mouth, as that can make it difficult to read lips (which we all do a little, even without training).

- Speak loudly, but don't shout. Increase your volume slightly, without raising your pitch.

- Use simple and direct sentences. When you are asked to repeat something, rephrase it. Different words may be easier for your parent to grasp.

- Use body language (touching, pointing, nodding) and facial expressions.

- Introduce the subject matter before starting a conversation. *Dad, about Thanksgiving . . .* If you switch topics midway through a conversation, make that clear: *Okay, now let's talk about your friend Ralph. . . .*

- If you go to a restaurant, ask for the quietest table. Avoid tables near the kitchen. Better yet, choose restaurants that you know are quiet, or go at off times.

- Do not ignore your parent or talk about him as if he were not present. This will only make him withdraw.

Clarity, Not Volume

Your father sits stony-faced at the end of the dinner table, missing most of the conversation, but then insists that he does not *need* a hearing aid, that he can hear just fine, and that if you weren't such an incurable mumbler, there wouldn't be a problem.

When he asks you to repeat yourself, and you raise your voice, he gets perturbed. *Don't shout! I'm not deaf, you know.*

Quite often—especially if your parent has only mild or moderate hearing loss—the problem isn't that your parent can't hear what you're saying. He does hear. It's that he can't *understand* what you're saying. It's not simply volume, but clarity, that's diminished. Sounds are muffled, voices in a crowded room blur together, a quiet person is impossible to understand.

Suggestions that he have his hearing checked or get amplifiers for the phone and TV are dismissed because he knows he can hear. In addition, people often think their hearing is fine because the loss typically develops so gradually that it is almost imperceptible. People don't wake up one day and say, *Hey, I can't hear.* Over the years, they turn up the television, need things repeated, and seemingly forget much of what has been said (or insist that no one ever told them in the first place because, of course, they didn't catch it the first time around).

Raising the Subject

If your parent is missing what you've said and resisting all offers of help, then you may be at your wits' end. But stay calm and approach this gently because it's a sensitive subject.

Ask your father if he thinks there is a problem rather than telling him there is one. And avoid criticism or accusations: *You never hear what I'm saying. You're deaf as a post.* Let him know that you realize he can hear but are concerned about how often he doesn't grasp what's being said. Ask him to think about the television volume and how often he asks people to repeat things.

Explain what he is missing by not dealing with his hearing loss and what he stands to gain by addressing it. Urge him to at least talk to an audiologist to get the facts and to learn what the options are.

For the sake of peace, take a little of the blame. *Perhaps I'm not speaking clearly and I need to work on that. Let's approach this together.*

Presbycusis

More than 90 percent of hearing loss is the result of presbycusis, also referred to as sensorineural hearing loss, nerve deafness, or age-related hearing loss. Noise, diet, hypertension, infections, illness, head injury, genetics, and just plain time all play a role.

Again, people don't lose volume as much as they lose clarity, so often they aren't aware that they are losing their hearing. Higher-pitched sounds, in particular, can become fuzzy (making it harder to understand women and children), and consonants, such as *s, f,* and *z,* may be indistinguishable from one another.

Presbycusis also makes it difficult to filter out background noise, so your parent may have more trouble hearing a conversation in a room full of people or if the television is on.

Tinnitus

Tinnitus causes a ringing, buzzing, clicking, or hissing sound in the ear, which is not simply annoying; it can hinder hearing and make it almost impossible for some people to get through the day. It is caused by loud noise, medications, illness, allergies, and hearing loss itself.

If your parent has tinnitus, she should see her doctor to find out if it is caused by something that is treatable. If it's not treatable, an audiologist can help find ways to alleviate it. Often, several approaches work better than just one.

A tinnitus mask fits on the ear and emits a "white noise" to drown out or soften the humming. Or your parent can create her own white noise by turning on a fan or listening to the static of a radio or fuzzy television channel on low volume. "Bedside maskers" are little boxes that do basically the same thing. Better yet, buy her some nature recordings of ocean waves, birds calling, crickets chirping, or the wind blowing, which will not only help soften the buzzing, but might also be soothing.

Relaxation techniques (stress seems to worsen tinnitus) and biofeedback, in which a person learns to control certain bodily functions by becoming familiar with them, can be helpful. Some medications are also used to alleviate tinnitus.

If other hearing loss is involved, then a hearing aid can help with the hearing loss and also, by amplifying other sounds, ease some of the tinnitus.

Finally, antidepressants are sometimes needed to ease some of the depression and anxiety that often accompanies tinnitus.

Solutions

Although hearing aids might seem to be the obvious solution, they aren't perfect, they are expensive, and they certainly aren't right for everyone. If your parent's hearing loss is not severe (and a doctor has ruled out treatable conditions), a number of sound amplifiers and other gadgets can help.

New technology has allowed for some impressive devices, and a number of them are surprisingly inexpensive. In fact, while shopping for your dad, you might find something that helps you as well, as a number of these products are perfect for boomers who are teetering on the edge of hearing loss.

PERSONAL SOUND AMPLIFIERS

Personal sound amplification products, or PSAPs, are the latest and fastest-growing entries into the market. They are considered "electronics," not "medical devices," so they do not require a prescription and they do not fall under the purview of the FDA (as hearing aids

do). However, several of them act much like a hearing aid.

At the low end of the scale ($20 or so), simple amplifiers, sometimes referred to as "ear readers," increase volume, which isn't terribly helpful unless there are only two or three people in an otherwise quiet room, because all noise is amped up indiscriminately.

Smartphone apps (free or maybe $10 to $20; more for a wireless version) can turn a phone into an amplifier. Sound comes into the phone, is enhanced and improved (based on the user's hearing needs) and then picked up on the user's earphones.

For about $100 to $150 you can buy a simple device that amplifies nearby sound and filters out background noise. These "pocket talkers," as they are sometimes called, are about the size of a deck of cards and easy to use. Your father can pull it out of his pocket, place it on the dinner table, and slip on a small earphone.

On the pricier side ($300 and up, so still significantly cheaper than hearing aids), are sophisticated gadgets that cancel out background noise, have directional microphones, and offer a choice of channels for different environments (restaurants, theaters, libraries).

A number of other products amplify a particular sound for a particular person, such as televisions, radios, mobile phones, answering machines, computers, and almost anything else that involves noise. This way, your father can hear the television, but the neighbors don't have to.

ASSISTIVE LISTENING DEVICES

While these are often grouped together with PSAPs, "assistive listening devices" typically refer to systems that are used in large group situations, like theaters and lecture halls, and are used as an adjunct to a hearing aid.

Basically, these devices amplify a specific sound (actors in a movie or play, a speaker at a lecture, a sermon) while reducing the volume of the other noise in the room. By placing a microphone close to the sound source, the device focuses on one sound while filtering out others.

Some are meant to be used alone; others can be used with a hearing aid or cochlear implant, improving the performance of the aid. (Don't let your parent think that a hearing aid is all he needs; the combination of hearing aid and a listening device can greatly improve hearing.)

Most assistive listening devices fall into three categories: FM systems, which are like miniature radios; inductive loops, which transmit sounds using magnetic fields; and infrared systems, which use invisible infrared light to transmit sound. Most places that have such systems advertise it, but it's always worth checking.

OTHER GADGETS

When you are trying to communicate from afar, amplified phones are great, but for some people, texting or talking via video online (Skype, iChat, FaceTime) is easier because then your parent can see your expressions and, at least in a rudimentary way, read your lips, which helps piece together a conversation.

Instead of amplifying, some products provide a visual signal, such as flashing lights. (You can make them flash in different ways to differentiate the phone ringing from the doorbell buzzing, for example.) Others provide a tactile signal, such as a vibration (strong enough that he actually knows his cell phone is ringing). Some send a signal through the television, advising your parent that the phone is ringing and announcing who is calling, for example (which is actually helpful for anyone).

You can get alarm systems that use especially loud noises or flashing lights. If you do nothing else, be sure your parent can hear his smoke and carbon monoxide detectors.

Although many of these gadgets can be purchased online or through catalogs, it's best to buy any complex or expensive device in person, so your parent can get expert advice, see and discuss the options, and possibly even try out a product.

HEARING AIDS

Hearing aids are most useful to people with mild to moderate hearing loss in both ears. They are not necessary in very mild cases, and are not terribly successful when hearing loss is profound.

The move to hearing aids, with the stigma that is attached to them, may be a tough one. Your parent will likely resist this with his heels dug in. But don't give up easily, because hearing aids could reconnect him to his world, his friends, family, and interests.

If your parent tried hearing aids in the past, got frustrated, and dumped them in the toilet, urge him to try again. The digital ones used today are far from perfect, but they're better than the analog ones your parent probably tried back when.

While you plead and prod, be sympathetic to your father's distaste for this idea, his insistence that they don't work,

FINANCIAL AID

Although Medicaid and the VA cover the cost of hearing aids, Medicare does not. However, local organizations and civic groups will sometimes help with the cost if your parent is not quite eligible for Medicaid. Check with the local senior center or the Better Hearing Institute (betterhearing.org).

or his concern that he'll look like an old man. Show him that many hearing aids today are barely noticeable. And let him know that he looks older and more conspicuous when he's constantly asking people to repeat themselves, leaning forward with a hand cupped behind his ear, and dozing at the dinner table because he's out of the loop.

Once your parent agrees to try a hearing aid, his doctor should recommend someone to fit it for him—usually a certified audiologist or a licensed hearing aid dealer. You can also search at the American Academy of Audiology's consumer website (howsyourhearing.org) or the Academy of Doctors of Audiology (audiologist.org).

Be sure your parent sees someone who is experienced and reputable and will spend a lot of time with him, because he will be extremely frustrated if a hearing aid is not properly fitted or suited to him—and most hearing aids are not fitted properly. (That is, they are not fitted well in terms of how much sound is amplified, not in how they fit around the ear.)

A specialist should do a complete exam, including hearing tests and evaluations, and then discuss various kinds of hearing aids. He or she should take time to listen to your parent and understand his particular needs, as the best hearing aid for one person is not necessarily the best for another. Sometimes, an audiologist will let a person try a couple of options to see which one works best for him.

Models range from tiny ones that sit completely in the ear canal and are virtually invisible, to ones that fit in the bowl of the ear, to ones that curl around behind the ear. Most hearing aids sold today are extremely small because the technology is so advanced.

Although the smallest models are less visible, they are also typically more expensive and can be challenging for stiff fingers to handle.

Most hearing aids these days are digital—they convert sound waves into digital signals, analyze the environment, and reprogram themselves automatically. These offer more precision and less feedback and whistling than the old analog aids.

A hearing aid should have a directional microphone, which will amplify sound that's in front of you and not the sound coming from behind you. It should also have feedback suppression, and direct audio input, so it can be connected directly to a TV, CD player, or computer.

A hearing aid should also have a T-coil, or telecoil, which enhances telephone conversations and works with any theater or auditorium that is set up for hearing aids. Basically, a wire loop

> " One night I took my mother to see a show in New York, figuring that even if she couldn't hear everything, she would enjoy the colors and lights and dancing. They had these plug-in amplifying headphones, and it was a miracle. For the first time in years, she could hear everything. She lit up."
>
> —Will B.

around the periphery of the room picks up the sound and delivers it to the T-coil. Such a loop can also be easily installed in, say, your parent's living room so he can hear the TV clearly when it's at a normal volume.

When buying any hearing aid, your parent should shop around, because prices and service vary. Medicare does not cover the cost of hearing aids, and the newer ones can cost more than $5,000.

Although price is a pivotal factor, don't forget to shop for good service—personal attention, adjustments, warranties, repairs, and maintenance for the life of the aid. The aid should come with at least a 30-day trial period, during which your parent can return the device for a refund. (Most suppliers will charge a minimal service fee, and often the cost of testing and of any custom parts is not refundable.)

Unfortunately, a hearing aid is not like a pair of glasses. Your parent will not walk out of the shop, suddenly have clear hearing, and say, *Wow, this is great!* It takes time to adjust.

But if your parent gets the right device and some training, goes back for readjustments when necessary, and can

be persuaded to wear it for, say, three to six months to get used to it, it is likely that he will adopt it for good and it will change his world.

COCHLEAR IMPLANTS

For people who are profoundly deaf, cochlear implants can be the answer. However, they require surgery, are expensive, and require some training while a person learns to interpret the sounds created by the implant.

A cochlear implant is made up of three parts: a microphone, which picks up sound; a speech processor, which converts sound into electronic signals; and a receiver, which sends the signals to the brain. The microphone is worn behind the ear; the processor is about the size of a beeper and is carried in a pocket or slipped onto a belt; and the receiver is a disk about the size of a quarter, which is surgically implanted under the skin behind the ear.

ⓘ FOR MORE HELP

Hearing Loss Association of America
hearingloss.org
301-657-2248

American Tinnitus Association
ata.org
800-634-8978

National Institute on Deafness and Other Communication Disorders
www.nidcd.nih.gov
800-241-1044

Better Hearing Institute
betterhearing.org
800-327-9355

Whereas hearing aids amplify sound, implants actually compensate for damage to the ear, replicating what an ear normally does—convert sound waves into electrical impulses and send them to the brain, where they are recognizable. Still, an implant does not replicate that process perfectly, and the sound is not what it would be normally.

Sleep

S leep, oh wonderful, wonderful sleep! It's an elusive state for many older people. More than a third of all elderly people say they have trouble getting to sleep and staying there. (Of course, we caregivers are also staring at the clock at 2 a.m., so read on.)

Although some sleeplessness is a result of the hormonal changes that come with age—for example, people often produce less melatonin, the hormone that helps us fall asleep—most serious sleep problems are caused not so much by aging itself as the ailments and habits that come with age: pain, illness, medications, depression, inactivity, and, particularly in men with prostate troubles, the need to urinate at night.

Heart disease, lung disease, or cancer will certainly turn daily patterns upside down. And dementia, which upsets a person's 24-hour clock, can drive wake-sleep patterns completely out of kilter. (See page 507 for more on dementia and sleep.)

But simply being less physically active, and spending the day sitting in an armchair, watching TV, and nodding off from time to time will lead to insomnia.

Having caffeine in the morning to stay awake and then a couple of drinks in the evening to help you drift off only exacerbates the problem.

If your parent complains of insomnia, be sure his assessment is correct. Sometimes people have misconceptions about sleep, believing they need more than they do. If your dad is dozing during the day, then he might need less sleep at night.

Not sleeping, whatever the underlying cause, can plunge your parent into a downward tailspin. Worrying about sleep is the surest way to stay awake. Alcohol, sleeping pills, napping, and going to bed early or lounging about in the morning—all intended to make resting more restful—just make matters worse.

Lack of sleep is associated with falls, confusion, depression, and forgetfulness. It will make both of you grumpy, distracted, and susceptible to illness.

Good Zzzzzs

If your parent isn't sleeping well, or if you are the one flopping about at 2 a.m., first check with the doctor to see if any underlying illnesses or medications are getting in the way of sleep. In addition to the aforementioned ailments, pain relievers, cold medicine, and medications for heart disease, inflammation, asthma, and Parkinson's all disrupt sleep. If your parent can't go without a particular medication, then see if it can be taken earlier in the day, the prescription can be changed, or the dose can be reduced.

Although they are tempting, avoid sleeping pills, or use them very, very sparingly. Instead, try these remedies, which will be more effective (and have no side effects). They won't work immediately—know that going in—but should be successful if your parent (or you) sticks with them.

GET PLENTY OF SUNSHINE during the day, or use a sunlamp. Broad-spectrum light triggers hormones that help maintain the body's internal clock.

EXERCISE, the elixir for so many problems, is a great antidote for insomnia. A brisk walk in the fresh air is sure to help with sleep problems. Exercising near bedtime, however, may only worsen the insomnia.

STICK TO A ROUTINE of going to bed and getting up at the same time each day, which will help regulate the body's clock.

ENGAGE IN A PRE-BED RITUAL. Bathing, reading, or listening to music may help your parent unwind and get her body in the mood for sleep. She should not discuss stressful topics, play competitive games, or watch upsetting late-night television just before bed.

AVOID "SCREENS" BEFORE BED. Computers, smartphones, tablets, and the like seem like nice bed companions, but the glowing "blue light" emitted by these devices interferes with the body's natural release of melatonin. Although TVs also emit blue light and can interfere with sleep, the effect is not generally as pronounced because people tend to sit farther from the TV.

ASSOCIATE THE BED WITH SLEEP. When sleep doesn't come after, say, 15 or 20 minutes, or if your parent is wakeful in the middle of the night, she should get up and read or knit or do something else, rather than lie in bed worrying about sleep.

STAY AWAKE. Seems like odd advice, but dozing off all day makes sleeping at night that much more difficult. Naps should be avoided, or if they can't be avoided, they should be limited to no more than one 30-minute nap each day. Naps taken around the middle of the day, about 2 or 3 p.m., are okay, but if your parent is nodding off in the late afternoon or early evening, it will definitely interfere with a good night's rest.

GET UP. Again, less time in bed will mean more productive sleep at night. When morning comes, get up and out. Making up for a poor night's sleep by lounging in bed all morning is counterproductive.

USE THE BATHROOM right before going to bed and limit fluids late in the evening.

RESERVE THE BEDROOM FOR SLEEP. Your parent (and you) shouldn't be getting in bed at 8 p.m. to read or watch television for an hour or two before turning the light out. She should wait until she is ready to sleep before she goes to bed.

MAKE THE BEDROOM CONDUCIVE TO SLEEP. It should feel safe, comfortable, and familiar. It should be dark (but leave a night-light on if your parent is apt to get up in the night), cool, and quiet. When noises are unavoidable, turn on some "white" noise, such as a fan, to cover up more intermittent noises. Make sure she has a supportive, comfortable mattress and good pillows.

KEEP DINNER LIGHT, low-fat, and not excessively spicy, and it should be served several hours before bedtime. It's fine for your parent to have a snack before bed if she is apt to be awakened by hunger. A glass of warm milk just before climbing under the covers helps some people sleep.

FORGO TOBACCO, ALCOHOL, AND CAF-FEINE, as they interfere with normal sleeping patterns. Caffeine, a stimulant, is obviously a bad idea. And although a stiff drink in the evening helps people relax, it also keeps them from falling into the deepest phases of sleep and causes them to wake in the middle of the night as the effects of the alcohol wear off. Nicotine is also a stimulant.

TRY RELAXATION. Buy your parent a soothing recording or teach her some relaxation techniques.

IF NONE OF THIS WORKS, ask the doctor for a referral to a sleep specialist. You can also get referrals from the National Sleep Foundation at sleepfoundation.org.

Sleeping Pills

Sleep medications, including over-the-counter versions, should be used only as a last resort, for no more than a few days at a time, and always under a doctor's guidance. Really.

Sleeping pills and anti-anxiety medications (Ambien, Sonata, Lunesta, Atican, Klonopin, Xanax, Valium) are known to increase the risk of falls and accidents, and to impair memory and judgment. If someone has dementia, such pills are apt to worsen the confusion.

Over-the-counter sleeps aids make you sleepy, but you don't get high-quality sleep. You think you slept beautifully but may feel oddly tired and "off" much of the day. They can cause other side effects as well, such as urinary problems and confusion.

Sleep Disorders

Our brains include an amazing biological clock that triggers the release of melatonin in the evening, which makes us sleepy, and cortisol in the morning, which makes us alert and ready to face the day. It's shockingly regular and accurate.

ⓘ FOR MORE HELP

American Sleep Association
sleepassociation.org

The National Sleep Foundation
sleepfoundation.org
703-243-1697

Willis-Ekbom Disease Foundation (formerly Restless Legs Syndrome Foundation)
rls.org
507-287-6465

American Sleep Apnea Association
sleepapnea.org
888-293-3650

This magical internal clock requires sunlight and activity, followed by dimming light and less activity. When we mess up that pattern—when someone is in a nursing home with few windows in the middle of the day or stares into the bright light of a computer at 10 p.m.—the clock runs amok and all bets are off.

As noted, medications, alcohol, illness, and pain also gum up the machinery. Grief and anxiety obviously play a part, but usually for a short period.

In addition, two common sleep disorders affect the elderly:

RESTLESS LEG SYNDROME. RLS causes a person's legs to feel fidgety, tingly, and eager to run or move—unfortunately, just as one is trying to fall asleep.

In a related disorder—periodic limb movement—the limbs jerk involuntarily after a person has fallen asleep, disturbing rest but not waking the person fully. The movements last for only a few seconds, but can recur often, every thirty seconds or so. (Periodic leg movements may disturb a spouse's sleep as well, so both your parents may be tired during the day. If so, they should move into separate beds.)

It's not clear what causes these syndromes, but they do have a genetic component. So if your mother is affected, you might well be, too. Caffeine, iron deficiency, stress, and certain diseases and medications all seem to play a role.

To ease the symptoms, try these tips:

• Limit, or better yet, avoid caffeine, tobacco, and alcohol.

• In case of iron or vitamin B12 deficiency, try supplements.

• Be wary of certain medications that can make RLS worse, such as those used to treat colds, depression, allergies, high blood pressure, and nausea.

• Massage the legs, stretch, use hot or cold compresses (or alternate them), or take a warm bath before bed. People find different approaches work for them.

• Exercise (but not right before bed).

• Try relaxation techniques, like meditation, yoga, or slow, deep breathing.

• Find activities that take your parent's mind off the RLS.

• Sometimes ibuprofen (Motrin, Advil) helps.

Although severe cases of RLS can be treated with medications, drugs should be a last resort and used only under the supervision of a doctor.

When restless leg syndrome is accompanied by periodic limb movement, as it often is, and your parent is not helped by other methods, doctors sometimes prescribe "transcutaneous electric nerve stimulation," in which electric stimulation is applied to the legs for 15 to 30 minutes just before going to bed.

SNORING AND SLEEP APNEA. If your father is snoring like a rhino all night and snoozing in his recliner all day, it's more than a mere irritation. It's potentially life-threatening for him, not to mention that he's probably keeping everyone else in the house awake.

For various reasons, some people stop breathing for a moment (usually 15 to 30 seconds) repeatedly through

HYPERTENSION

Your parent doesn't need to wait for the doctor to tell him that he has high blood pressure, or hypertension, to start doing something about it. Most older people have it, and the lifestyle changes one should adopt to lower blood pressure—stop smoking, lose weight, exercise, cut back on alcohol, cut back on salt—are good for everyone.

High blood pressure means that the heart is working hard—too hard—to force blood around the body. This undue force increases the risk of stroke and heart disease, as well as kidney disease, blindness, and other diseases.

If lifestyle changes alone don't do the trick (and be sure to give these a wholehearted effort—pun unintended), your parent's doctor will prescribe drugs. Often two or more are needed to bring blood pressure down significantly. Be sure your parent takes these as directed and, if he has trouble with side effects, see if the doctor can't modify the dose or the drug.

the night. The sleeper is jarred awake as he gasps for breath, but the awakenings are so brief that he usually isn't aware of them.

Obstructive sleep apnea, which is most common in overweight men, is often caused by an obstruction in the airway—the muscles in the throat relax and block the airway—so that air cannot flow out of the nose or mouth.

In a less common type of sleep apnea, called central sleep apnea, the brain fails to regulate breathing properly during sleep.

In some cases, people stop breathing 20 or 30 times per hour, leaving them exhausted the next day. They often have headaches in the morning and, with time, can develop high blood pressure, depression, irritability, and memory problems. Apnea also increases the risk of heart attack and stroke.

The most obvious symptoms are loud snoring and daytime fatigue. To get apnea diagnosed with certainty, however, your parent should visit a sleep clinic.

Apnea can be relieved through weight loss and avoiding (or at least limiting) alcohol, tobacco, and sleeping pills (sleeping pills make it more likely that the airways will collapse at night). Pillows can be used to keep the sleeper on his side, rather than his back.

Treatment commonly includes the use of an air pressure mask, called a CPAP (for continuous positive airway pressure). The mask is worn over the nose, and air is forced into the nasal passages to prevent the airway from closing.

Dental appliances are sometimes used to reposition the lower jaw. In extreme cases, doctors may recommend surgery to remove excessive tissue and increase the size of the airway.

If your father is keeping your mother awake, encourage one of them to sleep elsewhere until a solution is found. She needs her sleep!

Your Sleep

The work of caregiving, along with the worries and anxiety, all disrupt sleep. *Did I call the pharmacy? I don't trust that new aide. I've got to get grab bars installed. Why can't I sleep? I've got to get some sleep. Did Dad take his medication tonight? I can't remember. Maybe I should get up and check. No, I need sleep. I've got to get some sleep.*

Unfortunately, all the things that hinder sleep are particularly attractive now. After a long, long day, an extra glass of wine and an hour at the computer, and perhaps just a few more cookies, might seem like just the things you need, but fight the urge. They aren't helping. Sorry. But good sleep hygiene (see page 216) will help you sleep, which will reduce the stress, which will lead to even better sleep.

Of course, it might be your mother's lack of sleep that's keeping you and everyone else in the household awake. If she is pacing, tossing about, or wanting a snack at 3 a.m., no one will sleep well. And tiptoeing around in the middle of the day because she's finally conked out in the living room is not fun either.

Try the tips listed earlier in the chapter, and be sure your parent's room is set up so she can get whatever she needs— glass of water on the bedside table, a commode by the bed, and so on. Stop the napping by whatever means possible, and get her to get some fresh air and exercise.

If nothing helps, you may have to put your needs above hers. As a caregiver, you are pushed to your limit during the day; you desperately need your sleep at night.

Talk to her doctor. If nothing works, discuss the possibility of getting sleeping pills for her. Although it's far from ideal and careful monitoring is required, it might be necessary to take drastic steps so that the rest of the family can sleep.

If this is not medically advisable, consider hiring someone to cover for you during some evenings; alternatively, you may have to start looking into other housing options for your parent.

Temperature Regulation

Older people can become severely chilled simply sleeping in a cool room, or dangerously overheated in temperatures that the rest of us find quite comfortable.

Much of the problem is biological. Older bodies often have less protective fat and aren't as adept at constricting and dilating blood vessels, or shivering and sweating. Disease can further weaken the body's ability to warm or cool itself.

Also, in certain situations, an elderly brain, especially if it's confused, may fail to get the message that the body is too cold or too hot. As a result, your parent might stay out in the hot sun for too

RECOGNIZING A TEMPERATURE CRISIS

WARNING: Hyperthermia and hypothermia are medical emergencies that require immediate medical attention.

SIGNS AND SYMPTOMS	WHAT TO DO
Hyperthermia/ Heat Exhaustion Clammy, pale skin Heavy sweating Dizziness Weakness Nausea Headache Cramps Chills Rapid, shallow breathing Swelling of ankles and feet	Get your parent to a cool room or shaded area. Make him lie down, with his feet raised about 12 inches. Remove or loosen clothing and sponge his forehead and body with cool (not cold) water. Give him water or a sports drink. Do not bring his temperature down too quickly. Call the doctor.
Heatstroke Hot, dry, red skin No sweat Rapid pulse Body temperature above 104°F Unconsciousness or confusion	Get medical attention immediately. While waiting, keep your parent in a sitting position. Sponge him off and wrap him in a cool (not cold), wet sheet. Give him plenty of water. Do not bring his temperature down too quickly (because it can cause a heart attack) or overcool him.
Hypothermia Listless or drowsy Pale complexion Confusion Slow, shallow breathing Slurred speech Stiff movements Shivering (but not necessarily) Weak pulse Body temperature below 95°F Finally, unconsciousness	Get medical atttention immediately. While you are waiting (turn off any air conditioner or fan, of course), turn up the heat or move your parent to a warmer room. Do not warm him too quickly. Get him into sweaters and a hat and under blankets, or lie close to him and share your body heat. Do not rub him, however, because you might actually injure him. Offer warm (not hot) fluids. Do not let him go to sleep.

long, or fail to use a blanket on a cool night.

Some of the problem is also practical. If your father has a disability or painful ailment, he might not want to pull himself up out of a chair to get a sweater or to move into another room that's cooler. Or, in an attempt to save money, your parent may keep the thermostat low or forgo air-conditioning.

So when the snow is falling or the mercury is rising, remind your parent to dress accordingly and protect himself. When you are nearby, be aware of his comfort. It might seem silly, but this is serious stuff.

As a summer day heats up, give him plenty of cool drinks. He should avoid strenuous or prolonged physical activity and, obviously, long stretches in the sun. If he doesn't have an air conditioner or fan, get one. Contact the area agency on aging or local senior center about programs to help people pay for air conditioners.

If an air conditioner isn't possible for some reason, create as much ventilation as possible by opening windows and doors. Keep direct sunlight out with

> " When my father was very sick, near the end of his life, he was always freezing. I bought him arctic expedition long underwear. He lived in them day and night."
> —Charlie D.

curtains or shades. If his apartment is hot, your parent should spend the hottest part of the day elsewhere—in an air-conditioned library, mall, or senior center.

In winter, his house should be kept no cooler than 68°F. Be sure there are plenty of blankets, slippers, sweaters, long underwear, and hats on hand. Your parent might wear a light hat to bed.

Hyperthermia (when the body's temperature gets too high) and hypothermia (when it gets too low) are both medical emergencies. They are particularly worrisome in people who have dementia, stroke, or other neurological disorders, thyroid disorders, Parkinson's disease, diabetes, or cardiovascular disease, or are taking medications that make the body's temperature fluctuate. So be on the alert for symptoms.

Dehydration

Normally when a body is low on fluids, the kidneys go into emergency mode and hold on to water, and the brain screams out, *I'm thirsty. I need water. Now.*

But older kidneys are less efficient at conserving fluids, and the brain may not be receiving the kidneys' SOS cry, especially if a person suffers from dementia. And even when the message does get confused, tired, light-headed, and faint as his body dries out. Despite all this, or perhaps because of the confusion, he still might be completely unaware that he needs water.

Over time, ignoring the body's need for fluids can cause bowel problems, kidney trouble, urinary tract infections, and delirium.

Get your father to keep a glass of water (or some other noncaffeinated fluid) nearby at all times, and urge him to sip from it as often as possible. Unless the doctor wants your father to cut down on fluids for medical reasons, it is not possible for him to drink too much water.

Although people will tell you he has to drink eight glasses a day, the best indicator of whether he's drinking enough is the color of his urine. Dark yellow = not enough. Clear = perfect.

through, a person with a stiff knee or bad back might decide that a trip to the tap is not worth the effort.

As a result, an older person can become dehydrated easily and grow

Make sure that he isn't limiting his drinking because of incontinence. Consuming less water won't help; it will only cause new problems.

Skin Care

S kin announces the onset of old age with cracks, wrinkles, and spots long before any of us are ready for it, but usually the sags and blemishes are simply ego deflators, caused not simply by age, but by all that time in the glorious sun. When we become quite old, however, skin problems are no longer simple issues of vanity.

Older skin is thinner and less oily, so it tends to be drier and more susceptible to bruises, infections, and rashes. When injured, it doesn't heal as quickly as it once did, and minor irritations can become serious wounds. In other words, your parent's skin needs extra TLC.

The three most common skin problems facing the elderly, aside from skin cancer, are itchiness, bedsores, and fungal infections.

Itchy, Dry Skin

Dry skin is the most common skin complaint, especially in the winter when the air is less humid. It may not seem particularly important in the overall scheme of things, but severely itchy skin (known as pruritus) can be horribly annoying and, over time, make your parent irritable, weary, and tired (if it's hindering sleep).

Here are some ways your parent can ease the dryness and the itch:

- Take fewer showers or baths (two or three a week is fine) and keep them short and not too hot. Water and heat draw moisture away from the skin. Hot water is more irritating than warm.

- Use a minimal amount of soap, which removes the skin's natural oils.

- Avoid soaps containing alcohol, which is drying. Instead, use cleansers that contain glycerin, sunflower oil, or soybean oil (Dove and Olay both make emollient-rich cleansers), and then rinse well.

- Avoid deodorants and perfumed soaps, which contain chemical irritants.

- Avoid scrubbing harshly. Use a soft cloth or natural sponge instead of a brush or rough washcloth.

- Moisturize. After a bath or shower, your parent should pat his skin dry gently, leaving it moist, and then immediately apply a moisturizer. Find a moisturizer with petrolatum high on the list of ingredients. (Your father may not be in the habit of using lotion, but buy an unscented one and give him a nudge.)

- If your parent takes baths, she can add cornstarch or colloidal oatmeal to the tub water. Bath oils are lovely but use them sparingly because oily feet might make her fall and oily hands might lose their hold on any counter or grab bar.

- Apply pure petroleum jelly to very dry areas after a bath or shower. Your parent might wear pajamas, socks, or something else to protect clothing or sheets from the grease.

- Avoid bleaches, fabric softeners, and heavily perfumed detergents, which can irritate skin.

- Get your parent to wear cotton, which is less irritating than wool or synthetics.

- A humidifier will put moisture into dry winter air. But change the water regularly and keep the unit clean, as it can breed bacteria and other germs. Best bet: Get a humidifier installed as part of the heating system, if possible.

- Be sure your parent drinks lots of fluids.

- Steer him away from alcohol, spicy foods, tobacco, and caffeine.

- If itching becomes severe, try calamine lotion, cold compresses, or cortisone creams. Urge your parent to control his scratching (short fingernails and/or gloves will help), which may only aggravate the itch.

- If your parent's itching or dryness is severe and doesn't let up, or if itching becomes a nervous habit and is causing sores and bleeding, be sure he sees his doctor or a dermatologist.

Bedsores

Bedsores are a threat anytime your parent spends most of her time in bed or in a chair. The elderly are particularly susceptible to bedsores because their skin is thin and their circulation weak. Continuous pressure on a bony area, such as the heel, elbow, back of the head, or buttocks, blocks the flow of blood, which damages the skin and tissue, causing redness, blisters, or open sores.

Unfortunately, once again, you need to be vigilant. Don't assume the nursing home or hospital staff will be on top of this. Ask early on how they will prevent bedsores, and then keep your eye on it. If your parent is at home, this job might very well fall on you.

Some ways to prevent bedsores:

- If your parent is bedridden, he should be repositioned every hour or two, or should shift himself regularly if possible. Move him gently, because even being pulled across the sheets can harm his tender skin. Use pillows to raise his heels or elbows off the bed, or to relieve the pressure on his buttocks, hips, and knees.

- Get your parent to stand up, sit in a chair, or move about if he can. If he can't, get him to wiggle his toes, flex his arms, jiggle his legs, and rotate his neck—whatever movement is possible—to keep the blood flowing. This should help prevent not only bedsores, but also blood clots, which can form when the body is still.

- Be sure your parent's skin is clean and dry, as moisture adds to the risk of bedsores. His sheets should be changed regularly, especially if he is incontinent or sweaty.

- Dry is good, but not too dry, so a little lotion might also be necessary (consider giving him a gentle massage as you rub it on).

- If your parent is spending a majority of his time in bed, he should have a specialty mattress with alternating air pressure pockets. These can usually be obtained through Medicare, as can an electric hospital bed, which will make it easier to change his position.

- Likewise, special cushions—air, foam, gel—are available for wheelchairs. High-tech chairs tilt regularly to redistribute pressure points.

- If he's in bed, elevate your parent's head only slightly, because when the head is raised high, it puts pressure on the back.

- Pads of sheepskin or foam will help protect elbows, heels, and other vulnerable areas. You can also buy small trapeze-like gadgets that hold the feet up off the bed.

- Gentle massage will stimulate circulation (and is wonderful for physical and emotional comfort). But don't massage areas that have become slightly red, because the friction can damage the skin even more.

- At the first sign of any redness, alert a doctor or nurse. Untreated, bedsores can become infected and life-threatening.

ON THE ALERT FOR SKIN CANCER

Blemishes, warts, freckles, skin tags (tiny flesh-colored or brown flaps of skin), red dots, moles, and other markings are part of old age. Most are harmless results of sun damage and the aging process, but keep a watchful eye, especially if there is no spouse around who can check your parent's body.

Any moles or other markings that appear suddenly or grow rapidly, are larger than one-quarter of an inch across, bleed, or look unusual (for example, pearly round spots, gritty red patches, or irregularly shaped dark moles) could suggest skin cancer and should be seen immediately by your parent's doctor or her dermatologist.

A skin exam should be part of every physical, but because some doctors overlook this, it's worthwhile to ask if he or she will inspect your parent's skin. If anything seems suspicious, the doctor will refer your parent to a dermatologist. If your parent has a history of skin cancer, she should see a dermatologist regularly.

Fungal Infections

Fungal infections can crop up if your parent's immune system is weak or his circulation poor, if he has diabetes, or if he takes antibiotics or corticosteroid drugs.

Fungus grows in warm, moist pockets of the body, like armpits, under the breasts, skin folds, genitals, the scalp, the mouth, and the spaces around nails and between toes. It causes itchy, cracked skin, which can become infected. If your parent has a fungal infection, she should talk with her doctor. In the meantime, here are some ways to prevent or help get rid of fungal infections:

- Keep skin clean and dry. Use a hair dryer on a cool setting to dry hard-to-reach places.

- Wear loose cotton clothing, including underwear and socks (synthetics don't let air circulate as well). Avoid pantyhose.

- Change shoes and socks once or twice a day and, if possible, wear sandals or shoes made of mesh or woven fabric that lets air circulate.

- Use over-the-counter antifungal cream or powder.

Shingles

Shingles, or herpes zoster, is a disease of the nervous system that affects the skin. It is caused by the same virus that causes chicken pox. Small amounts of the virus sit dormant in the nervous system for years and then, because of a weakened immune system, stress, or illness, the virus is revived.

The virus travels along the nerves toward the skin, causing fatigue, headaches, and chills several days before the disease is visible—symptoms that can lead to misdiagnosis. Then, as with chicken pox, small blisters appear, but usually only on one patch of the skin, not over the whole body.

When the blisters open, shingles is extremely painful and debilitating, and the skin can continue to be sensitive for two to four weeks after the blisters have healed. Shingles may be so painful that your parent has trouble getting through her day and sleeping at night.

Antiviral drugs should be started immediately, as they can affect both the severity and duration of the outbreak. Nonsteroidal anti-inflammatory drugs (aspirin, ibuprofen, naproxen) will often ease the symptoms, as will a cool compress.

If shingles affects the eyes, it can cause blindness. Some people have neurological problems or pain that lasts long after the blisters have healed.

The good news is that a vaccine for shingles is reasonably effective and recommended for everyone over 60.

Skin Infections

A variety of skin infections are common in older people who are ill and quite frail, especially those who have poor circulation, diabetes, or edema.

The two most common skin infections—cellulitis and erysipelas—often start at the site of a scratch or wound, and grow into a red rash that is tender and warm to the touch. Erysipelas is often found on the face, has well-defined borders, can cause flulike symptoms, and can lead to serious eye problems as well as blood poisoning or clotting. Either type of infection requires a doctor's immediate attention.

Other Skin Issues

INTERTRIGO is an angry red inflammation that is caused by friction when the skin rubs against clothing or itself—for example, in the groin, under the armpits, between toes, or between folds of skin. Untreated, it can lead to oozing sores and bleeding.

It is best to avoid intertrigo in the first place by keeping these areas clean and dry, using powders if necessary, and wearing loose clothing. Once established, intertrigo can be treated with medication.

BRUISING is common in the elderly, even when they haven't banged into anything, because the walls of the blood vessels are so thin.

Avoid Motrin, Aleve, Advil, and other nonsteroidal anti-inflammatories, which can increase bruising. A cold compress might help reduce inflammation. If a bruise is excessive or if your parent is getting lots of bruises, talk to her doctor.

Also, be attuned to signs of abuse.

MEDICATIONS can cause swelling, burning, itching, blisters, allergic reactions such as hives or rashes, and a heightened sensitivity to the sun (unusual burning or staining after being in the sun). The

➕ ITCHING ALERT

If itching comes on suddenly and severely, it may be the result of a disease, such as kidney or liver disease, gallstones, or thyroid disorders. Severe itching on the hands, wrists, underarms, abdomen, and groin may be the sign of mites (scabies), which are found more often in people staying in a hospital or nursing home, and are usually treated with prescription medications (scabicides). Either situation should be checked by a doctor.

doctor may be able to change the medication, lower the dosage, or, at the very least, treat the reaction.

Such reactions may occur after your parent has stopped taking a medication, so keep those medication records handy.

Whether or not she is using medications, your parent should wear sunscreen (SPF 15 or higher) anytime she is in the sun for more than a few minutes.

Arms, Legs, and Feet

STASIS DERMATITIS. When fluids accumulate in the limbs it causes swelling. The skin becomes cracked and discolored, and varicose veins may appear.

Your parent should see her doctor because the problem can become severe. Treatment involves reducing pressure in the veins by using support stockings, elevating the legs, and, in some cases, using ointments to reduce the itching.

VARICOSE VEINS. The bulging blue veins that squiggle down your mother's leg aren't dangerous but they can be painful. Veins become distended because the valves that are supposed to keep blood that's supposed to be flowing up from draining down don't work. Blood headed for the heart flows back down the leg. Your mother should avoid standing for long periods of time and lie down from time to time with her feet elevated. Support hose (available from a medical supply store) should also help.

FOOT TROUBLES. After 70 or 80 years of pounding, stamping, and stomping, feet get pretty worn out, but caregivers and doctors alike often neglect them. Goodness knows, they aren't much to look at. But without proper care, the various calluses, corns, bunions, infections, and other sores that develop can become severe and make it difficult and sometimes impossible for your parent to get around. Make sure that your parent's feet are cared for (see box on next page).

PERIPHERAL ARTERY DISEASE (PAD). Although everyone talks about blocked and narrowed arteries leading to the heart, other arteries can also be damaged, preventing adequate blood flow, usually to the legs. In fact, PAD is common, can be dangerous, and is often undiagnosed or untreated in the elderly.

Sometimes a person's calf hurts when he walks, he has sores that fail to heal, or his leg or foot feels numb and cold.

Risk factors include old age, cigarette smoking, diabetes, high blood pressure, and obesity. Treatment usually begins with exercise, quitting tobacco, and weight loss, when necessary. Foot care is important. Medications may be necessary.

TLC FOR LEGS AND FEET

- It seems silly, but be sure your parent is wearing the right size shoes. Most elderly people wear shoes that are too small, causing untold problems. People think they know their shoe size, but feet expand with age (or, to be more accurate, the arch lowers and the feet flatten). Those 10-year-old shoes? Out with them!

- Shoes should have low or no heels, firm soles, good support, and preferably a wide cut across the toes.

- Your parent should rest with the legs elevated and avoid long periods of standing or sitting with crossed legs.

- Wash feet daily with mild soap and warm water, rinse, and towel dry, being sure to dry between the toes.

- Rub lanolin or lotion containing petrolatum on dry feet or skin.

- Keep feet warm and dry. Wear shoes made of a material that lets air flow (cotton, mesh, or real leather) and use cotton or wool socks—no synthetics,

please. Change socks as often as necessary to keep feet dry and clean.

- Walking or other exercise and foot and leg massages all improve blood flow.

- A warm foot bath is soothing for the soul as well as the soles.

- Keep toenails trimmed, straight across, to avoid ingrown nails.

- Never cut or shave off corns. Over-the-counter medications may help, but they can also burn the skin, so use them cautiously. Small, doughnut-shaped pads can relieve some of the pressure on corns. If they reappear, consult a doctor.

- Check feet regularly for cuts, infections, bumps, discoloration, bruises, and other signs of trouble. (Get your parent to take his shoes off for the doctor.)

- If your parent has diabetes, her feet will require special attention, as diabetes affects blood flow and puts the feet at extra risk of infections.

Teeth and Mouth

Just because your father is old does not mean he has outgrown the dentist's chair. In fact, older people are at more risk than ever for oral cancer, and people over 65 have more tooth decay than other age groups.

Dental problems are painful and can make chewing difficult, which can lead to poor nutrition. Furthermore, studies suggest that gum disease can increase the risk of heart disease, stroke, and a number of other serious conditions.

Apparently, bacteria from the mouth enter the bloodstream and cause all sorts of trouble.

Elderly people have more dental problems for a number of reasons. Visual and physical disabilities can make brushing and flossing difficult. With age, the gums recede, exposing vulnerable areas of each tooth to potential infection or decay. Also, older people often produce less saliva, which is needed to cleanse the teeth.

Brushing, flossing, and visiting the dentist regularly can reduce the risk of disease significantly. You or your parent should be sure to alert the dentist about any health problems your parent has, medications she is taking, or treatments she is receiving. Some medications, for instance, don't mix well with the painkillers, antibiotics, and anesthesia used by dentists. She should also alert the dentist to any pain or sores, or problems she has with swallowing, chewing, or dryness.

Wearing dentures is no excuse for skipping checkups or ignoring dental hygiene. False teeth, like glasses, need to be checked and refitted, and the gums, tongue, and insides of the cheeks still need some brushing to kill bacteria and keep the breath fresh.

Here are some tips on caring for your parent's mouth:

- See that your parent visits the dentist at least once a year.

- Be sure he brushes and flosses at least twice a day. Don't forget the floss!

- He should use a soft brush and replace it every three months.

- If your parent is having trouble managing a toothbrush, elongate the brush by taping a sturdy wooden or plastic stick to it, or enlarge it by attaching rubber or foam to the handle.

- An electric toothbrush is easier to use and might be more effective.

- Buy flossing gadgets with handles; they're easier to manage.

- If your parent's mouth is dry, ask his doctor if medication might be to blame. Maybe the dose can be lowered or the prescription changed. (Diuretics, antihistamines, antihypertensives, antianxiety drugs, antidepressants, antipsychotics, and drugs for Parkinson's disease all slow the flow of saliva.)

BAD BREATH

One final note: If you're gasping for air because your father has halitosis, you need to decide just how big a problem it is. Be sensitive. The odor may be caused by his medications or illness, so he may not be able to do anything about it.

If you can tactfully broach the subject, let your parent know that better oral hygiene can help kill some of the germs that cause bad breath. Your parent should brush or wipe the roof of his mouth, his tongue, and the inside of his cheeks, in addition to his teeth. Most breath mints and mouthwashes merely cover up odor, but gargling should help, as it loosens mucus lodged at the back of the throat.

➕ MEDICAL ALERT

Red or white spots, sores or lumps in the mouth, difficulty chewing or swallowing, or bleeding that does not go away within two weeks should be checked by a dentist, as they can be an early sign of oral cancer.

- Dry mouth can be relieved temporarily with sugarless candy or gum. Lip lubricants are a must, and chips of ice or sips of water will also help. Citrus fruits wet the mouth but also rinse it in harmful acid, so limit the lemons.

- If you brush your parent's teeth for him, ask the dentist or dental hygienist to show you how. (Again, using an electric toothbrush is easier.)

- If your parent has trouble swallowing, or if he is bedridden, skip or limit the toothpaste, because he may choke on the foam. Just use a wet brush, or wipe his teeth and gums with a damp cloth. You can also purchase oral swabs.

Chapter 12

The Body Imperfect

Part II

Bones and Joints • Incontinence • Constipation • Other Digestive Disorders • Anemia • Diabetes

---

S ometimes even serious health problems do not get the full attention of a busy doctor. Your parent might not mention a condition or symptom if she's embarrassed or believes it can't be treated. Your father might assume that stiff, achy joints are a condition he has to live with. Your mother might keep her incontinence a secret because she is ashamed. Or your parent might not realize that constipation is a serious matter. But most ailments can be alleviated, and adjustments to your parent's house and daily habits should make any remaining symptoms more bearable.

Learn the warning signs. If you suspect anything is wrong, urge your parent to talk with the doctor. Let her know that her complaints are important and not unusual. When the problem is severe or affects others (such as insomnia, depression, or incontinence), consult the doctor yourself. Your parent may not care if his illness is treated, but you have to find relief.

Bones and Joints

The human skeleton may look like a fixed, immutable frame, especially when it's hanging in a biology classroom, but skeletons are living organs that change with diet, exercise, body chemistry, and of course, age.

Be aware of this scaffolding, because when it breaks, the rest of the structure can quickly collapse. Older bones don't heal easily, and your parent may be laid up for months, putting him at risk for circulation problems, bedsores, pneumonia, lung complications, and death.

Osteoporosis

Osteoporotic bones look like termite-infested driftwood. Over time, the body's frame can become so brittle that tumbling off a step or tripping on a bathroom rug is all it takes to break a wrist or hip.

Osteoporosis is primarily a woman's ailment, because after menopause, when the production of estrogen slows, bone loss occurs rapidly. Women are also more affected because they start out with thinner bones and live longer.

But your father is not immune. Old age, along with the changes and inactivity that typically accompany it, whittles away at everyone's bones. About a quarter of people with osteoporosis are men.

Breaking a bone, particularly a hip, is serious business. About 25 percent of elderly people who fracture a hip lose their independence and require long-term nursing care. Nearly 25 percent die within a year of the accident.

The bones of the spinal cord can also collapse and compress from osteoporosis, causing deformity and crippling back pain.

The odds of your parent (and, gulp, you) having osteoporosis are staggering. Half of all women and a quarter of all men will fracture a bone because of osteoporosis in their later years. Thirty-two percent of women and 17 percent of men break a hip by the time they are 90, and osteoporosis is largely to blame.

SPOTTING OSTEOPOROSIS

Although stooped posture and a change in height are often signs of spinal osteoporosis, there are virtually no symptoms of osteoporosis in other areas until a bone is broken, which is why it is known as a "silent disease."

A number of factors increase a person's chances of having the disease:

- Old age

- Being a woman

- Having a small frame

- A family history of osteoporosis

- A diet low in calcium throughout life

- Early menopause (before age 45)

- A sedentary lifestyle

- Smoking

- Excessive use of alcohol

- Thyroid problems

- Long-term use of certain medications, such as corticosteroids (prednisone, cortisone), antidepressants, chemo-therapy, and drugs that treat gastric reflux

• Caucasian and Asian American women are more prone to the disease than are African American women.

Because there are now a number of treatments available to fight osteo-porosis, the National Osteoporosis Foundation recommends that all women over 65 have their bone den-sity tested. The recommendation is less clear for men, although many doc-tors argue that men should be routinely tested after age 80. The tests are expen-sive, however. Medicare covers the cost for elderly women and for men deemed to be at risk.

Although a bone density test is a good idea, risk alone merits preventive steps—and simply being old is a risk factor. If your parent needs convincing, have her talk with her doctor. A look at her medical history and a physical exam, along with some professional advice, should help her understand the impor-tance of prevention and treatment.

COMBATING OSTEOPOROSIS
The best time to fight osteoporosis is long before it sets in, by exercising reg-ularly, getting adequate calcium and vitamin D, avoiding cigarettes, and keeping alcohol use under control. Prevention of osteoporosis ideally begins in childhood, when bones are developing.

But the battle is not lost at age 70. With all sorts of new drugs on the market, along with lifestyle changes and precautions, people can strengthen their

ON THE LOOKOUT FOR SYMPTOMS

PROBLEM	SIGNS OF TROUBLE
Osteoporosis	Few symptoms until a bone is broken; risk factors include being a woman, old age, a family history of the disease, being thin, smoking, not exercising, and early menopause
Osteoarthritis	Painful joints; achy, stiff movement, especially first thing in the morning
Incontinence	Stains or odors, wet sheets, reluctance to go out
Diabetes	Fatigue, weight loss, blurred vision, itchy skin, frequent urination, thirst, sensations of tingling or numbness, confusion, depression
Anemia	Fatigue, headaches, chest pains, confusion, and in some cases, a sore tongue

bones and prevent fractures, even late in life. But do the work now, before there is an accident.

EXERCISE. Ironically, frail people, especially those worried about falling, tend to stay sedentary, safely propped up in the living-room chair. But that is the worst thing for them to do.

Walking, weight training, aerobics, and other exercise all strengthen muscles and bones; the bones actually get thicker and stronger. Most important, exercise enhances balance, coordination, and reflexes, which reduces the risk of falling. (Low-impact exercises like yoga and tai chi do not do much to improve bone density, but can improve balance and reduce falls.)

An exercise regimen should involve muscles throughout the body. Weight-bearing exercises (in which you're holding up your own weight, such as walking), as well as weight machines and weight lifting, can increase muscle strength and bone density in just 10 weeks. Yes, even for your parent.

CALCIUM, VITAMIN D, and healthful eating. Both calcium and vitamin D are needed for strong bones; calcium strengthens the bones while vitamin D helps the body absorb the calcium.

The best source of calcium is low-fat dairy products, but it is also added

> " My mother started going downhill after she fell three years ago and broke her hip. Before that, she had been very active, going up to Maine for the summers and going into the city on weekends. But the fall slowed her down tremendously. She lost her gusto for life. It's a constant effort to restore her confidence."
>
> —Kevin B.

to some juices and cereals. Calcium also comes from dark green vegetables (broccoli, kale, spinach, and others), canned salmon or sardines (with bones), and soy-based foods (such as tofu).

The best source of vitamin D is sunlight. Just 15 minutes of sunlight a day on unprotected arms and legs is usually adequate. It, too, is added to some foods, and is found in eggs, fish, and cod liver oil.

But one would have to eat a huge amount of dairy and forgo essential sunscreen to get enough of either one. Furthermore, elderly people are often deficient in these nutrients no matter what they eat, especially if they stay indoors.

Talk with your parent's doctor about supplements. Although evidence suggests that calcium and vitamin D supplements can lead to complications, such as heart disease and kidney stones, they are often recommended for people who have been diagnosed with osteoporosis, have a history of fractures, or are clearly deficient in these nutrients.

In general, for someone 70 and older, 800 international units (IUs) of vitamin D3 and 1,200 milligrams of calcium are adequate.

⊕ MEDICAL ALERT

Get your parent to a doctor immediately if she has a fall, allover body aches, numbness in part of her body, severe pain, immovable joints, or mild joint pain that lasts for several weeks.

Assuming your mother gets some of this from food and sunlight, she might not need to take the full dose in supplements. Also, any other vitamins she takes might include some calcium and/or vitamin D, so check the labels.

Of the many calcium supplements available, calcium carbonate is the cheapest, but calcium citrate causes fewer problems (like constipation) in elderly people. Any form of calcium is absorbed better in smaller doses, so if your parent takes 1,000 mg of calcium, divide it so she takes 500 mg with breakfast and 500 mg with dinner.

Adequate vitamin K intake is also important, as it is associated with decreased risk of fracture. Keeping sodium (salt) to a minimum also seems to reduce calcium loss. Research suggests that too much retinol, a form of vitamin A, can actually increase the risk of fractures.

SMOKING. Easier said than done, but nevertheless, your parent should give up cigarettes.

FALL PREVENTION. Even people without osteoporosis can stumble and break a bone, so regardless of your parent's bone density, her house should be "fall-safe." That means ample lighting, well-secured rugs, marked stairs, sturdy handrails, and nonskid shoes, among other things. (See page 123 for tips on preventing falls.)

DRUGS. A number of drugs are available to either prevent or treat osteoporosis. Your parent should talk with her doctor about these and other options.

Bisphosphonates, such as Fosamax, Boniva, Actonel, and Reclast, slow bone loss and increase bone density,

> ### ➕ MEDICAL ALERT
>
> If your parent faints, nearly faints, or has dizzy spells, get her to her doctor. Although fainting may be caused by something simple, such as reduced blood flow to the brain because of medications, it can also indicate more serious conditions.

and reduce fractures in postmenopausal women by more than 50 percent.

These drugs have been linked to rare, sudden fractures in the upper thighbone, and other complications, but only when taken for many years. These downsides do not mean that your mother shouldn't take them, but she should stop after three to five years of treatment.

Estrogen therapy combats osteoporosis, but is thought to increase the risk of cancer and possibly heart disease, especially when taken for any prolonged period. Furthermore, estrogen therapy is most effective at stopping bone loss in the first few years after menopause (when bone loss is most rapid).

Raloxifene (Evista), which mimics estrogen, strengthens bones without affecting the breasts and uterus, but it is not as effective as estrogen. It doesn't cause many of the unwanted side effects of estrogen, such as vaginal bleeding, breast tenderness, or increased risk of breast cancer, but it can cause hot flashes.

Teriparatide (Fortéo), a parathyroid hormone, actually triggers new bone formation and increases bone density in postmenopausal women (and in men). It is taken as a daily injection, is quite expensive, and is used only for very high-risk patients, as there may be serious side effects.

Denosumab (Prolia), which is also administered via injection, is often given to women who do not respond to other medications.

Ask the doctor about any drugs your parent might be taking that actually cause bone loss. In particular, glucocorticoid steroids can be to blame. These are found in some medications for arthritis, asthma, seizures, and insomnia.

Arthritis

Arthritis is not a single disorder, but a general term referring to sore or swollen joints. The word actually encompasses about a hundred different diseases, all of which should be treated early, so look for warning signs: swelling, redness, and pain at the joint; stiffness, especially in the morning; and restricted range of motion. If any of these symptoms last for more than two weeks, your parent should see her doctor.

OSTEOARTHRITIS, or degenerative arthritis, is almost universal after age 65, particularly among women, although some people have few or no symptoms. The cartilage in joints, which allows bones to glide easily back and forth without friction, becomes thin, cracked, and frayed. The joints become painful, and movement limited. It is most common in the hands, hips, knees, feet, and back.

Severe osteoarthritis can make everyday life exasperating and discouraging. Every movement hurts, and simple tasks, such as buttoning a blouse or holding a fork, are challenging if not impossible. Sometimes a hand will curl and twist into a deformed shape, and might develop knobby lumps, called

osteophytes (which look more painful than they actually are).

Osteoarthritis has a number of causes. When it strikes the hands or hips, it tends to be genetic, whereas osteoarthritis in the knees seems to be at least partially caused by the strain of obesity. The disease can also be the result of injuries or overuse.

RHEUMATOID ARTHRITIS also affects women more than men. For reasons not fully understood, the body's own defense system launches a misdirected attack on healthy tissue in the joints.

The disease is chronic, but there can be stretches when it's inactive, and then it strikes in waves, called flares. A flare usually begins with an allover achiness, stiffness, and fatigue. The joints become rigid, swollen, red, warm, and painful, especially first thing in the morning. Your parent might have a low-grade fever and lose her appetite during these flare-ups.

The feet and the hands—particularly the fingers—are often the first joints affected, but over time the disease can spread to elbows, knees, hips, and other joints. Usually, the joints are affected symmetrically. That is, the same joints on both sides of the body hurt. In some cases, pea-size lumps grow under the skin, and the joints become deformed.

Rheumatoid arthritis is one of the most difficult types of arthritis to control. It is critical that it be diagnosed and treated early, before bone and cartilage are damaged.

GOUT AND PSEUDOGOUT, two of the most excruciating types of arthritis, occur more often in men than women.

In gout, uric acid, which usually drains out of the body with urine, builds up and forms sharp crystals in the joints—often in the big toe, but also in the ankles, elbows, wrists, hands, or knees.

In pseudogout, the crystals are made of calcium pyrophosphate, and they usually affect the large joints (knee, shoulder, hip).

This assault on the joints happens suddenly, lasts for about two or three days, and then slowly fades over a week or two. The joint becomes painful, stiff, and swollen. The skin around the joint becomes dark red and very tender. Even a light brush with the bedsheets can be agonizing. Gout is sometimes accompanied by fever.

The sufferer often has another attack within a year and may experience several more episodes in following years, although some people have just one or two attacks and are never bothered by symptoms again.

MANAGING ARTHRITIS

Most types of arthritis cannot be cured, so the aim of treatment is to alleviate pain and increase mobility. If your parent's arthritis is severe, she should talk to a specialist, such as a rheumatologist or orthopedic surgeon.

Here are some ways to ease arthritis:

NONMEDICAL TREATMENTS. Warm baths and heating pads can relieve the pain and stiffness, and cold packs can reduce swelling and numb pain. (Your parent should try both and see what feels best.) Gentle massage can also help.

Although rest is important during a

GADGETS TO HELP ACHY JOINTS

Canes, walkers, and splints will give your parent support and a little more mobility. Shoes with shock-absorbing insoles can ease stress on sore joints. Poles and pulls help people get up from bed or a chair. Jar openers, toothpaste dispensers, large-handled flatware, faucet grippers, and other such devices will all make daily life easier.

You can find a wide variety of gadgets and tools at large pharmacies and in medical supply stores, or they can be purchased through catalogs or over the Internet.

---

painful attack, exercise in the interim can prevent joints from stiffening, increase range of motion and mobility, and ease inflammation and pain.

An exercise program should be comfortable, not overly strenuous, and preferably, recommended by a doctor or physical therapist. Weight-bearing exercises (in which a person carries his or her own weight, such as running, walking, dancing, hiking, or tennis) are recommended, although exercising in a warm pool is often easier on stiff joints. Tai chi also seems to be extremely helpful for people with arthritis, in terms of both easing pain and increasing range of motion. (See page 83 for more on exercise and the elderly.)

If your parent is heavy, losing weight will also ease the burden on her joints.

PHYSICAL AND OCCUPATIONAL THERAPY. Physical therapy should increase movement, strengthen muscles, and help people learn new ways to use their joints. Occupational therapists train people with limited motion to manage everyday tasks. Both therapies are often helpful in conjunction with other treatments.

MEDICATIONS. Your parent should check with her doctor before starting on any drug regimen.

- **Arthritis creams and gels,** rubbed directly on the joint, can ease the pain momentarily. Most are made with menthol or capsaicin (the stuff that makes hot peppers hot) and are harmless. Some people need to use them for several days before they help. Creams that contain nonsteroidal anti-inflammatory agents may be more helpful.

- **Acetaminophen** (Tylenol) and other analgesics, including tramadol and oxycodone, reduce pain, but don't affect inflammation.

- **Nonsteroidal anti-inflammatory drugs, or NSAIDs,** block the production of prostaglandins, the source of pain and swelling. These include ibuprofen (Advil, Motrin), naproxen (Aleve), and more powerful prescription versions of these drugs.

  Oral NSAIDs can cause bleeding in the stomach and intestines, ulcers, heartburn, vomiting, diarrhea, headaches, and kidney problems. They can also increase the risk of heart attack and stroke. Some forms of these medications, available by prescription, may have fewer of these side effects.

- **Corticosteroids** are a form of cortisone, a hormone produced naturally by the body. They too reduce swelling and pain. Corticosteroids, however, are potent and are usually prescribed only for brief periods. They can be given orally or injected directly into a joint.

- **Disease-modifying anti-rheumatic drugs,** or DMARDs (Plaquenil, Trexall), are usually the first line of defense for rheumatoid arthritis, because they slow the disease process and ease pain and stiffness. They can take weeks to kick in, though, so be patient.

- **Biologic response modifiers** (Remicade, Enbrel), a newer form of DMARDs, are injected and act more quickly, but they suppress the immune system, so are typically used only when the first line of drugs doesn't work. Combining the newer and older drugs is often most effective.

ⓘ FOR MORE HELP

Arthritis Foundation
arthritis.org
800-283-7800

National Institute of Arthritis and Musculoskeletal and Skin Diseases
niams.nih.gov
877-226-4267

National Osteoporosis Foundation
nof.org
800-231-4222

- **Glucosamine and chondroitin sulfate,** which are found naturally in the body, seem to help some people with mild osteoarthritis. They are made from shellfish shells and shark cartilage, and are sold as dietary supplements. Your parent should confer with his doctor before trying it.

- **Corticosteroids** (prednisone), and NSAIDS are sometimes used to treat gout and pseudogout. **Colchicine** can sometimes prevent a full-blown attack if taken early, but it can cause horrendous side effects. Doctors also try to reduce the level of uric acid in the body with drugs (such as allopurinol, sulfinpyrazone, and probenecid) or, if a large joint is affected, by withdrawing fluid from the joint and injecting corticosteroids to reduce inflammation.

SURGERY. If your parent is otherwise healthy, a doctor may recommend surgery to replace a badly damaged joint with an artificial one or to repair damaged cartilage. This can be very successful, but be aware that such surgery is a major undertaking, especially if your parent is old or very frail. Ask the doctor about arthroscopy, a less invasive procedure that requires local anesthesia and usually no hospital stay.

Incontinence

You've just noticed a large stain on your father's pants or a distinctive odor coming from your mother's laundry basket. There is a cold slap of shock. A wave of disgust. A stab of sorrow.

It's natural to be shaken, especially if you are left to clean up the mess. This is not a job a child ever expects to have. The odor alone can haunt you for days. Stay calm. If this is a one-time event, you can surely deal with it. If this is your future, then life just took a major turn. But don't despair. Read on.

The greatest shame of incontinence is not the problem itself, but the embarrassment and isolation associated with it, and the woeful lack of open conversation. You need to talk. It's a difficult subject, and you may meet with resistance or denial, but talking is the only way to ease the humiliation and find solutions. And there are solutions.

Be gentle, sympathetic, and tactful. Let your parent know that this is common (up to 30 percent of elderly people are completely or partially incontinent; more than 50 percent of those in hospitals or nursing homes have urinary incontinence), and that help is available.

Once the problem is acknowledged, get your parent to a doctor who will give the situation the attention it deserves. You may have to advocate with special persistence here. One study showed that 35 to 50 percent of doctors did nothing when told that a patient was incontinent.

" My mother got up from her chair in the living room to go in to dinner, and I noticed this spot on the cushion. She is a fastidious woman, and I think she was unaware that anything had happened. She had developed fluid in her abdomen from the cancer, and it was putting pressure on all of her organs, so maybe that triggered the incontinence.

I thought, 'Am I going to have to tell her, or will she notice it herself and try to hide it from me?' I wasn't offended by the problem. I was more worried that it would be just one more encroachment on her dignity. I really hurt for her."
—Ruth S.

If your parent's doctor is not helpful, she should see a urologist, gynecologist, gastroenterologist, or geriatrician. Some geriatric care centers and gynecological practices have special clinics devoted to incontinence.

Although urinary incontinence is common in old age, it is not normal, and it is almost always treatable with exercise, bladder training, surgery, and other techniques.

Bowel incontinence is another story, as it is far more upsetting and challenging for caregivers. But it, too, can be treated in many instances, and it can always be made more manageable.

Although incontinence can cause infections, it is not as much a medical crisis as it is a social one. Not only will it likely make your parent feel embarrassed, ashamed, and disgusted, but it can lead to withdrawal, isolation, and depression. And because it is so onerous for caregivers, it also leads to institutionalization.

You and your parent will fare much better if you each have a thick social skin and a ready sense of humor, as well as the determination to find adequate care.

Urinary Incontinence

Normal bladder routines run amok for all sorts of reasons. Urinary tract infections are a common cause of temporary problems. Constipation can cause urinary incontinence if it puts pressure on, or otherwise irritates, the muscles of the bladder.

Prostate troubles, hormonal changes, diabetes, dehydration (yes, oddly enough, dehydration), surgery, weakened or damaged muscles, and medications are all to blame. Stroke, dementia, and delirium can also lead to incontinence if the brain isn't sending or receiving bladder or bowel signals effectively. And of course, immobility can cause incontinence if getting up and to the toilet takes a lot of time and effort.

How incontinence is treated depends in part on what type of incontinence your parent has.

TRANSIENT INCONTINENCE comes on suddenly and acutely. A person who has never wet his pants starts having accidents because he can't physically get to the toilet or because of an infection, delirium, depression, medication, constipation, or alcohol use. The incontinence is almost always reversible and may even disappear on its own.

STRESS INCONTINENCE primarily affects women. They laugh, cough, strain, exercise, sneeze, or pick up a heavy box, and, oops. The culprit: The ring of muscles around the urethra, which usually holds in urine, is loose,

INPUT AND OUTPUT

Although it might seem logical that less input would mean less output, and perhaps fewer output accidents, it just doesn't work that way.

Your parent should not drink less in order to urinate less. This will cause dehydration and can make her incontinence worse, as highly concentrated urine can lead to infections.

Limiting fluids before bed makes sense, but otherwise, let her have her water.

often as a result of bearing children and the hormonal changes of menopause. As a result, small amounts of urine leak out when a woman exerts even the smallest pressure (or "stress") on the bladder.

URGE INCONTINENCE is characterized by a sudden and urgent need to urinate—so sudden that there is not enough time to get to the toilet. The bladder may empty on cue, when someone hears water running, touches water, drinks a glass of water, or even in anticipation as one nears a toilet. Bladder contractions run amok often because of damage to the nerves of the bladder, spinal cord, or brain, caused by Parkinson's disease, Alzheimer's disease, stroke, spinal cord injury, or diabetes. In **reflex incontinence**, a close cousin of urge incontinence, the bladder releases with no warning at all.

OVERFLOW INCONTINENCE occurs when the bladder is always full, and excess urine dribbles out. It is often seen in men with prostate troubles. When the prostate gland, which surrounds the urethra, is enlarged, it can block the passageway so urine can't drain out normally during toileting. Instead, the bladder remains full, causing minor leaks throughout the day.

Overflow incontinence is also seen in people who have diabetes, spinal cord injury, and other disorders that block the urethra or prevent the bladder from contracting normally. The buildup of urine can cause bladder or kidney infections if the disorder is not treated.

FUNCTIONAL INCONTINENCE is caused by physical limitations that prevent a person from getting to the toilet in time. Conditions that hinder mobility, such as severe arthritis or stroke, are often to blame.

MIXED INCONTINENCE, when two types of incontinence happen together, occurs in women more than men. Stress and urge incontinence are the most common combination.

MANAGING URINARY INCONTINENCE

Quite often, incontinence disappears on its own. When it doesn't, a doctor's first task is to treat any underlying problem—infection, obstruction, or illness. Medications such as diuretics, tranquilizers, sedatives, drugs for Parkinson's disease, psychotropic drugs, antihistamines, and calcium channel blockers can worsen incontinence.

After that, the best attack is a non-medical one—bladder exercises, bladder training, and regular toilet scheduling. These techniques require commitment and practice, but take heart; they are quite successful in treating stress and urge incontinence in particular. About 20 percent of people are cured, and almost all the rest are helped significantly.

Of course, you'll want to take some very practical steps, too. Make sure the path to the toilet is short, clear, and well lighted. Make sure your parent has elastic-waist pants or other clothing that is easy to get off. Invest in some waterproof mattress pads and sheets, and put disposable waterproof pads on chairs and beds.

KEGEL EXERCISES. No gym clothes. No sweating. These exercises require only a commitment.

Kegel exercises—also known as pelvic muscle exercises, or PMEs, strengthen the ring of muscles around the urethra, the exit tube from the bladder, and are particularly useful in treating stress incontinence.

The exercises entail squeezing the muscles of the vagina and anus. Your mother can get the feel of where the muscles are by stopping the flow while she is urinating. (She should not be tightening the muscles in her legs, fanny, or stomach, which are not involved in bladder control.) If she has trouble, a nurse or physical therapist can help her.

She should do these squeezes (holding each for several seconds) after every visit to the toilet, and at other times throughout the day, for a total of one hundred to two hundred squeezes each day. For stress incontinence, your parent should get in the habit of squeezing these muscles before lifting, sneezing, coughing, or, if possible, laughing.

Kegels can be done discreetly just about anywhere. However, like other workouts, they require dedication. It usually takes at least a month of doing Kegels before any real effect is noticed. Once there's some improvement, your parent should continue the routine to maintain bladder control.

You might want to join her. Coughing, laughing, and sneezing come with unexpected consequences for caregivers, too. (One in four adult women have occasional leakage. But don't let that stop you from having a good laugh. Just do your Kegels and get some paper towels!)

A SCHEDULE. Have your parent keep track of when she urinates or leaks for a couple of days, and then make a schedule that gets her to the toilet just before she typically needs to use it. She might sit on the toilet, say, every two hours whether she thinks she needs to or not. (Bathroom trips shouldn't be scheduled too frequently; that can actually cause incontinence, because the bladder learns to hold only small amounts of fluid.)

BLADDER TRAINING. Once your parent successfully schedules bathroom trips, she might be able to extend the time between trips. In bladder training, a person gets on a schedule of going to the toilet at set intervals, and then slowly lengthens the time between visits. Ideally, your parent should increase these intervals until she can wait two or three hours.

To practice, your parent should empty her bladder completely, and then suppress any urge in between scheduled trips by relaxing or diverting her attention. ("Holding it" during these intervals can strengthen the muscles around the urethra.)

BIOFEEDBACK. Used in conjunction with Kegel exercises, this technique can be very helpful, especially for stress and urge incontinence.

A person is hooked up to a device that informs him how well he is contracting and relaxing his sphincter, detrusor, and abdominal muscles—all involved in bladder control. People can also use a diary to track their progress. With this information as a guide, the person practices ways to manipulate these muscles and gradually gains better control over them.

DIETARY CHANGES. Limiting caffeine and alcohol should improve continence, and some studies suggest that avoiding spicy foods, tomatoes, and imitation sweeteners may help, too. Obesity also plays a role in some cases, so you might urge your parent to lose weight.

MEDICATIONS. Some doctors hear the word *incontinent* and immediately pull out their prescription pads. Watch out. It's important to determine the type and cause of incontinence, and change behaviors and habits first.

Some medications used to treat an overactive bladder (known as anticholinergic drugs) hinder memory and generally are not recommended for the elderly, particularly those with dementia. Other drugs affect blood pressure.

But when all else fails, certain drugs (and there are quite a number of options) can be used to stop bladder contractions,

strengthen the resistance of the urethra, or help relax muscles when emptying the bladder.

The bottom line: Try other approaches first. If nothing works, then you might have no choice. But start drugs at the lowest possible dose.

ELECTRICAL STIMULATION. The muscles of the urethra can be strengthened by short doses of electrical stimulation. Electrodes are placed (temporarily) in the vagina or rectum to stimulate the contraction of the urethra muscles and stabilize overactive muscles. This is useful in cases of stress or urge incontinence.

IMPLANTS, PLUGS, PATCHES. Doctors have had some success injecting collagen, silicone, or other materials into or around the urethra to narrow the opening and help control urination.

A stiff ring, called a pessary, can be inserted into the vagina to put pressure on the urethra and reposition it.

There are also inserts that plug the urethra (somewhat like a tampon) that are helpful for short periods (say, during a specific activity) in cases of stress incontinence.

SURGERY. Although a very serious and last resort, surgery is sometimes necessary to clear obstructions (for example, an enlarged prostate), to reposition the bladder (in cases of stress incontinence), or to repair or replace the urethra.

BEDPANS AND COMMODES. If your parent has trouble getting to the bathroom because of a physical disability or urge incontinence, put a commode, bedpan, or urinal by his bed or chair. Or if possible, have him sit or sleep near a bathroom that is not used by anyone else in the family.

PADS AND DIAPERS. These should be used only when all else fails, or for trips and other occasions that require extra security. Besides being uncomfortable, demoralizing, and inconvenient, diapers can lead to skin infections, and they typically worsen incontinence.

People learn to rely on them, and stop exercising their bladder muscles. Over time, the body can become desensitized to its own messages. (This is especially true when a person is in the early stages of dementia.)

Nevertheless, when necessary, adult diapers can be lifesavers.

The varieties and options fill drugstore aisles. For minor leaking, a menstrual "maxipad" or a similar pad that's made to absorb urine may be adequate. For men, a small patch of absorbent padding, called a "drip collector," is undetectable.

ⓘ FOR MORE HELP

International Foundation for Functional Gastrointestinal Disorders
aboutincontinence.org
888-964-2001

....

National Association for Continence
nafc.org
800-252-3337

....

National Kidney and Urologic Diseases Information Clearinghouse
kidney.niddk.nih.gov
800-891-5390

....

Simon Foundation for Continence
simonfoundation.org
800-237-4666

Otherwise, it's on to larger pads and full-fledged diapers (although "absorbent pad" is probably a better name, regardless of what you buy; it's less demoralizing). You can also buy waterproof underwear that fit over briefs or diapers.

Whenever your parent wears absorbent pads, take steps to avoid skin infections and rashes. Your parent should not sit in wet or dirty pants for any longer than absolutely necessary. The crotch must be thoroughly cleaned at every diaper change with *mild* soap and water and then, ideally, air-dried, as a towel or cloth can be rough on delicate skin.

A small amount of petroleum jelly or other ointment—no powders—helps prevent irritation. Boxes of nonalcohol "wipes," along with diaper rash ointment, can be found in the baby section of grocery stores, department stores, or pharmacies. Use diaper rash cream if necessary, and call a doctor if the irritation doesn't go away in a day or two.

CATHETERS. A catheter is generally not a good way to deal with incontinence because infections are so common, but when someone is largely immobile and bedpans aren't an option, it can't be avoided.

A catheter is basically a tube that runs from the bladder into a storage bag that hangs from a bed or is attached to the leg and hidden under pants or a skirt. It can be inserted into the bladder permanently by a nurse, or inserted according to a schedule by your parent. There are also catheters that attach to the genitals (a condom-like device for men and a somewhat less useful suction gadget for women).

Catheters are often used for overflow incontinence, or for brief periods after surgery or injury, or when someone is in a bed or wheelchair. Beware of infections. Catheters need to be checked and changed regularly.

Fecal Incontinence

Fecal incontinence is a less common but far more troubling problem, and may quickly become more than you can handle. Cleaning up messes, changing diapers, and protecting the house against damage is an enormous task, both physically and emotionally.

Try the treatments and approaches discussed here and talk with your parent's doctor. Fecal, or bowel, incontinence can be treated in most people. The problem might not be eliminated, but it can usually be improved, reducing "accidents" significantly.

If nothing works and you simply can't handle this, don't be hard on yourself. You might need to get outside help or consider whether it's time for an assisted living or nursing home.

Be very gentle with your parent, too. Few things are more mortifying than this. Assure her that it is not her fault, that she did nothing wrong, and it is not anything she should feel ashamed of. As you know, she really cannot help it. Let her know that this is the result of a medical problem, and that you and her doctor will work with her to get beyond this or at least make it manageable.

CAUSES

Oddly enough, the most common cause of bowel incontinence is constipation. When the bowel is blocked, liquid leaks around the obstruction. Diarrhea is also

> ❝ I had to clean up after her—the toilet, the tiles, the rug, her pants. I had to clean her bottom, thoroughly, with a wet cloth.
>
> I kept saying, 'It's okay, Mom,' 'Don't worry about it, Mom,' because I knew she was mortified. But honestly, I was fighting back the vomit. The smell was incredible. I was turning my head to the window and gasping for air.
>
> I would do anything for her. But this, this . . . I drove home, crying. I was so sad for her, and I was ashamed that I found it so revolting. I knew I couldn't take much more of it. This was not the first time I'd had to clean up like this."
>
> —Marge S.

a common cause of fecal incontinence in elderly people, as they are less able to hold on to soft or liquid stools.

Bowel incontinence can also be caused by surgery, medications, dementia, stroke, and cancer, as well as any injury to the anal muscles or the nerves that sense stool in the rectum (often caused by childbirth, frequent constipation, or prolonged laxative use).

Of course, if your parent is less mobile, simply getting to the toilet in time might be a problem, and if she is bedbound, then getting to a commode at all may not be possible.

TREATING FECAL INCONTINENCE

Try the suggestions for treating and managing urinary incontinence on page 243—setting schedules, exercising muscles, using commodes, waterproof pads, and so on—as many are useful in addressing bowel incontinence as

INCONTINENCE TIPS

- Clear a path to the toilet. If possible, make sure your parent has a private bathroom, so it's always available.

- Place night-lights and/or pieces of reflector tape along the path to the bathroom so your parent isn't stumbling around at night.

- Make sure your parent can use the toilet with ease. Install grab bars, buy a raised toilet seat, and put the toilet paper within easy reach.

- Get your parent clothing that can be easily removed (skirts or elastic-waist pants, Velcro or snap closures instead of buttons, knee-high stockings instead of pantyhose).

- Don't hurry your parent. She should take her time.

- If the toilet is far away or shared, buy a commode, bedpan, or handheld urinal. Get a portable urinal for traveling.

- Make sure your parent empties his or her bladder before going to bed.

- In any new place, locate the bathroom immediately. Avoid situations where there are no bathrooms, such as buses or shops without public facilities.

- Choose seats in restaurants, airplanes, theaters, and so forth that are near a bathroom. Call in advance and plan the seating.

- Use waterproof liners (disposable or washable) on the bed, in the car, and on your parent's chair. You can find these at a medical supply store or online.

- To reduce odors, deposit diapers and wipes in a small pail, equipped with a lid and a deodorizer. Ditto soiled clothing.

- A fan and an open window, whenever possible, will reduce odor problems. So will an open box of baking soda.

well. It's helpful to get a person to sit on the toilet about half an hour after breakfast, when the bowels are typically stimulated.

Any severe constipation or diarrhea needs to be treated immediately. If the incontinence remains, the doctor should search for other causes.

A high-fiber diet can help control bowel incontinence by restoring regularity and, in the case of diarrhea, giving the stool some bulk. (But talk to her doctor, as sometimes a low-fiber diet is used to reduce stool volume.) Be sure

she's drinking enough fluids, and avoiding greasy or spicy foods, cured meats, dairy products, caffeine, and alcohol.

A method of biofeedback, in which a balloon is placed in the rectum and the person learns muscle control by watching the results of his efforts on a monitor, is often successful in treating bowel incontinence.

When muscles aren't working properly—the person feels the need to go but can't hold on or get to a bathroom in time—electrical stimulation (using painless electrical currents to "exercise" muscles) can help strengthen the sphincter muscles (the ring of muscles around the anus).

When nerve damage numbs the normal sensations of an approaching bowel movement, enemas or suppositories can be used to empty the bowels on a schedule to reduce the chances of an accident.

Several drugs are also useful in reducing the number of "episodes." For example, stool-bulking agents can firm up loose stool.

As noted, when diapers are necessary, be sure your parent's skin is kept clean and dry, as fecal incontinence often leads to painful rashes. Soap can be drying, so keep it to a minimum. Go easy with the toilet paper, as his skin is thin and fragile. Use wipes (moist towelettes), but get the ones without alcohol (which is drying). Ointments will also help reduce rashes.

When all else fails, some surgical procedures can help. A torn or damaged sphincter can be repaired, an artificial sphincter can be implanted, or the rectum can be repositioned.

As a last resort, a colostomy is sometimes used to deal with fecal incontinence. An opening is made in the abdomen so stool can be diverted out of the body and into a bag.

Constipation

After about age 70, many people become concerned about their bowels. If they don't go to the bathroom for a day or two, they worry they will explode. The truth is, people don't need to move their bowels every day. In fact, once every three days will get your parent through the week just fine. So if he constantly complains of constipation, but has no symptoms other than irregularity, ask the doctor about it, but gently urge him not to worry so much.

True constipation, however, is miserable, and if left untreated, can become life threatening. If your parent has a bowel movement less than three times a week, stool is hard and dry, and/or your parent has gas or bloating, try the treatments listed here. If they don't work, consult her doctor.

Constipation may be the result of a number of underlying and often treatable conditions. The most common cause is simply inadequate amounts of fluids and fiber. Lack of physical activity, which is so common among the elderly, can also be at the root of the problem. "Holding it" (maybe because getting to the toilet is a lot of work) and, ironically, taking too many laxatives, can also be to blame.

Aging itself leads to physical changes that can cause constipation. It may be the result of hormonal changes or irritable bowel syndrome (also known as spastic colon or irritable colon syndrome).

> 66 I guess we all wish for the same thing—that our parents will be independent until they die. If they need help, it would be with a few practical things, like going shopping or taking care of the house, and you would include them in family affairs, and that would be it. You wouldn't have to hear about every bowel movement, which is where I am at with my mother. I don't really want to take care of her bowel movements. I'd rather take her shopping."
>
> —Barbara F.

Hemorrhoids or any other sore can block the anus or make a person avoid the bathroom, as can surgery in the abdominal area, though this is usually temporary. Immobility after surgery or simply a very sedentary lifestyle can also cause constipation.

Narcotics, antacids, antispasmodic drugs, antihistamines, antihypertensive agents, antidepressants, and tranquilizers can all cause constipation, as can some dietary supplements and a host of other drugs. Talk with the doctor about lowering the dose, stopping, or changing any drug that might cause a problem.

Damage to the digestive system from cancer, nerve disorders, Parkinson's disease, diabetes, and other illnesses can all obstruct the bowels.

If your parent is at risk of constipation because of illness or medications, act early and preventively.

Treating Constipation

FIBER, FIBER, FIBER. A good diet, for bowels and everything else, is packed with green, leafy vegetables, fresh fruit, beans, and whole grains. A high-fiber cereal eaten regularly is a quick fix, but it shouldn't replace more varied and natural sources of fiber.

On the flip side, high-fat meats, dairy products, eggs, rich desserts, and processed foods can all contribute to constipation.

WATER, WATER, WATER. Fiber aids regularity by absorbing fluids and softening feces, but it can't do this work in a dry environment. Your parent needs fluids, even if he isn't thirsty. Soda, juice, or herbal teas are fine, but drinks containing alcohol or caffeine won't help at all. He's drinking the right amount when his urine runs clear.

PRUNES. It's not totally clear why prunes are so useful at treating constipation, but daily intake of either prunes or prune juice can help tremendously. Prunes contain fiber (prune juice does not) and antioxidants, but their most potent weapon may be sorbitol, which is a natural laxative. Prunes are considered "nature's remedy."

EXERCISE. Physical movement helps keep bowels regular (along with its many other benefits). Your parent needs to get out for a walk or, if she's bedridden, do some stretching. Talk with the doctor about exercises and movements that your parent can do, even from a bed or chair, or call a physical therapist. Any exercise, no matter how little, is better than none. (See page 83 for more on exercise.)

BATHROOM ROUTINES. When it's time to go to the toilet, it's time to go. Make sure your parent doesn't "hold it," ignore the urge, hurry, or wait for a more convenient time and place. If your parent is in a new place, which can throw off her daily ritual, she should go at the same time of day she normally does and also stick with her regular diet as much as possible.

EASY ON THE LAXATIVES. Although it's tempting to seek solutions at the local pharmacy, beware. Your parent should use laxatives only when the above approaches don't work, and then, only sparingly and for short periods of time, as they can worsen the problem. Talk with her doctor before using any laxatives.

Up to 75 percent of elderly people use laxatives, many of them daily. But contrary to what the ads suggest—that with laxatives, your parent will stroll along a breezy seaside or bound over tennis nets—laxatives, when used routinely, can interfere with nature so severely that, over time, the body forgets how to operate on its own.

Fiber supplements (such as Metamucil and Citrucel), which are essentially laxatives, are okay, but your parent should begin slowly, as a big dose of fiber may leave her doubled over with stomach cramps. (Any initial bloating and gas should go away within a few days. She also should drink a lot of water so the fiber can do its job.)

Milk of magnesia and other saline laxatives, as well as osmotics (Miralax, Sorbitol), draw fluids into the intestine and are also a good choice for short periods. (Sorbitol is in some sugarless gum, so you may be getting your laxatives in tiny doses without even realizing it.)

Stool softeners (Colace, for example) should help, as they soften hard stools,

but they don't necessarily treat the cause of the constipation. The same is true of lubricants (like mineral oil), which do just what they say, lubricate. Lubricants may also hinder vitamin absorption.

Many laxatives come as suppositories—a small plug, usually in the form of glycerin, that is inserted directly into the rectum. While this might be intimidating, most suppositories can be easily used by your parent alone. (But if he needs help, yes, this job will fall to you or an aide.) They also come in the form of an enema, in which liquid is pushed into the rectum via a small tube. Speak with your parent's doctor before using enemas or suppositories.

Note that "natural," plant-based laxatives are not necessarily any safer than the others.

IF ALL ELSE FAILS. If none of the above helps, be sure the doctor is involved. A doctor might order prescription medications that increase fluid in the intestines and bowels.

Beyond that, a doctor may have to remove the obstruction manually or, in extreme cases, surgically.

Bowel Obstruction

In severe cases, the bowel can become completely blocked. This requires immediate medical attention, as the intestine can tear (or perforate) and toxins will seep into the bloodstream, an often fatal situation.

Bowel obstruction is more common in the elderly than one wants to imagine. But as we've noted, doctors are often focused on other medical issues, and constipation does not get the attention it deserves.

Symptoms of bowel obstruction (aside from lack of bowel movements) include nausea, swelling, and abdominal pain.

Surgery may be required at this point, but confer with the doctor about your parent's chances of surviving such surgery and, if she survives, what life will be like on the other side of it. If your

> ## ➕ MEDICAL ALERT
>
> Blood in stools, dark or oddly colored stools, a sudden change in bowel habits, or pain in the lower abdomen should be reported to the doctor immediately.

parent is severely ill, confer with a palliative care specialist or hospice.

Other Digestive Disorders

Diarrhea

An occasional bout of loose bowels is not a serious problem, although it can be upsetting. Severe or chronic diarrhea requires immediate medical attention.

Diarrhea is the body's way of getting rid of toxins in the digestive tract. It can be caused by bad food, laxatives, antacids, diuretics, antibiotics, chemotherapy, anxiety, or intestinal disorders. Dairy products can also cause diarrhea in people who are lactose intolerant. Most of the time, the problem disappears fairly quickly on its own.

If it is severe or chronic, or if there is blood in the stool, diarrhea may be caused by colon cancer, infection, diabetes, severe constipation (when liquid flows around the blockage), or other serious problems that need immediate medical attention.

Note: Be sure your parent is getting plenty of fluids, as dehydration is a common side effect of diarrhea. Sports drinks, which contain electrolytes, are also good. If things get serious, your parent will need fluids intravenously.

Over-the-counter antidiarrheal medications are not always advised, as diarrhea is a sign that the body needs to rid itself of bacteria or other toxins.

Difficulty Swallowing

Trouble swallowing (known as dysphagia) can be caused by a number of things, including weakened throat muscles, or illnesses such as cancer, stroke, or dementia, which disrupt the signals to and from the brain that control swallowing. Dry mouth caused by chemo and radiation can also cause dysphagia.

Dysphagia is common among the elderly, particularly among those in nursing homes.

Keep an eye out for clues, such as coughing, gagging, drooling, belching, and the like, while your parent eats. He might complain of having a "lump in his throat."

RX FOR CHOKING

If your parent has trouble swallowing, be prepared so you're ready if he chokes.

If your parent is able to speak, cough, and breathe, let him cough; this should resolve on its own. But if he is choking and unable to speak or breathe (in which case he may appear panicked, or grab at his throat), lean him slightly forward and, using the heel of your hand, smack him between the shoulder blades four or five times.

If this doesn't dislodge the object, perform the Heimlich maneuver. Stand behind your parent and wrap your arms around his chest. Make a fist just below the rib cage and above the navel, and clasp that fist with your other hand. With a quick, strong thrust of your hands, pull inward and upward. (Firmly, but not so hard that you break his ribs!) Repeat until the food is dislodged.

If your parent is lying on his back, straddle him and place one hand just above the navel in the middle of the abdomen. Place the other hand on top of the first hand and press in with a quick thrust. Repeat.

Meanwhile, someone should call for emergency help. For more information, contact the local chapter of the American Red Cross (redcross.org).

Consult a doctor. Unchecked, swallowing difficulties can lead to malnutrition, starvation, choking, or pneumonia (because fluid gets into the lungs).

A doctor will try to determine what is causing the problem and, if possible, treat that. A speech-language pathologist can teach your parent exercises to improve his swallowing skills and strategies to make swallowing easier.

Soft, moist foods and those accompanied by sauces may go down more easily than dry foods or thin liquids, like juice or water. If your parent is having trouble swallowing pills, try giving them in a spoon of applesauce or pudding.

Urge your parent to sit upright, to eat slowly, to take tiny bites, and to avoid chatting while eating. He should also avoid gulping a drink before a bite of food is chewed and swallowed completely. Sometimes a small change in the tilt of the head can help.

People with dysphagia are at risk of an oral infection called thrush, so brushing and rinsing is particularly important.

Heartburn and Acid Reflux

That burning pain in your parent's chest, a searing just behind the chest bone that is sometimes mistaken for heart disease (or being stabbed in the chest with a burning knife), might be heartburn.

A good name, but not an appropriate one, because it has nothing to do with the heart. It should be called esophagus-burn, because what's happening is this: Food travels down the esophagus to the stomach, and normally, it stays there, but when things aren't working exactly right, it can be pushed back up the esophagus, along with stomach acids and bile that eat at the lining of the esophagus. This is acid reflux. Heartburn is the pain one feels because of acid reflux.

The pain may become worse when your parent leans forward or lies down, as the esophagus fails to close completely and acid flows upward from the stomach.

If certain foods seem to trigger the trouble (chocolates or fried, spicy, or rich foods), your parent should obviously avoid them. Medications, caffeine, tobacco, and alcohol can all contribute. Also, he should eat smaller, more frequent meals rather than large meals; eat several hours before lying down; elevate his head at night; and avoid tight clothing.

Antacids can be helpful, but if this is not enough, he should talk to his doctor about other options, as there are stronger drugs that can help. Some people require surgery.

Most drugs come with warnings, and the drugs used to reduce stomach acid (such as Prilosec, Prevacid, and Nexium) are no exception. They interfere with the absorption of certain nutrients; long-term use can cause anemia (low iron), bone fractures, infections (particularly pneumonia and *C. difficile*, an infection found in many older hospital patients).

Studies also suggest that once someone starts taking these antacids, it's hard to stop. When you block the production of acid, the body compensates by trying to make more. So when you stop taking the antacids, you are in overdrive, and, no surprise, desperately need antacids.

Indigestion

Indigestion, or dyspepsia, is the Thanksgiving Day Dilemma caused by overindulgence at the dinner table—eating too much or too fast, or eating rich or spicy foods.

But persistent indigestion can also be a sign of a digestive tract disorder, like an ulcer or gall bladder disease. It causes heartburn, nausea, vomiting, bloating, and discomfort. Again, a change in diet should solve the problem, but if it doesn't go away, consult the doctor.

Ulcers

When the protective lining of the stomach fails to do its job, digestive acids, which break down food in the stomach, can eat away at the stomach lining, creating raw, painful sores called peptic ulcers.

Symptoms include a burning or gnawing sensation in the stomach, bloating, and/or nausea that comes on several hours after eating. Sometimes a person is awakened by vague pain and discomfort in the middle of the night (two or three hours after dinner). Symptoms may come and go for several weeks.

In most cases, these ulcers are caused by bacteria (*H. pylori*) in the digestive tract, which destroy the mucous coating the walls of the stomach and the duodenum, a short tube leading out of the stomach and into the small intestine.

Ulcers are also caused or worsened by long-term use of aspirin, ibuprofen, and other nonsteroidal anti-inflammatory drugs (NSAIDs). Drugs used to treat osteoporosis can also cause ulcers. In very rare cases, they are the result of cancer.

Stress and spicy foods are no longer thought to be culprits, although they don't help once an ulcer has formed.

Ulcers are common in the elderly, and they can be extremely serious, as they can cause internal bleeding, a blockage in the intestinal tract, and other complications. If you think your parent may have an ulcer, alert her doctor.

The most effective treatment is to kill the bacteria with antibiotics while taking other drugs to reduce the amount of stomach acid and protect the stomach lining. Unfortunately, this can mean taking up to 20 pills a day. Fortunately, the treatment lasts only a week or two.

Your parent should also stop using any NSAIDs and forgo smoking, caffeine, and alcohol. Meals should be small and frequent, rather than three bigger meals a day. Antacids are helpful, but they must be used with care, as some contain large amounts of sodium and can interfere with the absorption of other drugs.

To reduce the risk of ulcers in the first place, take any NSAIDs with food.

Diverticular Disease

Diverticula are small sacs that develop along the lining of the intestine for reasons that are not clear, although lack of adequate dietary fiber seems to play a role.

The presence of these sacs is called *diverticulosis*, a common ailment in elderly people. Half of all people over 65 have it, but only about 20 percent of them have any symptoms—cramps, bloating, constipation or diarrhea, and pain in the lower abdomen.

Usually the symptoms disappear with some rest, a diet high in fiber, plenty of liquids, and if these don't succeed, antispasmodic drugs or antibiotics.

Diverticulitis is a far more serious problem that requires immediate medical attention. In this case, the sacs become inflamed, often because stool gets stuck in the intestine, causing an infection or perforation. Diverticulitis causes pain, fever, and stiffness of the abdomen and can lead to a number of complications. It is treated with antibiotics, intravenous fluids, and, in some cases, surgery.

Hemorrhoids

Hemorrhoids can ruin an otherwise good day. Straining puts pressure on the veins around the anus, which distend outward and form small, painful protuberances. Hemorrhoids can also develop internally, in the lower part of the rectum.

They are often itchy and painful, and they may be bloody (which will be the only sign when they are internal). Older people may be at greater risk if they sit for long stretches of time, are constipated, or vomit, cough, or sneeze fiercely and repeatedly.

Usually fiber, fluids, and time will relieve the problem. Over-the-counter hemorrhoid creams, warm baths, petroleum jelly, ice packs, and cold witch hazel can ease the pain and itching. A doughnut-shaped pillow may make sitting more comfortable, but it should be used only for short periods, as it can cause pressure sores. Stool softeners will make defecating less painful. Heavy lifting and straining should be halted. If hemorrhoids persist and are severe, they can be removed or shrunk by several methods, all of them pretty simple. Talk to the doctor.

Be aware that rectal bleeding is not always caused by hemorrhoids, can be very serious, and should always get a doctor's attention.

Gas

Intestinal gas can be unpleasant for both you and your parent, but it is normal and not particularly worrisome—nothing a good sense of humor can't overcome.

As with constipation, older people sometimes become overly concerned about gas because they have some preconceived notion of what is "normal." (Healthy men ages 25 to 35 pass gas up to 20 times a day.)

Gas comes from swallowing air while eating, or from the production of bacteria in the bowels. Avoid dairy products, as lactose intolerance is common among the elderly. Other dietary culprits include beans, legumes, raisins, broccoli, cauliflower, Brussels sprouts, bran, and cabbage—all those high-fiber, low-fat foods that are so healthful. Rather than cut out these good foods, have your

➕ MEDICAL ALERT

Call the doctor immediately if your parent has sudden, sharp, and persistent stomach pain, or bloody or black vomit or stools. This could be a sign that an ulcer has broken through the stomach wall, broken through a blood vessel, or blocked the intestinal tract.

parent cut down on them, and then put up with a few bad odors.

Although gas can cause stomach pains and bloating, it is the ego that usually gets hurt. Elderly people often have little or no control over when or how gas is released. Your parent may be embarrassed, and you may be too, but try to ignore it, cover for her, or laugh with her about it.

FLU SHOTS

Your parent should get a flu (influenza) vaccine each year between September and mid-November, before the flu season begins. And because you are taking care of her, you should get one, too.

The shot is not foolproof. Your parent might still get the flu (and no, the vaccine cannot cause the flu), but the symptoms, duration, and risk of death will be greatly reduced.

Medicare and most insurers cover the cost of flu shots. Senior centers and local health departments often offer flu shots for free.

Be alert to signs of the flu—chills, fever, dry cough, stuffy nose, muscle aches, headache, and fatigue. There are medications that can reduce the severity and length of the illness, but they must be taken within 48 hours of the first symptoms.

Your parent should also have had a one-time pneumonia vaccine as well as a vaccination against shingles (recommended for everyone over 60).

Anemia

Anemia is a blood disorder that is common among the elderly, is often undiagnosed, and can have serious consequences.

When a person is diagnosed as anemic, it means that his red blood cells, which carry oxygen around the body, are damaged or in short supply. Anemia, once known as "tired blood," makes a person feel old and tired—even older and more tired than he already feels. Which explains why it's often overlooked; it looks like a bad case of old age.

But it can make life cumbersome for your parent, limiting his ability to do simple physical tasks and possibly shortening his life.

Anemia can also cause headaches, shortness of breath, irritability, apathy, cold hands and feet, chest pains, swelling, confusion, dizziness, depression, and, in the case of iron-deficient anemia, restless legs at night and, oddly enough, a sore tongue.

A simple blood test can detect anemia, so ask your parent's doctor about it.

Iron-deficient anemia, the most common type of anemia found in the elderly, is often caused by internal bleeding, which may be due to ulcers, cancer, hemorrhoids, and other problems in the digestive tract. Other types of anemia may be caused by chronic infection or inflammation, kidney or liver disease, low thyroid, cancer, or folate or vitamin B12 deficiency.

The doctor should determine the cause and treat any underlying disorder. Increasing the amount of iron in your parent's diet might help. Meat and poultry, especially liver, kidneys, and other organs, contain iron, as do egg yolks, dark green leafy vegetables, dried fruits, and dried beans and peas. But iron supplements or injections are usually necessary.

Diabetes

More than a quarter of the population over age 60 has diabetes, a condition in which the body loses its ability to regulate glucose, a simple sugar that acts as fuel for the body.

If not managed properly, diabetes can lead to heart disease, stroke, kidney failure, blindness, nerve damage (and the amputation of extremities), and death.

The pancreas makes insulin, a hormone that regulates the use of glucose in the body. When the body doesn't make insulin or doesn't use it effectively, glucose builds up in the blood, causing an array of problems.

Normally, early signs of the disease include thirst, frequent urination, fatigue, weight loss, blurred vision, and, sometimes, tingly, itchy skin. But the elderly often have very different symptoms. They might become dehydrated, confused, incontinent, and/or depressed. As a result, the diagnosis is sometimes missed until things get serious.

The first line of treatment is a controlled diet, exercise, and, for most people, weight loss. When insulin and/or hypoglycemic agents are necessary, they should be managed carefully, as these drugs are extremely dangerous for the elderly.

Controlling diabetes can be complicated, especially in an elderly person, so it's best approached by a team that includes an endocrinologist, a nutritionist, and a diabetes educator.

If your parent has diabetes, he will need to pay special attention to his skin care, his oral hygiene, and his feet (check daily for sores, blisters, infections, and heavy calluses).

For more information about diabetes, contact the American Diabetes Association (800-232-3472 or diabetes.org).

Chapter 13

Matters of
the Mind

Depression • Delirium • Anxiety Disorders • Delusions and
Hallucinations • Hypochondria

Growing old is not easy, and at times it is just plain dreadful, but it does not, by itself, cause depression, anxiety, or other mental illness. Despite all the losses and disabilities elderly people face, most adapt pretty well. Indeed, many find joy and peace in this final chapter of life.

When sadness turns into despair, when simple worries become paralyzing, when your parent no longer finds joy in the things she used to love, it is time to seek professional help. Hopelessness, surliness, and constant worry are not "just a part of growing old."

The challenge lies in finding the cause. It makes sense that hearing loss and incontinence are associated with high rates of depression, because these problems are isolating. But in the elderly, heart attack, stroke, infection, and surgery are also precursors of depression; some physiological change occurs that makes otherwise resilient people unable to bounce back.

The reverse is also true. That is, mental illness can cause physical ailments and make it more difficult to recover from illness. For example, studies suggest that about half of all complaints of gastro-intestinal pain in the elderly—heartburn, diarrhea, nausea, gastritis, and so on—have a psychological component. That is not to say that these problems are invented. They are real. But they are sometimes caused, in part, by anxiety, paranoia, or other mental distress.

Now throw into this mind-matter muddle the death of a spouse, the loss of mobility, or a move, and things can get complicated. Is your father staying to himself and feeling glum because his old friend died, or because he is suffering from an infection? Does he need antide-pressants or antibiotics?

What do you treat, how do you treat, and how do you, as the caregiving child, cope?

Depression

Your father doesn't want to play bridge anymore, and he won't even look at a crossword puzzle. He turns down his favorite mint chocolate Girl Scout cookies. He dresses in the same clothes every day and refuses to go out. *What's the point?* he says, staring vacantly at the television set. *I'm just an old man. I'll be dead before you know it.* Then he calls you by the wrong name and goes to bed.

You may think that he's just being ornery, causing you untold worry and exasperation, but in truth he may be suf-fering from depression.

The rate of depression rises after the age of 65, as does the rate of suicide, especially among men. Studies suggest that up to 15 percent of people over 65 suffer from some degree of depression.

In nursing homes, that rate jumps to somewhere between 30 and 50 percent.

What's alarming, however, is not the number of elderly people who are depressed, but that so many elderly people suffering from depression are never diagnosed or treated. They slog through old age carrying this unbearable weight until they die (which is usually earlier than it would have been had they been treated).

Depression is overlooked in the elderly for a whole host of reasons. They themselves ignore the blackness that has overcome them because they were brought up during a time when depression was considered a weakness, a character flaw, something one should be able to control.

ON THE LOOKOUT FOR SYMPTOMS

PROBLEM	SIGNS OF TROUBLE
Depression	Withdrawal, apathy, fatigue, feelings of worthlessness and hopelessness, vague physical complaints (headache, stomachache), change in sleep habits, confusion, memory loss, irritability, poor hygiene, unreasonable fears, change in appetite, difficulty concentrating or making decisions, nervousness
Anxiety disorders	Excessive worry or fear, agitation, insomnia, muscle tension, irritability
Delirium	Inattentiveness and confusion that come on suddenly, often accompanied by grogginess or anxiety
Dementia	Confusion, chronic forgetfulness, and other mental lapses that get progressively worse. (See Chapter 23 for a full discussion of memory loss and dementia.)

It goes unnoticed because family members and caregivers assume that being antisocial and grumpy is just part of growing old. Indeed, even many doctors are guilty of this ageism.

Depression is also overlooked because the complex stew of illness, medications, and grief that commonly affects elderly people complicates any diagnosis. For example, depression in the elderly is often triggered by an illness, particularly heart disease, stroke, certain cancers, chronic lung disease, infections, arthritis, vitamin B12 deficiency, Alzheimer's disease, and Parkinson's disease. It can also be the result of medications, particularly blood pressure medications, anti-ulcer medications, muscle relaxants, steroids, and drugs for Parkinson's.

Confounding things further, older people who are depressed often have atypical symptoms. Rather than feeling sadness or hopelessness, they complain about sleepless nights, backaches, headaches, or stomachaches, or they simply become irritable.

Finally, many of the more common symptoms of depression—fatigue, apathy, weight loss, confusion, a change in appetite—can easily be attributed to some other illness or ongoing treatment. It doesn't occur to anyone that the symptoms are part of a treatable psychiatric disorder.

Such neglect is a shame, because depression is not normal at any age, and it is virtually always treatable with medication, counseling, or both.

Untreated, it increases the risk of stroke and heart disease, causes confusion, and exacerbates dementia. Your parent might not take care of himself

SUICIDE

Suicide is more common among people over the age of 65 than in any other age group. Of elderly people who commit suicide, 75 percent have seen their doctors within a month of killing themselves. Many saw their doctors on the same day.

If your parent talks about harming or killing himself, get help. If you think he is in immediate danger, call 911. If your parent resists help, saying that he's fine or he'll handle it himself, be assertive. Contact his doctor. Or for more immediate help, take him to the hospital emergency room. Remove or lock up pills, knives, and other weapons.

If you are concerned about suicide and your parent refuses help, you might have to get a "certificate of involuntary commitment" from a judge, psychiatrist, or other physician. This forces your parent to have a brief psychiatric evaluation (which can sometimes be done at home) and may result in institutionalization for a period of time.

or get out to see others. Engulfed by despair, he might not follow his prescribed treatments or show up for medical appointments, thereby derailing all efforts at recovery. His physical illness gets worse, as does his mental illness.

In a nutshell, depression will make these "golden years" miserable for your parent and everyone around him.

> " My father had to be hospitalized twice because of severe infections in his feet. We were all so concerned about his diabetes and his infection that at first we failed to see the real problem: depression. Because he was depressed, he wasn't taking care of himself. He wasn't controlling his diabetes, he wasn't eating well, and he didn't call anyone when he first noticed trouble. I guess he figured it didn't matter."
>
> —Katherine S.

Know the signs of depression in the elderly, and if you have any concern at all, ask your parent's doctor about the possibility that your parent may suffer from it. If the doctor doesn't take this seriously—doctors can be biased or ill informed—get an opinion from another doctor or a psychiatrist, preferably one with experience in geriatrics.

Even if your parent doesn't meet the strict psychiatric criteria for depression—if he is just mildly depressed, perhaps a bit lethargic or unusually restless—he should still seek help. Mild depression like this usually sorts itself out with time, but counseling, support, and other treatments are available and can be very helpful.

Depression and Grief

Depression can creep into a person's life without any particular trigger. However, the loss of a loved one or a series of friends, the loss of physical or mental abilities, or a move to a nursing home can cause untold grief that, unabated, can evolve into full-blown depression.

Grief is a normal reaction to loss, not an illness. But when severe grief—sleepless nights, loss of appetite, crying bouts, and fatigue—lasts for more than two months, doctors typically consider it depression.

The problem is that when losses pile up—a spouse dies, a friend dies, your parent's arthritis gets worse, she moves into a nursing home—there is no clear starting point for this artificial clock. Use your judgment. If her grieving drags on, get your mother to talk with her doctor or a psychiatrist.

Depression and Dementia

Your father may be forgetting luncheons and names, leading you to fear the worst. But before you call the Alzheimer's Association, have him evaluated by a doctor. Depression is often mistaken for dementia and therefore left untreated.

Even if your parent is in the early stages of dementia—and depression often occurs, understandably, during those first glimmers of forgetfulness—any depression needs to be treated, as it will only exacerbate the confusion.

Have your parent evaluated as soon as possible. If he has dementia, you both need to know. If he is suffering from depression, regardless of what else is happening with him, it needs to be treated. That should alleviate some of the confusion.

Broaching the Subject

Before you talk with your parent, it's important to fully understand that

> " After Marjorie died, Dad cried a lot. For months he would weep anytime her name came up in conversation. His legs hurt. He was tired all the time. And he repeated himself. He'd tell me the same story over and over.
>
> He's 90, so we weren't surprised. But he used to be really interesting, so bright. He read the paper cover to cover and could talk about current events. That was gone.
>
> A psychiatrist at the center where he lives suggested he try antidepressants. He didn't want to and fought it for months, but finally he tried them.
>
> Honestly, it was amazing. Within about six weeks, he was himself again. Still sad about Marjorie. His knees still hurt. But he was engaging and smart again."
>
> —Susan P.

depression is not a mood, nor is it a moral failing; it is a medical illness. The chemistry in the brain has changed and needs rebalancing.

Why it comes on is not clear. Some people inherit a genetic vulnerability to depression. Personality traits developed early in life—low self-esteem, poor coping skills—play a role as well. Medications, illness, hormonal and biological changes, inactivity, poor diet, grief, fear, boredom, worry, loneliness, and, as mentioned, a loss or move to an institution can all contribute to depression.

Whatever the cause or causes, your parent cannot "snap out of it" any more than he can snap out of cancer or Parkinson's disease. This is not "just the blues"; it is an illness. Although your

DEPRESSION AND YOU

Caregiving, all by itself (never mind taking care of a parent who is depressed or anxious), can lead to depression. Take good care of yourself, or you might well end up in the same hole as your parent. Your father's irritability or your mother's incessant worrying will drain you quickly. Get away from this situation regularly, see friends, exercise, eat well, get some sleep, find a support group, and laugh as often as you can. Most important, don't take your parent's comments, criticisms, or moods personally.

impulse may be to try to propel your parent out of this despair, it's not helpful to tell him to "cheer up" or to "look on the bright side." Attempts to convince him that life isn't so bad will only send the message that this is something he can control and, that because he is not controlling it, he is a failure.

Instead, listen to his concerns and acknowledge his fears and misery. Don't change the subject. If he pauses, wait and let him continue. Rather than giving him advice or reasons why he should feel differently, confirm that you hear what he's saying.

Let him know that you are there for him and that you care, that you want to help. *I know you feel lonely right now. It must be very difficult. We're going to get through this thing together.*

Be as patient as you can with any irritability, sullenness, or criticism that might come your way. This is the disease talking (or refusing to talk), not your parent.

Make it clear that his despair might be the result of medications or infection, and that depression is a biological illness that can be treated; it is not a reflection of character. You don't even have to use the word *depression* in the first conversation. Simply explain that attending to "whatever this is" will help him remain independent; failing to treat it will certainly lead to more dependence, illness, and disability.

If he still won't budge, tell him that it would be a great relief to you if he at least spoke to a doctor about it. You might get a trusted friend or member of the clergy to initiate a discussion with him. Or talk to his doctor yourself about it.

If the prospect of seeing a psychiatrist makes your parent uncomfortable, a family doctor who is savvy in such matters can treat the depression. But be sure the doctor takes this seriously; don't be deterred by a physician who suggests this is natural at his age. No one should have to live with the deep pain of clinical depression.

Treating Depression
The first step in treating depression in the elderly is to identify any underlying cause or contributing factors (such as medications, dementia, vitamin deficiency, loneliness, or loss).

After that, experts recommend a multipronged approach of antidepressants, therapy, and lifestyle changes. If the depression is recent and mild, your parent should try therapy and lifestyle changes before taking any medications.

LIFESTYLE. Exercise, social activities, sleep, community involvement, intellectual stimulation, a good diet, and an understanding and loving family will not, by themselves, cure depression. However, they are potent in keeping depression at bay. Those patients who take care of themselves and have support and encouragement from friends and family fare better than others.

Be sure your parent gets good medical care. Keep an eye on his diet, exercise, and sleep. Note that while alcohol might provide temporary relief, it actually worsens depression.

Gently encourage your parent to get back into activities that he once enjoyed and to join social gatherings. Creative outlets—drawing, painting, sculpting, music—can help reduce stress and ease feelings of hopelessness.

OTHER SUPPORTS. Your parent might find strength in support groups, either in person or online. Talking to others who struggle with the same issues can make a person feel less alone. Pastoral counseling and spiritual support can also be enormously helpful. Having a pet can be a powerful elixir for depression, as well as for anxiety and other mental illnesses.

ANTIDEPRESSANT DRUGS. Although antidepressants can help, any medications, including antidepressants, should

DEEP IN DEPRESSION

Brief bouts of sadness and grief are normal, and most people with very mild depressive symptoms get better on their own. But if your parent has several of the following symptoms for more than two weeks (or more than two months after a major loss or move to an institution), press his doctor for action or get him to a psychiatrist.

- Dejection and sadness without any apparent cause

- Feelings of hopelessness, helplessness, guilt, or worthlessness

- Lack of interest in activities that were once considered enjoyable

- Social withdrawal

- Unusual restlessness, irritability, or hostility

- Frequent crying spells, weeping, or tearfulness

- Change in appetite or weight

- Insomnia or change in sleep habits

- Fatigue and lethargy, loss of energy

- Lack of concentration, forgetfulness, indecisiveness

- Excessive worry

- Vague complaints of physical aches and pains

- Unusually poor grooming and personal hygiene

- Increased use of alcohol, drugs, or tobacco

- Talk of death or suicide

GETTING HELP

Because mental illness is so complicated in the elderly and is often linked to physical illness, medications, and issues that are specific to elderly people, you should look for a psychiatrist (or psychotherapist, for therapy) who has a good deal of experience in dealing with elderly clients. Ask what percent of the practice comprises clients over 65. Ideally, it should be at least 25 percent. Some psychiatrists are certified in geriatric psychiatry, although they are few and far between. You can get a referral from the American Association for Geriatric Psychiatry (aagponline.org).

be used judiciously when treating an elderly person. They should be part of a comprehensive treatment plan (including lifestyle changes and therapy). And they should be started at a very low dose (and increased gradually, if needed).

These drugs affect certain chemicals in the brain, called neurotransmitters (because they "transmit" messages between nerve cells). Depression is often the result of an imbalance in these chemicals.

It usually takes about four to eight weeks before they are effective, possibly longer.

Because recurrence is common, the drugs are often continued for at least 6 to 12 months after the symptoms have subsided. Depending on the severity of the depression, a doctor might recommend that your parent stay on a medication for several years.

Common side effects include dry mouth (sip water), drowsiness (take the medication at bedtime), insomnia (take it in the morning), restlessness (talk to the doctor about reducing the dose), nausea, diarrhea, dizziness, or constipation (these should subside after a few weeks). More serious (but uncommon) side effects include stroke, falls, fractures, and in some people, an increased risk of suicide.

If a medication causes unpleasant side effects or, after several weeks, does not seem to be helping, your parent should alert his doctor. Sometimes a person needs to try a different antidepressant, change the dose, or try a combination of medications.

Be sure your parent sticks to any regimen. Skipping medications or stopping early may make them ineffective and lead to relapse or other problems.

PSYCHOTHERAPY. Drugs can relieve the severity of depression, bringing a person out of the pit of despair, but they do not resolve any issues that might have contributed to the depression. Therapy, individually or in a group, can help your parent address these issues.

Your parent might have to try several therapists before she finds the right fit. Once she does, encourage her to stay with it for at least 10 weeks, preferably longer.

ELECTROCONVULSIVE THERAPY. When depression is very severe and antidepressants and counseling don't help, electroconvulsive therapy, or ECT, is often effective. It is particularly successful in treating severe depression in elderly patients and has fewer side effects than medications.

Although there used to be plenty of horror stories about ECT, the procedure has been fine-tuned and is considered to be an effective, fast, and safe way to reverse depression. It usually works faster than drugs, but the effects don't last as long. (Medication will sometimes help lower the rate of recurrent bouts of depression.)

In the procedure, a patient is given anesthesia and a muscle relaxant, then padded electrodes are placed on the head. A small machine sends an electric pulse through the electrodes into the brain until the patient has a minor seizure in half of the brain. The seizure triggers neurons to release chemicals that are necessary for a healthy, functioning brain. People often need 6 to 12 treatments over a few weeks.

The procedure is not painful, but many people experience mild short-term memory loss; this should subside within a month or two. However, ECT may be a poor choice for a person with dementia.

Your parent, or you, should discuss all the pros and cons with the doctor. Understandably, the idea may frighten your parent (and you), so by all means get a second opinion.

UNCONVENTIONAL MEDICINE. There are numerous alternative or complementary therapies that may be useful in alleviating depression and anxiety. They include acupuncture, massage, meditation, yoga, tai chi, and breathing exercises.

Biofeedback seems to be more helpful in treating anxiety than depression, but some studies suggest it may be effective for depression as well. In biofeedback, a person learns to control his or her bodily reactions—muscle tension, heart rate, breathing—to stressful or upsetting situations.

Guided imagery, or visualization, which involves going into a deep state of relaxation, is often used to treat depression, addiction, and anxiety.

You can find information about these and other therapies at The National Center for Complementary and Alternative Medicine's website (nccam.nih.gov).

> " After my father moved into the retirement home, he went to a very dark place. He didn't want to do anything. Nothing pleased him. He stayed in his room, refused to see people, and just didn't care about anything. When I suggested that he get help, he became angry.
>
> Finally, I couldn't stand it anymore. I marched into his room and told him to get in the car, and I took him to the geriatric psychiatry unit at our local hospital. I've never been forceful with my father, but something just got to me. I couldn't bear to see him like that.
>
> He had ECT for several weeks, and now he's in a day program where he meets with the psychiatrist and goes to a support group. It's made a difference. He's not jumping about, all excited about life, but he's definitely better."
>
> —Eleanor R.

Delirium

Your father, who was always competent and able, is insisting that he is in his sister's house and not at the nursing home. His speech is garbled, he can't seem to read the lunch menu, and now he is screaming that there are owls in the room. Is this it? Has he completely lost his mind? What is happening?

Delirium is common in the elderly, but is, sadly, often unrecognized or misdiagnosed. Unchecked, delirium often leads to other serious medical problems, even death. It's essential that you be on the lookout and treat it immediately.

Delirium typically is characterized by confusion, inattentiveness, anxiety, memory loss, aggression, disorientation, and hallucinations. However, some patients become apathetic, quiet, and sleepy. The key characteristic is that it comes on suddenly and severely, over the course of a few hours or days.

Although delirium is most common in hospitalized elderly patients, it is increasingly seen in nursing homes and even private homes, largely because people are sent home so quickly from the hospital.

Illness, such as stroke, heart failure, kidney or thyroid dysfunction, or internal bleeding, can precipitate delirium, as can a move to a new environment, dehydration, infections, poor eyesight or hearing, alcohol withdrawal, or severe urinary or fecal retention.

Delirium is often caused by medications, especially when a new medication is started, a dose is changed, or a medication is stopped. Psychoactive drugs, such as sedatives, antidepressants, opioids, and anticholinergic drugs (as well as many other prescription and nonprescription drugs) are all likely culprits.

Diagnosis and Treatment

As the person who best knows your parent, you may be the first to spot the symptoms. Anytime you notice a significant, sudden change in your parent's behavior, alert a doctor immediately and ask about the possibility of delirium.

Since it's often not possible to identify a single cause, doctors attack this on many fronts. Any infections or illnesses need to be treated, and certain medications—particularly any sedatives—should be stopped. Physical restraints should be avoided. The doctor should take steps to treat bedsores, urinary and fecal

> " While my mother was in the nursing home, she became very confused and started to act oddly. She refused food and water and would wander about like she didn't know where she was. I was scared, and definitely more concerned than the nurses were, so I was the one who called it to the doctor's attention. He said she was delirious, and he put her through dozens of tests. They found that she was dehydrated, had a urinary tract infection, and was taking too much of an antipsychotic drug. As soon as they adjusted the dose and dealt with her other problems, she returned to normal."
> —Gloria C.

disorders, malnutrition, dehydration, and other problems that often accompany delirium.

Help reorient your parent by surrounding him with familiar objects. Put clocks and calendars where he can see them. Close the curtains at night and open them during the day to help reset his biological clock.

Assure your parent that he is safe and try to keep him calm. Keep movement and noise levels low. Speak softly to him, reassuring him that things are okay. You know best what might calm your parent, but soft music, gentle massage, and relaxation techniques are sometimes useful.

Make sure your parent has his glasses and hearing aids. Sometimes physical therapy or some light exercise can help.

Delirium, once properly diagnosed, is usually reversible, although there might be some residual confusion for a few weeks.

Anxiety Disorders

Has your mother always been a worrywart, or have her anxieties reached new heights? Is your father suddenly afraid of closed spaces? Does your parent panic when you leave the house?

Although elderly people are often more cautious (with good reason), they can suffer from a number of anxiety disorders, including the following:

GENERALIZED ANXIETY DISORDER. About 5 percent of the elderly suffer from generalized anxiety disorder. The defining symptom is excessive worry that lasts for at least six months.

People with generalized anxiety disorder often know that their worries are overblown, but still they can't relax. The worry or dread can be so great that it gets in the way of daily activities.

Generalized anxiety disorder is usually accompanied by agitation or restlessness, irritability, exhaustion, insomnia, difficulty concentrating, and/or muscle tension. A person might also suffer from shakiness and trembling, dizziness, shortness of breath, nausea, hot and cold flashes, and frequent urination. They often have exaggerated responses when startled and may be extremely vigilant and edgy.

Of course, nothing to do with the elderly is simple. Several ailments can cause anxiety, including hyperthyroidism, and heart or lung diseases that cause palpitations and/or shortness of breath. Anxiety and agitation may also be symptoms of delirium, depression, or dementia.

It's possible that your parent is reacting to justifiable fears (for example, running out of money or being trapped in his wheelchair) and has no psychiatric disorder. But if he has an anxiety disorder, the fear far exceeds reality and is unabated when the cause of the fear is addressed.

PHOBIAS. Many elderly people suffer from phobias—irrational and intense fears of a person, place, or thing. Although phobias often focus on heights, spiders, and flying, elderly people are often afraid of death (not so irrational, actually), a family crisis, or, interestingly, dental procedures.

They sometimes develop social phobias that are grossly exaggerated, yet also understandable. A person who is losing his memory or is unable to bathe and dress himself might become terrified of being in public because he is afraid of making a fool of himself or looking unkempt.

While the basis of the fear might make some sense, the reaction—sweating, panicking, breathing rapidly, shaking, chest pains—is out of whack.

OBSESSIVE-COMPULSIVE DISORDER, another type of anxiety disorder, is characterized by intrusive and unwanted thoughts, often about something silly, scary, or disgusting, and strong urges to do something repeatedly. These rituals—hand washing is common, but a person might repeatedly fix her hair, relock the door, or check to make sure the light is off—ease the obsessions.

OCD doesn't usually crop up suddenly in old age. A person typically suffers from it earlier in life as well.

People in the early stages of dementia might seem to have OCD if they compensate for losses by being unusually fastidious, checking and double-checking that the stove is off, that tasks were

completed, that plans are set. Then, of course, minutes later they forget that they checked, and need to check one more time.

HOARDING is related to anxiety and OCD, and the symptoms are self-explanatory. These people don't just have clutter; they have an avalanche of "stuff," so much that it is nearly impossible to move around or find a place to sit.

Like other mental illnesses, hoarding does not respond to logic. You cannot use reason to stop your father from collecting and storing more stuff. Furthermore, his house isn't packed to the gills because he's too lazy to throw things out; indeed, just the opposite. Hoarding is a lot of work.

Hoarding often stems from a host of anxieties, and efforts to reduce the clutter can exacerbate these worries and cause untold grief. You might have to simply clear a safe walkway and then let it go. Talk to his doctor.

Treating Anxiety Disorders

Anxiety disorders are usually caused by a combination of legitimate concern or fear, chronic grief, genetics, other mental illness, disease, trauma, medications, caffeine, vitamin deficiency, and withdrawal from alcohol or sedatives. Dementia is one of the most common causes of anxiety among the elderly—both because of physiological changes and because forgetting things and losing control is terrifying.

Obviously, any contributing factor (medications, disease, infection) should be addressed first.

Anxiety is often alleviated with antidepressants, but you should always be

BIOLOGICAL, NOT LOGICAL

It is natural that you want to talk your parent out of any irrational feelings. *Dad, you just need to stop worrying so much. Everything is going to be fine.* And when that doesn't work, it's natural to be frustrated, even angry.

It's incredibly hard to accept that your parent can't think reasonably, overcome his fears, or cheer up. But if he is suffering from a mental illness, he cannot. And no matter how hard you try, you cannot convince him otherwise. (And your irritation might only escalae his worries or depression.)

If your parent had a huge wound on her leg and was in a wheelchair and in terrible in pain, you would not say, *Stop moaning. Get up and walk!* No, you'd say,

That must be awful. I'm sorry you hurt so much. What can I do to help? Well, mental illness hurts, too. It just doesn't bleed.

Recognizing the biological basis of this, and accepting the illogical aspect of it, should ease your frustration and help you find a more positive and useful approach.

Let him know that you hear him, acknowledge that this must be hard for him (*Dad, I'm sorry you're so worried. That must be exhausting for you*), find out what, specifically, he is anxious about, and address his fears, if possible. Reassure him that you will remind him when it's time to go, or set an alarm for him. And of course, talk to his doctor or someone versed in geriatric psychiatry.

---

leery of adding drugs to your parent's regimen. Antianxiety drugs like Valium, Xanax, Klonopin, and Ativan should generally be avoided because they increase the risks of falls and accidents, and decrease memory and cognition.

Treatment also includes counseling to deal with specific causes of concern, family support, exercise, pets, massage, biofeedback, and relaxation techniques. See the discussion of treatments for depression on page 264, especially the paragraphs about psychotherapy and lifestyle changes, as these are all extremely useful in treating anxiety.

In all of these anxiety disorders, you may have to simply learn to live with

some behaviors. Medical professionals generally don't agree with this line of reasoning, but we are dealing with reality here.

If your 90-year-old father is a hoarder and not bothered by it, you can take him to a psychiatrist, give him medications, and start cognitive behavioral therapy, or you can say, *What the heck*, step over the piles, and give him a hug. If your mother is worried that someone will steal her jewels, but functions pretty well otherwise, buy a lockbox and put the key around her neck. In other words, if the problem is causing you more pain than it is causing your parent, acceptance may be the best medicine for everyone.

Delusions and Hallucinations

Delusions are beliefs that are simply not true, like thinking that someone is trying to kill you or is reading your mind. Hallucinations are visions that don't exist, like seeing an elf on your bed or a camel in the corner.

Delusions and hallucinations are often symptoms of depression and/or

ⓘ FOR MORE HELP

National Institute of Mental Health
nimh.nih.gov
866-615-6464

National Alliance for the Mentally Ill
nami.org
800-950-6264

Depression and Bipolar Support Alliance
dbsalliance.org
800-826-3632

Geriatric Mental Health Foundation
gmhfonline.org
301-654-7850

dementia. They can also be the result of delirium, infections, poor hearing or vision, overmedication, dehydration, and a variety of other factors.

Get your parent to a doctor who has a lot of experience with elderly patients. Be sure he or she doesn't simply prescribe antipsychotic medications without first looking for an underlying cause.

Although a number of medications are effective in treating excessive paranoia, delusions, or hallucinations, these drugs are also quite dangerous in the elderly and can worsen the psychosis and cause other problems. If your parent's doctor prescribes one, be sure it is absolutely necessary, and that the dose is low.

If your parent has psychotic symptoms, as always, stay calm. Listen. Be empathetic. Do not try to reason with him or argue. Let him talk about his concerns. Let him know that you hear him. *It must be very frightening to feel that way. What else worries you?* If there is a giraffe in his room, don't tell him it doesn't exist; ask what it wants for lunch.

Hypochondria

At least 5 percent of people over 65 suffer from hypochondria or a related problem called "undifferentiated

somatoform disorder." In the first (which is technically known as hypochondriasis), a person is obsessed with the idea that he has a serious illness. In the latter, a person complains about symptoms (such as fatigue, abdominal pain, and loss of appetite) that have no medical basis.

Obviously, you must be sure that your parent isn't actually sick. Once this is determined, then the most effective treatment is a form of psychotherapy known as cognitive behavioral therapy (CBT), which teaches people to identify irrational beliefs and unhealthy reactions and change these responses.

Again, be cautious with medications. Your parent's doctor should gently steer her away from unnecessary tests and treatments, but still treat certain symptoms, such as insomnia or pain.

Keep in mind that even though symptoms might not have a biological basis, they are still real to your parent. Be sympathetic, but don't reinforce the behavior.

Chapter 14

In the Hospital

Avoiding It • Choosing a Hospital • Admission • Following His Wishes • Tests, Surgery, and Treatments • At the Nurses' Station • Providing Comfort • When You Are Far Away • Hospital Dangers • Resolving Disputes • Preparing for Discharge • Bills, Bills, Bills

No matter what hospitals do to look more welcoming and genial—put large plants in the lobby, colorful prints on the walls, friendly volunteers at the door—they are still scary, especially when the patient is elderly, frail, and vulnerable.

Your parent needs plenty of love and reassurance now. She also needs a strong advocate, someone who will be informed, honor her wishes, and ensure she is getting proper care.

That being said, if you've been handling the lion's share of your parent's care and this is not a dire situation, then this hospital stay might be a much-needed break for you. Keep tabs on her care, but try to get others to check on her so you can take advantage of this time.

When you are not at the hospital, get your mind off your worries, spend time with friends, and catch up on your sleep. You need it. Remember, you'll be of no use to your parent if you don't take care of yourself.

Avoiding It

An odd note to start on, but if at all possible, don't let your parent go to the hospital in the first place. A minor hospital stay can quickly turn into a major disaster for an elderly person. Frail bodies can quickly succumb to dehydration, a fall, infections, over-medication, and other common risks of hospital life. Nursing home residents (or those eligible for nursing home care) are especially vulnerable.

Surgery, in particular, is often more than elderly people can handle, as their reserves and ability to heal are already compromised. Many don't survive, or don't survive for long. Others return home, but never regain their physical function or mental capacity.

Ask a lot of questions and be sure this is the best course of action, even when a hospitalization seems urgent and unavoidable. Talk with the doctor and, if possible, your parent. If your parent is quite frail, find out if there is any way to get him the care he needs at home instead.

Choosing a Hospital

A doctor can work only in those hospitals where he or she has admitting privileges, so if your parent is committed to a particular doctor, there may be little choice in selecting a hospital. Also, her Medicare plan or other insurance might require that she go to certain doctors, hospitals, or rehab centers. In an emergency, your parent may have to go to the nearest hospital (once she is out of danger, she can usually be transferred).

If your parent doesn't have a choice about which hospital to use and some time to make the decision, she (or you) should select both the hospital and the doctor.

EXPERIENCE. Choose a doctor who has a lot of experience with the particular procedure, surgery, or treatment your parent needs, and a hospital that specializes in it. If it's a common procedure, like bypass surgery or a hysterectomy, then the surgeon should have performed close to 100 such surgeries in the past year. (If it's a less common procedure or your parent lives in a rural area, that number will be lower.)

SIZE. Generally, large medical centers have high-caliber specialists, dedicated clinics, and more sophisticated technology than small community hospitals. Thus, they have higher volume and

✚ MEDICAL ALERT: DELIRIUM

Elderly patients, particularly those who undergo surgery or stay in the intensive care unit, often wind up with delirium. Many of them never fully recover simply because they are misdiagnosed or not diagnosed in time, so learn the signs.

Delirium comes on suddenly and causes severe confusion, inattention, disorientation, garbled speech, forgetfulness, agitation, and hallucinations. Report any sudden changes in your parent's personality or behaviors to the staff.

Delirium and other hospital risks are discussed later in this chapter. It's best to know about them in advance and act preventively.

more experience with many procedures. They are also generally better equipped to treat unusual ailments and perform risky procedures.

But large-scale can also mean that patients get less attention and TLC than they would in a smaller hospital. So if a particular surgeon has privileges at more than one hospital, your parent might be happier in the smaller hospital.

AFFILIATION. A hospital run by a religious organization will generally offer more compassionate care than, say, a large city hospital, although it might also have policies about end-of-life care and medical decisions that may or may not fit with your parent's wishes.

A hospital that is affiliated with a medical school will be focused less on the soft side of patient care and more on teaching and research. However, a research hospital, affiliated with a large university, will offer more state-of-the-art treatments.

Teaching hospitals train young doctors, using patients as teaching models, which can be disconcerting and, when five or six young doctors are standing around the bedside, embarrassing. However, physicians-in-training ask a lot of questions, and this brings important matters to the attending doctor's attention.

Many hospitals are linked to specific nursing and rehab facilities. If your parent is likely to need rehab or nursing care, ask which facilities are linked to which hospitals.

If your parent is a veteran and there's a VA hospital in the area, the Department of Veterans Affairs (va.gov or 800-827-1000) can tell you about eligibility and benefits. VA hospitals, which are often affiliated with a university hospital, can be good, and are certainly less expensive.

> ❝ My father always went to the same hospital, but when I called 911, the ambulance took him to a different hospital. Here my father was in a strange place, with a new doctor who didn't know him at all, who didn't have any personal relationship with him.
>
> It took me more than a week, but I finally got them to move him. They kept saying that he was too weak to make the move, that he was fine where he was. But I knew he wasn't.
>
> He was moved, and he died about two weeks later. But I know that he was more comfortable in a familiar place, with doctors and nurses who knew him and where his friends could visit him easily. He couldn't tell me so, but I believe that I did the right thing."
>
> —Chris D.

COST. Although people don't typically shop around for the best price when heading to the hospital, you might want to start. Hospitals charge widely different rates for the same procedure. For example, surgery at a not-for-profit community hospital might be 25 percent cheaper than at a large, for-profit hospital. Depending upon your parent's health care coverage, price might be surprisingly important.

THE REPORT CARD. You can look at a hospital's "report card" at the Medicare website (medicare.gov/quality-care-finder). These report cards are only moderately helpful because the results are similar across most hospitals (very few patients find it quiet at night, about half say staff explained medications, most get some instructions upon leaving, and so on), but they will let you know which hospitals to avoid.

Admission

The hospital will want a range of information and documents signed before your parent is admitted. They will want her Social Security, Medicare, Medicaid, and other health insurance cards. They will need to know about medications, allergies, and previous hospitalizations and injuries. They will also want copies of any advance directives.

If you know in advance about the hospitalization, ask what documents are needed and if the paperwork can be done early so your parent doesn't have to deal with a lot of questions on an already tense day. Also, see if someone can drop you and your parent off at the hospital so she doesn't have to wait alone while you park.

If your parent will be in the hospital for some time, find out if there is a choice in rooms, because once your parent is assigned to a room, the staff will be reluctant to move her (it requires paperwork, as well as physical work). If there is any choice, ask for a bed near a window. Natural light and a view—even if it's a view of a rooftop—can boost the spirits. You can also ask about roommates, privacy, and anything else that concerns your parent. She may not be given a lot of choice, but it's certainly worth asking.

At the same time, inquire about a telephone and television, as it can take a day or two to get these services up and running (of course, if she's bringing her cell phone, then having a phone in the room is not an issue). If this will be a long stay, find out about other amenities, such as newspaper delivery, barbers and hairstylists, Internet access, and book and magazine carts. Patients often aren't told about these services unless they ask.

- Books and magazines

- Kindle, iPad, or other tablet, but only if there is a safe place to store it

GUILT, AGAIN?

Your parent is not in the hospital because of something you or anyone else in the family did or failed to do. Don't torture yourself with guilt. *I knew I shouldn't have left her alone. . . . I should have told the doctor he was having chest pains. . . .* Life is so clear in hindsight, but there was no way you or anyone else could have predicted this accident or illness. And doing things differently might not have changed the outcome.

This hospitalization is not anyone's fault, so focus your valuable energy on taking care of your parent, and leave the guilt in the garbage can by the door.

- iPod or other music player, and headphones, but again, only if there is a safe place to store it

- Toiletries, including toothbrush, toothpaste, deodorant, shampoo, soap, razor, lip balm, and moisturizer

- Clock, watch, calendar, and/or appointment book

- Any special pillow, if your parent has a preference (best to put it in a colored case so it doesn't get mixed up with the hospital laundry)

- Crackers, dried fruit, cereal, or other nonperishable foods, if allowed

- Earplugs and an eye mask

- A small amount of cash for vendors— no more than $20 or $30

Packing a Bag

Your parent needs very little in a hospital. Jewelry and other valuables should stay at home. Label all items clearly. A hospital bag might include:

- List of medications (including supplements and over-the-counter meds), dosages, allergies, and medical history. (If you're rushing, throw all pill bottles into a bag and bring it all to the hospital.)

- Copies of a living will, a health proxy form, and other advance directives

- Hearing aids, eyeglasses, dentures, cane, or walker

- Slippers with rubber soles, or better yet, rubber-soled socks

- Robe and/or bed jacket

- Cell phone and charger

Planning Ahead

As soon as you know your parent's prognosis, talk with the hospital's discharge planner, especially if there's any chance your parent will have difficulty returning to his former life.

The discharge planner will help you prepare for your parent's return home, lining him up with community services, home care, and medical equipment, or making arrangements for him to move into a rehabilitation center, nursing home, or other living situation. All of this planning takes time, and you want everything to be in place when your parent is ready to leave.

It's helpful to talk to the discharge planner even if you think your parent will be just fine returning to his own home. First of all, he might not be as fine as you'd hoped. Second, discharge planners often have a wealth of information about community services and supports that, if they are not needed now, might be needed in the near future. Use this service while it's at your disposal and you're right there, wandering the hallways in search of a cup of coffee.

Where's Her Doctor?

Your parent's primary doctor may relinquish control once your parent enters the hospital. Usually this is because a specialist is now overseeing her care or because her doctor focuses only on office-based care. Sometimes doctors prefer, or insurance plans or hospitals require, that designated hospital doctors (called "hospitalists") oversee inpatient care.

If this switch is disconcerting, talk with your parent's doctor. It may be that he or she can remain involved. At the very least, all doctors should be in close communication.

A Question of Cost

In any other part of life, we ask what something costs before we say yes or no. But when it comes to medical care, this somehow seems inappropriate. It is not.

The price of various tests and treatments might or might not affect any decisions, but you should know up front what things cost, what Medicare, Medicaid, or other insurance will cover, and what your parent will have to pay out of pocket.

Be sure to get the full cost, as there will be separate bills from the hospital and individual practitioners. Ask about other costs, too, because those little

INPATIENT OR OUTPATIENT?

Any time your parent is in the hospital, ask if he is an inpatient or an outpatient, as this affects Medicare coverage.

Even if he stays overnight, he might still be considered an outpatient. In fact, patients can spend several days in a hospital room on "observational status," and be considered outpatients. So check.

If your parent is an inpatient, Medicare (Parts A and B together) will cover most hospital and doctor bills after a deductible is met. But as an outpatient, your parent is responsible for copayments and routine drugs—prices that can add up quickly.

Furthermore, his inpatient/outpatient status will affect whether Medicare covers any nursing care that is needed once he gets out of the hospital. He needs to be an inpatient for three days to get coverage. This does not include any time spent in the emergency wing or as an outpatient; it must be three days logged into the computer as an inpatient.

things—the routine test, the quick visit, the stuff they hand you as if it were nothing—all have price tags. A single pill that costs $2 normally might cost $50 or $100 in the hospital (and most don't allow you to BYOP). That bath? $40. A special meal? $15. When asking a nurse for a little extra, find out just how much that "extra" is going to cost.

You're overwhelmed already, but if possible, keep a list of what was provided each day. Even a partial record will help when it comes time to decode a hospital bill.

Following His Wishes

Once in the hospital, your parent is in a river that runs fast and furiously in one direction: Diagnose and treat. Before you know it, your parent is in the ICU with half a dozen machines keeping him alive.

If your parent does *not* want all medical treatment possible at any cost, then you need to be persistent, all along the way, to be sure his wishes are followed.

Be sure your parent has signed advance directives (a living will and health care proxy), and remind the medical team throughout the process of your parent's wishes. Ask questions about his options, the likely outcomes, and the goals of any treatment. That is, is this procedure being done in an effort to give him more time, more lucidity, more mobility, or more comfort? If it's simply a matter of prolonging life, then at what cost to his independence, comfort, and competence? Is this in line with your parent's instructions?

If you are making medical decisions, keep your parent's needs ahead of your own. Although you might want to just keep him alive, no matter what that means, that might not be what he would opt for. Ask yourself not what you want, but what he would want.

If your parent is very ill, don't hesitate to call the local hospice to get another opinion. Sometimes doctors will tell you that surgery is the only option, when in fact it is not. You won't cause your parent to die sooner simply by learning the options. (Indeed, in some cases, people who opt for palliative care live longer than those who receive aggressive medical care.)

Also, ask the doctor about writing up a POLST (Physician Orders for Life-Sustaining Treatment), which is not simply a vague directive, but a medical order outlining precisely what treatments are wanted and unwanted. Or, get your parent a Do Not Resuscitate (DNR) order. It might sound terrifying, but the fact is that restarting a heart that has stopped functioning is a brutal procedure that is rarely successful in elderly people and can lead to an array of awful outcomes.

Tests, Surgery, and Treatments

Some studies suggest that up to one-third of all medical procedures are unnecessary, some of them dangerously so. That percentage is even greater among the elderly, who are sicker, less likely to fare well, and often don't want everything that medicine can dish out.

Doctors overprobe, overscan, and overtreat because they are used to certain routines, fearful of malpractice lawsuits, enamored of technology, or baffled by a profusion of unusual symptoms. (Sadly, some overtest and overtreat because they make money doing it.)

Impose safeguards by asking plenty of questions, making informed decisions, and getting a second opinion whenever you have doubts. Medicare covers most costs of second opinions, any extra tests required, and, when there's dispute, a third opinion as well. (But check first.)

If your parent is quite ill, see the chapter "Nearing the End" on page 524, which includes a section on decision making when life is in the balance.

Here are some of the questions you might want to ask the doctor. (Be sure to write down the answers, because with all that's going on now, you are apt to forget the details.)

- Why is this test/treatment/surgery recommended?

- What is the goal of this procedure?

- What are the risks?

- What is the likely outcome? How will it affect her health and lifestyle?

- What other options exist, and what are the risks and benefits of each? (Are there other approaches that might be

TRUTH TELLING AND DECISION MAKING

Unless your parent has given directions to the contrary, he should be given honest information about his health, and he should be involved, to whatever extent possible, in decisions about his care.

Although it's natural to want to protect your parent by keeping bad news from him or even lying about a diagnosis, it's likely this will only add to his fear and isolation. Patients usually know, at least on some level, what is happening.

If you are uncertain about how much information to pass on, then let your parent tell you how much he wants to know. *Dad, I spoke to the doctor about your illness. Is there anything you want to know?* Let him lead the way, asking questions. Give as much information as he requests.

If your parent is confused, assume that he can understand what is being said. Give him basic information and reassure him that he is in good hands and that any previous instructions he gave are being followed.

> " When the two of us brought my father to the hospital, my sister asked about the room selection, and I was completely embarrassed. It didn't occur to me that there would be a choice, and I thought she was being frivolous and pushy. But just as I was searching for something conciliatory to say, the woman at the admitting desk said that she could arrange for Dad to be in a private room with a window, even though his insurance covered only a semiprivate room. It had to do with their occupancy level. I guess I learned my lesson."
>
> —Katherine S.

tried first, such as changes in diet or exercise?)

• What will this test tell us, and where will we go from there? (If it won't affect treatment, why bother with the test?)

• Where will it be performed? How long will it take? Will you be doing this procedure?

• How long will it take for my parent to recover?

• How much will it cost? Is it covered fully by Medicare, Medicaid, or my parent's private insurance?

• Are any experimental treatments available, and what are the risks and benefits of those?

Preparing for Surgery

If your parent is headed for surgery, ask about the surgeon's credentials and experience—in particular, how many times he or she has done this procedure.

Find out when the surgeon and your parent's doctor will visit your parent after the surgery and how to reach them if there is a question.

Before any surgery, you or your parent should talk with the doctor about the aftermath. What sort of care will she need during her recovery? What kind of pain might be involved, and how will that be addressed? What other problems should she expect or hurdles might she face? How mobile and functional will she be once she is discharged?

At the Nurses' Station

In the hospital, a doctor will oversee your parent's medical care, but it is the nurses who will actually tend to his needs and monitor his health. It is the nurses who will (hopefully) notice if a medication is having side effects, if your parent has a new symptom, or if his mood or mental abilities change.

Unless your parent is in the hospital for a very brief stay, make an effort to get to know the nurses who care for him. They are important allies.

SHOW RESPECT. No matter how urgent your concerns may be, no matter how unraveled you feel, avoid the urge to bark orders. *I don't want my mother waiting for her pain medication! She was supposed to get it at 2 o'clock! What kinds of idiots are running this place?*

Protect your parent, guard her rights, and advocate firmly on her behalf, but treat the staff as friend, not foe. Recognize the pressures that nurses and other staff are under. When there is a problem, work with them to find solutions. *I know you're busy and I don't mean to be a pest, but my mother is supposed to get her pain meds at 2 p.m. and today she didn't get them until after 4. Is there anything I can do to be sure she gets them on time?*

When you treat nurses with respect, they will be far more willing to treat you and your parent with respect.

If you do lose your cool, and most likely you will, apologize later.

ASK QUESTIONS. Don't withhold important questions and comments for fear of "bothering" the nurses. Most nurses do not consider questions or comments from family members a bother. Your questions may bring an error or an oversight to their attention.

PROVIDE INFORMATION. Be sure the nurses know about any allergies or sensitivities, any other medications your parent is taking, and any symptoms she may have. If you are worried about something in particular, tape a large note by the bed—"Mrs. Parker is severely allergic to all seafood." Also, be sure the nurses know about any special needs, habits, quirks, or preferences that will help them care for your parent. They are usually open to reasonable requests.

If your parent has dementia, has become extremely crotchety in her old age, or can't communicate, tell the nurses what she used to be like, or bring in a couple of photos of her in her younger days and put them over her bed. Let people see the person behind the illness.

PICK YOUR BATTLES. Remember, your parent is not in a hotel and nurses are not maids, waiters, or janitors. Your parent might have asked for a baked potato instead of mashed or, once again, be left without a spoon, but the nurse has far more important demands on his or her time. Ring for the nurse when your parent really needs help, and be patient when it's not urgent. If you need a spoon, go get one.

....

6 6 The rehabilitation therapist got very frustrated with my dad because he wasn't cooperating. But he wasn't cooperating because he didn't know what the hell he was doing. He has dementia, and he gets anxious and ornery when things are new or when people push him to do things he doesn't want to do.

I learned that at some point, it's the habit of the rehab people to stop trying. I guess they deal with people like this all day long and it gets to them after a while. I told the therapists that I understood it probably was demoralizing for them, but also how grateful we'd be if they could keep trying with my dad. I had to cajole and encourage and push to get them to keep working with him, but they did stick with it and Dad did, finally, go along with it."

—Jacqui L.
....

WHITE COATS

Who is the person checking your father's stitches? Who is that new young man reading your mother's chart? And where, pray tell, is your parent's regular doctor?

"Attending physicians" are doctors with admitting privileges to a hospital, like your parent's personal doctor. These days, however, many doctors don't visit their patients in the hospital. They relegate that job to a "hospitalist," a doctor who specializes in the care of hospitalized patients. (Don't panic. Many of them are very good at what they do.)

Members of the "house staff" have medical school degrees but are still in training and are not yet certified in a specialty. The house staff is composed of "interns," who are one year out of medical school, and "residents," who are several years out of medical school. Teaching hospitals also have medical students who wear white coats (short ones) and might perform some minor tasks, although they do not yet have medical degrees.

You and your parent are unlikely to know who's who, but feel free to ask.

UNDERSTAND THEIR MOTIVES. Sometimes nurses refuse to help a patient not because they are mean or lazy, but because they want the patient up and moving. Or perhaps they want to see how your parent fares when trying to feed herself or get out of bed.

Likewise, a nurse or therapist might ask you to, say, feed your parent because she or he feels that your father will eat better when someone familiar is there with him. Or she might want you to learn how to get him out of bed because she wants to know that when he returns home, someone is able to care for him.

> **"** My trick was to learn the nurses' names and something about them. That always softened them."
> —Anne B.

KINDNESS COUNTS. Anxiety can make you forget all the usual social niceties, but thoughtfulness can be enormously important to an overworked nurse, aide, or orderly. When things are done well, when an extra task is undertaken, express your appreciation.

If your parent is going to be in for a long stay, go a step further. Bring in a bowl of fruit, some cookies, or a jug of coffee. If one person has been especially thoughtful, send a small gift or write a letter to a supervisor.

Kindness to the staff is especially important if your parent is withdrawn, confused, or a bit of a curmudgeon. It's hard for nurses and aides to be pleasant or helpful when a patient is rude. Remind the staff that your parent's attacks are nothing personal, and keep letting them know that you appreciate what they are doing.

Providing Comfort

I t's unusual to be happy in the hospital, but there are ways to make life more comfortable.

Meals

Although some hospitals are sprucing up their menus, hospital food is still notoriously bland and unidentifiable. It's also served at odd times or left to grow cold in front of a patient who can't lift a fork.

Your parent's diet isn't simply a matter of comfort; the rate of malnutrition among the hospitalized elderly is estimated to be as high as 50 percent. A poor diet will make your parent's recovery extremely difficult.

Although hospitals don't always advertise it, many offer an array of foods and special meals—kosher, vegetarian, low-salt—and options that aren't on the usual menu, such as omelets and sandwiches. Also, snacks and drinks are often available between meals.

You can also ask that meals be brought at different times if that would help your parent eat more. (They might not do it, but it's worth asking.)

Whenever possible, visit during mealtimes so you can check on your parent's eating habits and, if necessary, help him eat. Bring him an occasional home-cooked meal, as long as it's within his diet.

If you can't be there, ask other visitors to come at mealtime, or ask the hospital's patient advocate about volunteers who might help your parent dine. Simply having company may encourage your parent to eat more.

Sleep

Just when your parent needs a good night's sleep to heal, he is woken up at all hours. The hallway is noisy and bright. His roommate watches TV at odd times. Someone comes in to take his temperature at 4 a.m., and just as he falls back to sleep, someone comes in for a blood sample. Although you can't create a nighttime oasis, you should be able to stop the commotion a bit.

Typically, vital signs are taken as nurses change shifts, which is usually at an ungodly hour. But sometimes, if vitals aren't critical, a doctor can put orders in a patient's chart that he is not to be woken.

Talk to the staff about ways to reduce noise and dim lights at a reasonable hour. (When there's a choice, the bed farthest from the door is usually the most peaceful.) Buy your parent earplugs and an eye mask.

Visits

Visitors are the best first aid. However, they should call first, as an unannounced visit, especially when someone is wearing a backless gown, can be awkward for everyone. They should space out their trips so they come one at a time or in small groups, and for only a brief interlude (less than thirty minutes is usually more than enough), as your parent will tire easily now.

You are the gatekeeper. Give visitors guidelines, if necessary, about how long to visit, what sort of visit your parent is up for (balloons and hearty cheer, or a quiet time for two), and whether to bring young children or not.

At times, your parent may be too tired for visitors but may not be willing to tell people for fear of hurting their feelings. It's your job to tell them, as tactfully as possible, to come another time. In fact, there may even be times when your parent doesn't want you to visit. Don't take it personally.

Some things to keep in mind when visiting:

BE PREPARED. If your parent has had a sudden and severe illness or accident, you may be shocked by his appearance on your first visit. He may not only look different, but he may be confused, weak, in pain, or attached to a lot of machines. Brace yourself so you don't gasp in horror or burst into tears as you enter the room.

Understand that if your parent is in the intensive care unit, it doesn't mean that he is close to death, only that he is being watched closely. Elderly people are often put in ICUs after surgery, stroke, or accidents.

BE YOURSELF. Hospitals and illness breed discomfort. *What do I say? Should I be cheery? Should I talk about what the doctor found or avoid mentioning her illness?* All of this is especially awkward if your parent is near, or seems to be near, death.

Relax. Your embarrassment will only make your parent ill at ease—and she is already ill enough. Be yourself. It's okay to ask about her ailments, her pain, and her feelings, if that's something you want to know about. In fact, she may welcome such honesty and an opportunity to talk about her situation. Take your cues from her.

Then move on to other topics. Hearing about day-to-day things—the weather, the grandchildren—is a welcome escape from constant talk and thoughts about illness.

ARRANGE FOR SOME PRIVACY. Interruptions are a way of life in hospitals. Someone comes in with medication, then it's time for a blood sample, and just as you and your parent start talking, her temperature must be taken.

If your parent shares a room, pull the curtain around his bed. If his condition allows it, get him into a wheelchair and move the conversation into a lounge. Otherwise, ask the nurse if you can have some uninterrupted time and put a note on the door.

"WHY DON'T YOU EVER COME SEE ME?"

If your parent suffers from dementia and doesn't remember that you have visited every day for the past week, or doesn't seem to know who you are, keep in mind that your visits are crucial nevertheless. They are comforting, even if he doesn't remember them. And, more important, they allow you to make sure that your parent is being well cared for (vitally important now because of his confusion). Your visits also show the staff that you are concerned about his condition and care, and will act if that care is inadequate. In other words, don't visit less just because your parent doesn't remember that you came.

SILENCE IS GOLDEN. If your parent can't speak or if she is too confused or tired for conversation, you might read to her, watch a movie together, or just let her lie peacefully while you read or do some work. There's no need for conversation. Your presence alone is powerful and will relieve her fear and ease her loneliness.

GET PHYSICAL. Don't let tubes, monitors, or injury deter you from touching, stroking, kissing, and holding.

Human contact is potent medicine. Hug him, hold his hand, stroke his cheek, caress his arm—touch whatever body parts are available. If there are a lot of machines in the way, ask the nurse if there isn't some way to make physical contact easier.

FIND THINGS TO DO. If your parent is relatively alert, his hospital stay will

> " When my mother was in the hospital after her stroke, she turned to me and said, 'Pizza.'
>
> I said, 'What?!'
>
> And she said, 'I really want some pizza. And a chocolate milk shake. It's all I can think about.'
>
> My mother is not a pizza eater. She usually eats like a bird. So I drove around town looking for pizza and a chocolate shake. She didn't eat much of it, but she ate enough. I guess it was just a craving. Her body was crying out for something caloric and filling, and I was glad to see her eat something with such gusto."
>
> —Fran M.

SPREADING THE NEWS

If your parent (or you) has a wide circle of family and friends who all want to keep abreast of what's happening and know when they can visit or how to help, create a group email list so that at the end of a busy day, you can write just one email and send it to the group. Or, set up a Facebook group, or use a web service like CarePages (carepages.com) or CaringBridge (caringbridge.org) to spread any news.

seem awfully dull. Look for things that will entertain him—games, books, magazines, puzzles, playing cards, materials for a hobby, art supplies, music, and audiobooks.

If your parent has a laptop or tablet, he can watch movies or play games without disturbing a roommate. Scan family photos and send them to him. Skype when you can't be there in person.

PAMPER HER. If possible, do something to make your parent feel special and pampered—wash or comb her hair, massage her feet, or paint her nails. You might bring in some favorite foods or simply jazz up the hospital tray with a red napkin and a few flowers. Give her a bright bed jacket or new slippers.

RESPECT THE RULES. Enforcing visiting hours allows patients to get some rest. Stay within the rules whenever possible. If the only time you can visit is after hours, or if your parent is extremely ill and needs someone nearby all the time, the staff will usually adjust the rules. (If your parent is in an intensive care unit, the rules will be stricter.)

> " Quite often we'll see a family come, six or seven of them at one time. They all cram into the person's room and chat with each other, and the grandchildren run around, and there are a lot of gifts and food and flowers. It's all very hectic and very exciting. And then they all leave. And no one comes to visit for two weeks. That's very sad."
>
> —Lorraine N., R.N.

DON'T FORGET THE CHILDREN. In most cases, a child is a welcome visitor, adding vitality and sparkle to a dreary hospital day, singing songs, asking funny questions, stroking Grandpa with tiny fingers. Children sometimes see beyond the ugliness of illness and don't fear the things that adults find worrisome (they may be more absorbed by an IV bag than by Grandpa's paralysis).

Your instinct may be to protect children from seeing Grandma ill, but children learn from seeing life and death and all that falls between. However, if Grandma doesn't seem pleased at the prospect of a child's visit, or if your child is afraid or hesitant, don't press the matter.

Of course, there's always Skype or iChat, so grandchildren can be seen from a distance.

Gifts

Flowers are always nice, but a framed photo, child's art project, small pine-scented cushion, and cheerful cards are great gifts. The smallest thing can mean a lot when one is facing the four walls of a hospital room. You don't have to spend a lot of money. In fact, some of the best gifts are a story, a special poem,

or a prayer. Anything at all that is made by a grandchild is wonderful.

If your parent is going to be in the hospital for some time and you are able to spend a little more money, buy a robe, new slippers, a pouch that attaches to a walker or wheelchair, or a soft, downy pillow.

If your parent is confused, bring pictures, photo albums, and items from home that will make the room seem more familiar and help orient her.

Religion and Counseling

Whether or not your parent was religious before her hospital stay, she may have some spiritual thoughts now. Someone from her church or synagogue should be willing to visit her. Otherwise, hospital clergy will gladly stop by a patient's room.

Hospitals also have counselors, social workers, or psychologists who will talk with your parent about particular issues—fears about dying, family relationships, a diagnosis—as well as practical matters such as housing, finances, and community services.

Dignity

It's hard to find dignity in a backless gown.

Do what you can to protect hers. It might not seem important in the face of a stroke or hip surgery, but these are the little things that devour some people.

A short sweater or jacket, or even a cozy scarf wrapped over her shoulders, will provide a little more coverage. If she'd like it, comb her hair, rub in some lotion, snip her nails, or give her a little makeup, if that's what she's used to.

REST FOR THE WEARY

Sometimes a parent's hospital stay is anything but a break from your caregiving role. As advocate you might be micromanaging your parent's care—which can be a rigorous test of your endurance. Deeply worried about your parent, you return to the hospital every free moment you have. Then, when you finally drag your weary body home, you're deluged by messages from family and friends. There isn't a minute when you aren't living and breathing your parent's hospital experience.

Protect yourself. Make one phone call and ask a sibling or relative to relay information to others in the inner circle. Or create a group so you can send one email easily to all.

When others are visiting your parent, get away, even if only for a walk outside or a cup of tea in a nearby café. Ask one of the nurses if there is a lounge or an empty room where you can lie down. Take a day off and go out with a friend and talk about something—anything—else.

It's vital to take care of yourself now. Your parent will need your strength when he returns home.

Ask the staff to address your parent by whatever title she chooses—Mrs. Asher, Professor Madison, or, if she prefers, a nickname. Likewise, if someone is calling her Sweetie, and she hates it, just ask him kindly to use her name instead.

Roommates and Rooms

If a roommate's habits or his visitors are keeping your parent awake, talk to the roommate or a nurse about setting up a schedule of "quiet time." Then, get your parent some earplugs and/or a music player with headphones to muffle any loud snoring or chatter.

If a roommate is obnoxious, see if you can't leave a curtain drawn permanently between the two beds. If all else fails, request a room change. It involves some paperwork, but sometimes it is necessary.

When You Are Far Away

It's hard enough having a parent in the hospital when you're near, but when work or miles keep you away, the worry can be overwhelming.

If you can't be there in person, do what you can by phone. Call the nurse manager on your parent's floor and explain your dilemma. Find out if there is a primary nurse overseeing your parent's care who will speak with you on a regular basis.

Collect information early—whom to call if there's trouble, names of doctors and their phone numbers, numbers for insurance carriers. Talk with the hospital discharge planner early about when and how your parent will be discharged so you can make all necessary arrangements.

Check in with the doctor, too, as regularly as possible. Be sure he or she knows your parent's symptoms and concerns, ask as many questions as you need to, and be sure the doctor can reach you at any time of the day or night if there is a change in your parent's health (thank goodness for cell phones).

Reminder: One family member should be designated to speak with nurses and doctors, and that person should relay information to other family and loved ones. Dealing with more than one spokesperson is difficult for care providers, and can lead to misunderstandings.

When you are far away (or busy at work), make sure your parent has company as often as possible. See if a relative or friend might check in with your parent from time to time. A local senior center or religious organization might know of volunteers who will visit. Or, if you can afford it, hire a companion to visit and monitor your parent's care.

When you can't be there, call and write. Send your parent cards and family photos. Video chat. Mundane, day-to-day things—what happened at the bus stop, what the kids did in school, what the dog brought home—may seem trivial, but for someone alone in the hospital, these can be wonderful stories that temporarily bring him home and help him forget his pain.

Hospital Dangers

Unfortunately, hospitals are not safe havens, not in the least. In fact, a hospital is one of the most dangerous places your parent could be. Doctors and nurses frequently work at, or beyond, capacity, so mistakes are made and patients are neglected. And by the very nature of the beast, germs are rampant, so people contract infections and illnesses they didn't have when they walked in.

You can't eliminate all the risks, but you can reduce them significantly simply by being aware. The information given here is not intended to heap yet more work on your weary shoulders or to frighten you; it is simply meant to alert you and, in the long run, make life easier.

Delirium
Elderly patients who show no signs of confusion at home often become

disoriented, argumentative, and forgetful in the hospital, and those who already
suffer from dementia can become even
more muddled. If you see any sudden
change in your parent's personality or
behavior, bring it to the doctor's attention immediately, as this is an emergency.

Delirium is one of the most common
and most dangerous side effects of hospitalization for the elderly, largely because
it so often goes undiagnosed. Ignored,
the problems can become irreversible
and even fatal. However, if delirium is
spotted early and treated, the symptoms
can disappear almost immediately.

It is most common in people who
have surgery (particularly emergency
surgery) and those who wind up in the
intensive care unit, although all elderly
patients are at risk. It is usually triggered
by infections, trauma, illness, or medications, but can also be brought on by
stress, disruption of daily routines, poor
diet, and dehydration.

One of the key symptoms of delirium
is inattention. Your parent might veer off
subject or be unable to focus on what's
going on around him. People often
become agitated, confused, or unable to
recognize familiar faces. Their speech
can become garbled and their words
nonsensical. Some become anxious or
angry. Many hallucinate or become
paranoid.

Complicating matters, some people
do quite the opposite, becoming sleepy,
quiet, unresponsive, and withdrawn.
You know your parent best; trust your
instinct if you feel something's not right.

Unlike dementia (and the two are
often confused), delirium comes on
quickly, often within days or hours. Also,
it can come in waves. While someone

> ❝ She broke her leg and spent five days in the hospital. Then four days in a rehab place.
>
> Then they said they needed someone from the family to come in and speak the language. I thought, 'My mother doesn't speak any other languages.' I thought they had the wrong person.
>
> I got there and she was speaking something else. They couldn't under-stand her. She was making no sense. She needed someone familiar. When I got there, she kept saying, 'What happened to me?' over and over. It turned out she'd had an overdose of the pain medication.❞
>
> —Maggie B.

with dementia might have better and
worse times of day, his or her skills are
relatively constant; someone with delirium can be fairly lucid at one moment
and quite confused another.

If you're unsure or if you suspect trouble but your parent can't speak because
he's on a ventilator, here's a quick test that
involves only a nodding of the head. Ask
your parent these simple questions: Are
there fish in the sea? Is one pound heavier
than two? Will a stone float on water?
Then, hold your parent's hand and ask
him to squeeze your hand every time you
say the letter A. Slowly spell out "SAVE A
HEART." If he makes two or more mistakes in this test, get the doctor's attention
right away.

TREATING DELIRIUM

Treatment begins with eliminating or
reducing certain medications. Note that
the focus should be on *reducing* medications, not increasing them. Sedatives,

> " My mother started talking about a high school friend of hers, a woman she hasn't seen in at least 50 years. Here I was, thinking my mother was very sick and these might be our last moments together. I wanted her attention. I said, 'Mom, why are you doing this?' but she looked up at me as though she didn't have any idea who I was.
>
> I was so crushed that I left. I walked the halls for a while and tried to calm down. I was so hurt and angry. I felt betrayed. Then I spoke to this wonderful nurse who helped me realize that I had to take what I could get, that being angry or trying to force her wouldn't help either of us. So I went back in and I just sat there and stroked her hair and listened to her ramble. I learned to meet her wherever she was, not where I wanted her to be."
>
> —Carol P.

painkillers, sleeping pills, and other medications, which are often (and erroneously) used to calm delirious patients, will only make the situation worse. Likewise, tying an agitated patient down (in an effort to avoid falls and keep him from pulling out tubes) will also exacerbate things.

Of course, any other underlying cause, such as an infection or dehydration, needs immediate attention.

Beyond that, a calm and supportive environment is the best remedy. Unfortunately, hospitals are anything but calm and supportive, so you'll have to fight the system.

Reassure your parent that he is safe. Do not argue or disagree with him. *I'm not actually sure why there's a cow in the room, but I'm sure he's a nice one.* Keep conversations simple. Don't ask a lot of questions or give a lot of instructions.

Be sure your parent has any eyeglasses or hearing aids. Provide ample reminders to help him orient himself—a clock, a calendar. Bring in familiar objects and family photos. Tell him patiently (the caregiver, ever patient) what day it is, where he is and why, and say the name of anyone entering the room. *Dad, your daughter, Sally, is here to see you.*

Although it's not easy in a hospital, try to keep the room quiet and mostly dark at night, in an effort to get his natural cycle back on track. Ideally, meals should also occur on his usual schedule.

Sometimes music or massage helps. Get your parent moving if he can. Even small range-of-motion exercises in bed will help his circulation and lung function. Ask if a physical therapist might work with your parent.

Medical Mishaps

It happens far more than anyone can imagine: A patient is given the wrong medication, the wrong treatment, or, yes, treatment to the wrong part of the body. *(It was her left knee, not the right, that required surgery.)*

Although hospitals are working hard to make the system foolproof, iatrogenic diseases and injuries—problems that are caused directly or indirectly by the medical staff—are a serious hospital problem. An injury or ailment may be caused by a doctor's neglect or incompetence, or it may be the result of acceptable medical care. For example, a necessary treatment for one illness may cause another, less serious illness. The elderly are at high risk of iatrogenic disease because their medical care is so complex.

Again, the single most important thing you can do is ask questions. *Why is my parent getting this medication? Is this treatment necessary? Are you sure those pills are for my parent?*

Ideally, every time your parent is given a medication, someone should ask what it is and if it is for her. Sometimes people get drugs that are meant for a roommate.

And it's best not to be chatty while a nurse is preparing medications or doing tests, because you're only redirecting her or his much-needed attention.

Falls and Restraints

When you visit, take a look around for things your parent might trip over or that might cause her to fall—furniture on wheels, chairs without arms, waxy floors. Fix what you can (for example, buy a rubber runner for the stretch between the bed and the toilet, take the faulty chair out of the room), and if she is well enough, make her aware of the dangers. Tell her not to lean too heavily on the pole holding her intravenous drip, and show her how to lower the bed and raise the head end so she can rise out of bed more easily.

To guard against falls and to keep patients from pulling out tubes, meandering away, or crushing a delicate wound, hospital staff sometimes restrain patients either physically (with armbands, vests, bed side rails, full body straps, or wheelchair trays) or chemically (with sedatives, tranquilizers, and other drugs). Be wary of restraints, because they are not necessary in most cases, and can be dangerous for an elderly person. Federal and state laws impose a variety of restrictions on the use of restraints.

" My father was in a car accident and was taken to the hospital. I called him as soon as I heard. I knew immediately that something was very wrong. His words were hard to understand and he wasn't making any sense. He started telling me that he was visiting his brother and that he was in another state. And then he'd start talking about something else.

I went into a panic. I just kept saying, 'Daddy, I'll be there as soon as I can. Hang on. I'm on my way.' I was shaking.

My father is very competent, smart. Old and sick, yes. But never confused. I couldn't stop crying on my way there.

By the time I arrived, maybe three hours later, he was fine. It was so bizarre. I don't know if it was the accident or the ambulance and the rush into the hospital, but something happened, and then he was fine. I was sure he'd never be the same again. Thank God I was wrong."

—Tina R.

Know what sedating drugs your parent is being given and why. If your parent is being physically restrained, ask the doctor if it is absolutely necessary and what else can be done. Restraints are not as useful as people expect, and can themselves cause injuries and accidents (people have actually been strangled wiggling to get free).

Bedsores

Although the nurses should work to prevent bedsores, be watchful for any red, tender, or raw spots. Pressure on an area—a hip, a heel, a shoulder—impedes the flow of blood, creating a tender spot that will develop into an open wound if not treated immediately.

> " My father spent so much time in bed that the nurses and I thought it would be good for him to sit up in a chair for a while each day. But he was so weak that he would just fall onto the floor unless he had some support. This strap, it's a seat belt really, works quite well. He doesn't stay in the chair long, but at least it's a change. I don't think it's dangerous or confining for him—I think it's freeing in a way because it allows him to get out of bed."
>
> —Sasha L.

Be sure your parent is being routinely repositioned to alternate the pressure on vulnerable areas, and alert the nurses to any suspicious-looking marks. (See page 226 for more on bedsores.) Various pillows and special mattresses with alternating air pressure can relieve the strain.

Hospital-Acquired Infections

Studies have found that up to 10 percent of patients develop infections while in the hospital. And these infections, called nosocomial infections or hospital-acquired infections (or HAI), tend to be virulent.

You've got sick people infested with bacteria and viruses living with patients who have weakened immune systems, open wounds, and tubes in their bodies—it's a volatile mix.

Hand washing is the best weapon against hospital infections. Doctors, nurses, and staff are supposed to wash before touching or examining a patient, but they sometimes fail to do it. Don't hesitate to ask the person handling your parent to please wash his or her hands first and, preferably, to wear gloves. It's a little awkward, but most health care providers won't mind.

You should wash your own hands frequently, as well, when caring for your parent.

Urinary tract infections are one of the most common nosocomial infections, especially among older women, and catheters are the major offender. If a urinary catheter is recommended, find out if it is absolutely necessary (they are often inserted without great thought, especially in the emergency department), and if it is essential, ask that it be removed as soon as possible. (The longer it is in, the greater the chance of infection.) A catheter should be changed regularly and checked often to make sure that it is draining smoothly.

If your parent has symptoms of a urinary tract infection—a persistent urge to urinate, burning during urination, and pain in the lower abdomen—alert the doctor or nurse. Urinary tract infections are treatable with medications, but they can lead to serious problems if ignored.

Pain Relief

Pain will not only make your parent cranky, tired, and generally miserable, but will limit his ability to function and heal. The conundrum is that pain medications can cause problems, such as nausea, drowsiness, and constipation.

Talk to your parent's doctor, who should be able to select a low dose of an appropriate medication.

Relaxation exercises, peaceful music, reassurance, massage, visualization, biofeedback, and other nonmedical approaches can all reduce pain also.

CONVALESCING: UP AND AT 'EM

When your parent is recuperating from illness or surgery, your instinct might say "rest" while the doctor is saying "move." Trust the doctor here.

In most cases, people need to get up and move about in order to get all the bodily systems functioning again (and to avoid constipation, stroke, lung infections, muscle wasting, and other complications). They also need to do simple tasks, like feeding themselves or combing their hair, to regain movement, coordination, and independence.

It may seem as if the nurses and therapists are being cruel if they are forcing your mother to move in ways that she doesn't want to move, or being lazy if they leave her to do certain things for herself, but often they are just practicing good medicine.

The process may be painful for you to watch, especially if your parent is struggling, complaining of pain, or spilling her food. But let her do it herself and encourage her to keep going. Restrain yourself from helping too much. It will allow her to recover faster and more fully.

The interesting thing about pain is that although it stems from an illness or injury, it is exacerbated by fear, anxiety, and depression. All these things become intertwined, making the original pain that much worse, which leads to anxiety, more pain, and so on. For your parent, just knowing that someone is paying attention to this and taking steps to treat it will, by itself, be a great relief.

Also, pain is much easier to fight when it is treated before it sets in rather than when it has become well established.

If your parent is limiting pain medications because she doesn't like the grogginess or other side effects, talk to the doctor about switching to a lower dose or to some other drug that might not be so sedating.

If your parent is skipping pain medications because she feels that taking the drugs is a sign of weakness, she fears addiction, or she doesn't like to complain,

> " After the operation, I tried to help my father get his teeth back in. I struggled for a time and they finally went in. Then I looked at him and thought, 'Pop, you look weird.' I tried again with that cushion stuff, but nothing made it better.
>
> Finally, I realized these weren't his teeth. They were someone else's! I went traipsing to the room he used to be in, to the doctor's office, and even to the operating room—all over the hospital—looking for the right teeth, but I never found them. It was really kind of funny, because here I am looking for a set of teeth and realizing that somebody else must be wearing Pop's teeth. Luckily, he thought it was funny, too."
>
> —Jacqui L.

talk to both the doctor and your parent. Your parent should be counseled on the benefits of pain management (comfort, sleep, more mobility, less anxiety) and the risks of not treating pain (discomfort, distress, insomnia, irritability, poor mobility, more illness).

If her pain and your concerns are not addressed adequately, ask the doctor if there is a palliative care or pain specialist in the hospital.

If your parent is in the final stages of life, then he should receive all the pain medication necessary to be comfortable. Fight for it.

Resolving Disputes

If you are facing an urgent problem and need immediate results—the nurse is abusive, the doctor reeks of alcohol, your parent's Do Not Resuscitate order is being violated—go straight to the hospital's administrator.

If you or your parent has a less severe problem with a doctor, nurse, or other staff member, talk with that person directly, if possible. Do your best to use your Kind Person voice, not your Frazzled Angry Caregiver voice. Be specific about your concern and cite an example of the problem. Many problems are caused by a lack of communication—the nurse didn't know that your parent is allergic to lactose because it hadn't been entered in her chart, or you didn't realize that the doctor had ordered her regular medication stopped.

If the problem isn't resolved, go up a step on the ladder to the head nurse on the unit or the hospital's director of nursing. If it's a medical issue, the next step is the medical director of the hospital; if this is a question about bills, see the financial administrator.

You can also use these channels:

PATIENT ADVOCATES. Most hospitals have patient advocates, or ombudsmen, who serve as a link between patients and the hospital system. Their job is to represent the patient, making sure that questions are answered and any problems are resolved. Your parent (or you) can ask a patient advocate to help with practically anything—disputes with staff, lost hearing aids, billing questions, faulty plumbing, late lunch trays, roommate problems, or inadequate insurance coverage. Of course, some patient advocates are more helpful than others, but the good ones are godsends.

Patient advocates should be listed in the hospital brochure or directory, or their phone number may be posted on the hospital room wall. If you don't see it, ask the nurse.

HOSPITAL COMMITTEES. If a dispute is over a medical decision—you and the doctor disagree about when to withhold treatment or you believe your parent has received the wrong treatment—many hospitals have ethics committees that review such dilemmas. Ask the hospital's patient advocate, a nurse, or an administrator how to appeal a medical decision.

QUALITY IMPROVEMENT ORGANIZA-TIONS. If you believe that your parent has received inadequate care or unnecessary treatment in the hospital, if she is refused admission, if she is being discharged too soon, or if you believe Medicare coverage is being denied unfairly, contact the state Quality Improvement Organization.

A QIO is a group of physicians and other health care professionals who are contracted by the federal government to ensure that Medicare patients receive proper care from hospitals, doctors, nursing homes, and home health care agencies.

To reach the QIO in your parent's state, talk to the patient advocate or discharge planner, or contact Medicare (medicare.gov/contacts or 800-699-8873) or the American Health Quality Association (AHQA) (ahqa.org). Hospitals are required to give your parent a pamphlet about Medicare, patients' rights, and the appeals process.

Note: Every state calls their QIO something different—a Peer Review Organization (PRO), a Quality Health Foundation (QHF), a Health Services Advisory Group (HSAG)—but don't let this get you in a muddle. The AHQA list of QIOs and PROs will make your head spin briefly, but you're actually in the right place.

STATE BOARDS AND AGENCIES. Although they may not be that helpful, it is important to notify the appropriate state licensing board if your complaint involves the skills or conduct of a nurse, doctor, or other licensed professional. This way, you protect the next person.

Preparing for Discharge

The hospital discharge planner should help arrange your parent's return home or move to a facility. He or she can order necessary medical equipment, help you get in-home care, or arrange for institutional care. The planner or a nurse should also review all medical and practical information.

Before your parent leaves, be sure she has written (and legible) information about everything—medications, dosages, when and how to take them, potential side effects, diet, rehab, precautions, symptoms to watch for, and whom to call in case there's a problem. She should also have a follow-up appointment.

Find out what daily activities your parent can do on her own and what she'll need help with. Don't make assumptions. *Can she climb the stairs? Can she take a shower? How do we care for her wound? Is it okay if she goes to her granddaughter's wedding in two weeks?*

The planner, who usually knows a fair amount about local home care agencies and senior residences, can be very helpful, but be aware that his or her primary job is to get patients out with speed. Take time to study the options and make a careful choice, if at all possible.

Is It Too Soon?

Hospitals discharge people in pretty miserable states. (Of course, most are eager to depart.) If you do not believe that your parent is ready for discharge, or if you simply need to buy an extra day or two while you make housing arrangements, talk with the doctor or the patient advocate, who may be able to convince Medicare or other insurance carrier that your parent needs coverage for a longer hospital stay. Or, you can usually squeeze an extra day out of Medicare by appealing the discharge decision.

When your parent entered the hospital, she should have been given a pamphlet on Medicare rights regarding discharge and the appeals process. If not, ask for it. Quite often, the discharge planner or the patient advocate (ombudsman) will help with appeals.

DEPARTURE CHECKLIST

It's wise to talk with the discharge planner long before your parent leaves the hospital, so you can begin making plans for your parent's departure. Some things to consider:

• Where will your parent live?

• What help will he need—bathing, dressing, eating, climbing stairs, remembering medications?

• What services will he need (for example, aides, nurses, physical therapy, meal delivery, transportation)?

• What medical equipment might he need? Where can you get it? Will insurance cover it? What do you do with it when you no longer need it?

• What should you do to prepare for his return home (for example, move his bed downstairs or buy specific foods or supplies)?

• How will you get your parent from the hospital to his home or other residence?

• What skills do you need to properly lift him, move him, feed him, or help him in other ways?

• What medications will he take? When does he need to take them? What side effects should you look out for? What should he do if he misses a dose?

• Whom should you call if there's a question or problem?

• What can he do to improve his health or heal more rapidly?

• What should you expect up the road? How fast might he heal? Or how might he get worse?

• When is his next medical appointment?

• Is there a support group nearby for family caregivers, or a social worker available to support your family?

You'll need to contact the state Quality Improvement Organization. You must ask for the review before noon on the first working day after the hospital has given you what's known as a "Notice of Non-Coverage." The appeal process usually takes at least 24 hours and can take up to three days. (If you appeal on Friday, for example, it's likely that little will happen before Monday.) During the appeal process, you don't have to pay for the hospital stay. So even if the QIO rejects the appeal, your parent will get a little extra time in the hospital.

Of course, your parent can stay in the hospital without coverage, but she will have to pay for it herself.

Bills, Bills, Bills

Hospitals have perfected chaos when it comes to billing. They use so many codes, abbreviations, and notations that it is almost impossible for a mere human being to figure out what a bill actually covers.

And your parent will not receive just one bill, but a seemingly endless series of bills—from the hospital, the surgeon, the anesthesiologist, the radiologist, the physical therapist, the laboratory.

The U.S. General Accounting Office has found that nearly all hospital bills include overcharges. According to a survey by *Consumer Reports*, people are frequently charged for medications, lab work, tests, and procedures that were not given or performed; charged for more time in the operating room than actually took place; and charged for the day they were discharged even though hospitals are not supposed to do that. They are also charged for more expensive services and procedures than the ones they received.

If possible, save every bill or receipt for your records. If a bill is confusing or some expense is questionable, call the hospital's billing department and ask for an itemized bill, including explanations of any notations.

Scan the itemized bill for duplications, charges for services that your parent never received, or unauthorized tests or procedures. If anything seems out of place, ask for an explanation.

If you need help, every state has a State Health Insurance Counseling and Assistance Program, or SHIP (shiptalk .org). Counselors assist Medicare clients with all sorts of insurance questions, including help with billing. There are also private companies (which you can find online) that will sift through hospital bills, keeping some percentage of what they recover.

For questions and concerns about Medicare coverage, contact Medicare (medicare.gov or 800-633-4223). For questions about Medicaid coverage, contact the state medical assistance office (medicaid.gov).

Handling the Paperwork

Chapter 15

Paying the Way

Talking About Money • First Steps • Dipping into Your
Own Funds • Financial Planning • Benefits and Discounts
• Getting Cash Out of a Home • Tax Tips • Professional Help

Certainly, life is a whole lot easier if your parent has ample funds, but no one is free from financial headaches. If you are not concerned about a stack of current bills, you may be worried about your parent's future security, taxes, or a dwindling inheritance. Some parents refuse to let go of a penny, pocketing breadsticks at every opportunity, while others will hand a check to any stranger with a pitiful story to tell.

Of course, siblings will join the fray, wrangling over how finances are handled and what is being spent, saved, or given away.

Money is a private and often touchy subject, and the mere mention of an annuity or reverse mortgage might make your eyes glaze over, but you need to talk and plan, because it will save you a lot of time, money, and headaches down the road.

Be sure that your parent can cover her expenses, both now and for the future; that she isn't hiding financial problems from you; that she is getting all the benefits to which she is entitled; that she has adequate (but not too much) insurance; and finally, that she is not seduced by scam artists and other slippery sorts. Help her simplify her finances and take steps so that someone can take over when needed.

You also need to think about the effect your parent's care is having on your finances. What are you willing to pay for, if anything? How much are you able to give up in lost wages to care for your parent? Can you share the burden with your siblings or get paid for this work?

This chapter lays out the financial groundwork.

THE MONEY THAT GOT AWAY

Your parent might qualify for any number of free or low-cost services, small monthly payments, and help paying for health care, prescriptions, food, utilities, and taxes. Millions of older Americans who qualify for benefits fail to take advantage of them. Go to benefitscheckup.org to find out if your parent is eligible for public or private benefits. You can find additional information about programs and services for your parent at eldercare.gov and govbenefits.gov.

Chapter 17 looks specifically at paying for medical and personal care, which will be by far the biggest expense. And Chapter 18 looks at legal issues, many of which concern your parent's finances. Whatever the situation, the best solutions require advance planning, so don't delay.

Talking About Money

Whether your parent is financially savvy or naive, a saver or a spender, you need to talk. At the very least you need to find out where relevant documents are kept; determine how you (or someone else) will assume responsibility if the need arises; and be sure your parent is able to pay for the daily care that most elderly people need at some point.

But tread gently. As you well know, money is a deeply private matter. Your parent might not wish to talk with you or anyone else about his financial situation. He might not want you tampering with his hard-earned savings or to listen to your advice. Your mother may be reluctant to divulge her spending habits. You walk a fine line between respecting their privacy and ensuring their financial security.

Consider the issue from your parent's perspective as this may give you a little insight and patience. Not only did your parent grow up in an era when money wasn't discussed, but also much of his identity may be invested in his role as a provider. He may feel that talking about his finances will strip him of that role. He might worry that you will think less of him when you see how little there is, or that you might get greedy when you see that his savings are significant.

Furthermore, your parent's view of saving and spending may be quite different from your own. If he lived through the Depression, watched prices rise astronomically throughout his life-time, and now faces an unknown future on a fixed income, he may be fiercely protective of every penny. He may not be willing to spend now to save later, to hire a lawyer, to buy adequate insur-ance, or to pay for necessary home health care.

Ironically, the worse things get, the more your parent may keep her finan-cial situation secret. She may be deciding between buying groceries and medica-tions because she simply can't afford to pay for both. She may be turning off the lights and turning down the heat to save on utilities, putting herself in a danger-ous situation and not want you to know about it.

Whatever the details may be, you need to talk.

Broaching the Subject

If being direct doesn't get you any-where—*Mom, I'm worried about the cost of long-term care. Can we talk about ways you might pay for this if you need it?*—then approach it from the side. Mention your own financial planning and ask for advice, and then shift the focus to them. *Dad, I've been putting money away, but I'm not sure how much I'll need. Did you save when you were my age? Do you feel you have*

> " I have a joint checking account with my mother, but I still pay for a number of her expenses out of my own pocket. She examines the statements carefully and would have a fit if she knew what some things cost. I've hired extra help and paid for a few minor repairs on the house. I also paid some of her lawyer bills because otherwise she would never have hired a lawyer.
>
> Anytime I do this, I keep receipts so I can show my brother what I've spent. He's not apt to challenge things like that, but you can never be sure how people are going to react and I'd much rather be safe than sorry."
>
> —Rhoda B.

enough now? Or talk about the financial hardships of a relative or acquaintance, or mention a news story (on, say, the cost of nursing care), and then lead into ques-tions about whether your parent feels financially secure.

Whatever approach you take, remember to listen to your parent's thoughts—her view of what the problems are, her priorities, and her plans—before offering your own opinions. (For more on difficult, but essential, conversations, see page 4.)

As you talk, let your parent make her own choices whenever possible. That's not easy, especially when you feel you know what's best, but remember, it's her money, and her life, that is at stake.

Hitting a Wall

If your parent resists, don't throw in the towel. Proceed slowly, but proceed. You might discuss basic financial tools

and ways to make things simpler—
direct deposit or automatic bill-paying,
for example—without prying into the
specifics of his situation right away.
Then, with time, move further into the
conversation.

If he won't speak with you, urge him
to speak with a financial planner, which
he should do in any case. People are
often more comfortable talking with
someone outside the family.

If nothing works and your parent
simply refuses to confront any of
this, consider the gravity of the situation. If your parent is facing a serious
and immediate problem, spell out the
consequences. Tell him calmly and
clearly that if he doesn't refinance his
mortgage, he will have to move out of
his house, or that if he doesn't pay his
health aides, he will be left to manage
on his own.

If you still come up against a brick
wall, you might be able to do some of
the work on your own. Contact the area
agency on aging (eldercare.gov), which
should have counselors who are familiar with these difficulties and are versed
in various benefit programs and special services to protect elderly people
from eviction, utility cutoff, starvation,
or other danger.

Depending upon the situation, it
might make sense for you to speak with
a financial planner or elder law attorney yourself.

If the situation isn't dire, and your
parent is clearly competent, you might
have to back off on certain issues. Your
parent might not spend his money
exactly as you think he should. He
might fall down the stairs because
he's too cheap to install a ramp, or the

"When my mother was still able,
we created a revocable trust. She
chose me to be co-trustee, and we added
my name to her checking account. At
times, I have transferred funds from my
account to hers if she was in danger of
overdrawing, and then transferred the
money back into my account when funds
were deposited into her account.

My siblings have entrusted me to do
this. It occurs to me over and over that it
would be very, very easy to take advantage of the situation. In some ways it's
an overwhelming responsibility. Should
anything go amiss, the buck stops with
me. I do not even want to think what the
consequences might be, should distrust
arise."

—Diana R.

government may get the family home
because your parent didn't plan ahead.
There may be little you can do but live
with his decision (and make sure there
are sturdy handrails along those stairs).

If you believe your parent is making
irrational decisions because he is cognitively impaired (as opposed to plain
foolish—a tricky distinction to make)
or under the influence of a scam artist,
you will have to step in more forcefully.
Talk to his doctor. Find out if depression,
dementia, substance abuse, overmedication, or another problem is getting in
the way of rational thinking. If he has
any sort of cognitive impairment and is
mishandling his money or if someone
is exerting undue influence, you may
need to petition the court for financial
authority. (See page 381 for information
on guardianship.)

First Steps

If he hasn't done so already, your parent should sign a durable power of attorney so someone has the legal authority to handle his finances and property when he no longer can. Check with his financial institutions, because most have their own forms that they will want signed as well (this will make life much easier, as financial offices are not apt to question their own forms).

Although it might seem sensible for your parent to name someone else as a joint owner of a bank account, enabling that person to sign checks, be careful, because a joint owner is, well, a joint owner. He or she will have full access to the funds. And when your parent dies, that account will go to this person, raising tax questions as well as other obvious issues (*Mom* gave *you that money?!?*). Also, if the co-owner has financial troubles, that account will be subject to creditors. One possibility is to create a joint account but then have it automatically funded each month with a small amount—just enough to cover your parent's monthly bills.

Your parent also might choose to establish a trust, naming you as a trustee, which allows you to manage everything in the trust. (See page 374 for more on trusts.)

Make It Easy

With all that you have to do, and all that your parent may not be able to do (now or in the future), now is the time to simplify.

TAKING THE FINANCIAL REINS—GENTLY

If you are taking over some or all of your parent's finances, do so gently and with the utmost respect for the power entrusted to you. Not only do you need to be extraordinarily careful with your parent's money (if you want her expenses to be covered and your siblings to ever speak to you again), but you also need to be sensitive to your parent's feelings. Personal financial control is a source of independence and pride; turning it over to someone else can be painful.

Whenever you take over a new task, do so with your parent's consent, if possible.

Don't tell him you are doing it; ask him if it would be okay—a subtle, but important difference. Proceed slowly, keeping him in charge to whatever extent possible.

If he wants to stay in the driver's seat, let your parent retain whatever financial powers he still can—or at least the sense that he maintains control. If he can't handle the important bills, he might continue to write checks for his weekly groceries, donations, small gifts, and other expenses. Or, he might simply sign or approve the checks you write and review his statements from time to time.

> *Until you get brought inside their financial life, you may not know how damaging the situation is.*
>
> Both Mom and Dad fell prey to credit card offers. This might not have been a signal of financial desperation, but rather a sign that they were less able to manage their affairs on their own.
>
> By the time we moved them out of their house, we learned enough to know they couldn't cope any longer, and they knew it too. But it was a process—it didn't just happen by flipping a switch. It took time. They, and we, reached a point where we all knew they needed us to start taking control."
>
> —Dan M.

- Consolidate her accounts and, if possible, get them all within one financial institution so there is one statement, one set of forms, and, ideally, one person overseeing the accounts.

- Consider selling any real estate beyond her own home, so that she is not playing landlord or worrying about other properties. (Of course, if the property has risen considerably in value, someone needs to assess the tax consequences and weigh that against any tax deductions.)

- Bills can be paid automatically, giving her, or you, one less thing to think about. It will protect her so that her utilities are not shut off, her insurance policies don't lapse, and her credit is not jeopardized. (If your parent doesn't want her bills paid automatically, and you are concerned that she may forget to pay them, get duplicate statements or ask the creditor to notify you or another family member if bills become overdue.)

- Social Security, pension, and other income can be deposited automatically so that checks don't pile up or get thrown out accidentally. Your parent can authorize you to be her representative, or you can apply directly (if she is not able to do so). Contact the local Social Security office or the Social Security Administration (ssa.gov or 800-772-1213). They can also help you oversee her Medicare bills.

- Direct deposit and automatic bill paying should take care of most day-to-day financial chores, but if your parent's routine finances are still more than you and your siblings can handle, you can hire a "daily money manager." This sort of manager (as opposed to one who oversees investment portfolios) will pay bills, make deposits, balance checkbooks, organize tax records, deal with creditors, and handle medical bills and insurance claims. Obviously, this is costly and you need to be cautious. Keep a close eye on things.

  You can find a daily money manager through the American Association of Daily Money Managers (aadmm.com or 877-326-5991). They generally charge between $30 and $100 an hour, depending upon the area.

- AARP, in conjunction with several states and financial institutions, has volunteers who help low-income elderly people budget their money, pay bills, make deposits, and keep track of finances. To learn more, contact AARP (aarpmmp.org or 888-687-2277).

Dipping into Your Own Funds

The costs associated with your parent's care can sneak up on you slowly—you're buying your mother groceries occasionally, paying to have a ramp installed, paying for gas so you can see her regularly, and cutting back on your hours at work.

Or, it can come at you suddenly. Your father's had a stroke and needs his home renovated and an aide, and he has no way to pay for any of it.

Either way, you might find yourself spending large sums on your parent's care. How do you regulate the smaller expenses, and should you pay the larger ones?

Before you do anything, learn about benefits, services, and programs that can help your parent at benefitscheckup.org. Quite often, families pay a parent's way without realizing that they might have been able to tap into public or private programs.

Learn about Medicare, Medicaid, Veterans Affairs benefits, benefits for

> My mother-in-law lives on her Social Security payments, which come to less than $900 a month. She managed on it, sort of, but now she needs help at home and can't afford it. My husband thinks we should pay for it, but his income and mine together barely cover our expenses, with the kids and all. I'm so angry. I feel like we shouldn't have to do this, but if we don't, I can't imagine what will happen."
>
> —Kathy P.

government employees and their families, and work-related benefits that might extend to others in the family. Find out about adult day care, transportation, meals-on-wheels, legal aid, and other community services that are provided free or on a sliding scale.

If your parent might be eligible for Medicaid at some point—and even those with a decent nest egg can end up on this federal health insurance for the poor because personal care is so expensive—you certainly don't want to spend your money. Your parent should be "spending down" so she can get on this government program ASAP. (So let her treat for dinner.)

If you are still tempted to spend your own money, look carefully at your own financial resources. What do you need to live, to retire, to care for your children? What can you afford to spend? Are you really willing to spend it?

If you decide to spend your own money and you have siblings who are willing to share the burden, you might create a fund to which all of you contribute and then appoint someone to keep track of all expenses from the fund.

If you are the only family member willing or able to help, talk with your siblings about how to move forward (and how to remain friendly). A sibling who can't afford to pitch in financially might help in other ways.

Talk about ways to get reimbursed, at least in part, at some later date. For example, you might give your mother a

FILIAL DUTY

Ancient law required that children take care of their parents (because, after all, they took care of you). And in fact, the vast majority of care of the elderly today comes from family members. However, much of the financial responsibility was shifted to the government with the passage of Social Security, Medicaid, and other entitlements.

Despite this realignment, about half the states still have "filial responsibility" laws, and more than a dozen states can impose penalties—fines and even imprisonment—if children fail to care for their parents and foot their bills.

By and large, states don't enforce these laws, and even if they did, the laws typically come with "outs." That is, you are exempt in most states if you can show that you can't afford to pay your parent's bills or that your parent was abusive or neglectful. However, states have the option and can, out of the blue, exercise it.

Legal scholars continue to debate the merit and legality of such laws, but for the time being, it's worth finding out what's happening in your parent's state before flat-out refusing to pay any of his bills.

---

loan that will be paid off, with interest, upon her death. Or you might buy her house and let her remain in it until she moves or dies, which would provide her with more spending money.

Or, you can simply keep track of all expenses and make arrangements to be reimbursed from your parent's estate after her death. In this case, send your siblings regular financial reports and keep meticulous records, including all receipts, bills, and canceled checks.

If the problem is not expenses, but income lost because of caregiving, again, talk with your parent and siblings to come up with a plan so you don't end up in financial trouble yourself. You might get reimbursed for some of the lost income. (See page 66.)

Whatever the details, be clear with your parent and siblings up front, write up a statement that defines the terms of the arrangement, and have it signed by both parties, as well as your siblings. If you are dealing in large sums, a deed or title, or anything that might affect taxes or Medicaid eligibility, get a lawyer involved.

You are not betraying any assumptions of goodwill by being businesslike about these matters. Even the closest family relationships can be torn apart by financial issues. There will be less

> " It was very stressful. I was trying to care for my mother and take care of my business. But I couldn't put in a full day. Every time I went to see a client, I had to find someone to stay with her. I had received a big fellowship and it was a big opportunity, but I couldn't put in the hours or stay late."
> —Angela S.

CAREGIVER COMPENSATION

Yes, most care and assistance is provided out of love and family duty, but when caregiving becomes extended and laborious and the work falls largely to one sibling, it is reasonable for the primary caregiver to receive some compensation, especially if this task is jeopardizing his or her career and income. Done correctly, such compensation can help your parent "spend down" for Medicaid eligibility. See page 66 for more on caregiver compensation.

division and contention if everything is decided in advance and handled in a businesslike manner. In fact, you should be more businesslike when dealing with family members than at any other time, because the risk (losing these relationships) is enormous.

Also, keep track of your expenses, because you might be able to deduct some of them from your taxes, declaring your parent as a dependent.

At the end of the day, the decision to dip into your own funds is a personal one. There is no right answer. What you decide to do will depend upon your own financial security, your parent's financial situation, your relationship with your parent, and your personal views. Do not compare yourself with others. Do not feel either righteous or immoral for the decisions you make.

It is perfectly reasonable not to want to jeopardize your own finances to pay your parent's bills. And you should think very seriously before taking on debt, quitting a job, or otherwise getting yourself into financial straits to cover your parent's expenses, as you will only be passing this burden on to your own children.

Medicaid is a very welcome safety net; use it.

Financial Planning

Regardless of the size of your parent's estate, she should do some financial planning. Advance planning is the best way to avoid a financial crisis, at any income level.

Basically, financial planning means reviewing one's worth, income, budget, and future needs, and then creating a plan that will increase income, decrease spending, and protect assets, as necessary. It also means developing a strategy to pay for future expenses and care. If your parent has a relatively large estate, she will need to review her investments and insurance and think about protecting her assets from taxes, and she will probably need a professional involved. Someone with a smaller net worth might be looking into low-income benefits and Medicaid eligibility.

The Financial Planner on page 651 will help you get started. But someone who knows about state laws and is savvy about financial issues, especially issues facing seniors, will be of enormous help. You can hire a financial professional or lawyer, or ask the area agency on aging (eldercare.gov) about free or inexpensive guidance.

It shouldn't take an inordinate amount of time to create a comprehensive financial plan, and it will be time well spent. The following guidelines will help your parent (and you) get started. Begin by collecting information you will need, including tax records, bank statements, and financial reports.

. . . .

❝ My mother loves to travel, to go out to eat, to buy new clothes. She hasn't saved much, and she's spending what she has. I don't know what's going to happen when she needs help, when she has medical bills or needs nursing care. I have saved and skimped my whole life. I have put away money for retirement. My wife and I don't think it's right that we should have to pay for her care when she's lived this high life and been so irresponsible. Yet I know my sisters will think it's my duty. It makes me angry."

—Carl R.

. . . .

If you are doing this with your parent, restrain the urge to take over completely, unless your parent wants or needs you to. Although it's far easier said than done, respect her privacy, autonomy, and right to make her own choices.

Assess the Current Situation

Make a list of all your parent's assets (savings, investments, real estate, and so on) and then calculate her debts (mortgages, loans, outstanding bills). This will show her "net worth" and an overall framework to consider as you move forward.

Once you have done this, add up all sources of income (pensions, Social Security, and so on). Then figure out her monthly expenses (mortgage, rent, utilities, groceries, etc.). Reviewing past entries in a checkbook or bank statement should reveal some of her regular expenses.

If she is spending more than she is taking in each month, how is that gap being covered? Is your parent building up debts on a credit card? (Put an end to this right away. For help, contact the National Foundation for Credit Counseling at nfcc.org or 800-388-2227.) Is she going through her savings? How long can she continue this way?

Are there expenses that can be trimmed or eliminated? Are there other sources of income she might tap into (a home that can be used as collateral against a loan, a life insurance policy that might have cash value, properties or other assets that can be sold)? Are there programs and services for senior citizens, particularly those living on a low income, that she might use?

PREPAID FUNERALS

The primary reason to prepay for a funeral is for Medicaid eligibility, and in this case, it makes some sense. Although the rules vary state to state, most states allow this purchase, up to a limit, without penalty. (In fact, some states allow prepayment for family members as well.)

The other reason to prepay is to limit the excessive funeral spending that can go on when family members are drenched in grief. A parent might want to keep things simple by arranging it all in advance.

But for the most part, prepaying is not a great idea. So many things can go wrong—the funeral home goes out of business, your parent moves, the funeral home later insists that the money won't cover all the expenses, and so on.

If your parent still wants this paid for in advance, he can set up a trust or put money into a "payable on death" account and leave explicit instructions.

Any bank can set up a "payable on death," or POD, account. The money will be solely his, and then, upon his death, be immediately available to the other person named on the account, in this case, for funeral expenses. Of course, he needs to trust this person, and he needs to be very clear with everyone in the family what this account is for and how it is to be spent, as the cash will belong to this other person upon his death. (It may be best not to put too much into it.)

If your parent insists on buying a prepaid funeral, he should ask a lot of questions—what happens if prices rise, if money is left over, if he changes his mind, if the funeral home closes, if he moves, and so on.

If your parents are anywhere near Medicaid eligibility, or would be near if either one of them needed extensive care, then they need to learn about how to protect the surviving spouse, "spending down," and other issues of Medicaid (see page 354).

Look at your parents' insurance policies. Do they have enough coverage? Is the coverage redundant? Be sure that policies have not lapsed or that they are not paying for an old policy that is no longer necessary.

Study any investments or savings. Are they invested aggressively enough to provide growth and yet conservatively enough so that your parent will have money for the future?

You'll also need to know how assets are held—in whose name and under what sort of ownership—and the cost basis of any investments or holdings (the cost at the time of purchase).

Anticipate the Future

What do you anticipate your parent's income and expenses to be up the road?

The big question is what sort of care might your parent need? If he needs home care, nursing home care, or some other long-term care, which can cost more than $70,000 a year, how might

" My parents have done nothing to prepare for their old age. They have simply spent whatever money they had without thinking of the future. They never listened to us when we told them to save. Now they are running out of money. Neither one of them is healthy, and they are both growing helpless. I'm sure one of them, and probably both of them, will need nursing care at some point soon. And they won't be able to afford it.

My brothers and I are wondering who's going to pay for this. I probably have the most money of the three of us, but I also have four children. I can't afford to pay for nursing care, nor do I think I should. I feel for them and I want to help, but I'm also angry at them for dumping this responsibility on us."

—Diane P.

he pay for it? Again, might he be eligible for Medicaid? Can he (and should he) get some sort of mortgage to help cover his expenses? If he has long-term care insurance, how much of his care will it truly cover?

Are there tax credits or deductions, or any free or low-cost services that he might be eligible for in the future?

If both your parents are alive and you are helping them with their finances, explore how each of them would fare financially if the other became ill or died. Determine how each spouse's income and expenses would change and how they might protect themselves.

Your Parent's Priorities

As you and your parent create a financial plan, talk about his goals and priorities. What does he need money for, and what is most important to him? Does he want to enjoy these years as much as possible, or is he committed to keeping a family house or setting aside money for his children? Is it possible to do both? Is he adamant that he pay all his bills without going on public assistance or borrowing?

WHOSE MONEY IS IT?

You may find that, as much as you want the best for your parent, you are also eyeing her assets with some thought to yourself. *How much is there? How much might be passed along? How can this money be protected?* To some extent, these are healthy thoughts—conscientious, not greedy. Your parent should protect whatever he can. Certainly, it is better that his money goes to his heirs than to the government.

But be very careful not to overstep the boundaries of helpful financial planning.

This money belongs to your parent, not to you. It should be used, first and foremost, for his comfort and care, even if that means spending every last dime on aides and special medical equipment.

If your parent's money is disappearing, you might have to simply resign yourself to the situation and accept the fact that you will not inherit anything. You will save yourself from aggravation now and from disappointment when everything is gone.

Encourage your parent to consider these issues so that he can arrange his assets to meet his goals.

Develop (and Follow) a Plan

Once you have a picture of your parent's financial strengths and weaknesses, come up with a plan to meet her needs. This may include changing her spending habits, buying a new insurance policy, renting out a room in her house, setting up a trust, selling some assets, or revising her investments to include more bonds and fewer stocks.

Be sure your parent follows the course that's been laid out. It does no good to spend hours figuring out ways to save money if the cost-cutting measures are ignored. Give your parent encouragement and support while she tries to alter fixed habits. And keep after her, because waiting is a dangerous game.

Review the plan in six months or a year, or any time there is a change in your parent's circumstances—illness, disability, injury, divorce, or financial windfall.

Benefits and Discounts

Find out right away what services, discounts, and programs your parent might be eligible for. Far too often, people spend, worry, struggle, do without, and borrow from family when, in fact, help is available. So look into this before your parent spends more than she needs to or you dig into your own pockets.

Of course, there's Medicare and Medicaid (both discussed in Chapter 17) and various programs that help people sort through health care coverage and insurance questions. And there's Social Security, which provides income to workers after they retire. But there are other, less known benefits that your parent should tap into.

Start by filling out the questionnaire at benefitscheckup.org, which is run by the National Council on Aging. This will give you a list of programs and benefits to which your parent is entitled. You can also fill out the questionnaire at the government's site, govbenefits.gov. These are fairly inclusive. Nevertheless, you might also want to contact the area agency on aging, which may know about other state and local programs (eldercare.gov).

Most programs are aimed at people living on low incomes, but some programs are available to all seniors, regardless of income—programs that will lower her monthly bills, offer tax relief, or provide services and consulting at a discount, such as legal and insurance guidance, prescription drugs, home maintenance and repairs, health care savings programs, and more.

Supplemental Security Income

Elderly people (or blind or disabled people) on very limited incomes and with few assets are eligible for monthly payments of several hundred dollars a month from the federal program Supplemental Security Income, or SSI. (This is not the same as Social Security.)

Income limits vary from state to state. Usually, a person's assets (excluding their home, clothing, furnishings, a car, and a small burial fund) cannot exceed about $2,000 for an individual or $3,000 for a couple.

To learn more about SSI or apply for it, contact the local Social Security office or the Social Security Administration (ssa.gov or 800-772-1213). Your parent will need her Social Security number, birth certificate or other proof of age, proof of where she lives (such as a property tax bill or lease agreement), bank book, and/or payroll stubs.

Food

Although the Supplemental Nutrition Assistance Program has the catchy acronym SNAP, it is still commonly known as food stamps, from the days when people actually received coupons, or "stamps," to buy groceries. Nowadays, you get an Electronic Benefits Transfer (EBT) card, or debit card, which is replenished automatically each month. The average benefit is less than $100 per person per month, which isn't much, but it helps.

Eligibility for food stamps varies from state to state. In most cases, a person cannot have more than about $3,500 (this does not include the value of a home, furnishings, and so on) and a monthly income of about $1,000 (after most medical and household expenses are met). Anyone receiving SSI benefits, regardless of assets, is eligible.

For information, contact the local food stamp office or the national SNAP office (fns.usda.gov/snap or 800-221-5689).

Meals on Wheels (food delivery programs have a variety of names, but this has come to be the generic name) provides meals to seniors, either at senior centers or community centers, or directly to the senior's house if he or she has trouble getting out. Contact the local senior center or the Meals of Wheels Association of America (mowaa .org) to learn more.

In addition, local food pantries provide basic foods (and often, fresh fruits and vegetables) for free. The Senior Farmers' Market Nutrition Program allows seniors to buy fresh, local farm goods with coupons. To learn more about these and other food programs, contact the area agency on aging or call the National Hunger Hotline (866-348-6479).

Energy Assistance Programs

The government's Low Income Home Energy Assistance Program (which has the unmanageable acronym LIHEAP) helps pay energy bills so your parent can stay warm in the winter and cool in the summer, which is critical for elderly people, who are very susceptible to both overheating and hypothermia. LIHEAP programs are federally funded but managed locally, so eligibility and benefits vary. Some LIHEAPs also offer weatherization and energy-related home repairs. To find out if your parent is eligible,

DISCOUNTS AND SPECIAL SERVICES

Businesses and professionals of all types sometimes offer special services and discounts to elderly customers. These are some of the popular marketing programs aimed at seniors:

- Grocery stores: free deliveries, senior discount days

- Veterinarians and other pet services: house calls, discounts, and pet-walking services

- Pharmacies: free deliveries and discounts

- Hairstylists and manicurists: house calls and discounts

- Phone and utility companies: discounts and other services, including amplified phones, large-button phone pads, and large-print bills. Also, call several providers to be sure your parent is getting the best deal based on her calling habits.

- Local utilities: discounts, rebates, or help aimed at getting the elderly to insulate and otherwise "weatherize" their homes; lower utility bills; special programs to help elderly and low-income customers with heat and power bills

- Health clinics, hospitals, and public health departments: free health screenings and shots, and some discounted services

- Dentists and hygienists: discounts and services for low-income seniors and the homebound

- Restaurants: discounts for seniors on certain nights or at particular times

---

contact the National Energy Assistance Referral project (which has the far better acronym NEAR). NEAR can be reached at 866-674-6327.

To apply, your parent will need recent copies of utility bills, recent proof of her income (including Social Security, payroll, pensions, disability, and so on), proof of address, and her Social Security number.

Phone Bills

Lifeline is a government program that helps cover the cost of monthly phone bills (wireline or wireless). It is available to anyone eligible for Medicaid, Supplemental Security Income, food stamps, or energy assistance programs.

Lifeline provides a monthly discount, which, with matching state funds, may be between $10 and $15 a month. Only one discount is allowed per household.

For information, go to lifeline support.org or call your parent's local telephone company or department of human or social services.

Housing

The U.S. Department of Housing and Urban Development (HUD) has a number of programs to help people on limited incomes stay in their own homes or find low-cost housing. Programs vary from state to state. For information, contact HUD at 800-569-4287 or hud.gov (click on "Topic Areas" and then "Information for Senior Citizens").

Transportation

The area agency on aging (eldercare.gov) can tell you about van service for the elderly and other accessible transportation, as can the American Public Transportation Association (apta.com/resources/links or 202-496-4800).

Tax Help

Tax Counseling for the Elderly is a program funded by the Internal Revenue Service that offers free tax help to older people. The counselors (who are volunteers) are trained in issues pertinent to the elderly, such as Social Security benefits, tax credits, and rebates. The volunteers set up shop each year in early February in public libraries, senior centers, and banks (some will make house calls).

To speak with a volunteer, contact a local senior center or IRS office, the federal IRS office (irs.gov or 800-829-1040), or AARP (aarp.org or 888-687-2277). As part of the IRS program, AARP sponsors volunteer tax counselors through its program, Tax-Aide.

Getting Cash Out of a Home

Although your parent can get cash out of his home by borrowing money and using his home as collateral or by getting a mortgage, he needs to be *extremely* cautious.

Borrowing is a complex business. A bad deal can get your parent into serious trouble. He should consult a lawyer to make sure that any arrangement is a safe one. And he should be sure that a loan will actually cover his financial needs, now and in the future, because once he has used the equity in his home—and some of these loans have high fees and expanding interest rates—he may have little else to use for his expenses or to offer as collateral.

Your parent needs to consider how any mortgage will affect his income and taxes, and particularly his eligibility for programs such as Medicaid and SSI. For example, he might be able to go on Medicaid and keep his house, without any need to draw cash from it. (In fact, drawing cash from his house might make him ineligible.)

If he needs cash, consider the benefits explained above and other ways to improve his financial situation. It might be better for him to take in renters or downsize to a smaller home. He might also be able to refinance any existing mortgage to get a lower rate.

Reverse Mortgages

Reverse mortgages have become increasingly popular, but that's largely because financial institutions have realized their value and are pushing them heavily. Advertisements gushing about the "tax-free cash" are springing up all over.

But many people are finding their money gone, their homes in foreclosure, and their mortgages in default. Regulations are getting stricter, but still, be very careful.

Basically, a reverse mortgage can provide your parent with a lump of cash to renovate his home, a flow of money to pay ongoing bills, a line of credit to cover unpredictable medical expenses, or some combination of these things. Unlike a typical loan or mortgage, which has to be repaid in monthly installments, these loans do not have to be repaid until the home is sold, or the homeowner moves or dies.

Closing costs and upfront fees, which may be substantial, can be financed within the mortgage. And because money from the loan is just that, a loan and not income, it isn't taxed.

Reverse mortgages can be useful if done properly, but be sure your parent understands all that is involved, weighs upfront and annual fees, considers the value of fixed interest rates, finds out what happens if the value of the home drops, and determines whose name should be on the loan (if your father dies, your mother shouldn't be forced to sell their home).

FEDERALLY INSURED PLANS. Most reverse mortgages are known as Home Equity Conversion Mortgages (HECM). They are provided by private lending institutions, and backed by the federal government. This guarantees that your parent will be allowed to stay in her home for as long as she likes, and generally the lender cannot claim any other assets or leave a family with debt if the house depreciates. Payments to your parent are guaranteed—a reassuring advantage. However, a fee is tacked on to the loan to pay for this insurance.

To receive an HECM loan, your parent must be 62 or older; the house must be her primary residence; the house must be owned outright or have only a small mortgage balance that can be paid off with proceeds from the loan; and your parent must meet with a counselor from an agency that is approved by the U.S. Department of Housing and Urban Development (HUD). Her house can contain no more than four housing units, and she must, obviously, occupy at least one of them.

....

“ We looked into a reverse mortgage and thought, 'This is ridiculous.' I said, 'I'll just loan you money.' Basically, we just ran a tab. I wrote it up with an attorney. I put a lien on the house, just as you would with anyone else. My brothers all knew. I charged a fair rate of interest. And when my parents sold the house and moved into an assisted living facility, they paid me back.

It was all on the up-and-up. There were no fees beyond what it cost to have an attorney draw up the paperwork.

None of my siblings were in a position to do it. The alternative was to sell the house or get a reverse mortgage and lose $10,000 in fees."

—Mark S.

....

Because upfront costs can be high, the government now offers an "HECM Saver" mortgage, which has lower fees for people needing a smaller amount of cash. These loans tend to be 10 to 20 percent smaller than standard HECMs.

To find a HUD counselor, call 800-569-4287 or go to hud.gov and click on "Topic Areas" and then "Information for Senior Citizens."

PROPRIETARY REVERSE MORTGAGES. Loans that are not insured by the Federal Housing Administration (FHA), but instead are privately owned and backed, are referred to as "proprietary," or privately backed, reverse mortgages. When the housing market crumbled, these loans largely disappeared, but if prices improve, the loans should become more available.

These reverse mortgages are not subject to the same regulations as HECMs, and there are no limits on the amount of money one can receive, so they tend to be offered only on more expensive homes.

Although the loan amount may be larger than one your parent can get from an HECM, be sure cost comparisons are accurate. Look at all costs and changes in the loan over time. Some credit lines grow with time; some do not. Sometimes the lender will want, in addition to the amount owed, a percentage of the appreciation in the value of the home. Be sure your parent knows what he is getting into and that he has compared the options thoroughly.

Home Repair Loans

Home repair loans, which are typically offered by government housing agencies

ⓘ FOR MORE HELP

Be leery of websites providing information on reverse mortgages (or any other financial advice), as many are run by the very institutions doing the lending or by scam artists. Unfortunately, even many news reports have been fed by lenders and are not terribly accurate.

For information, go to hud.gov and click on "Topic Areas" and then "Information for Senior Citizens" and then "Reverse Mortgages." AARP has good information at aarp.org/revmort, including a booklet called "Borrowing Against Your Home."

or nonprofit organizations, are terrific if you can find one. They provide a one-time lump sum for home repairs (fixing a roof, repairing plumbing, weatherstripping, insulating) or renovations that make a house accessible for people with disabilities (installing ramps, grab bars, a lift, or lower cabinets). Home-repair loans cannot be used for cosmetic work or additions judged to be unnecessary.

These loans, sometimes referred to as "single purpose loans," are usually offered without interest or at a very low interest rate, and with no or low fees and closing costs. Sometimes, if a person lives in his home for a designated length of time, the loan is forgiven, meaning that your parent owes nothing. And the cherry on top of all of this is that the construction might increase the value of the home so much that it covers the loan or even leaves a profit. These loans, however, are usually available only to people with moderate or low incomes.

Home-repair loans are often set up as reverse mortgages so that nothing is paid on the loan until your parent dies or sells her house.

To find out about such loans, call the area agency on aging or the local housing department.

Property Tax Deferral Loans

In many states, elderly people who meet certain income limits can defer paying property taxes. Again, the amount owed, plus any interest, is paid off when a person sells his house, moves, or dies. For more information, call the area agency on aging or the local tax collector.

Sale-Leaseback Plans

Unlike other plans, which are offered by government agencies or private lenders, sale-leaseback deals are usually made between individuals—often between family members. Your parent sells his home to another person, but remains in it indefinitely as a tenant with a guaranteed lifelong lease. Although your parent gets cash and no longer bears the burdens of home ownership, he also relinquishes some control over his home.

Tax Tips

- Some older people are not required to file federal tax returns, so make sure of your parent's tax status before doing unnecessary work.

- People over 65 are entitled to a tax credit and a higher standard deduction.

- Even if your parent does not need to file a federal tax return, call the local tax office about state tax laws. Individual states offer various tax-relief programs and tax credits for seniors.

- Elderly people are not required to pay taxes on most public assistance, such as mortgage assistance, improvements paid for by the state to reduce home energy costs, nutrition programs, and veterans' benefits. They may be required to pay taxes on part of their Social Security income, however.

- You can claim your parent as a dependent and get an exemption under the following circumstances: No one else claims him as a dependent; your parent's gross taxable income is less than a few thousand dollars (the exact amount changes from year to year); and you pay for more than half of his care and living expenses for the year. If you and your siblings share this cost, you can all agree to declare one sibling, who's footing at least 10 percent of the cost, for the exemption (fill out the Multiple Support Declaration form). If your parent does not live with you, then you have to pay half the cost of keeping up his home for that year to declare him as a dependent.

- Your parent can deduct medical expenses that exceed 7.5 percent of his adjusted gross income (if he doesn't take the standard deduction and instead itemizes his deductions). This includes all medical and hospital care not reimbursed by insurance, dental care, health insurance premiums and copayments (including a portion of premiums paid for long-term care insurance), prescription drugs, nursing services, eyeglasses, hearing aids, medical supplies, and transportation to medical appointments.

  The entire cost of nursing home care (including room and board) is deductible as long as the stay is medically necessary. (With such a large deduction, this would be a good time to consider IRA withdrawals or taking capital gains.)

  Your parent can also treat as a medical expense the cost of any home improvements that have been made because of a disability or medical condition, such as installing ramps or widening hallways and doorways to accommodate a wheelchair. If the work increases the value of the house (say your parent installs central air-conditioning because of his asthma), then he can deduct the amount spent minus the amount the property increases in value (which has to be determined by an appraiser).

- If you are paying your parent's medical bills, you can add them to your deductions if you paid more than half

of his total living expenses in that year (whether or not you claim him as a dependent on your tax return). Again, you can deduct medical expenses only if they exceed 7.5 percent of *your* adjusted gross income.

- If several siblings are sharing the costs, you might still be able to deduct medical expenses if you all sign the Multiple Support Declaration mentioned above.

- Tax credits are available for certain home services, adult day care, and supervision. If, for example, you hire someone (and pay their Social Security contributions) to care for your parent while you work, you can take a credit of up to 30 percent of the cost of the care.

- Your parent may not have to report the sale of his home (his primary residence) on his tax return unless the gain was more than $250,000 ($500,000 if he is married and filing a joint return).

....

" After my father died, I had to file his tax return. My father was incredibly orderly. But I have never seen such a disorganized mess as his tax information, including masses of past tax forms and receipts. I hired an accountant to help me, and we sorted through papers for months. Dad always hated the IRS and taxes. He died on April 15, which has become a little joke in our family—maybe, lying in that hospital bed, he started thinking about his taxes and the IRS and it was just too much for him to bear. Taxes: It should be on his death certificate as cause of death."

—Gloria C.

....

For answers to tax questions, go to irs.gov, or call your local IRS office or the IRS tax information number, 800-829-1040.

Professional Help

Friends, colleagues, and neighbors, sometimes even doctors and social workers, are eager to offer financial and legal advice and share their own experiences. Be wary. Even people who are trained in these matters have a hard time keeping up with the fine print and the ever-changing rules. And each individual's situation is different.

Unless your parent's situation is exquisitely simple, seek the advice of reputable and experienced professionals. Although it is expensive, the savings and protection provided are usually worth the price.

Also, be careful about taking a broad spectrum of financial guidance from one person. You don't want investment advice from an insurance broker or insurance advice from a tax adviser. Most people need to speak with an accountant, an attorney, and if they have significant savings, an investment adviser.

Who Are All These People?
Here's a quick rundown of the professionals your parent might consult:

FINANCIAL PLANNER is a generic term for anyone offering financial advice. If your parent (or you) wants a financial plan, take the time to find someone who specializes in this work, preferably an

independent adviser who is a fiduciary and is paid only (or primarily) through fees.

Explanation: A fiduciary has a legal obligation to put your interests first (not his own). A fee-only adviser is not getting commissions to sell products, such as investments or insurance.

Financial planners come with a variety of letters after their names showing that they have taken courses and passed the exams and requirements of a particular organization. Most are Certified Financial Planners (cfp.net), and a few are Chartered Financial Consultants (chfc higheststandard.com). The National Association of Personal Financial Advisors (napfa.org) represents financial planners who work on a fee-only basis.

ACCOUNTANTS handle taxes and audits. Most are Certified Public Accountants (CPAs), which means they have passed an exam and are licensed by the state. Those who are not actually CPAs may have been in the business before licensing laws went into effect. Some accountants have additional training in financial planning and so carry the title Personal Financial Specialist (PFS).

LAWYERS come in all stripes, but two are most apt to deal with the elderly.

Estate attorneys generally focus on estates, wills, trusts, and the like. Elder law attorneys help with Medicaid and other public benefits, probate, guardianship, and long-term care planning.

BROKERS, INVESTORS, AND MONEY MANAGERS buy and sell stocks, bonds, and other investment tools. Be careful that someone isn't pushing your parent to buy or sell investments just to make a commission. Again, it's best to find one with fiduciary obligation.

For information about brokers, firms, and any disciplinary action against them, or to file a complaint, contact the Financial Industry Regulatory Authority (finra.org or 800-289-9999) or the U.S. Securities and Exchange Commission (investor.gov or 800-732-0330).

Hiring a Professional

Get recommendations from trusted friends or from other professionals whom you like—lawyers, financial planners, accountants.

Once you have the names of three or four people who seem promising, make an appointment to talk with each one. Some issues to consider and questions to ask:

EXPERIENCE AND EXPERTISE. What is your specialty—estate planning, investing, taxes, insurance, health care? How long have you been practicing? (With few exceptions, it should be at least three or four years, preferably more.) What percentage of your clients are elderly or the families of elderly people?

HOLDING ON TO THE PURSE STRINGS

Although it is tempting to throw your hands up in the air and assign the whole financial mess to a professional, finances are too important to relinquish completely to someone else. Financial and legal advisers should be used for just that—advising. Your parent, you, or another family member should oversee what a professional does. You should have regular meetings, and if you don't understand something, keep asking until you do.

TRAINING AND CREDENTIALS. What degrees, certification, or special training do you have? (Several organizations test and certify financial planners and require continuing education.)

SERVICES PROVIDED. What, exactly, will you do for my parent and/or family? Determine what you want done and be sure you are getting at least that. If more is being offered, is it something your parent wants to pay for?

Are these services personalized? That is, does a financial planner simply put your parent's financial information into a computer and then hand you a printout, or does he or she consider the specifics of your parent's situation and her priorities? Likewise, do you get the feeling that a lawyer is going to fill in the blanks on generic forms or tailor advice and legal documents to meet individual needs?

COST. How do you charge—an hourly fee, a flat fee? What is your estimate of

TOO MANY COOKS

If your parent or family is dealing with more than one professional—an estate lawyer, accountant, and investment adviser, for example—be sure they are able and willing to work together. In the best of circumstances, such professionals should work as a team, talking every year or two to review a plan. Otherwise, a financial planner may be dedicating certain assets for future use while a lawyer is protecting them in an untouchable trust and an insurance agent is advising your parent to use the money to buy a new policy.

Your parent, or you, should talk with each person involved and choose one to oversee everything (although none should have the right to make important decisions without your parent's or your approval).

the total cost? What happens if the cost exceeds this estimate? (The professional should get written permission before exceeding the estimate.) Are bills itemized? Is an advance payment required? How often do you bill?

Fees are almost always negotiable, so once you find someone you like, compare prices and ask if he or she can bring the price down. Then get a written agreement concerning bills, payments, penalties, and services provided.

COMMISSIONS. Are you getting commissions for any services you provide? If so, consider whether this person will be acting in the best interests of your parent or simply working to sell a policy, an investment, or another financial or legal tool.

REFERENCES. If possible, get the names of two or three clients, preferably people in a similar situation, and then call and find out how long they have used this professional and how helpful, open, and knowledgeable they have found him or her to be.

THE TIME FRAME. What needs to be accomplished, and how long do you estimate it will take?

OTHER HELPERS. Who else in the office will work on this matter? If it's an assistant or associate, will his fees be lower, and how much supervision will he receive?

COMPATIBILITY. As you talk, get a sense of the person's character and personality. Do you and your parent like him or her? Do you share a basic approach or philosophy? Do you sense that this person will be honest and direct? Does he or she answer questions so that you and your parent can understand the situation clearly?

Chapter 16

Avoiding Fraud

Who's at Risk? • Common Scams and Scoundrels •
Preventing Exploitation • Signs of Trouble • What to Do

Loneliness, illness, fear, and a comfortable nest egg, coupled with old-fashioned good manners, make your parent the perfect target for financial exploitation.

This might seem like something you don't need to worry about, something that happens to other people, but think again. Financial exploitation of the elderly occurs with heartbreaking regularity. It is thought to be the most common form of abuse, robbing the elderly of their hard-earned savings and forcing many of them to rely on Medicaid and family members when the money is gone. Furthermore, such exploitation is often a precursor to emotional and physical abuse and neglect.

Scammers come in all shapes and sizes, from global networks to, alas, a family member or friend. Some have elaborate schemes, while others slip inadvertently into this role.

Be aware of common scams and protect your parent *before* there's trouble. If you suspect there's already a problem, take action immediately.

Who's at Risk?

Your parent, no matter how capable he might seem, is at risk. Truly. Even if he has never bought into this kind of nonsense before, even if he has always been guarded with his money, even if he is a financial wizard, he is susceptible.

First of all, as people age, even if they are otherwise quite competent and independent, they often lose the ability to make sound financial decisions. It might be because they are in the very earliest stages of dementia, or because of medications, loneliness, or grief. Whatever the reasons, their financial sense may not be what it once was.

In addition, your parent may have time on his hands—time to attend a free lunch, to listen to a stranger on the phone, or to make a new friend.

Bored and lonely, he might be thrilled to have anyone's attention and companionship—at any price.

Fear also may be tossed into this mix—fear of running out of money, of being abandoned, of being a burden, or of ending up in a nursing home. Scammers prey on these fears. *How are you going to pay for adequate care? What will happen when you run out of money? Let me tell you about a safer bet. . . .*

One of the biggest risk factors of all is isolation. If your parent is out of view of friends, family, and community, he's an easy target.

The point is, don't assume that your parent wouldn't buy in. Everyone is vulnerable. And quite often, people are swindled without even realizing their money is disappearing.

Common Scams and Scoundrels

The best defense is knowledge. If your parent is warned about common scams, he'll know what to look out for.

Financial abuse comes in a variety of packages, but it can be broken down into two broad categories. (For this discussion, we are not looking at blatant crimes—break-ins, purse-snatchings, robberies, and the like.)

The first is large-scale, organized fraud, such as sweepstakes, investment scams, telemarketing rip-offs, and identity theft. These are often done by phone, through the mail, or over the Internet.

The second is personal, face-to-face exploitation. The culprit may be a stranger who suddenly steps into your parent's life, a repairman, a trusted caregiver, a lawyer or social worker, or, more often than we want to imagine, a family member.

Industrial Fraud

Some common examples from the industrial fraud basket:

- A call or letter announces that your father has won a sweepstakes! Hooray! He just needs to send a fee so they can process his winnings. Of course, the fee is gone and the winnings never arrive.

- A "nonprofit" group solicits a donation, but once your mother donates, the calls keep coming, and more "donations" are sought. The caller might become threatening if your parent stops donating.

- Your parent is invited to a free lunch and seminar. He's got nothing to do, and what sane person would turn down a free meal? There, all his worst fears about money are spelled out, but a solution is offered, a "can't lose" financial product. Act now, they tell him, and you get a $500 bonus! Of

> ❝ My dad was always buying lottery tickets, even if there was no money in the checking account.
>
> My mother took care of all the bills, but when she was having knee surgery, he sent $69 to the Australian lottery. Once you do that, you are on every list, every lottery.
>
> My mom called me one day and said, 'This check bounced, and I thought we had money in the account.' So I went to the bank. He had written a check on an old, closed account, and the Australian lottery was going to take action against them.
>
> We got together and decided they couldn't live alone anymore, couldn't be independent, needed watching over, because of the driving and financial decisions."
>
> —Maggie B.

course, he either loses all his money or it is now tied up in some 20-year, terrible investment that he can't touch.

- In what's known as "phishing," your parent gets an email advising him that

EVEN A TOUGH NUT CAN BE CRACKED

Interestingly, submissive, trusting people are not the only victims of financial exploitation. Bossy, opinionated, tough guys are easy to dupe, too.

Your father might be a resolute skeptic. He might insist that it's "my way or the highway." But a trained scammer will know exactly how to prey on this sort of thinking: Give him everything "his way." That is, agree completely, with everything. *You're a staunch conservative? So am I! You hate the city? Me too! You love to fish? So do I!*

It makes for a very fast friendship with the gruffest curmudgeon. A small loan or new investment is just part of the deal.

" Mum succumbed to some appeal supporting firefighters or police. I had to write a nasty note to get them to cease and desist, to stop calling her. . . . At one point we changed her phone number, and now it's not readily available to people.

If my mother gets a bill in the mail, she believes she owes money. If it is in black and white, it is true. And solicitations often are set up to look like bills.

Eventually, we created a revocable trust with me as co-trustee, and we added my name to Mum's checking account. I can access her account online, which helps me keep a close eye on her expenses."

—Diana R.

his bank or another institution needs him to update some information. A link takes him to a seemingly reputable website where he is asked to fill out his name, password, and other private information, which is then used for a variety of illegal purposes.

• In one of the cruelest schemes, your mom gets a call in the middle of the night from a desperate voice claiming to be her grandson (they use his name and perhaps other family names and identifying information, often taken from a newspaper clipping or social networking site). He's in serious trouble and needs her to wire money to him immediately. But, he explains, because he's in jail or the hospital or otherwise indisposed, she has to wire it to "a friend."

In addition to these, there are bad loans, worthless products, cheap vacations, free prizes, and Ponzi schemes. There's also Medicare fraud and, because no subject is off limits, deception involving prepaid funerals.

Relations, Helpers, and New "Friends"

The majority of these crooks aren't strangers. Sadly, they are people our parents know and trust—a son or daughter, companion, caregiver, adviser, or new friend.

Many "up close and personal" abusers make a living out of cheating the elderly. They seek out vulnerable prey and have a methodical ruse.

For example, people prowl coffee shops and diners looking for lonely older people whom they befriend. Then, after the friendship has taken root, they coax them into financial schemes or bad investments.

Others drive around neighborhoods looking for elderly homeowners. They offer cheap supplies or a helping hand, and quickly uncover things that need to be repaired *immediately*. They sound knowledgeable and incite fear—*That roof is going to come down on your head if we don't reinforce it.* Perhaps some work is done, perhaps nothing is done, but the bills are enormous.

Then there is the insidious "sweetheart scammer," who seeks out lonely old people and quickly becomes a mate—and beneficiary. They search want ads looking for companions, or obituaries listing the surviving spouse of a long marriage. What 87-year-old man, drowning in grief, wouldn't love to have a devoted 50-year-old woman at his side?

Often, elderly people are targeted

by the very people meant to protect them. For example, sometimes when an elderly person is declared incompetent, the court names a guardian—usually a family member, but sometimes a "professional guardian," who is a stranger—who is given full control of the senior's life, including all of his assets. A perfect setting for abuse. These criminals can easily make off with all or most of a person's assets and leave the senior in dire straits.

Many exploiters don't set out to swindle and might not even see their actions as such. They are simply involved in your parent's life and become the beneficiaries of his generosity or see an opportunity that's too good to ignore.

In fact, a common source of financial exploitation is a member of the family, the inner circle, who abuses power of attorney or guardianship. This person writes checks to himself, swindles your parent into altering a deed, or coerces her into changing a will.

These people aren't necessarily deviant criminals. In fact, many start out with good intentions. But caregiving is draining, and easy money is just too tempting.

Perhaps a sibling who is handling your parent's finances runs into a little financial trouble herself. What's a check here or there? It's so easy to justify, given all she is doing for your parent. Indeed, she is quite sure that your parent would want her to have it, and perhaps she would. But the checks add up, and suddenly it's not a couple of hundred dollars

SHOCKING BUT TRUE

The most common thief: a family member, adviser, caregiver, or trusted friend. A pot of unwatched money is simply too alluring, especially when someone feels overburdened by the care they have to provide.

You have to trust people or you'll drive yourself nuts, but when someone bears responsibilities or has access to funds, be clear about the rules from the start. Establish safeguards.

for some groceries, but tens of thousands of dollars that are moving from one bank account into another.

Or maybe it's that lovely aide you hired. She has become friends with your parent, and what a relief that is for you! Your mother is overjoyed to finally have some companionship. So when Mom hears of her new friend's hardships, it's only natural that she wants to help, to write a check or give her a raise. It's just a little at first, but it grows. More checks are written. Gifts are purchased.

> My mom hired this 'very nice' man to do some work on her house. None of us particularly like him. He was too friendly with her. He stopped by a lot, had meals with her.
>
> It turned out that he convinced her it would be easier to do the work if she just gave him her ATM card and some signed blank checks. We still don't know exactly what he took, but it was bad."
>
> —Tina R.

Trips are underwritten. A car's title is transferred.

The question becomes, what constitutes a crime, especially if your parent has bonded with this person. Is this an acceptable relationship, or have things run amok? The line between help and heist can be fuzzy. How do you know what's happening, when enough is enough, or how to stop it?

The fact is, it's often hard to know. That's why it's best to start out on the right foot, with checks and balances in place. Then be on the alert, and if you smell even a whiff of rat, take action immediately to protect your parent.

Preventing Exploitation

Just alerting your parent to the more common scams should head off trouble. Discuss common scams listed above and some basic dos and don'ts (heavy on the "don'ts") with your parent early on:

- Avoid anything that sounds too good to be true. This includes easy money, surefire investments, and lofty promises to improve memory, increase libido, cure disease, or add muscles, love, or years to your life.

- Be wary of anything that is "free." (If your parent insists on going to the free lunch, go with him.)

- Don't be pressured into buying anything. Be leery of any salesman who ignores your refusals or urges you to make a quick decision. "Act now!" and "Only good for a limited time!" should set off warning bells.

- Never give out important information (address, credit card number, passwords, Social Security number) unless you initiated the contact and know exactly with whom you are dealing. Give health insurance or Medicare information only to your doctor and other health care providers.

- Check bills and statements regularly, looking for unfamiliar charges.

- Don't open unsolicited email, and never open attachments on emails unless you know who sent it.

- Give donations only to established, reputable charities or to local causes with which you are personally familiar.

- Sign up with the federal "Do Not Call" registry (donotcall.gov). Tell any callers that you are on the list and make it clear you do not want to be called again. If you continue to be harassed, complain to the Federal Trade Commission (ftc.gov or 877-382-4357).

- Beware of "free" or "trial" medical equipment and tests.

- If salespeople come to the door, do not let them in.

- Always get receipts, avoid paying in cash, and never send cash in the mail.

- Steer clear of contests, lotteries, and sweepstakes. The odds of winning are ridiculously low, and many involve hidden fees, taxes, and other costs. Also, your parent's name then goes on a sucker list and is passed on to other, similar groups.

- Rip up any preapproved credit card offers, which can be filled out by someone else. Similarly, be careful when discarding credit card receipts and statements, which might hold all the information necessary for new charges.

- When using an ATM, do so in private, and hold your hand over the keypad when entering your PIN. Never let strangers help you with a transaction. Thieves can actually install a device that reads your card's encoded data, use a hidden camera to get your PIN, and then drain your bank account. Review statements and report any unauthorized withdrawals immediately.

- Never wire money to someone you don't know, under any circumstances.

- Don't leave repairmen or other workers unattended in your home or give a stranger the house key.

- Never give financial authority to a new friend or caregiver.

- Do not lend money without ample legal documentation.

- Get anyone who is overseeing your parent's funds (even siblings) to provide detailed accountings and copies of bank statements on a regular schedule.

- Lock away all valuables and never leave money lying about.

Watchful Eyes

One of the best ways to avoid scams is to be sure your parent isn't isolated. Cut off and alone, he's easy pickings. Visit, call, video chat, get other people involved in his life; get him out to a volunteer job, a senior center, or adult day care. For so many reasons, not just scams, he should not be sitting alone all day.

This is not so easily done, of course. See page 104 for ideas on keeping your parent, even your very ill and frail parent, active.

Financial Prep

Certainly, if your parent hasn't already done so, he should update his will and assign power of attorney to someone he trusts implicitly. At the same time, address any financial concerns your parent might have. Assuage his worries, and/or get him to a financial planner.

If your parent will allow it, get the password to certain accounts so you or someone else in the family can review his statements (and be on the watch for unusual withdrawals). Or, find out if the bank will send copies to family members.

Clear Rules

When a new caregiver shows up, or anyone new comes into your parent's life, be clear about the rules from the start. He or she is not to accept extra money or elaborate gifts, for any reason, at any time, no matter how adamant your parent might be.

Of course, if your parent is largely in charge of her own life, you need to talk with her about this first. Explain that exploitation is common, and that clear rules will help everyone feel safer.

Likewise, if your parent moves in with a sibling or sets up a joint account with a sibling, everyone should be very clear from the start what is happening, how things will be managed, what is to be covered, what is not to be covered, and what sort of oversight there will be. You can do this respectfully and without accusation. Explain that it's always best to make everything clear so there are no misunderstandings. Depending upon the situation, a monthly accounting might be helpful.

> " My brother said he and his wife would buy a house that had two living areas so my parents could live with them. They would pay $500 a month in rent to help out with the mortgage.
>
> It was a good solution until we found out that my sister-in-law was stealing money from my parents. She had convinced my mother to open a joint checking account so she could help pick up her groceries and stuff. But then she was using Mom's money to pay her own bills.
>
> We found this out by chance because my mother wrote a check to my nephew and we saw that my sister-in-law's name was on the account. We went through the statements and found about $2,000 for dog grooming, her daughter's school, etc."
>
> —Ann M.

Signs of Trouble

The first sign of trouble is a particularly vulnerable parent. Beyond early dementia, which clearly puts someone at risk, all sorts of things affect judgment and decision making: age, medications, lack of sleep, immobility, grief, depression, boredom, and pain, to name a few. As mentioned earlier, loneliness—simply being on one's own—is one of the biggest risk factors for financial manipulation.

Even if you think your parent is immune, be on the lookout. A few worrisome signals:

- Any change in your parent's behavior regarding money (Is he suddenly having trouble covering routine bills or uncharacteristically silent about financial issues?)

- Unfamiliar charges or withdrawals from your parent's bank account

- Items suddenly missing from the house

- Any changes in a will, power of attorney, property titles, or insurance policy

- A collection of free mugs, 12 new magazine subscriptions, sweepstakes envelopes, or an unusual number of solicitations in the mail or by phone

- A handyman or mechanic who finds multiple things that need fixing

- New credit cards

- A change in financial managers, lawyers, or accountants

- Anyone who is suddenly dear "friends" or romantically involved with your parent

- A caregiver who talks about her own financial problems

- Any caregiver who readily accepts generous gifts, tips, bonuses, or financial help from an elderly person (They might not be scammers, but they certainly don't understand boundaries or the vulnerabilities involved.)

Undue Influence

If a suspicious friendship has recently evolved, be aware of the common tactics of coercion and what's known as "undue influence."

People who financially exploit the elderly often start with promises (spoken or implied) of abundant care and companionship, thus creating a bond. With time, they isolate the victim by limiting phone calls, canceling appointments, and making excuses for why he can't go out. Perpetrators don't want family and friends snooping about.

Abusers might incite fear and dependency by making family members out to be the enemy (*Your children don't really care about you. They just want your money.*) and/or threatening abandonment (*If you're not good to me, I'll leave, and you'll end up in a nursing home*).

They might also induce shame, telling the older person, for example, that no one could love him or that he's made a mess of things. They might also over-medicate, making the elderly person weak and vulnerable.

If you notice these signs, get help immediately.

" A caregiver ingratiated herself to my mom. My siblings and I all had a sense of uneasiness about her, but we all lead busy lives and we overlooked certain signals.

Mom loved her, and she seemed fond of Mom. But she lost her sense of boundaries. She guilted Mom, and managed to get several raises. She entertained her friends in Mom's house when she was supposed to be cleaning or caring for her. We found out she was leaving Mom alone during the day, and then she would stay late and say that she worked extra hours.

It was hard for us to see how bad it was, and to finally fire her. But when we did, we changed the locks and the phone number, and we had to get a restraining order.

Mom was confused, but eventually she understood that she had been taken advantage of."

—Dan M.

What to Do

I f you think that something's amiss, don't delay, because this sort of situation can deteriorate rapidly.

First, talk to your parent. Use kid gloves, though, because if you are angry with him, you might very well send him further into the realm of the perpetrator. Or, he might refuse to talk to you because he's ashamed of what's happened.

Start by asking him if he has any concerns about the situation. Gently hint at your concerns, but refrain from passing judgment or saying anything that will cause him to feel he has erred. Let him know that what's happening is completely understandable, that he's not alone, and that these things are common. Talk about what to do about it, giving him the opportunity to find his own solution.

Then act quickly to protect him and his assets. Encourage your parent to cancel any credit cards to which the abuser might have access, change passwords, and alert the bank to problems. Cancel checks that have already gone out but have not yet been cashed.

Call any organization involved and, in no uncertain terms, let them know that you want your parent off their call list or mailing list. If the scam involves a lot of money (or the possibility of a lot of money), talk to a lawyer about how to protect your parent's assets.

Call Adult Protective Services or abuse hotlines in your parent's state. You can find contact information for state APS offices through the National Center of Elder Abuse (ncea.aoa.gov) or the National Adult Protective Services Association (napsa-now.org). You can ask that your complaint be anonymous, if you wish.

The Senate Aging Committee also has a fraud hotline. Staff should either help you resolve the problem or lead you to sources that can assist (aging.senate .gov/fraud-hotline or 855-303-9470).

Contact the local police department for immediate help with a crime, or, if your parent is in a nursing home, talk with the long-term care ombudsman (ltcombudsman.org).

The National Consumers League has a toll-free consumer protection line (800-876-7060) and a helpful website (fraud.org). The FBI also has information about fraud directed at seniors (fbi .gov/scams-safety/fraud/seniors).

Finally, talk with your parent's doctor, as poor financial decisions can be an early sign of dementia.

Breaking Off Emotional Ties

If you are concerned about a new "friend," for heaven's sake, get involved.

BE THERE. Isolation is what gets people into these messes, so step one is to make sure your parent isn't alone all day. Get

> " There was a Ponzi scheme. The guy got $10,000 from my father. It was absurd. I saw it and said, 'You can't do that.' And he said, 'I already have.'"
> —Lou Ann W.

everyone involved in your parent's life—as many people and as often as possible. Ask family and friends to visit, stop by unannounced, call regularly, and email.

It's hard for a perpetrator to, well, perpetrate under all those watchful eyes, and most will skedaddle.

TALK. Now more than ever, you need to be highly sensitive to what's going on in your parent's life, why this relationship is important, why he might feel embarrassed or ashamed by the situation, and why he might feel trapped.

As always, listen first. Be open and calm. What does your parent feel about the relationship? What does he get out of it? What does he think the other person wants? What worries him? Talk to him about trust, loneliness, companionship, and what constitutes abuse.

Difficult as it may be, make this a conversation, not a lecture. Try to understand that this is painful for him, that he is vulnerable and perhaps scared, even though he might not admit it.

You might let him know that if he is happy and well cared for, he should keep the relationship but protect his money, or at least protect the bulk of it—enough so that he will be able to pay for his own care (including any nursing home or in-home care) for the rest of his life. Be clear that this isn't about you or your needs (or your inheritance), but his well-being.

MEET. Hold a family meeting, preferably with a geriatric care manager, family mediator, or elder law attorney, to discuss everyone's concerns. Yes, the perpetrator must be invited; that's the whole idea. Even the suggestion of such a meeting might send the abuser packing, or at

> " After my mom died, my father was alone in the house, and he cried a lot. He hired a housekeeper/companion 30 years his junior, and about six weeks after she arrived, he announced that they were getting married.
>
> We knew this was trouble, so we met with a lawyer. We told Dad, 'Go ahead and marry her, but before you do, please take some precautions—lock up your assets and see if she sticks around.' He willingly set up a trust and changed the deed to his house.
>
> She is still there, living with him, and they still plan to get married. She moved all her stuff in, and she's taken down the family photos. She usually leaves as soon as we arrive. Sometimes she disappears for more than a day. She rarely walks with him, and he sees his own friends much less than before.
>
> I worry all the time, but I'm not sure there's a lot more that we can do. I'm afraid that the more I push, the more I alienate him. We just have to keep a close eye on things, but I'm sick over it."
>
> —Lynette R.

least get him or her to realize that poor behavior will not be tolerated.

RECORD IT. Keep a log and any emails that reflect your concerns (and those of others). Note dates and describe actions that are improper. If things get ugly—if you have to go to court or argue for guardianship or sue someone—such a log will help your case.

Let's say your father has fallen in love. Keep track of when and how they met, how the relationship progressed, and any suspicious comments or actions you and others have noticed. *On June 8, he was left alone for four hours. On June 15, she called to say he couldn't have lunch with me. On June 22, she said he couldn't come to the phone.* And so on.

CONSIDER A TRUST. A power of attorney, giving someone the authority to make financial decisions on your parent's behalf, is a critical document; however, it isn't that useful if your parent is rewriting it and renaming his agent on every whim. If this is the case, a well-written trust, assigning a trustee to oversee finances, might be a better tool, as it is generally more difficult to revise.

GUARDIANSHIP. If things aren't resolved, and your parent's competence is in question, consider seeking guardianship. It's a last resort, but sometimes the only choice.

Be extremely careful about handing over authority to a guardian, however, as this person will then be in a perfect position to exploit your parent. (See page 381 for more on guardianship.)

ACCEPTANCE. If your parent is fully competent and capable (this can be a massively difficult thing to judge), and you've tried everything you can think of, then you might have little other recourse than to accept the situation. Stay involved as much as you can, keep an eye on things, and get him to protect whatever assets he has. But he's made his own decision, and you (and he) might have to live with it.

Chapter 17

Paying for Health Care

Medicare • Medicaid • Long-Term Care

If medical, nursing, and home care bills** are not pouring in now, the prospect that they soon will be lies ominously ahead. Premiums, deductibles, copayments, prescriptions, and other expenses not covered by insurance can quickly consume a nest egg.

The biggest quandary, even for those with a comfortable savings account, is how to cover the cost of long-term care—the day-to-day help that is needed when someone has a chronic illness or disability. Although families provide much of this care, people often need to pay for some services—home care, day care, or assisted living or nursing home care, and the price tag can be significant. The problem is, Medicare and other health insurance cover very little of these costs.

As a result, people pay out of pocket, and when they use up their funds, they go on Medicaid, government insurance for low-income people, which does cover long-term care.

If he hasn't done so already, your parent and/or you should review his finances, evaluate his insurance, and consider how he might cover such expenses. Act now, because your parent will become ineligible for certain types of insurance as he grows older, and he might be able to protect some of his assets before going on Medicaid. He should also consider his living arrangements and evaluate local programs and services so that he can get the best care possible within his budget.

PROGRAMS AND OPTIONS, IN BRIEF

MEDICARE. Federal health insurance for people over 65.

MEDICARE ORIGINAL PLAN. Part A covers inpatient hospital care, hospice care, and a limited amount of skilled nursing care and rehabilitation. Part B covers 80 percent of the cost of doctors and other health care providers, medical equipment, and hospital outpatient care (after a deductible is met).

MEDIGAP. For those with Original Medicare, this is a *supplemental* policy offered by private insurers that fills some of the gaps, such as copayments and deductibles.

MEDICARE ADVANTAGE. Private insurance companies offer these plans, also known as Medicare Part C, as an *alternative* to the Original Plan. They typically provide more coverage than the Original Plan, but limit coverage to a specific network of doctors and hospitals.

MEDICARE PART D. Prescription drug coverage. This is included in most Medicare Advantage plans, but if it's not part of a plan, it can be bought separately.

MEDICAID. Government health insurance for low-income people. Medicaid covers medical costs and a good deal of long-term care. Specifics vary from state to state.

EMPLOYEE OR RETIREE COVERAGE. Your parent might have some health care coverage from a former employer.

FEDERAL EMPLOYEE HEALTH BENEFITS. Health coverage, including prescription drug coverage, for federal employees.

VA AND MILITARY BENEFITS. Veterans and those with TRICARE coverage (expanded coverage for uniformed services retirees and their families) receive generous medical and long-term care coverage.

STATE PROGRAMS. States have various programs to help people who have low incomes but are not eligible for Medicaid.

FEDERALLY QUALIFIED HEALTH CENTERS (FQHC). Low-cost health care at a community clinic.

LONG-TERM CARE INSURANCE. Private insurance that covers some of the cost of long-term care (nursing home, assisted living, and in-home care).

MEDICAID WAIVERS. In an effort to keep people out of nursing homes, states get waivers so they can use Medicaid funds to pay for a variety of home and community-based services (HCBS). They also have programs that allow recipients to determine how money is spent and who provides care.

Medicare

Medicare is federal health insurance for people over 65 and for certain disabled people younger than 65. The program is run by the Centers for Medicare & Medicaid Services (CMS).

Anyone who receives Social Security benefits gets a Medicare card when they turn 65. If your parent doesn't receive Social Security benefits, she can still apply for Medicare. To do so, she should contact the local Social Security office or the Social Security Administration (ssa.gov or 800-722-1213).

Fortunately, but also unfortunately, Medicare offers choices, and sorting through them can make your eyes glaze over. We'll keep it simple. For detailed information, go to medicare.gov.

The Original Medicare Plan
The Original Medicare plan is divided into two parts. Part A covers inpatient hospital care, hospice care, and some nursing home care and medically necessary, "skilled" home care. Part B, the medical insurance portion, covers most doctor's fees, medical equipment, diagnostic tests, outpatient care, and some mental health care and rehabilitative therapy.

Most people do not pay anything to receive Part A (because this was paid through payroll taxes), but they are responsible for deductibles, coinsurance, and copayments once they need care.

If your parent has to buy Part A, she should enroll right away, because if she waits until she is hospitalized, she (or, most likely, you) will face a mountain of paperwork and bureaucratic delays at an already difficult time. (The premiums are about $450 a month.)

For Part B, the medical portion, there is a monthly premium (about $100 for most people; more for those with higher incomes), which is taken directly out of Social Security payments. An annual deductible (about $150) must be met, and then, after the deductible is paid, your parent pays a "coinsurance" of about 20 percent of the cost of most covered services. Many preventative services are free.

Part B is optional. If your parent doesn't want Part B (because she is adequately covered by another policy), she needs to contact the local Social Security office and let them know.

> **"** A woman from the hospital called and said that my father had used up his Medicare hospital days.
>
> I didn't even know that was possible. He'd used them up 16 days earlier and no one had said anything. The bill was enormous. We didn't know what to do.
>
> He could use the 60 lifetime days, but then he'd be done with Medicare hospital coverage, and that's a big leap.
>
> It forced us to reevaluate his care. We would never have made a decision based solely on price, but it forced us to evaluate whether staying in the hospital was the best option, which it wasn't. Eventually, we got hospice involved, which was the best decision we ever made."
>
> —Kim K.

IN BRIEF: Medicare Part A, Hospital Insurance

This chart outlines basic information about the Original Medicare plan.
Coverage will vary under Medicare Advantage plans.

	COVERED (once the deductible is met*)	NOT COVERED
Hospital stays (including stays at rehab and mental health facilities)	• Semiprivate rooms, meals, nursing, drugs, and medical treatment • The first 60 days in a benefit period** • The next 30 days require a copayment (about $300/day) • The copayment doubles for any additional days (only 60 of these "reserve days" are allowed in a lifetime).	• Private duty nursing • Extra cost of a private room, unless medically necessary • Television or phone • All costs after the 60 "lifetime reserve days" are used up • Care in a psychiatric hospital is limited to 190 days in a lifetime.
Nursing home care	• "Skilled" nursing and rehab care that follows an inpatient hospital stay of at least three days*** • The first 20 days in a benefit period** are fully covered • A copayment (about $150) is required for the next 80 days (after which time, care is not covered) • Medications, meals	• Custodial care (help with bathing, dressing, eating, etc.) that is not part of "skilled" care services • Any care that is not related to a hospital stay of three days or more • All costs after 100 days per benefit period** • Extra charges for a private room
Home health care	• Part-time or intermittent "skilled" care (nurses, therapists, and aides) when ordered by a doctor for treatment or rehabilitation. A patient must be largely homebound. Services must be provided by a Medicare-certified agency. • 80 percent of the cost of reusable medical equipment (such as walkers, wheelchairs, and hospital beds) ordered by a physician	• Custodial care (help with bathing, dressing, eating, etc.) that is not part of "skilled" care services
Hospice care	• All medical, nursing, and social services • Drugs for pain and symptoms • Medical equipment • Spiritual and grief counseling • Short-term hospital care • Respite care (to give caregivers a break)	• A small copayment for drugs (less than $5) • 5 percent of the "Medicare approved" cost of inpatient respite care

* The deductible changes annually, but it's generally about $1,200.

** A benefit period begins on the day your parent is admitted to a hospital or nursing home, and it ends when she has been out of any such facility for 60 straight days. There is no limit to benefit periods.

*** Your parent must be formally admitted as an inpatient at the hospital for three days. Be sure she is not staying at the hospital as an outpatient.

IN BRIEF: Medicare Part B, Medical Insurance

	COVERED (at 80 percent, after a deductible is met)	NOT COVERED
Doctor and other health care providers	• "Medically necessary" care from doctors who accept Medicare's approved rates • Care also from physician assistants, nurse practitioners, and other providers • Limited chiropractic care	• Charges in excess of the approved fees • Routine physical exams • Routine dental care, some chiropractic care and foot care • Cosmetic surgery
Outpatient hospital and mental health care	• Most medical services and supplies, including emergency-room visits, one-day surgery, and some rehabilitation • Outpatient mental health care	• 20 to 40 percent of the cost of outpatient mental health services
Nursing care and therapy	• "Medically necessary" outpatient skilled nursing care, physical, occupational, and speech therapy • No limit if therapy is provided by a hospital outpatient facility • Some nutrition therapy • Certain weight-loss and smoking-cessation counseling	
Diagnostic and laboratory services	• Blood and urine tests, X-rays, scans, EKGs, biopsies, some screening tests	
Medical equipment and supplies	• Durable equipment, including hospital beds, wheelchairs, walkers (from approved suppliers)	• Hearing aids, dentures
Ambulance service and emergency care	• Ambulance transport, when medically necessary • Emergency care	
Preventive care (Most of this is fully covered, and no deductible or coinsurance is required.)	• Mammograms, Pap tests, and pelvic exams; pneumonia, hepatitis B, and flu shots; bone mass, colorectal, prostate, heart disease, HIV, and glaucoma screening; diabetes screening and services; alcohol abuse and depression screenings • Annual "wellness" visit	• Most other preventive care
Drugs	• Coverage for a few (very few) prescription drugs	• Most prescription drugs (unless you have Part D)
Other	• Dialysis services and supplies	• Any medical care outside the United States • Routine dental care • Acupuncture

Medicare Advantage

Private insurance companies contract with Medicare to provide plans called Medicare Advantage, which is an alternative to the Original Medicare plan. These are also referred to as Medicare "Part C" or "MA Plans."

The good news is that they cover the same services covered in the Original Medicare plan, and usually include additional coverage, such as vision, hearing, and dental care. Most include prescription drug coverage. The bad news is that under most Advantage plans, your parent will be restricted to a network of doctors and other health care providers.

Your parent can switch plans every year between mid-October and early December. Under special circumstances (say, he moves, loses his Medicaid coverage, or a plan changes its contract with Medicare), he can change plans at other times of the year. He can also switch to a five-star plan (based on surveys of members and providers) pretty much any time of the year (from December 8 to November 30). And he can return to the Original Medicare Plan during the first six weeks of the year. It's all oddly complicated.

Most Medicare Advantage plans fall into one of these categories:

HEALTH MAINTENANCE ORGANIZATION (HMO). Under most of these managed care plans, your parent can go only to hospitals, doctors, and other providers who are part of the plan's network. Also, her primary care doctor may have to make a referral in order for her to see a specialist. Be aware that doctors can leave the plan at any time. If your parent is happy with her current doctor, be sure he or she is in the network and has no plans to leave it.

PREFERRED PROVIDER ORGANIZATION (PPO). These work much like managed care plans, except that people

PARTICIPATING PHYSICIANS

Medicare keeps costs down by determining in advance what it will pay for medical procedures and supplies. When a health care provider or equipment supplier accepts this fee as full payment—called "accepting assignment"—your parent pays only the deductible and any coinsurance.

Although some doctors accept assignment for some procedures and not others, doctors who are "participating physicians" accept assignment on all Medicare claims.

If a doctor does not accept assignment, your parent will have to pay the difference between the doctor's fee and Medicare's approved rate. Also, he might have to pay the bill in full at the doctor's office and then get partial reimbursement from Medicare later (although the doctor should submit the claim).

You can find a participating physician either by calling doctors' offices or by going to medicare.gov/physiciancompare.

GAINING ACCESS

You'll need authorization to access your parent's Medicare records and bills. Get this permission early, while your parent can still sign the forms. Contact the local Social Security office or the Social Security Administration (ssa.gov or 800-772-1213).

are allowed to see doctors and specialists who are not in the network; they simply have to pay a bit more.

PRIVATE FEE-FOR-SERVICE (PFFS). These plans operate much like the Original Medicare Plan, except that a private company, rather than Medicare, determines the "approved fees," premiums, deductibles, coinsurance, and copayments. Your parent can go to any doctor or hospital that is approved by Medicare and accepts the plan's fees as payment.

SPECIAL NEEDS PLAN (SNP). These plans provide basic Medicare coverage plus any specialized care that is needed because of a specific situation: a disease or disorder (such as end-stage renal disease, congestive heart failure, dementia, or diabetes); someone who needs nursing care; and people who are eligible for both Medicare and Medicaid. Patients generally have to stay within a network of providers.

POINT OF SERVICE PLANS let your parent go to doctors and hospitals not in the plan's network, but he may have to pay higher deductibles and coinsurance to do so. Some Medicare Advantage plans—although very few—offer this option.

MEDICAL SAVINGS ACCOUNTS are offered by a few companies. These plans have a high deductible, but Medicare puts money into a savings account that can be used to pay any health care costs. Money that isn't used immediately can be saved for medical expenses in future years.

MEDICARE COST PLANS are private plans that are bit more flexible, accepting people who have only Medicare Part B. They allow people to sort of bounce between the private plan and the Original Plan, and allow them to join and leave the plan outside the normal time frames. They are not widely available.

PILOT PROGRAMS, in which new plans and programs are tested, are available for short times in specific areas of the country.

> " I ordered a lightweight wheelchair that I could lift into my car and use to maneuver the sloped streets of our town. But Medicare denied it, saying that we should have ordered a standard wheelchair. It cost $3,000. I appealed many times, but was denied."
> —Walker L.

MEDICARE RESOURCES

Medicare Part A, B, C, and D? Medicare Advantage? Medigap? Appeals? Special exceptions? How does anyone figure it all out? To ease the head pounding and confusion, there are several sources of help:

MEDICARE. You can get most of the information you need, including the annual "Medicare & You" booklet and information about state organizations, at medicare.gov or 800-633-4227. The website also has a "Plan Finder," which helps people find the plan that best fits their needs (medicare.gov/find-a-plan), and a coverage search that allows you to see if a particular treatment or service is covered by your parent's plan (medicare.gov/coverage).

STATE HEALTH INSURANCE ASSISTANCE PROGRAMS (SHIP). State counselors help people sort through the medley of insurance options, decode bills, and appeal Medicare decisions. Find SHIP programs through the National SHIP Resource Center (shiptalk.org).

THE CENTER FOR MEDICARE ADVOCACY. In addition to advocating nationally, this nonprofit organization has a wealth of information about Medicare on its website (medicareadvocacy. org) and can often help individuals with specific questions or problems.

MEDICARE SAVINGS PROGRAM. These programs help people living on low incomes pay Medicare premiums and sometimes deductibles. Again, the

Medicare site (medicare.gov/contacts/) can guide you to the MSP in your parent's state.

STATE INSURANCE DEPARTMENT. This should be a good source of information on Medigap plans in your parent's state. Medicare can link you to the appropriate insurance department.

SOCIAL SECURITY ADMINISTRATION. For more information about Medicare, or to get a replacement card, ask about eligibility, or get help paying for prescription drug costs, contact the SSA (socialsecurity.gov or 800-772-1213).

COORDINATION OF BENEFITS CONTRACTOR. If your parent has coverage from more than one source, generally any other source must be billed first, before Medicare. If there is uncertainty about where to send bills, contact the Coordination of Benefits Contractor (800-999-1118).

MYMEDICARE.GOV. By creating an account at this site, your parent can check his benefits and access claims information.

VA AND TRICARE. For information about veterans' benefits, contact the Department of Veterans Affairs at va.gov or 800-827-1000. For questions about TRICARE, expanded medical benefits for those retired from uniformed services, call 886-773-0404 or go online to tricare.mil/mybenefit.

Medicare Supplement Insurance (Medigap)

Medicare Supplement Insurance, also known as Medigap, is private health insurance that fills some, but not all, of the holes in the Original Medicare plan. To get a Medigap policy, your parent must have both Part A and Part B of the original plan. She will then pay the Medigap premium and the monthly Part B premium.

Typically, Medigap pays the cost of copayments, coinsurance, deductibles, and sometimes physician bills that exceed Medicare's approved charges. Some plans cover care outside the U.S. They do not cover long-term care and plans purchased after 2006 do not have prescription drugs coverage.

If your parent wants to fill some of the gaps in her Original Medicare plan, she also has the option of switching to a Medicare Advantage plan.

Anyone enrolled in a Medicare Advantage plan or other health plan that provides ample coverage should not get a Medigap plan. Also, anyone who is nearing financial eligibility for Medicaid should not buy a Medigap policy. (In fact, it may be illegal for a company to sell your parent a Medigap plan in these situations.)

MEDIGAP PLANS

To make shopping easier, insurance companies must offer only certain, standardized plans, starting with Plan A, the core plan, which covers basic benefits and is available in all states. Plan names then skip sporadically through half of the alphabet. (It's not that our government doesn't know the alphabet, it's just that some plans, such as H, I, and J, were dropped.) By law, these plans cannot vary from company to company or state to state. The language and format used in the policies are also standardized.

But—yes, there is always a *but*—some states do not offer all of the plans, and a few states (Massachusetts, Minnesota, and Wisconsin) have their own version of these plans. So although these plans are meant to help you comparison shop, your mother in Minnesota may not be able to buy the same plan that her sister bought in Illinois.

Also confounding things is the fact that any of the standardized plans can be sold as "Medicare SELECT" policies, which work like managed care plans. This means that clients are required to use a designated group of doctors, clinics, and hospitals, but they usually pay less for the plan.

Finally, insurers are allowed to add benefits to a standard plan, making it, alas, no longer standard.

And oh yes, the prices are *not* standardized, so two companies can offer precisely the same policy and charge different premiums—a good thing to know.

The bottom line is that despite all these efforts at standardization, you or your parent should read any policy carefully to understand exactly what is covered and what, if any, exclusions or restrictions exist. Ask the company for a clearly worded summary, which insurance companies are required to provide.

By and large, your parent will be comparing apples with apples, so she should be able to decide with relative ease which type of plan she wants, and then shop around for the best price and service and the most stable and reliable company. Medicare offers a helpful booklet, "Choosing a Medigap Policy," which is available at medicare.gov /publications.

MEDIGAP SHOPPING TIPS
Although the standard policies are essentially the same across companies, the prices can vary widely, so do some research. Below are some tips to keep in mind when looking for a policy:

EXAMINE YOUR PARENT'S NEEDS. Determine how much your parent spends on health care each year (premiums, deductibles, copayments, excess charges, and so on), how a policy might affect these costs, and what her future

STANDARD MEDIGAP PLANS
(except in Massachusetts, Minnesota, and Wisconsin)

BENEFIT	PLANS									
	A	B	C	D	F*	G	K**	L**	M	N***
Part A coinsurance, and an additional 365 days of hospital coverage	✓	✓	✓	✓	✓	✓	✓	✓	✓	✓
Part B coinsurance or copayment	✓	✓	✓	✓	✓	✓	50%	75%	✓	✓
First three pints of blood	✓	✓	✓	✓	✓	✓	50%	75%	✓	✓
Part A hospice care coinsurance or copayment	✓	✓	✓	✓	✓	✓	50%	75%	✓	✓
Nursing home coinsurance			✓	✓	✓	✓	50%	75%	✓	✓
Part A deductible		✓	✓	✓	✓	✓	50%	75%	50%	✓
Part B deductible			✓		✓					
Part B excess charges					✓	✓				
Emergencies in foreign countries			✓	✓	✓	✓			✓	✓

✓ = 100%

* Plan F also has a high-deductible version.

** Plans K and L include an annual out-of-pocket limit (about $5,000 for Plan K and $2,500 for Plan L).

*** Plan N requires a copayment of $20 for some office visits and $50 copayment for emergency room visits (unless they result in an admission).

health care might entail. (Okay, that last part is a bit difficult to do.)

DON'T BUY MORE THAN NEEDED. Duplicate coverage is expensive and unnecessary. (It's also widely prohibited.) And don't pay for features your parent doesn't need (for example, coverage for emergencies in foreign countries, unless she's traveling).

DON'T BE PRESSURED. Take time to pick the best policy. Your parent shouldn't be forced or frightened into buying a policy, or into switching from one policy to another. (Pressuring prospective buyers is against the law.)

KNOW THE COMPANY YOU'RE DEALING WITH. Check with the state insurance department to make sure a company or agent is licensed. Beware of any claims that a policy is sponsored by a state agency, or that an insurance agent represents Medicare. Neither is true.

CHECK FOR PREEXISTING CONDITION EXCLUSIONS. Don't be misled by the phrase *no medical examination required.* If your parent has a health problem, the insurer might not cover treatments related to that problem until the policy has been in effect for six months.

COMPLETE THE APPLICATION CAREFULLY. Do not believe an insurance agent who says that the medical history on an application is not important. If your parent leaves out any of the medical information requested, coverage could be refused for a period of time for any condition that wasn't mentioned. The company could also cancel the policy.

USE THE "FREE-LOOK" PROVISION. Insurance companies must provide at least 30 days to review a Medigap policy. If your parent changes his mind during this time, he can cancel the policy and get a full refund of any premiums paid.

BE CAREFUL WHEN REPLACING AN EXISTING POLICY. Your parent should not terminate an old policy until he is all set with a new policy, even if this means paying two premiums for one month.

DON'T PAY CASH. Use a check, money order, or bank draft payable to the insurance company, not to the agent. Be sure to get a receipt that includes the insurance company's name, address, and telephone number.

Medicare Prescription Drug Coverage

Medicare offers a prescription drug plan called, you guessed it, Medicare Part D. Your parent can get drug coverage as a separate plan or as part of her Medicare Advantage plan. The cost of these plans will vary depending upon the plan and your parent's income.

Numerous companies offer Medicare drug plans, and each offers different discounts on individual drugs. Because your parent can have only one Medicare drug card, she needs to choose wisely. Your parent (or you) should make a list of the medications she takes and how much she pays for each, and then plug those into the "Plan Finder" at medicare.gov /find-a-plan. The search will not only show the best insurance plan, but should also show the cheapest pharmacy or mail-order company for her drugs.

Plans should be reviewed every year during the open enrollment period, as her prescriptions will change, premiums

A NOTICE, NOT A BILL

Your parent will get a Medicare Summary Notice (MSN) every three months. While it looks bill-ish, this is not a bill. Do not pay it. It is simply a summary of medical services received. Look it over to be sure it is accurate. If something is not right, call the number on the statement.

change, and the prices a plan charges for a particular drug can change. Drastically. An annual review can save her thousands of dollars.

If your parent is part of a Medicare Advantage plan, she might have no choice in discount cards; she might have to use the card offered by the plan.

Note: If your parent doesn't sign up for drug coverage when he is first eligible for Medicare or if he goes for more than two months without some sort of drug coverage, he might be charged a penalty.

THE DONUT HOLE

For the time being, most drug plans have a gap, a moment when coverage is limited, commonly known as "the donut hole." However, this gap is shrinking rapidly and should be gone by 2020.

Basically what happens is this: Your parent pays for her drugs until her annual deductible, which is usually a couple hundred dollars, is met. Then she pays a copayment for any prescriptions covered by her plan. Once her *total* prescription drug costs—what she has paid and what the insurer has paid, combined—equal

some predetermined amount (about $3,000), she falls into the donut hole.

While in this "hole," she still gets a sizeable discount on her drugs, but she pays more out-of-pocket than before. Once her out-of-pocket expenses exceed a ceiling (about $4,000), she arrives at the other side of the hole, called "catastrophic coverage." At this point, she is well covered and pays only a small amount for each drug. This cycle starts anew each year.

Some plans have no deductibles and/or less of a "donut hole" but charge higher premiums.

HELP COVERING THE COST

Medicare helps people who have meager resources and income pay for prescription drugs through a program aptly named Extra Help. (It's also known as the low-income subsidy, or LIS, which isn't as snappy.) The program helps cover premiums, deductibles, and other costs associated with a drug plan, and does away with the donut hole.

If your parent did not get a purple letter (yes, it is actually purple) informing her that she automatically qualifies for Extra Help, she can get more information about the program and an application form through Social Security (800-772-1213 or socialsecurity.gov /prescriptionhelp).

DRUG DISCOUNT PROGRAMS

Medications can be so wildly expensive that older people skimp on their doses or skip the pills completely—obviously a bad idea. Others forgo groceries to pay for medications. Also not ideal. There are ways to save.

Numerous public and private programs provide free or discounted prescription drugs. While most of these programs are aimed at people living on very limited incomes, some do not have any eligibility criteria. For example, most states have prescription drug cards that offer hefty discounts at large chains.

Far more people are eligible than use the programs, so it's worth checking to see if your parent might fit the bill. Check out these websites:

- The National Council on Aging runs benefitscheckup.org.

- Medicare has a similar search tool at medicare.gov (or 800-633-4227). The Medicare site also directs you to state programs that help cover drug costs, known as State Pharmaceutical Assistance Programs (SPAPs).

- Pharmaceutical companies sometimes offer discounts or free prescriptions, which you can learn about through the Partnership for Prescription Assistance (pparx.org).

- Many state and corporate discount programs can be found at rxassist.org.

- The Together Rx Access Card (togetherrxaccess.com) provides discounts to people who do not have prescription drug coverage.

OTHER WAYS TO SAVE
- Ask the pharmacist if there is a generic version of the drug. The Food and Drug Administration requires that generic drugs be as effective and safe as their brand-name counterparts, and they are usually much less expensive.

- Shop around. Pharmacy prices vary widely, even within one area. Although it's ideal to have one pharmacist who has a record of all the medications your parent takes, it might be cheaper to have a few sources. One supplier may have the lowest price on asthma medication, but another may have less expensive hypertensive medication.

- If a particular prescription is not included in your parent's drug coverage plan, ask the doctor if an equally effective drug is on the list of those covered. If not, see if the doctor might get an exception granted from the insurer.

- Ask the doctor about splitting pills. Sometimes, if your parent needs 40 mg of a particular drug, it is cheaper to buy the pills in 80 mg tablets and split them in half.

- Ask the doctor for free samples. Drug companies often leave samples with physicians who can offer them to patients.

ONLINE DRUGS

Although it's generally okay to get prescriptions filled online, be cautious. Some sites will swindle you, selling medications that are contaminated or fake. For a list of reputable online drugstores, some of which may offer discounts, go to the National Association of Boards of Pharmacy website (nabp.net) and click on "Consumers."

- Find out if a larger prescription might cost less. Often a bottle of 50 pills is cheaper than a bottle of 25. Be sure they will keep, however.

- If your parent is in a nursing home, keep tabs on the cost of medications—both prescription and over-the-counter drugs. Many nursing homes charge wildly inflated rates—sometimes two or three times what a drug would cost elsewhere. If that's the case, demand the right to buy your parent's medications yourself.

- Associations and foundations connected to specific illnesses (such as Alzheimer's, Parkinson's, and arthritis) often know of ways to get drugs pertaining to that illness at a discount. Check their websites.

Medicare for Less

If your parent has little in the way of income and assets, but is not quite eligible for Medicaid, he should be able to get under the Medicare umbrella at a discount—no premiums, and sometimes no deductibles or copayments. States have various programs, called Medicare

> " The hospital was going to discharge my mother simply because Medicare allowed only so many hospital days for her procedure, and then they wouldn't pay anymore. But I knew she wasn't well enough to leave, so I told the discharge planner that I was keeping her there and contesting the decision.
>
> It was a battle, but in the end Medicare paid the additional hospital bill, about $5,000. It was definitely worth the trouble. You can't let these guys get the best of you—you have to fight for what's right."
> —Lucille L.

Savings Programs, which are part of the Medicaid system, to help cover these costs.

The rules are a bit different in every state, but if there is any chance that your parent might qualify, apply. Many people who are eligible never apply and end up spending hundreds of dollars each year needlessly.

To learn more about such programs and to see if your parent is eligible, call the state Medicaid office, which you can find at medicaid.gov.

THE BLUE BUTTON

If she hasn't done so already, your parent (or you) should go to mymedicare.gov and register. That will let her (and you) keep track of her personal Medicare information and look up claims, deductibles, and services.

Once she registers, the "blue button" on the Medicare website lets her download her personal health information to a file on her personal computer. She can use this to update any other online health management tools, and she can print it out and bring it with her to her next medical appointment.

A WORD OF CAUTION

Before your parent has any medical procedure or buys a medical device, find out if his insurance covers the cost and if it doesn't what the out-of-pocket charges will be. Don't hesitate to shop around or try to negotiate a lower fee. In the end, you might decide that the procedure is not worth the expense. Make an informed decision; don't get stuck with unexpected bills.

If his insurance does not cover a procedure and a provider offers a line of credit or loan (via some sort of medical credit card, usually) to pay for it, be wary. Often, these procedures are not necessary, and the loan, which might start out with an alluring promise of zero interest, will eventually have a hefty interest rate, leaving your parent to pay for the service years into the future.

Appealing a Medicare Decision

Don't think for a minute that it's not worth challenging the bureaucracy of Medicare. It is. Well over half of all appeals are successful, at least to some extent.

If you disagree with a decision—if coverage has been refused or stopped or is inadequate, or if there is some other problem—first talk with the doctor and be sure needed services have been ordered, and speak with the hospital or agency involved.

If your parent has the Original Medicare plan, find the Medicare Summary Notice (which she should receive every three months) and follow the instructions on the back. Your parent has 120 days from the date she receives the notice to file an appeal. She should get a decision within 60 days. You can also find appeal forms at medicare .gov/medicareonlineforms.

Other Medicare plans must tell your parent, in writing, how to appeal

a decision. (If a medical decision threatens her health, demand "fast action" on the appeal.) If the private plan does not decide in your parent's favor, the appeal is then sent on to an independent organization for review.

If your parent is in the hospital, she should be able to remain in the hospital, receiving care, while Medicare reviews any appeal.

If your appeal concerns prescription drug coverage, your parent or her doctor (or you) can contact the company issuing the plan and request an exception. Again, you can specifically request fast action on a claim.

> " Our father told us years ago not to pay for expensive caregiving if he began to suffer from severe dementia the way his father did. He protected his assets so he would be eligible early for Medicaid. It all happened the way he'd imagined. I'm grateful he had such foresight."
>
> —Fred S.

For more information on filing these appeals, contact the insurance company directly or visit medicare.gov or the Center for Medicare Advocacy's website medicareadvocacy.org.

Note: If your parent has Original Medicare, she might get something called an Advance Beneficiary Notice (or ABN), which is a warning that Medicare won't pay for a certain service. This is not a final denial. She can still choose to get the services, file the claim, and if it's denied, appeal it.

Medicaid

Don't wait to learn about Medicaid— also referred to as "medical assistance" or Title 19, or a litany of other state names, like Medi-Cal and MassHealth. By any name, this is generous government insurance for people who have very little money. It covers, among other things, the cost of home care and nursing home care when a recipient can no longer care for himself.

Unlike Medicare, which is fully regulated by the federal government, Medicaid is a joint program of both federal and state governments. The federal government sets guidelines, and states establish their own rules and programs within these broad parameters.

Broadly speaking, to qualify for Medicaid, a person's monthly income can't be more than $2,000 or $3,000. His assets (not including a home, personal belongings, a car, and a few other things) can't be worth more than $2,000 to $15,000, depending upon the state.

Learn the rules that apply to your parent, because they're complicated and vary not only by state, but sometimes by county.

In many states, if a person has meager assets, but his income is above the eligibility limit and below the cost of care, Medicaid will cover the difference. In other words, if the state's income limit for Medicaid is $2,000 a month and your parent's income is $3,000 a month, but the cost of nursing home care is $5,000 a month, then Medicaid would pay the difference (being sure to leave him with a small spending allowance).

Also, most states are careful to protect a spouse who is living independently

> " My mom became eligible for Medicaid about two years before she died. She was entitled to the maximum amount of care, about eight hours a day. But there was no one in this area who would do it because they pay so little.
>
> So we hired Anna and paid for her ourselves."
>
> —Angela S.

USING FUNDS *YOUR* WAY

Once upon a time, Medicaid paid for care in a nursing home, with few options. Then, states realized it was cheaper for them and better for recipients if care was provided at home. So they gave people the option of staying at home and using home health aides, adult day care, meal delivery services, and other local programs, known as Home and Community Based Services (HCBS).

Then states went a step further, granting people even more control over how these funds are used. For example, instead of having an aide for six hours each day as prescribed, your father could buy a scooter, build a ramp, and have an aide for three hours a day. Or instead of hiring an aide from a certified home care agency, your mom could hire a friend, neighbor, or, in most states, even you.

The details vary from state to state, but generally a caseworker sorts out how much care is needed, and then your parent decides how money will be spent and who will provide the care. A fiscal manager or home care agency oversees the money, payroll, and accounting (no, the state is not going to hand you a chunk of cash). And, of course, there are limits and rules to prevent abuse.

These programs, generally known as participant-directed services, are referred to by different names in every state—Personal Choices, My Choice, Personal Attendants, Elders Waiver, and so on. Some states refer to them as consumer-directed, person-directed, or self-directed services.

(By the way, it's best not to call and say, "I've been caring for my mom for years and now I want to be paid." Understandably, states do not want to pay family members for care they have been providing for free. Simply call and say you need help. They will likely send a caseworker over to investigate and make a plan.)

To find out about these programs in your parent's state, contact the area agency on aging (eldercare.gov), the local Medicaid office, the National Resource Center for Participant-Directed Services (participantdirection.org), or the Aging and Disability Resource Center (adrc-tae.org).

Note for veterans: The Veterans Administration has its own HCBS and patient-directed services programs. The Veterans Affairs office or national resource center cited above (under the link for Veteran-Directed Resources) should have more information.

---

from becoming indigent. In most cases, a spouse can keep the couple's home and a significant chunk of the couple's income and assets.

Elderly people who qualify for Medicaid are considered "dual eligible," meaning that they are eligible to receive both Medicare (because of their age) and Medicaid (because of their finances). Between those two programs, most health care costs are covered, including premiums and deductibles, prescription drugs, hospital care, outpatient care, nursing home care, and home care, as well as eyeglasses and hearing aids. Medicaid often covers transportation to medical appointments, assisted living care, home care, community programs, and case management.

But there may be a price to pay. Some health care providers and nursing homes won't take patients on Medicaid, or will accept only a limited number because the reimbursement rates are low. In some areas, it may be difficult (or impossible) to find aides or other home care workers who will take Medicaid. As a result, Medicaid patients may have to settle for fewer choices and lower quality care. (Of course, in many facilities Medicaid recipients live side by side with people paying full freight, and no one would ever know there was a difference.)

Furthermore, Medicaid has largely switched over to managed care plans, which means that your parent has to receive care from a particular list of providers. Her doctor and many specialists might not be in that group.

Any time Medicaid has refused to cover what you or your parent think are necessary services, contact the state Medicaid (or "medical assistance") office.

Despite any downsides, Medicaid is a vital and welcome safety net. Learn more about it by talking with a counselor from the area agency on aging (elder care.gov or 800-677-1116) or from the State Health Insurance Program (ship talk.org). You can also contact the state Medicaid office (medicaid.gov).

Note: State counselors can advise you on how to get Medicaid only if you are eligible; they cannot advise someone on how to protect assets before going on Medicaid.

Protecting Assets to Qualify for Medicaid

Your parent saved diligently so he could live out his days comfortably and perhaps pass a little something on to his

WHEN IS A HOUSE NOT A HOME?

When determining a person's eligibility, Medicaid does not include the value of his home (up to a certain limit). But that all changes when a home becomes merely a house.

As long as your parent, a spouse, and/ or any dependents live in his home, most states will not include it as part of his assets when he applies for Medicaid (again, up to a limit). However, if he has no spouse or dependents, and he moves out of his home—either because he sells it, moves permanently into a nursing home

or other facility, or dies—the empty house (or what he received for it) becomes fair game. He will lose his Medicaid eligibility and/or the state will go after the equity in the home to recoup what's been spent on health care. (The specifics vary from state to state.)

If an adult "child" lives in his parent's home and cares for that parent for more than two years, some states allow the home to be transferred to the caregiver without penalty. A house can also be passed to a disabled child without penalty.

children. Maybe he wanted a family home or a piece of land to stay in the family. But faced with the prospect of nursing home bills, his savings, and perhaps the house or the land, are in jeopardy.

Your parent may be able to protect some of his assets and still become eligible for Medicaid, but to do so, he has to plan in advance. The sooner he acts, the more he will be able to protect.

Of course, the notion of protecting one's assets and then going on Medicaid raises troubling moral questions. Medicaid and other public programs are meant for those who are truly needy. What your parent saves, other taxpayers must pay. Your family has to be guided by its own moral and political code.

Every state has its own rules, and those rules are complex and ever changing. The opportunities to protect assets are becoming narrower and may eventually disappear; what is permitted today may not be permitted tomorrow. If your parent wants to protect some assets, he should speak with a Medicaid planner, typically an elder law attorney, to sort it all out. You can find an elder law attorney at the website of the National Academy of Elder Law Attorneys (naela.org) or the National Elder Law Foundation (nelf.org).

SPENDING DOWN

The most common way that people protect their assets before applying for Medicaid is known as "spending down," which means that they spend money on items that Medicaid doesn't count as an asset. Purchases that are not counted in Medicaid equations in most states include a home, a car, home furnishings and other personal belongings, prepaid funeral expenses (a common tool in Medicaid planning), home renovations, or any payments to homemakers or aides. If someone is near, but not quite

---

FOR VETERANS ONLY

If your parent is a veteran, he may be eligible for additional pensions and generous medical and long-term care. Call the local Veterans Affairs office for more information on services and coverage, or contact the U.S. Department of Veterans Affairs at va.gov or 800-827-1000.

" When the lawyer talked to me about putting Dad's house in my name, I thought it was a great idea. Then I got home and I began to feel it was wrong. Dad believed in paying his own way. I didn't think he would want me to do this.

The more I thought about it, the more confused I felt. I know he wanted us to have his house, but I also know he wouldn't want to be on welfare or have us do anything dishonest. Here I was, choosing between these two horrible things, and he couldn't express his opinion because he was too sick. In the end, I didn't put the house in my name. I just felt it was wrong. We still have it now, but the lawyer tells me that the government will come after it eventually."

—Mark P.

> **"** My sisters think that my father should be in a nursing home because it would be cheaper, and they say he doesn't know or care where he is anymore. I think he should stay in his home with private nurses because I believe he does know the difference.
>
> It's true, we're spending a tremendous amount for his care. All of his money is disappearing. I know what they're feeling, because I'd planned on having some inheritance, too. But I think we have to make his life as comfortable as possible. I don't want the inheritance if it comes at such a price. **"**
>
> —Katherine S.

at, the eligibility limits, sometimes he can, well, just start spending his money (what fun!). Of course, gifts to others are not allowed.

LOOK-BACK PERIOD

For the time being, in most states, your parent can protect his assets by giving them outright to others or by putting them in an irrevocable trust. But this has to be done very early in the game—five years early, to be specific.

When a person applies for Medicaid, officials examine his financial records for the past five years to see what, if any, gifts or transfers have been made. Anyone who has given a gift or otherwise transferred assets during this penalty, or "look-back" period, won't qualify for Medicaid right away. (Transfers to a spouse or dependent do not count.) Usually, the person must wait the number of months it would take to spend the amount that was given away on nursing-home care. (The exact

amount is determined by each state.) In other words, if someone gives away $60,000 and nursing home care costs $6,000 a month, he would have to pay for his own care for 10 months.

If your parent chooses to give away his assets, set up a trust, or transfer property so that he can go on Medicaid, he shouldn't be overly zealous about it; he doesn't want to be left penniless (and depending on his children to honor any deal that was made). He might also want to keep enough money so that he can apply to a nursing home as a self-paying resident for several months (which generally improves his odds of getting into a better facility).

WHEN THERE'S A SPOUSE

Under the Community Spouse Resource Allowance (CSRA), Medicaid will allow a spouse to keep the couple's house, car, belongings, and, in some states, more than $100,000 in assets.

Medicaid also allows the spouse to keep all of her own income and, if her own income is not enough to cover her bills, some amount of her spouse's income as well. If her income is dependent upon certain assets, sometimes these become exempt, too.

Let's say a husband earns $3,000 a month and a wife earns $500 month, and the husband enters a nursing home. The problem is, she needs $2,000 a month to pay her living expenses. In this case, Medicaid might allow her to keep $2,000 a month, leaving her husband with $1,500 a month (and thus eligible for Medicaid).

And finally, in some states, all assets can be moved into the "well" spouse's name and then that spouse simply refuses to contribute to nursing home bills. This can be done immediately before applying for Medicaid, with no "look-back" or exemption period. (However, the state might sue the spouse for reimbursement at some point.) And in some cases, a spouse might be able to pour all the excess assets into an irrevocable annuity.

So you see, it is complicated. Talk to a lawyer. People often make poor decisions and "spend down" more than necessary because they don't know the rules.

Long-Term Care

The missing piece in Medicare and most other health insurance plans is coverage for long-term care, and as we've noted, it's a very large piece indeed.

Medicare pays for short stints of nursing home care after a hospitalization that's at least three days long. The first 20 days are fully covered. The next 80 days require a co-pay (about $150).

Medicare also covers some skilled care (nurses and therapists) in the home when ordered by a doctor and when a person is largely homebound (he can get out, but only with great difficulty). Other than aides associated with this skilled care, it does not cover help with basic daily tasks, such as dressing or bathing.

Medicaid covers most long-term care costs, but someone has to use up virtually all of his assets to be eligible.

The average cost of nursing home care is almost $80,000 a year nationally. Care in an assisted living facility is about half that—less than $40,000 a year—and having aides and homemakers at home costs about $20 an hour.

So what's a family to do if a parent doesn't qualify for the Medicare benefit and is not nearing Medicaid eligibility? Learn about community programs like adult day care. Consider having your parent move in with you. And, use your imagination. If your parent has a spare bedroom and her needs aren't terribly demanding, get someone to help her out in exchange for free rent. Or hire an unemployed family member to care for Dad for a fraction of what a home care agency would charge. Or get a group of seniors together and share the labor costs.

There are other ways to foot the bill, but none are ideal. People get reverse mortgages on their homes, but this doesn't make sense if Medicaid is on the horizon. Sometimes a family member lends Mom or Dad the money, which can work nicely if everyone in the family is on board.

Some life insurance policies allow for "advanced" or "accelerated" benefits, which are paid out early (but usually at a fraction of the original value of the policy). In a slightly different twist on that idea, a company or individual will

MEDICARE HOME HEALTH CARE

Medicare covers part-time or intermittent nurses, therapists, and aides when ordered by a physician for someone who is homebound or able to leave the house only with great difficulty.

"Part-time or intermittent" means that a person needs skilled care for a brief, predictable period (usually fewer than 21 days), or needs such care fewer than 7 days a week or fewer than 8 hours a day.

Your parent does not need to be on the path to improvement to receive such services; she can get coverage to maintain her current condition or to slow deterioration.

If coverage is denied, contact your parent's doctor (to be sure the order for care is clear) and the home care agency (which should work things out so your parent is covered). The agency should tell you how to request a Medicare determination.

For more help, contact the local health insurance counseling agency (shiptalk.org). The Center for Medicare Advocacy also has information at medicareadvocacy.org.

buy an individual's insurance policy for a fraction of its value (known as "viatical settlements").

Before considering any of these options, talk to a lawyer or accountant. As mentioned earlier, your parent might be able to protect some assets *and* receive Medicaid.

Long-Term Care Insurance

If your parent has long-term care insurance, now is the time to use it. If she doesn't have a policy, it's probably too late to buy one. These policies are not a viable option for most people after age 80 or if a person has already gotten a diagnosis of a debilitating illness.

If your parent might be eligible, long-term care insurance is certainly worth investigating. Or, if you are looking 50 or 60 square in the eye, consider it for yourself. For more information on buying long-term care insurance, see page 588.

If your parent has long-term care insurance and claims are being denied or you feel she is otherwise being treated unfairly, the first step is to complain directly to the company and call the broker who sold her the policy. You should also contact the state insurance department. You can find the insurance commissioner in her state through the National Association of Insurance Commissioners (naic.org or 816-783-8300). If you continue to wrestle with this, contact an attorney who specializes in insurance or elder law.

Chapter 18

Legal Issues

Where There's a Will . . . • Power of Attorney •
Advance Directives • Trusts • Reducing Estate Taxes •
Probate • A Question of Competence • Legal Help

W hether your parent has $1,000 or $10 million, legal issues arise. How do you gain access to your father's accounts if he is too ill to pay his bills? Who will make health care decisions for him when he can't? Can your mother avoid expensive probate proceedings or protect her savings from hefty estate taxes? How do you take over if your parent is showing signs of dementia but refuses to relinquish control?

Whatever the specifics, your parent should do a little estate planning. If that conjures up images of wide rolling lawns, pillared porches, and polo fields, don't be put off. In a legal context, an estate is simply a person's property and possessions, however grand or modest. Estate planning ensures that your parent's affairs will be taken care of, that he will be cared for properly, that his savings and other assets are protected, and, when he dies, that his belongings and assets are distributed according to his wishes.

As we've said, your parent should have an up-to-date will, directives regarding his health care, and a durable power of attorney. These documents don't cost much (if his estate is simple, you can get them for free), and they will help guard your family against costly legal proceedings and bitter arguments.

This chapter describes these essential documents along with other basic legal tools. Obviously, the information here is meant to serve only as a broad guideline; your family should work with a lawyer who is knowledgeable about the laws in your parent's state and experienced in issues concerning the elderly.

Where There's a Will . . .

Any adult with children or assets—a house, a savings account—should have a will. Drafting a will, along with other basic legal documents, will cost anywhere from a couple hundred dollars to several thousand. But it's money well spent.

Typically, a will explains how a person's finances, property, and other belongings are to be doled out after the person dies. Most wills include a general bequest, giving all assets to a spouse or dividing them among children. Some dictate that assets are to be put in a trust for children or grandchildren or some other person, either to reduce taxes or to hold money for a disabled relative or young child. A will might include specific instructions, assigning certain items to individuals (a ring, a medal, a painting). An executor is named who will pay taxes, bills, and other debts out of the estate, and be sure that money and other assets are

distributed in accordance with the will's instructions.

Legally, a will affects only that part of the estate that goes through probate. Anything that is jointly owned, in a trust, or passed directly to a beneficiary (such as life insurance proceeds) does not go through probate and so is not bound by the terms of a will.

If your parent is drafting a new will, he should discuss it with his lawyer alone (most lawyers will ask other family members to leave the room), and ideally, no one else (aside from a spouse) should see the will until it has been signed. Why? Because if there are any disputes later, someone could argue that anyone who sat in on these discussions influenced your parent's decisions (which he or she might well have done).

A properly drafted will ensures that your parent's belongings will be divided according to her wishes. It can prevent, or at least diminish, family squabbles,

GENERIC AND ONLINE LEGAL FORMS

Many of the forms that your parent needs—a will, power of attorney, advance directives, and even the papers to set up a trust—can be found at stationery or legal supply stores, public libraries, and on the Internet. You can also buy interactive software that allows your parent to answer questions and set parameters to create a document that meets her particular needs. But is this a safe bet?

In some cases, these forms are fine. Advance directives from the Internet, for example, are commonly used and widely accepted. Just be sure they are specific to your parent's state and include any special instructions she might have. (You can find state-specific forms at caringinfo.org.)

A computer-generated will may be sufficient as long as your parent's estate is small and simple and the document is specific to her state. Your parent should hire a lawyer to write a will if there's any reason to believe that it might be challenged, if your parent owns a business, or if the estate is worth more than a million dollars.

Likewise, you can use a generic power of attorney form, but as a precaution, get additional forms directly from any financial institutions your parent uses, as many have their own versions.

Although generic is better than nothing, it is often worth the money to have a lawyer draft these documents. If the language in a generic document is loose, or if a small detail, such as the date, is missing or wrong, the entire form may be declared invalid.

Also, because generic forms are not customized, they may not accomplish what your parent hopes they will. Lack of clarity can lead to family arguments and even lawsuits over the terms, language, and validity of the document.

reduce the time and cost of probate, and minimize taxes.

If your parent dies without a will, the court will decide how his property is to be distributed and appoint someone to oversee the final details of the estate. (And that person can charge a fee—in some states, up to 5 percent of the value of the estate.) When your parent dies, you will have a lot on your mind; a clearly drafted will can make this period easier for everyone.

If both your parents are alive, they should each have a will, as a joint will can complicate matters. If your parent already has a will, be sure it is up to date.

A will should be reviewed every couple of years and whenever there is a significant change in your parent's assets, his family (a death, a divorce), his living situation (he moves to another state), or his beneficiaries.

Of course, once a will is written, your parent's assets must be set up so that the instructions in his will can be carried out. A will is of little use if, say, his assets are held jointly or held in a trust and therefore do not fall under the jurisdiction of a will.

Be sure you know where your parent keeps the original will, codicils (amendments) to the will, and any letter of instruction that accompanies the will. (Copies of a will aren't valid; you need the original.) If he doesn't already have a safe spot for it, suggest that he keep it in his lawyer's office, in a strongbox, or with a state registry service. Check with a bank representative or lawyer before tucking it away in a safe deposit box, as some states order these sealed at the time of death and require a court order to open them. (He can also add a joint owner to the box.)

Letter of Instruction

Your parent's will explains in broad legal terms how his estate is to be passed on, but does anyone know what is to be done with his beloved cat? Or who should get the family's photo albums? Or which of his colleagues should receive the books, files, and computer in his office?

Beyond the scope of a will, there are often a number of practical matters that need attention. Get your parent to write a letter of instruction, which is an informal, nonbinding (and easily changed) document that explains any personal matters not mentioned in the will.

The more comprehensive it is, the better, especially if your family is prone to disagreements or your parent has failed to talk with family members about these issues in advance. A letter of instruction might include the following information:

- Names and addresses of lawyers, doctors, brokers, accountants, and other advisers

- Names and addresses of people to be notified after your parent's death

- The location of important financial and legal documents, such as a will, financial statements, insurance policies, birth certificates, deeds, and so on, as well as the location of any safe deposit box (and key)

- Inventory of assets and debts, including savings and investment accounts, life insurance policies, pensions, real estate holdings, military benefits, loans, and mortgages

- List, and possibly an appraisal, of valuable personal belongings

- Instructions on what to do with business files, equipment, and computer software

- Account PINs and passwords

- Any special funeral and/or burial instructions

- Explanations or instructions regarding investments, income tax returns, outstanding debts, credit card accounts, other properties, mortgages, renters, insurance policies, and death benefits

....

❝ My mother-in-law was worried about her children bickering over who got what, and she talked all the time about how she wanted this one to get this painting and that one to get her silverware. Finally, I couldn't take it, so I had her write down all her specific bequests on a sheet of paper and sign it, right across the whole thing, and then I tucked that in with her will. It wasn't terribly official looking, but it worked in her case. Everyone honored her wishes.❞

—Nelly O.

- Special instructions on how to operate or maintain a house or other property, and a list of regular maintenance workers

- Personal wishes, such as thoughts on how beneficiaries are to use their inheritances or how children should

divide belongings not mentioned in the will

- Special messages to an individual or last comments to the family (although personal thoughts to an individual might be better conveyed in a private letter)

Power of Attorney

More important than a will is a power of attorney. This doesn't give anyone the power of a lawyer, of course. It is a document by which one person (the "principal") authorizes another person (the "agent" or "attorney-in-fact") to take care of his business affairs—to write checks, transfer funds, sign contracts, and buy and sell properties, for example.

A power of attorney won't strip your parent of her own legal powers. She can still make decisions, vote, and control her own legal and financial affairs. It simply names a deputy who can handle some or all of these matters, if necessary—for example, if your parent is unable to handle them herself, or if she simply wants someone else to take on certain jobs for her, such as paying bills.

It is an essential document. It is easy to draft. It costs virtually nothing. And it can save your family from awful legal battles. If there is no power of attorney and your parent becomes unable to handle her own affairs—and most

people do become unable to handle their affairs at some point—then your family will have to petition the court to have someone named as her legal guardian. This is a lengthy and often humiliating process that, even if it's uncontested,

> " My mother-in-law's will was so poorly written and rewritten that we couldn't make any sense out of it. We asked her lawyer about certain sentences, and even he didn't seem exactly sure what it meant. I mean, that's scary— he wrote the darn thing. It seems that she wanted certain things to go to certain people, but anytime she was upset with one of us, she'd call him up and tell him to change it. In the end, there was one desk that was actually given to two of us. We don't even live in the same state. How could a lawyer let that happen? Looking back, I'm sure we should have sued him or reported him or something. It was a mess."
>
> —Peg G.

A LEGAL LEXICON

DECEDENT: a person who has died.

PERSONAL REPRESENTATIVE: the general name for anyone overseeing the estate of a decedent—paying taxes and bills, and then distributing property according to the terms of the will.

EXECUTOR: (also known as a "personal representative") a title used in many states for the person who is named in a will to manage an estate. (A female executor used to be called an executrix, but no one really uses that word anymore.)

ADMINISTRATOR: a person named by the court to manage the estate when no will exists, no executor is named in the will, or the executor named cannot serve.

FIDUCIARY: someone who is entrusted to act on behalf of another person. In the case of wills, the executor is acting as a fiduciary. In the case of trusts, the trustee is a fiduciary.

PROBATE: a legal process that involves confirming a will's validity, creating an inventory and appraisal of the deceased person's property, paying any debts, and distributing the remaining assets and property.

GRANTOR: a person who establishes a trust.

BENEFICIARY: a person who is designated to receive money, property, or other assets from an estate, trust, or insurance policy.

TRUSTEE: a person who manages a trust for the beneficiaries.

AGENT OR ATTORNEY-IN-FACT: a person who has the legal power to act on behalf of another person.

PRINCIPAL: the person granting the power of attorney. An agent must act on behalf of a principal's best interests.

---

can take months and cost thousands of dollars.

As usual, don't wait. Once your parent is ill or confused, and cannot fully understand the legal ramifications of the document, she will no longer be permitted to sign one.

Your parent should execute a document known as a *durable* power of attorney, which will remain in effect when she needs it most—when she is incapacitated. A regular power of attorney is useful if your parent wants to give someone short-lived legal authority, such as paying her bills while she is

on vacation. But if she becomes incapacitated, this power will be revoked. A durable power of attorney remains valid until she dies.

Power of attorney documents should be written to suit the specific needs of your parent and the laws of her state. Typically, the form includes the name of the person granting the power; the name of the person who will serve as the agent; the name of a backup person to serve if the first person can't; a list of the duties and powers being granted; an explanation of when, for how long, and under what circumstances the power is valid;

and the signatures and seals required by the state.

If your parent has assets in more than one state, she needs a durable power of attorney for each state.

Your parent, the agent, and any backup person should all have copies of the documents. The original should be filed with a county recorder's office, with your parent's attorney, or in an office file to which you both have access.

To be sure that nothing goes wrong, she should also get a power of attorney form from individual financial institutions. Understandably, banks and brokerage firms are uncomfortable giving money and accounts to someone not named on an account. To ease any doubt, most will provide their own versions of these documents. Although a state form is perfectly legal and should be honored, it's best to have all the bases covered.

Defining the Power

Make sure your parent's wishes are very clear. Some states limit the powers of an agent unless specific provisions are written in, such as the authority to give monetary gifts, to deal with the IRS, and to transfer assets into or out of a trust.

Your parent can give his agent broad powers, including the authority to handle all financial, business, real estate, and legal matters, as well as all personal matters, such as housing decisions. Or he can turn over limited power, such as the authority only to sign checks from a single account. He can also decide when the power goes into effect (say, when he becomes incapacitated) by signing a springing power of attorney, which

"springs" into effect at a predetermined time in the future.

In general, a straightforward, durable power of attorney is best. First of all, who's to say when your parent is incapacitated? Perhaps the document says that a particular doctor has to make this decision, or maybe even two doctors, but what if her doctor is out of town, or the two doctors disagree? One might think your parent is completely incompetent, and the other feels that she is still able to make certain decisions for herself. Even if they agree, a bank might question this, wanting more proof of incapacity.

Also, if your parent turns over only limited powers to, say, one bank account, what happens if you need broader power? What if you need to deal with his taxes, or sign a contract, or gain access to another account? You'll end up in court doing just what everyone wanted to avoid.

If your parent trusts someone enough to give them this power, he should trust

> 66 I told my mother how important it was for her to sign a durable power of attorney, and she said no. That was it. No more discussion. She has always been controlling, but now that she is sick, she is clinging more desperately to that control. She can't handle the idea that anyone else would ever manage her money or anything else in her life. But I'm afraid that this will all end up on me, that I will pay the price of her decision, that I will have to deal with the mess when she can't take care of things herself. But she is adamant. She won't budge on this. It makes me crazy."
>
> —Diane P.

YOU, TOO

This is a good time to get your own affairs in order. Do you have a will, a durable power of attorney, a living will, and a health care proxy? Have you thought about ways of protecting your estate from taxes and the future costs of long-term care? Do it now. Everything here applies to you as well.

them to know when to use it and how to use it. A wide berth will cover all angles and ensure that you don't have to go to court.

If your parent doesn't trust anyone with such power, then so be it. But he should know that, if someone needs to handle his finances, a judge will name a guardian—and this could be a total stranger. The court is supposed to monitor all dealings, but courts are busy and abuse is not uncommon.

Choosing an Agent

Your parent should think very carefully about whom to designate as her agent, because this is a powerful tool. Having access to another person's money can be tempting even for the most trustworthy souls. In fact, a power of attorney is sometimes referred to as a "license to steal"—here's the checkbook and here's a pen. While most people are honest, it's best to have a few checks and balances in place.

Ideally, her agent should be someone whom she trusts completely, someone whom others in the family trust, and someone who has basic financial sensibilities. When there's uncertainty, it's better to pick the peacemaker in the family over the bossy financial expert.

Although parents are often tempted to name several or all of their children as agents, be careful. Will they be able to act separately, or will all financial dealings require both (or all) of their signatures? If they disagree, how will decisions be made? Having two agents might make sense if the financially savvy child lives far away (but can handle the taxes and more complex financial issues), and a second child, who lives near, can simply sign papers or pay bills.

It's not a bad idea to set things up so that other siblings (one other, or maybe all of them) receive copies of bank statements and other financial documents, just to be sure everything is on the up-and-up. In some states, you can appoint a "monitor," who gets copies of all financial documents. Sometimes a backup agent can request financial statements, or you can make arrangements with a financial institution to send statements to another person.

Your parent should be sure to name a second person as a backup, in case the first person named is away or otherwise unavailable.

An agent is required *by law* to act in the best interests of the principal (your parent). He or she has a legal obligation to deal with your parent's finances and affairs responsibly.

If you suspect trouble or feel that your parent's agent is not acting in her best interest, call the state department on aging (in the state where your parent lives); each state has its own rules and procedures. You can also call Adult Protective Services if you suspect any sort of abuse (financial exploitation is abuse). You can find the local office through the National Adult Protective Services Association (napsa-now.org). Another option is to call a lawyer and find out about gaining guardianship over your parent through the courts.

Advance Directives

A straight power of attorney covers pretty much everything, with one exception: decisions about health care. This is why your parent needs two other documents that are easy to get and absolutely vital.

When a person is too ill or confused to make medical decisions or to communicate his preferences, doctors usually confer directly with family members and rely on them to make decisions. Some states allow this by law; others permit it by practice. But all too often, family members disagree with each other or with the doctor, or they simply don't know what the patient would want in a given situation. These decisions become particularly vexing at the end of life.

To avoid court battles, family conflicts, and, most of all, a horrendous and painful death for your parent, several things need to happen. And they need to happen now, before your parent is too sick or confused to discuss her wishes.

Step One: Sign

It's easy to put this off or to assume that advance directives are not necessary. But these forms are not for the rare occurrence, the freak incident. The majority of deaths in hospitals occur after a decision is made to forgo life-sustaining treatment, and in most of those cases, it is not the patient but the family who makes the decision. Furthermore, family members routinely make many other treatment decisions that do not have to do with end-of-life care.

Advance directives must be signed while your parent is competent, so don't wait. They are easy to get. Easy to fill out. Easy to file. And they are free. So there are no excuses.

"Advance directives" refers to two documents: a living will and a health care proxy.

A LIVING WILL outlines your parent's wishes regarding life-sustaining medical care. Typically, it says that a person does not want aggressive medical treatment when the end is in sight and there is little chance for recovery. Usually the terms are broad, but your parent can list specific treatments that are either wanted or unwanted in various situations. For example, in some states, wishes to forgo artificial nutrition and hydration must be expressly written into the document. (It goes against all logical thought, but forcing fluids and nutrients into a dying person only makes the process more painful.)

A HEALTH CARE PROXY (or power of attorney for health care) allows a person to appoint someone else to make medical decisions on his behalf. Of the two, this is the more important document to have because the choices can be murky, and a knowledgeable person can weigh pros and cons. The form should include a list of specific instructions and the powers that are granted.

Of course, one needs to think carefully about whom to appoint. A spouse might seem like the logical choice, but if your father is frail and elderly himself, or if he wouldn't be able to think clearly at a time of grief, your mother might want to choose someone else. The key is to choose someone who will be able to talk to doctors, consider the options thoughtfully, and then make tough decisions.

You can get state-specific advance directives from a lawyer, the public library, or through Caring Connections (caringinfo.org or 800-658-8898). If your parent spends time in more than one state, he needs advance directives for each state.

He should keep the originals in a safe place—an office file or strongbox—that is easily accessible, and inform the rest of the family of its location. Copies should be given to family members, agents, doctors, lawyers, and others involved in your parent's care. He should also include contact information for his health care agent on a card, with other vital medical information, in his wallet.

Step Two: Talk

Please don't stop with a signature, because these documents alone will do very little to protect your parent. Advance directives should serve primarily as a springboard for ongoing discussions, so that when you have to step in, you have a good understanding of what she would want and how to handle the situation.

Oh, you say, you know what your parent wants. She doesn't want to be hooked up to machines or have her death dragged out. But what, exactly, does this mean? If your mother has severe Alzheimer's and needs constant care and supervision, and she gets a potentially fatal infection, one that would allow her to leave this world peacefully, would she want antibiotics? If she breaks a hip at 87 and needs surgery, but has only a modest chance of surviving the operation and getting out of the intensive care unit, would she opt for the procedure? If a simple transfusion might give her a few more months of life, albeit not terribly comfortable ones, would she go for it?

Simply saying that she doesn't want to be hooked up to a lot of machines is way too broad a statement applied to a vast number of possibilities, all of which are inconceivable to a relatively healthy person.

Unfortunately, expressions like *terminal illness* and *futile treatments* suggest that some clean dividing line separates normal illness from the deadly sort, or beneficial treatments from frivolous ones. When someone is elderly and has numerous ailments, most medical decisions, even seemingly mundane ones, are "end-of-life" decisions.

You will probably have to make some extremely tough calls. To do that, you need to know everything you can about her views and her wishes.

Obviously, this is not an easy topic to bring up. You can begin by asking your parent if she has advance directives, and then letting her know that the documents alone won't protect her; she needs to talk to her health care agent. Or, let her know that you have signed your directives and it got you thinking about how to avoid excessive medical treatments.

However you approach it, know that this is an ongoing conversation. The first time you bring it up is the hardest, but keep the conversation going, bringing it up as her health changes. *(Mom, remember how we talked about this before? Do you still feel that way?)*

What you talk about depends on your parent. Some issues you should discuss:

- In terms of illness and age, what does she most fear, dread, or worry about? (Being immobile? Being a burden? Being alone? Being in pain?)

- How can you ease these fears (learn about pain control, talk about comfort care)?

- What does she find comforting when she is sick, or what would she want if she were dying (physical touch, music, readings from a religious text, to be alone, to have company, or something else)?

- What are her beliefs about life and death, and how does that affect her feelings about dying?

- Talk about someone else's situation. How does your parent feel about the decisions that were made? How does she think things should have been handled?

- What are her thoughts on receiving life-sustaining medical treatment—ventilators, surgery, or even something as simple as antibiotics—when she is terminally ill or permanently incapacitated? Would she want to try a treatment to see if it got her through a crisis, or would she want to focus instead on comfort care and the gentlest exit possible?

- What disability, treatment, or situation would be unacceptable to her?

- Which is more important to your parent, to be free of pain or mentally alert? (You may have to make decisions about the quantity of pain medication she receives.)

- What are your parent's feelings about receiving artificial hydration and nutrition? (See page 535 for more on this.)

> My father had a bout in the hospital last year when things didn't look good for him, and after that I got much firmer. When he got out of the hospital, I said, 'Listen, Dad, there are several things that we have to face head-on, and one of them is a living will.'
>
> My brother had said that we had to be delicate, but I said, 'I don't think we're going to have to be careful. I think we're going to find him ready for this.'
>
> And he was. Ready, and even relieved to talk about it."
>
> —Eleanor R.

DNR AND POLST

Talk with your parent and his doctor about the possibility of getting a Do Not Resuscitate (DNR) order. Resuscitation—pumping on the chest or using electric shocks to jolt the heart, and putting a tube into the airway to provide oxygen—is a brutal procedure that can lead to a variety of painful consequences, such as broken ribs, perforated airways, and punctured organs, not to mention brain damage.

Sick, elderly people are unlikely to survive these efforts to restart the heart or lungs once these organs have stopped functioning, and the few who do survive rarely leave the hospital or survive more than a few months.

A DNR can protect your parent from all this. Or he can get Physician Orders for Life Sustaining Treatment (POLST), which are more detailed medical orders outlining exactly what procedures are to be used or avoided. In addition to resuscitation, they address tube feedings, antibiotics, transfusions, hydration, and other treatments, as well as instructions about whether or not a person should be hospitalized at all.

- Under what circumstances would she want to be put on a ventilator? Feeding tube?

- Does she want medical orders (a DNR or POLST) now to protect her from unwanted treatments?

- What are her feelings about hospice programs, which focus on keeping people comfortable instead of battling death—that is, on quality of life rather than quantity? (Would she like to talk with a hospice provider to learn more about it?)

- If you face a wrenching decision about odds and possibilities—for example, a painful treatment holds a 20 percent chance of giving her another three to six months of life—what would she want you to consider at such a moment?

- Has your parent expressed her philosophy and feelings about medical intervention and end-of-life care to her doctor? Does the doctor understand her wishes, and is he or she prepared to abide by them?

- Do other family members understand her wishes?

Step Three: Prepare

Step three is critical.

Your parent has signed the papers and you've had the talks, but are you truly ready? Do you understand what's involved? If your parent were in the emergency room struggling for air, could you refuse a respirator and ask for pain relief instead? When the doctor recommends surgery despite your mother's already very poor health, could you really say no?

We think we are prepared, but death pulls us up short. The decisions are too complicated, the emotions too acute, the loss too large. Our hearts want to believe that this isn't the end, not really, not yet, not now.

We trust the doctors to tell us the best course, but the medical system tends to flow, rapidly and aggressively, in one direction—toward more treatment. And so we go with it. We follow the tide, accepting one procedure after another, until our loved ones die in agonizing pain, distanced from the very people they need most.

It doesn't have to be this way. Death can be gentle. But you have to be prepared. Extremely prepared.

If your parent has a particular illness, speak with her doctors about her prognosis, what choices are likely to arise, and how you might handle them. Doctors are not great guides on this particular voyage, so you will have to push. *Why would we do that? What are the chances she'll survive? What does that survival look like? What happens if we refuse that treatment?*

When making decisions about treatments, don't hesitate to call a local hospice to get another opinion. Then think carefully about what your parent has told you. And think not only about what you won't do, but what you will do. How will you provide comfort and care at the end? How will you say good-bye?

For more on avoiding a protracted death and understanding the issues that often arise at the end of life, see Chapter 26. It may seem morbid and as though you are tempting fate, but learning about death doesn't make it happen. It only relieves fears and makes for a gentler passage. Learn about it now, talk, and prepare, *before* decisions must be made.

Trusts

A trust is merely a way of holding money, property, or other assets. Rather than having a bank account in your parent's name, for example, the account is held in the name of a trust (for example, the John Parker Trust). A trustee, which can be a person or institution, oversees the trust on behalf of another person (the beneficiary).

Trusts are not just for the rich. Yes, they are commonly used to protect large estates from taxes, but they have other important uses as well:

TO AVOID PROBATE. Probate, the legal proceedings in which a person's will is settled, can be time consuming, costly, and public. The contents of a trust, however, are not subject to the terms of a will, and therefore do not pass through probate. (They are still subject to taxes, though.)

Setting up a trust does not always save money, as establishing the trust costs money, of course, and lawyers are typically needed to manage an estate even when assets are in a trust. Also, to avoid probate completely, absolutely everything must be in the trust, which is difficult to do.

However, establishing a trust to avoid probate is useful in states that have onerous probate proceedings; when something about an estate would make probate particularly complicated; or when a person has property in several states, requiring multiple probate proceedings.

Avoiding probate is also useful when there may be disputes over an estate. All potential heirs must be notified of probate proceedings, and anyone can show up and dispute its terms. This battle can prolong hearings, which are paid for out of the estate. If, instead, there is a trust, potential heirs do not need to be notified, and if someone wants to make a fuss, they have to initiate any legal action.

Finally, people sometimes want to avoid probate for privacy reasons, as probate proceedings are public record.

TO AVOID GUARDIANSHIP PROCEEDINGS. A trust can be used somewhat like a power of attorney, giving someone access to property, financial accounts, and any other assets held in the trust.

A trust, in this instance, allows your parent to dictate, in advance, exactly how certain assets are to be managed, and to monitor the actions of a trustee. As your parent loses his ability to manage these matters, the trustee steps in and gradually takes over. Your parent can name a bank or law firm as a secondary trustee, to oversee the primary trustee.

In most cases, a power of attorney is the preferable tool. The advantage of a trust is that it's almost impossible to

dispute. The advantage of a power of attorney is that it can cover absolutely all assets.

Even when a trust exists, your parent should still assign power of attorney because some assets (such as cars or cash) might not be in the trust, and there may be issues and decisions that fall outside the realm of the trust.

TO HOLD MONEY UNTIL A CERTAIN TIME OR FOR A SPECIFIC USE. Trusts are often established to hold money until an heir reaches maturity, or to care for a family member who is disabled and needs someone else to oversee his finances. If, say, you have a brother who is disabled, your parent might put money into a trust that is to be used for his care and needs. Or, your parent may hold money in a trust for a grandchild, and then dictate that he can have the money when he reaches a certain age, graduates from college, or reaches some other benchmark. Or, a man might want his second wife to have access to a certain percent of the value of an account, but then have the remaining money go to his children.

TO PROTECT ASSETS. Because a trust is private and only the trustees need know about its assets and terms, people use them to protect money from creditors. They are also used to protect money so someone can get Medicaid coverage before they would normally qualify. This is extremely difficult, though, because the trust must be set up many years in advance and written so that your parent cannot have access to the principal.

TO REDUCE TAXES ON LARGE ESTATES. There are a number of ways trusts are used to shelter an estate and reduce federal and state estate taxes. These are described on page 374.

Three Basic Types

Trusts fall into two broad categories: *testamentary trusts*, which are set up after a person dies, under the terms of a will; and *living trusts*, which are established while a person is still alive. Living trusts are either "revocable," which means that the person who set it up maintains control over it and can change it at any point, or "irrevocable," which means that the person has no power to revoke or alter the trust in any way.

Your parent, the "grantor," appoints a "trustee" to manage the trust—often a family member and/or a professional. The "beneficiaries" are the folks who get money or assets from the trust.

A trustee has a legal responsibility (known as a "fiduciary duty") to manage the trust carefully and in the best interests of the beneficiaries. If the beneficiaries question the actions of the trustee, they can challenge him or her in court.

TESTAMENTARY TRUSTS. A testamentary trust is described in a will and created after the grantor's death. Such a trust is often set up to hold assets for a specific purpose, such as a child's education or the care of a disabled relative, or until a specific time, say, when an heir matures. They are also commonly used to reduce estate taxes.

REVOCABLE LIVING TRUSTS. A revocable living trust is set up during the grantor's lifetime and can be changed or canceled at any time. The grantor usually acts as the primary trustee, retaining full control of the assets. A secondary or successor trustee steps in when the primary trustee becomes incompetent, relinquishes control for some other reason, or dies. This person now manages and distributes the assets according to the terms of the trust.

Such trusts are used to avoid guardianship proceedings, to reduce the cost and time of probate, to protect a person's privacy (because probate is public), and to hold assets until heirs mature.

IRREVOCABLE LIVING TRUSTS. Setting up an irrevocable trust, which can be neither changed nor destroyed, is a serious step that requires a good deal of thought.

Irrevocable trusts are sometimes used to reduce estate taxes. As long as your parent is not a beneficiary of the trust and has no control over it, she is no longer considered the owner of the assets, and they are not considered part of the estate. The trust would still be subject to gift and capital gains taxes, but these may be less than estate taxes.

Irrevocable trusts are used to shelter life insurance policies so the proceeds are not included in the estate, or to keep assets that are expected to appreciate significantly out of an estate. A house can also be put into an irrevocable trust, allowing your parent to take his house out of his taxable estate.

Choosing a Trustee

A trustee, like an attorney-in-fact, should be a family member who is respected and trusted by the beneficiaries of the trust and is at least somewhat savvy or capable financially. Or the trustee might be a professional trust manager or financial adviser. A relative can be appointed in conjunction with a professional, which makes a good mix—the heart and soul of a family member combined with the business instincts and neutrality of an outsider. (For an irrevocable trust to be excluded from an estate, the professional trustee must be able to outvote a spouse who is named as a trustee.)

Reducing Estate Taxes

If your parent has considerable assets, he might want to consider more extensive legal wrangling to dodge hefty estate taxes.

The federal government taxes estates valued over a certain amount at a high rate, usually between 35 and 55 percent. States also add a tax, which can bring the total to well more than half of the estate. The amount that can be passed on before these taxes kick in changes from year to year, ranging anywhere from $1 million to more than $5 million.

> ❝ I was the executor of my mother-in-law's estate, and it was an eye-opener, seeing how much money is paid out in taxes unless you do something to protect yourself. It's shocking. More than half of her estate went to Uncle Sam. Having been through all that, my husband and I have made sure that our affairs are in order. We each have a will and a durable power of attorney, and we have started to give our money to our children each year. We learned the hard way, and we don't want them to have to go through what we did.❞
>
> —Nelly O.

Although it may seem that your parent's estate isn't anywhere near those numbers, the total value of all assets—a house, life insurance, a business, a retirement account, and savings—can be surprising. Furthermore, states typically have lower, or no, exemptions.

Below are a few of the most common ways in which people shrink larger estates to minimize taxes. But be careful. Don't let your parents be overly zealous about giving money away to reduce estate taxes. They shouldn't give away so much that they jeopardize their own financial security, and they shouldn't give away items that they still use and enjoy.

GIFTS. Your parent can give several thousand dollars to any number of individuals without paying gift taxes (the amount changes from year to year, but is generally around $13,000). He can make tax-free gifts in excess of this amount to an individual if the additional money is paid, on behalf of this other person, directly to an institution for medical care or education.

BYPASS, OR CREDIT SHELTER, TRUST. This type of trust, also referred to as a family or A-B trust, is one of the most common and effective ways of avoiding estate taxes when holdings are large. It actually doubles a family's tax exemption, potentially saving them hundreds of thousands of dollars.

Normally, when a person dies, all his assets go to his spouse, tax-free. Then, when the spouse dies, all the assets go to the children or other heirs. Anything over the amount of the current tax exemption will be heavily taxed. But it's possible for both parents to pass on the maximum amount tax-free, doubling the exemption.

There are two ways to do this. One is to give the money outright to the next generation, either during one's lifetime or through the terms of a will. But this should be done only when an estate is quite large and the surviving spouse will still have plenty of money left. The other way is to put money into a bypass trust.

When the first parent dies, his will says that a specified amount is to be put into a bypass trust for his children, but the money can be used by the surviving spouse during her lifetime. He has effectively given the money to his children (tax-free) but given his spouse access to it. As an added bonus, even if the money in the trust grows, it is still free from estate taxes (although not free from capital gains taxes).

IRREVOCABLE LIFE INSURANCE TRUST. Putting any life insurance policy into a trust is one of the most painless ways of shrinking an estate. Ordinarily, the benefits of a life insurance policy are included in the taxable estate of the owner. By putting a life insurance policy into an irrevocable trust, your parent removes

it from his taxable estate. This means that he can no longer borrow against it or change the beneficiaries. But it saves on taxes, the proceeds can be used by the next generation to pay any estate taxes, and it provides them with quick cash, which is useful when most of the value of an estate is in real estate or a business.

(*Note:* Once the trust is set up, the premiums will be considered a gift to beneficiaries. Also, if an existing policy is transferred into a trust and your parent dies within three years, the benefit will be included in his estate.)

QPRT TRUST. A Qualified Personal Residence Trust (referred to as a "Q-pert") allows a person to give his house to his children, thereby removing it from his taxable estate, but he can remain in it during his lifetime. This is particularly beneficial if the value of the house is expected to appreciate significantly. If that is the case, then by all means, get it out of the estate. This requires some serious advance planning, however.

The advantage is that the IRS values the house at far less than its true value because your parent will continue to live in it for a certain number of years, and you and your siblings won't take possession of it right away. So a house that is actually worth $500,000 might be valued at, say, $300,000.

The problem is that the trust must set some time frame, say 10 years, at which point the house is turned over to the children. If your parent dies before the 10 years are up, then the trust is void and the full market value of the house at the time of death is included in the value of the estate. If, on the other hand, your

A LIVING TRUST IS NOT A WILL

Some people call living trusts "substitute wills" because a trust dictates how assets will be distributed, just as a will does. However, it is virtually impossible to put all assets into a trust; some part of an estate is usually left out. Therefore, regardless of any trusts that are established, your parent should still have a will as well.

Likewise, although a living trust mimics a power of attorney, it should not replace a power of attorney. Your parent should still sign a durable power of attorney, giving someone the authority to manage assets that are not in the trust, sign contracts, and handle other legal and personal affairs.

parent outlives the trust period, then he must either move out of the house or pay fair market rent to his children. This is fine if you have friendly family relations. In fact, by paying rent, he further reduces his estate. However, if the kids are feeling nasty, Dad could, in theory, be pushed out of his home.

CHARITABLE REMAINDER TRUST. Of course, anyone can shrink an estate by giving money to charities, either during one's life or after death. This is particularly useful when an asset has appreciated significantly, because you don't pay tax on the gain, and you get a tax deduction on the gift. But then, of course, the money has been given away.

Another option is to put an asset into what's known as a charitable remainder trust, which removes the asset from the estate and creates a tax deduction while also providing income for your parent during his life.

Let's say your father bought a stock 10 years ago for $5,000. That stock is now worth $50,000. If he puts the stock into a charitable trust, the trust can sell the stock tax-free, and then, depending upon the terms of the trust, it would pay your parent some percentage of the value of the principal (say 6 percent of $50,000, or $3,000 a year). This way, he removes the stock from his estate, doesn't pay capital gains taxes, gets a deduction for the charitable gift, gets annual income, and feels good about giving to charity. The trust can be set up to give to one charity or any number of charities. However, this is useful only if your parent wants to give money to a charity; it's not the best money-saving tool.

Ownership

Ownership should be a simple matter; something belongs to one person or it belongs to another. But by law, an item can belong to one person, to another, or to two or more people in a variety of ways. The way in which a person owns a house, a stock, an account, or other assets affects how vulnerable the property is to creditors, how it is passed on, and, most important, how it is taxed.

SOLE OWNERSHIP is fairly straightforward, but even here there are gray areas. For example, if your parent puts her house in your name, but remains

> **"** My mother-in-law died almost a year ago, and I am still in contact with the lawyer almost weekly. I thought her financial situation was simple, but it turns out she made a number of gifts years ago and never paid any gift taxes. And she has property in a couple of states. It's a nightmare. I think she named me as her executor so she could torture me even after she was gone."
> —Susan V.

in the house as a tenant, some states, along with the IRS, might still consider the house part of her estate. Likewise, if an item is in your parent's house, it is usually considered hers. That is, in most states, your parent can't write notes on the back of valuable objects ("This painting belongs to Jane," "This silver belongs to Ann") and assume that the objects are no longer part of her estate.

JOINT TENANCY WITH RIGHT OF SURVIVORSHIP means that two people jointly own something, but when one dies, the property becomes owned solely by the second person. The advantage is, the property does not go through probate.

The concern in any joint ownership agreement is whether one owner trusts the other. When a bank account is owned jointly, all owners can draw on the account (even empty the account) without the approval of the others. Joint assets are also vulnerable to all owners' creditors.

Also, if a parent makes a child a joint tenant, half of the value of the assets will be considered a gift, for tax purposes.

TENANTS IN COMMON means that the parties own property jointly, but there is no right of survivorship. Each person owns a specific share that is passed on directly to his heirs. For example, your father might own a business equally with two partners. When he dies, his third would be passed on to his heirs, not to the other business owners.

Probate

Probate, the legal process of distributing assets to heirs, has a nasty reputation, much of which is deserved. It often involves enormous amounts of paperwork and thousands of dollars in legal fees. The process usually lasts at least 6 to 12 months, but it can go even longer.

Probate itself isn't that expensive. The court might charge a couple hundred dollars. The bills start coming in when the lawyers get involved, and lawyers are often necessary. A lawyer will fill out paperwork (which must be done precisely), notify family members, and get permission to pay bills or sell a house, for example, during this time. Appraisers and accountants might also be involved, adding their bills to the total.

The cost and time involved depends largely upon state law, but also upon the whims of the presiding judge, the complexity of the estate, the clarity of the will, the efficiency of the executor, and whether the will is contested. If property is owned in more than one state, each state will conduct its own probate proceeding, adding to the time and cost.

Having said all that, in some instances, probate, or "estate administration," as it is sometimes called, isn't so onerous, and, depending upon state rules and the size and complexity of the estate, it may be far easier and cheaper than anyone expects. Small estates, or those that contain only a small amount of probate property, may qualify for a streamlined version of probate, called "small estate administration" or "summary administration." In this case, the transfer of assets is handled through an affidavit, or court order, that takes no longer than a few months to complete.

Although experienced local attorneys can usually expedite probate proceedings, it is possible, in some states and some situations, to do it yourself. A probate clerk can guide you through the process.

A Question of Competence

Your mother has a diagnosis of Alzheimer's, and just this morning she confused the coffeemaker with the blender, but she wants to change her will. Is she competent to do so?

Your father hasn't received any kind of dementia diagnosis and seems lucid, but he has given some unusually generous gifts to his housekeeper. Should you intervene?

Your parent has to decide whether to have chemotherapy, but he's in pain and just nods in agreement anytime the doctor makes a suggestion. Is he really making an informed decision?

These are not easy questions because there is no clear dividing line between competence and incompetence, no simple test to determine your parent's ability to make decisions and handle her own affairs.

Even someone with Alzheimer's might be competent at certain times of day, say early in the morning, or someone who's heavily medicated might be competent when the painkillers wear off.

Likewise, someone who seems capable might not be fully functioning, especially when medications, grief, and loneliness are at play.

Questions of competency also depend on the matter at hand. Someone might be deemed competent to sign a standard will but not competent enough to turn over the deed to his house. Someone who cannot handle his bills

THE GRIEF OF GUARDIANSHIP

Your father, who represented strength and vitality, who guided you through much of your life, is now unable to make basic decisions for himself. It's painful to see a parent become confused and vulnerable, and even more painful to have to go to court to have him declared unfit. When it's over, you may feel uncomfortable in the position of chief decision maker.

- Be gentle with yourself. A lot is being asked of you right now. Take time off, if possible, to handle this new workload and to give yourself a chance to grieve.

- Move slowly, keeping your parent informed and in control as much as possible and for as long as possible. When you make big decisions, explain to him what is happening and why, even if you think he cannot understand you.

- Remember, this might be harder on you than on your parent. He may be relieved to let go of his duties and concerns, or he may be unaware of what is happening.

- If, on the other hand, your parent is angry with you for taking over, it's completely understandable. He is losing control of his life. Reassure him that you will do your best to honor his wishes. Keep in mind that his anger may be a symptom of any dementia. Remind yourself daily why you are doing this and what would happen if you didn't take on this responsibility.

might be perfectly able to decide where he wants to live.

Competency is defined as the ability to receive and understand information, evaluate choices, make a decision that is consistent with a set of personal values and goals, and communicate that decision to others. Certainly, just because your parent makes decisions that you consider foolish—he refuses a medical treatment or climbs on the roof to fix a gutter—does not mean that he is incompetent.

If you have concerns about your parent's competency and are not sure how to proceed or whether you should step in and act on his behalf, talk with your parent. If questions remain, ask his doctor, lawyer, or a geriatric care manager for guidance.

Also, see page 27 for a discussion of when to intervene aggressively and when to let your parent make his own decisions.

If your parent has assigned someone durable power of attorney and health care proxy, that person might be able to make, or oversee, some decisions.

However, if no one has been assigned durable power of attorney, or if your parent insists that he is perfectly capable of handling his own affairs, when he clearly isn't, then you might have to petition the court to have your parent declared incompetent. You or someone else will be named his legal guardian (sometimes known as a conservator).

People often seek guardianship to gain access to an ill parent's funds so

GUARDIANSHIP ABUSE

Obviously, stripping an elderly person of his rights and giving someone control over his life and assets is an extremely serious act and it sets the stage for exploitation.

Guardians are perfectly positioned to write generous checks to themselves or otherwise profit from the situation. In some cases, a family member is the perpetrator. But in others, professional guardians sap an elderly person's funds and leave him in dire straits.

A stranger (usually a social worker or lawyer) can be handed full or partial control for all sorts of reasons: when there is no one in the elderly person's life who is capable or available, or when the situation is considered an emergency.

Unfortunately, most of these stories will never be known because the victims have no voice. Once it is determined that they

need supervision and the court appoints a guardian, they lose most or all of their rights, including the right to hire a lawyer or otherwise seek redress.

If your parent needs a guardian, think very carefully about who will have that power. Do not hand it over to anyone without establishing oversight and safeguards—limits around what can be spent, ways to monitor bank accounts, guidelines for when others can step in—anything to make abuse more difficult.

Be on the lookout for signs of trouble: someone is overeager to become a guardian; a guardian isolates your parent (blocking visits and phone calls); a guardian refuses to talk with family members; financial accounts are changed; items go missing; or your parent seems lethargic or dazed (possibly overmedicated). See page 333 for more on abuse.

they can pay his bills, to have a severely confused parent admitted to a nursing home, or to handle a business or sell a house.

People also seek guardianship when they feel a parent is succumbing to "undue influence"—that is, someone is taking advantage of your parent and exploiting him in some way. (See page 326 for more on fraud.)

Mediation

Before heading to the courthouse, consider mediation. Quite often, a neutral third party—usually professional mediators, family therapists, geriatric care

managers, or elder law attorneys—can settle the matter privately, with less expense, pain, and disruption than a court.

Mediation is useful when you question a parent's competency, but also when siblings disagree or when there's any other dispute. Perhaps you feel that your dad should move and he strongly disagrees, or maybe two siblings feel a third is misappropriating Dad's money, or siblings can't agree on medical decisions.

Rather than hiring lawyers and arguing it out in court, the dispute can be heard and discussed in mediation. Views are heard, new options offered, and compromises made. Of course, down the road, guardianship might still be necessary, but this is often an effective first step.

To find a mediator, contact the National Association of Professional Geriatric Care Managers (caremanager .org), the Area Agency on Aging (elder care.gov), or the Association for Conflict Resolution (acrnet.org).

Gaining Guardianship

Going to court to become a surrogate decision maker is, obviously, a grave step and therefore a last resort. If your parent is declared incompetent by the court, he will lose some or all of his legal rights— the right to make decisions about his medical care or living arrangements, to handle his own finances, to buy or sell property, to vote, to marry or divorce, and to drive.

It is a time-consuming and expensive process that can be draining for everyone involved, especially if your parent puts up a fight. But sometimes going to court is unavoidable and truly in your parent's best interest.

States have different rules about guardianship, most of them, understandably, stringent. In most cases, you must retain a lawyer to petition the court. A hearing date is set, and an attorney is assigned to represent your parent, who is now referred to as "the proposed ward." A judge, or in some cases a panel or jury, interviews family members, doctors, and others involved in your parent's life to determine if he is truly unfit to handle his own affairs and to what extent.

Anyone interested in your parent's well-being can seek guardianship—

> *"After my mother died, my father's dementia got much worse. He started doing bizarre things, and a couple of times he became violent. Eventually, I had to establish a guardianship for him, and I can tell you, doing it was horrendous. My father has always been very proud and independent. He would never accept help from anyone. He fought the guardianship, and the court proceedings dragged on for almost five months. During all of that time he argued with me, screamed at me, and once he even threatened to kill me.*
>
> *All the way through it I kept telling myself, over and over, 'This is for him. This is my gift to him. I am doing this for him.' Some days I believed it, some days I didn't. Some days it felt as though I was punishing him. He certainly saw it that way. But I know now that it was the right thing to do."*
>
> *—Rona S.*

relatives, caregivers, neighbors, and friends. A guardian can also be a professional (usually a social worker, geriatric care manager, or attorney who is registered by the state) or even an agency or corporation. A court might also name two people to share the duty.

Guardians can be granted total or limited authority. For example, you may be given the authority to handle your parent's personal affairs, and a bank trustee will be assigned to oversee his finances.

In most states, a guardian must report to the court at specific intervals or whenever a major decision is made, to show that he or she is acting responsibly.

Legal Help

M ost people get referrals to lawyers from family, friends, and respected professionals. You can also get information and referrals from the following:

- **The State Bar Association** or the state agency that licenses them, often called the legal, or bar, examining agency

- **The American Bar Association** (findlegalhelp.org)

- **The National Academy of Elder Law Attorneys** (naela.org) gives referrals from its list of members, as does the **National Elder Law Foundation** (nelf.org). Elder law attorneys specialize in the needs of elderly—long-term care, Medicaid planning, nursing home rights, Medicare, guardianship, elder abuse, Social Security, and estate planning.

The process of hiring a lawyer and some questions to ask are described on page 323.

Free and Low-Cost Legal Help

Local offices on aging sometimes offer free legal help to people over 60. Although these services are available to all seniors, most states gear programs to people who are living on lower incomes, and give legal advice primarily about public benefits. To find these services go to eldercare.gov or call 800-677-1116.

Legal aid societies throughout the country also offer free or low-cost help to low-income seniors. These are sometimes referred to as LSC services, because federal funds are funneled into the programs through an organization called Legal Services Corporation. To find a legal aid society and other legal help, visit lawhelp.org.

ON THE WEB

The Internet is loaded with all sorts of free legal advice. Be careful. Use only sites set up by well-respected organizations and check several sites, rather than relying on one. Not only is there a lot of inaccurate information, but every state has its own laws. What's good advice in one state can get you in trouble in another.

The Internet also offers scads of ways to find a lawyer. Heaven help the person who searches "find a lawyer." These are largely moneymaking sites that charge a fee directly, get a fee from the lawyer, or make money by selling downloadable forms. Or they ask clients to explain their situation, and then lawyers bid for the job. Steer clear.

Home Away
from Home

Chapter 19

Moving Out, Moving In

Launching the Discussion • Is It Time to Move? •
Should Mom Move Closer? • Should Dad Move In? •
Under One Roof • Separate Quarters

Home certainly is where the heart is, and it is probably where your parent wants to stay, but at some point it may not be feasible for him to remain in his own home. He might not be able to care for his house on his own anymore. He may be isolated and lonely. His needs may be too extensive. Finances might necessitate a move.

Whatever the reasons, when your parent can no longer stay in his own home, it's a major turning point for everyone. For your parent, it means leaving a familiar place and giving up some independence and privacy. It might also represent a final move, a last stop.

For you, it's a time of doubt, worry, and, once again, that old familiar friend, guilt. *Does he have to move? Is this the best place? Will he be all right? Are we doing the right thing?* You may find yourself sparring with siblings, and even with your parent if he sees you as the force behind a move he doesn't want to make. And if he's moving in with you, well, you have a whole other set of concerns and worries.

A move might come slowly after years of caregiving, renovations, home care, deliberations, and waiting lists. Or your parent, who was independent a nanosecond ago, is now lying in a hospital bed while you frantically fix up the den in your house or tour nursing homes.

However this move happens, once the dust settles and everyone adjusts, a new living arrangement can provide social and mental stimulation as well as the physical care your parent needs.

This chapter focuses on the decision to make a move, and some guidelines for living together under one roof. The following chapters look at other housing options and the move into a nursing home.

As always, don't put this decision off because such a seismic shift takes time. Typically, people need to move long before families address the issue, and by the time they take action, fewer options exist. Talk with your parent. Contemplate his needs and preferences, think about what his future might hold, and learn what's out there. Planning ahead and becoming familiar with the options will help both of you navigate this difficult terrain.

Launching the Discussion

Quite often, there is an assumption that when a parent needs care, he will move in with you or one of your siblings. No discussion, just an assumption. It might be your assumption. It might be his assumption. The problem is, it might not be a shared assumption.

You might assume that when your father needs care, he will move in with you, but the fact is, he has no intention of ever moving in with any of his children. Or your parent might assume that

she's moving in with you one day. The problem is that she's demanding and self-centered and you can barely share a meal, much less a roof.

Don't make assumptions, and don't make promises. Don't tell your parent that she can move in with you when the time comes, or that you'll never put her in a nursing home, because you simply don't know what the future holds.

Instead, talk—openly and often. As was discussed in Chapter 1, start by

" My parents were having difficulty keeping up with the house and yard, but they were reluctant to get help. My dad had heart problems for years, but he would climb on the roof and sweep stuff off. He was used to doing everything himself in the yard.

We said, 'You have a choice. You can stay in your house and get the support you need and pay for it, or go into a facility of some sort, or you are welcome to live with us.'

I was fine with it, until right when they were going to come, and then I was like, 'What am I getting myself into?'

I went for a walk in the woods, a walk I've done many, many times, and I got lost. I was so stressed about my parents coming to live with me."

—Margaret O.

listening. *Mom, are you happy living in this house? What are some of the problems? Do you think you will be able to stay here indefinitely? If you had to move, what would matter most to you?*

Ask her about her needs, both current and future. Find out what is most important to her as far as housing goes—staying in her own home, privacy, companionship, activities, a garden, proximity to family? Talk about what her finances will allow. Discuss the options—what modifications might be made to her home, local services, and what other housing options exist. Talk about the future, and what would happen if she needed more supervision or more complex medical care.

As you talk, keep in mind that your parents' home, no matter how grand, modest, or messy, means the world to

them. Your parents worked hard to buy this house and pay the mortgage. They spent many hours fixing that old stoop, painting that room, and weeding that garden. It is where they built their life together, raised a family, and welcomed their friends. It is the container of their life and their memories.

More than perhaps anything else, this house represents your parents' independence and privacy. Leaving it, especially to go to a place that is earmarked for the elderly, may be devastating.

Even if this old home doesn't look like much to you, even if it's loaded with risks and problems, understand what it means to them and what this move represents. If your parent skirts the subject, delays a decision, and, in general, clutches defiantly at the status quo—frustrating you to no end—just know that what you perceive as stubbornness or foolishness may be a perfectly normal desire to stay in her own home, and a deep-rooted fear of what lies ahead.

So be gentle and compassionate, even if you must be urgent.

" My mother wasn't happy living at home, and there were issues with her caregivers getting along, as well as trust issues. It was difficult dealing from afar. In fact, it was impossible.

So Dan and I talked about taking her in. My mother had a nice personality. She wasn't a difficult person.

We knew we couldn't afford a big enough place in the city, so we had to move to the country. That was hard for us. Really hard. But you make it happen. You just make it work."

—Anne L.

Is It Time to Move?

Before you pack your mom's bags, be sure that she can't stay in her own home, if that's what she'd really like to do. Think about ways to renovate and rearrange her home to make it safer and more accessible (such as wider entryways, first-floor bedrooms, wheelchair accessible bathrooms). Look into community services and home care. And study some of the financial options that might free up some cash, reduce her costs, or provide public benefits. (All of these issues are discussed in other chapters.)

Newer "aging in place" technologies (such as medication dispensers, fall detectors, and sound amplifiers) also make living at home more feasible.

If time is on your side, your parent should weigh the reasons for moving and for staying, visit a few residences, and then let the idea sit for a spell before making a decision. Although her personal wishes are the top priority, there are other issues to consider:

HER SAFETY. Your parent may need more medical care and supervision than visiting nurses and aides can reasonably provide at home. Or, she might need full-time help but not have space for a live-in helper. Her house might not be an option if there are, say, narrow flights of stairs or hallways that can't accommodate her wheelchair.

YOU AND YOUR SIBLINGS. Of course, you and your siblings are a big part of this equation—how near you are, how much help you can offer. Should a parent

move closer? Should a parent move in? Should she move into a group home or assisted living facility near you? Be realistic about what is best for her, and what is doable for your family.

Perhaps you and your siblings have cared for your parent for some time, but it's become too much. You might not have the ability, time, or stamina to tend to his needs, especially if he has dementia or incontinence, or if he is immobile. Even when private home care is involved, someone has to juggle schedules, oversee services, and fill in when workers cancel. This is your parent, and you need to be sure he is well cared for. But you also have to consider your own limits.

COSTS. Property taxes, a mortgage, home maintenance, and hiring aides and nurses might be too much for your parent's purse. If finances are the only problem, ask someone at the area agency on aging about programs that help older homeowners stay in their homes, save on property taxes and utility bills, and get affordable help.

Assisted living or nursing home care may very well cost more than staying at home. It all depends upon your parent's needs, how much family help is available, and whether your parent is eligible for Medicaid and other assistance.

LOCATION. If your father lives halfway across the country from his children and other relatives, a move might be imperative. Or if your mother lives in the country and cannot drive because

WHOSE DECISION IS THIS?

It's time for a move, no doubt about it, but your father insists, absolutely insists, on staying put. Who has the final say?

If he lives with you, in your home, then you decide if he can stay or it's time for a change. If he has dementia and cannot make a reasoned decision, then you have to consider his best interests and decide. But if he lives on his own and is essentially competent, then the choice is his.

Alert him to the risks, discuss the costs, be clear about what you can and can't do to help, examine the options, consider the future, and get others to talk with him about it. But at some point, if he insists that he is never leaving, despite the steep stairs and the icy stoop, despite his trouble operating the microwave, despite the loneliness, then you have to take a deep breath and accept it.

But, you say, he's going to hurt himself. He's going to starve. You can't stand by and watch that happen.

Of course you can't. It's an unbearable situation for a child. But you don't have much of a choice. You can prod and cajole, but at the end of the day, he's an adult who has the right to make his own decisions, however foolish those decisions might seem to you. And if he dies a bit sooner because of it, well, you gave him a great gift—the freedom to choose and the right to stay in his own house, where he wanted to be.

Do what you can to make the situation safe and get him the help he needs, but then take a step back—take a long, deep breath—and try to let go. Impose a little sanity on your own life. This was his choice. Someday, perhaps your kids will honor yours.

---

of poor eyesight, she might need to move closer to public transportation. If winters in Maine are too hard on your father's ailing heart, he may want to head south or find a housing situation that doesn't require scraping windshields or shoveling snow.

LONELINESS. Your parent may love his home, but it might be a little hollow and quiet these days.

Companions and community visitors might fill the void for a time. Your parent could also have someone move in with him, or he might move into an apartment or a group living situation. If he shuns communal living, he might simply move into town so he is closer to people, activities, and shops.

THE OPTIONS. If there are terrific senior housing options nearby, that will certainly affect this decision. Find out what exists. Talk to residents and families. It's hard to know what's what until you see it firsthand.

Likewise, what are the stay-at-home options? If there are great community programs, adult day care, transportation, and home care, then home might be a more viable option.

HIS FUTURE. A diagnosis of Parkinson's, Alzheimer's, or another debilitating disease means it's time to prepare for a future when your parent will need a lot of help.

Generally, it's better to move sooner rather than later, while your parent is well enough to take part in activities and get to know people. With dementia in particular, it's often better to move while your parent can be part of the decision and adjust to the change.

If your parent will soon be eligible for Medicaid and a nursing home is on his horizon, it may be better for him to move while he still has some funds and can pay his own way for six to nine months. He'll have more choices if he can self-pay for a time, and once he's in, he should be able to stay (the rules and situations vary, but typically, getting in is the hardest part).

> " When Dad moved in, he was okay physically. But I know he'll get worse. What did I get myself into? At what point will he need more care?
>
> My brothers are supportive, but my sister doesn't want me spending his money, even on him. That's all she really cares about. She doesn't want me hiring help.
>
> It hurts. They don't understand the burden of the day-in-and-day-out care, of not getting any personal time or time off."
>
> —Pat N.

Should Mom Move Closer?

In most instances, the answer is yes. When your mother needs to move, it's ideal if you can find a place that is near you or other family members. That way, you can keep an eye on things, and she gets to see some of her family.

But there are exceptions. For example, if your parent has been living in the same community for decades, what will she lose by moving away? Are you uprooting her from dear friends, a longtime doctor, a beloved congregation, paths she knows, and people she trusts?

If your parent lives in an area with plenty of good housing choices and senior services, that might be preferable to living near you if you live in a rural area with little in the way of options for seniors.

Before suggesting she move near you, be sure it is really the best thing for her, that there are decent options in your town, and—very important—that you will be available to visit and help. There's no reason for her to move if you won't see her often. Finally, you might not want to move her nearby if you have any thought of moving yourself (thereby leaving her, again, on her own, or forcing her to make yet another move).

Should Dad Move In?

This is a biggie. When a parent can't live alone any longer, you might have an instinctive response to take him in. He's your parent, for Pete's sake.

It's a generous thought, certainly, and if it can work, then it's wonderful. Your parent gets terrific care. You get time with your parent. Your children have a relationship with a grandparent and learn the importance of caring for a family member. But it's not always the best option, and sometimes it's an enormous mistake.

Having your parent move in with you is a serious commitment, so think it over carefully before extending the invitation. It entails a lot of work—more than you probably realize—and can strain your marriage, career, budget, family, and sanity.

When in doubt, test the waters for a time. Ask your parent to visit for several weeks or move in for a couple of months, being clear about the trial nature of the arrangement, and then see how it goes.

If you've had a successful trial run, and your parent wants to do it, go for it. Living together works for many families, and it can be a wonderful arrangement.

Some things to consider as you ponder the possibility of long-term togetherness:

CAN YOU GET ALONG? It's not worth trying this if your blood pressure rises at the mere thought of it. Think about your relationship with your parent. What was your most recent visit like? Did you enjoy a pleasant afternoon together, or did you watch the clock until you could leave? Is your parent capable of respecting your privacy, your lifestyle, and your authority in your home? While you might develop a closer relationship, it's also quite possible that old problems and annoyances will be more pronounced when you are under one roof.

WHAT ABOUT THE REST OF THE FAMILY? How do your spouse and/or children (or other housemates) feel about having your mother move in? Do others in the house get along with her? Listen to each family member's views. Everyone should be heard (although children should not call the shots).

....

❝ My mother moved in with us at age 95. I bought a reclining chair for our guest room and a television set and flowers, and I bought her a beautiful nightgown and robe so that she looked lovely all the time. She started to accept herself again, and her spirits came back.

It was very draining, though, because I was getting up during the night to change my mother's colostomy bag. And from the very beginning my husband and I missed our privacy.

I brainstormed with my sisters, and we decided to split up the care. Now Mother goes to one sister's in May and June and to another sister's in July and August. The moving around is a little tough on her, but otherwise it works pretty well."

—Margaret F.

....

FINANCIAL COMPENSATION

Mom is moving in, and among the many issues that have arisen is that ever so touchy subject: money. Maybe she is footing the bill to turn the den into a bedroom. But should she also contribute something monthly to the family budget? And if so, how much?

Should she chip in some percentage of the grocery and utility bills? Should she pay a chunk of the mortgage each month? Should she pay the going rate for an apartment locally? Should her contribution be generous enough to compensate you for the time you are putting into her care?

You are not doing this to make money, but you are giving (and giving up) a lot here. A contribution to the household would certainly ease the strain on your family and alleviate any resentment. It might also appease any guilt your parent (and siblings) might have.

Sort this out in advance and get your siblings on board. Explain what it will cost if your parent moves into some sort of facility instead, and let them know how you will keep the finances transparent.

Be sure that they are supportive and won't, later in the game, pounce on you for the financial arrangements.

DO YOU HAVE THE SPACE? This seems like an obvious question, but it's one that many people fail to consider fully. Intergenerational living is far more successful in homes that have a separate apartment or a bedroom that's set off from the rest of the house. Tight quarters will exacerbate everyday problems and strip everyone of their privacy.

IS YOUR HOUSE EQUIPPED FOR THIS? Ample space won't do any good if the extra room is upstairs and your father can't climb stairs (although you can buy conveyors to get him up and down the stairs).

Take a good look at your house in light of your parent's needs and disabilities. Are the hallways, doorways, and at least one bathroom wide enough for his wheelchair? Can you make needed changes, such as installing handrails, ramps, or whatever else might be necessary?

HOW MUCH CARE DOES YOUR PARENT NEED? Consider his daily needs—meal preparation, transportation, help getting showered, dressed, and to the toilet. Can you meet his needs yourself? Are there community services? Can he afford home care? Will you be able to coordinate and oversee workers? Are you willing to have strangers in your house?

What about entertainment? Will he roost in the center of the living room every day with nothing to do, waiting for you to come home? Can he get out and see friends or go to adult day care or volunteer?

HOW MUCH CARE WILL HE NEED IN THE FUTURE? Perhaps you can give him what he needs now, but what about down the road? What sort of care might

A VERY PERSONAL DECISION

Having your parent move in with you is a major proposition. Everyone has to dig deep to find his or her own way on this one.

Sure, if your parent needed a few months of care, she should pack her suitcase and come on over. But years? Perhaps many years? In your home? What if your parent's care will rock your marriage or threaten your career? What if your mother was abusive or your father was a drunk? What if she's confused or incontinent? What if the whole thing is simply too much for you, for whatever reasons?

You have a duty to be sure that your parent is safe and sheltered. You should stay on top of things and visit. But beyond that, you have to decide what's right for you. No one else can make this call. And there is nothing wrong with deciding against having your parent live with you if it will wreak havoc. Start looking for a different solution.

---

he need in the future? Will you be able to provide that?

If not, it still might make sense to have him move in with you, at least for a while. You might make other provisions for help later. But this should all be part of the discussion, as moves are stressful.

WHAT ABOUT MONEY? If you have to renovate a basement or make a bathroom wheelchair accessible, what will that cost? If you have to cut back on work hours, what will that do to the family budget? If your parent needs more help—a companion or aide—what will that run?

As you weigh the pros and cons of sharing your roof, think long and hard about the cost. If your parent is financially solvent, he should, of course, pay for his own care and any needed renovations, and he should contribute to general household expenses. Ideally, he should also cover any lost income to you and your family or compensate you in some way for all the work you do. (See page 66 on caregiver compensation.)

If your parent can't pay for much, then any siblings should be asked to cover expenses (since you are already contributing your home and your time to this effort).

....

❝ My father has always been a big drinker, and sometimes he likes to smoke a cigar after dinner. That was fine in his own home. But Mary and I don't like it.

When we invited him to move here, I told him right away that the drinking and smoking would have to stop, or at least be cut back. I was amazed at how well he took it. I'm not sure I've ever stood up to him like that. I think it caught him off guard. But he listened and, so far, he's respected our wishes."

—Ben W.

....

If your parent is eligible for Medicaid, then Medicaid should cover the cost of renovations, home care, and other long-term care expenses. In fact, in some states, Medicaid will even pay you, the family caregiver, for the hours you put in. Contact the area agency on aging (eldercare.gov) for more information.

DO YOUR LIFESTYLES MELD? Do you sleep late, but your parent gets up with the sun? Does your teenager listen to loud music in the afternoon when your parent likes to nap? Will you have to make meat-and-potatoes meals even though everyone else in the family is a vegetarian? Is your parent a chain-smoker and your husband asthmatic? If your lifestyles clash, is there any way of living together in peace?

DO FRIENDS AND FAMILY LIVE NEARBY? Are there friends and family members in the area who might be able to help or even take your parent in occasionally so you can have a break? Are they willing to get involved? Extra hands will certainly make living together easier.

Or, will relatives whom you're not all that fond of be congregating at your house?

If none of your parent's friends or family lives in your community, will she be dependent upon you for all her daily needs? It's not a deal-breaker; just something to consider.

CAN YOUR COMMUNITY MEET HER NEEDS? Will your parent be moving from an urban area that has a plethora of senior services into a town that has little to offer? Are there volunteers, companions, adult day care services, home care agencies, and other senior programs?

> " The pros are that logistically, it is a lot easier to have my parents closer. When they were in Texas, things would come up and I'd have to go take care of them.
>
> The cons are, you enlarge your family. How do you maintain boundaries, and an identity as a nuclear family?
>
> And if I'm invited to dinner, do I bring my parents? How do you incorporate them into your life?
>
> It's also the constancy of it. The little things are hard. Since they moved in, we've had quinoa quite often. And every time I serve it, my mother says, 'What's this?'"
>
> —Carol P.

If your parent loves gardening, moving her into a 10th-floor apartment might not be a good idea. If she loves art, music, and city life, she might be miserable in your country home.

WHAT ARE THE PROS? This can be a perfect arrangement for your parent, because she does not have to be alone; she does not have to maintain a property; she does not have to be in an institution; she can be with her family; and she will have supervision, as well as a trustworthy person overseeing her care.

You also stand to gain by caring for your parent during these last years of her life. Although the task is exhausting and consuming, and will certainly take you away from other things (job, kids, friends, hobbies, vacations, sleep), there might be precious moments, intimacy, and laughter, and a certain sense of pride. It is a gift you will be glad you gave. Your children can also benefit from time spent with a grandparent and from learning about how families pull together.

There might also be tangible advantages to this arrangement, as well. Your parent might pay some rent and/or compensate you for the hours of care you provide, helping your family financially. If your parent is still in relatively good health, she may be able to help around the house, do some shopping, or stay with the children when you're out. Don't hesitate to have her chip in if she can.

WHAT ARE THE CONS? Certainly you'll have less privacy (maybe none). You'll have less time for your spouse and children and friends. You'll have less sleep and exercise and downtime. You'll have more worry and stress.

ARE SIBLINGS SUPPORTIVE? This will be a whole lot easier if other family members think it's a great idea and are willing to support you in any way they can. One sibling who thinks Mom should have gone elsewhere, or is angry about this arrangement for any reason, can make life miserable. It's not enough of a reason to forgo this plan, but it's certainly an issue to keep in mind. This is a big job, and it is nice to have siblings on your side, offering you support by phone, days of respite, help with daily tasks, and other assistance.

Should You Move in with Him?

Sometimes the tables are turned and an opportunity arises in which it makes sense for an adult child or grandchild to move in with an elderly parent. This can be a great option on many levels. You or

> " Twenty years ago my mother was alone, so we told her to sell her house and come live with us.
>
> She is pretty easy to live with, except that she complains a lot. As the kids got older, the complaining got worse. It caused a lot of conflict. 'You should do this with the kids. You shouldn't do that.' I said, 'I'm the mother here. You're not their mother.'
>
> But it didn't work. So we sold our house and bought one with an in-law apartment. I see her in the afternoon, drop off her meals, and drive her around, but we also have our own, separate lives. It's much better this way."
>
> —Lucille L.

another family member gets room and board in exchange for providing care, and your parent does not have to leave home.

Plus, if your parent is headed for Medicaid, some states allow a family caregiver to take ownership of a house if he or she has lived there for at least two years, and has provided care that kept the parent out of a nursing home for at least two years. (The transfer of property will have tax consequences, so talk with a lawyer and/or tax adviser.) The state will probably require documentation that the care was necessary and a log showing the level of care provided.

Review the issues raised earlier in the chapter regarding family living. If you're moving to share a home with Dad, you want to be sure it has a decent chance of working out. And you have to remember that as much as this is going to be your home, it will always be his, and he will always be the boss.

Under One Roof

When an elderly parent moves in with a grown child, whether by choice or by default, there can be warmth and humor, and wonderful memories for the future. But the stage is also set for friction. You are giving up space not just to any boarder, but a boarder who needs your help and supervision on a regular basis. More problematic, this is a boarder whose opinions matter to you, who may be able to paralyze you with a simple comment.

For your parent, he is becoming not only dependent, but dependent on his child, a person who has depended on him and looked up to him. In addition to the pain of leaving his own home, he might feel embarrassed by this living situation and his own inabilities. He might connect you to his loss of independence and blame you for it, however illogical that might be.

As a result of all this, his gratitude may be mixed with resentment. So rather than feeling thankful for all that you are doing, he might fight you and criticize you as he clings to any remaining bits of autonomy.

Understanding his irritability or anger, and even anticipating it (sort of like knowing that a teenager needs to rebel and putting up with it) might help you cope—some.

Discussing these issues and setting down clear house rules should also help. Even the closest of families should establish some rules and routines right away. Work out any guidelines with your parent, spouse, and children, if possible.

WHO'S IN CHARGE? Your parent used to rule the roost, but this is your house. Will your parent have equal say in everything or do you (and your spouse) ultimately decide what's what? Make your roles clear from the start.

Likewise, if you have children, set some boundaries if your parent might usurp your job or undermine your authority.

ESTABLISH RULES AND JOBS. If you are concerned about a specific issue—noise, meal times, smoking—discuss this early on. Determine when it should be quiet, where people can smoke, when meals will be served, what will happen when you have other dinner plans, and so on.

So that you don't end up as butler, cook, and bottom-washer, make a list of chores on day one, so everyone in the household contributes. Many of the jobs you used to do will have to be farmed out to others, because your job description is about to grow.

> " When she moved in, I said, 'This is not going to be like when you come visit. This isn't like Christmas and we're home all the time. This is going to be our everyday life.'
>
> She knows I'm not available all the time. I have a full-time job and a part-time job and my boys and lots of activities. She knows I'm not there to be her companion, but there's part of her that wants me to be."
>
> —Carol P.

All of this might sound formal or difficult, but it's actually much easier if everyone knows what is expected of him or her. There's no reason for you to take on the whole load, even if it is your mother (and especially if it is *not* your mother). Don't start this journey as a martyr.

PROTECT EVERYONE'S PRIVACY. Devise a way to give everyone in the household some privacy. Be sure your parent has a space where he can shut the door and be alone without being disturbed. Naturally, you will need a similar space. If you plan to go out to restaurants or away on vacations without your parent, make that clear from the start. Clarity will not only preserve some of your

> " Mom loves to sit in our family room in the late afternoon and read, but within minutes, she falls asleep. When the kids come home from school, I race out to let them know that Grandma is sleeping. Then we all tiptoe around whispering. They can't stay and chat or watch the news. I can't start dinner.
>
> I told Mom several times that she'd have a much better nap if she lay down in her room, and she said, 'Oh, but I like it here. I'm fine, really.'
>
> Finally, I said, 'Mom, I know you like it here, but it's hard on the rest of us.'
>
> She did go to her room to sleep the next day, but after that, she was back in the family room, conked out.
>
> Now I head her off the minute she sits down. I feel awful, shepherding her out when I know she wants to stay. But I have to think of the rest of the family."
>
> —Lorraine R.

privacy, but also allow your parent to enjoy your time together without worrying that he is intruding.

LET HIM CONTRIBUTE. Ideally, if your parent lives with you, he will pay some sort of rent or contribute to the monthly bills. If at all possible, give your parent chores to do, even if they are menial. He might make the morning coffee, set the table, or water the plants. If he can't get around, then give him some paperwork to do, or laundry to fold.

He'll be happier if he feels useful and knows what is expected of him, and you will feel less resentful if he helps out, even a little bit.

CHOOSE YOUR BATTLES. When things don't work out, consider what you can live with and what is truly unbearable. Everyone will have to make compromises. Decide which battles are worth fighting, and try to solve others. If your parent is yelling into the phone because he's deaf, get an amplifier for the phone. If your mother falls asleep with the television blaring each night, buy yourself some earplugs and program the TV to turn off at a certain time.

CREATE A FORUM FOR COMPLAINTS. Problems should be aired before frustrations reach a breaking point. Talk about this in advance. How will each of you approach conflicts and problems? Perhaps you can have a family dinner once a month in which the living situation is reviewed and disagreements are discussed (kindly).

REMEMBER YOUR LIMITS. So simple, and yet so difficult to do. Once your mother is situated in your house, resist the urge to do everything for her, to

SIBLINGS, WORKING TOGETHER

When a parent moves in with one child, it is time for the siblings to have a very frank talk.

First of all, siblings need to understand, in some way, what is involved. This is a life-altering move that will require a great deal from the sibling who is opening her home. She, and any spouse and children there might be, are giving up their privacy, family time, work time, and well, pretty much everything else. Yes, they might have wonderful times with a grandparent (or two), but the day-to-day grind can be overwhelming.

The rest of the siblings need to find ways to share the duties and to support the one who's housing Mom. Maybe another sibling can handle the finances and oversee medical issues. Or perhaps other siblings can contribute financially. Some people share duties by having a parent move back and forth regularly between houses. This may be hard on a parent, but if it's the only way to make this work, then so be it.

If they aren't sharing the daily work, then siblings should either take your parent for a chunk of time or come stay in your house with your parent, so that you can take breaks and vacations.

If you are not the one living with Mom, if you are the sibling on the sidelines, be very supportive. Know that even a parent who is kind and relatively independent can strain a household. Offer respite, be there for consoling phone calls, and send an occasional surprise gift of support. (A certificate for a massage? A gift card? A new sweater?)

Distant siblings also need to realize that what they see in a weekend visit is most likely not what happens day to day. Your parent might be excited about your visit, prepare everything so it will be just so, and be terribly attentive to a child whom she sees in two-day slots. She is not expecting a visiting child to do her laundry and make her meals and take care of her mail. Being there, on the ground, is very, *very* different from an occasional visit.

disrupt everything for her, to anticipate her every need. Recognize the limits to what you can do for your parent. Accept that problems will arise, and make room for your own needs.

GIVE IT TIME. The beginning may be turbulent, but in a few months you should all settle into a routine. Don't pack your parent's bags before you've allowed ample time for adjustment.

KNOW WHEN TO QUIT. If you've given the arrangement a good dose of time

and a reasonable chance, and your instincts are telling you it's not working, pay attention. Any number of issues can bring family togetherness to a painful, grinding halt. Confusion, wandering, incontinence, and immobility are among the top reasons. There may be no simple reason, no single moment, just a realization that the situation is not working. You can try to ignore it, and the arrangement may last a few more months, but eventually you will have to speak up and make a change.

If this situation is damaging your marriage and ruining your career, or making your heart race, see what can be done to solve the problem. Talk with a family counselor, if necessary.

Then, when you've done what you can, act. Don't wait until you are physically sick or abusive toward your parent. Start looking into alternatives. Talk with your parent about the move and begin preparing for it. The transition will take time, and it will be smoother for everyone if it is done before you're a total wreck.

> " As soon as I come in the house, I get hit with questions. Like, 'This lamp is broken. What should I do? This bill came.' I'm bombarded by stuff that needs to be done.
>
> I have a time when I do the bills, a time I do the groceries. If she has a bill that she has a question about, I say, 'We'll deal with it on Monday. Monday is our day to do your books.'
>
> I have to have boundaries. And I have to feel okay about that."
>
> —Sue W.

Separate Quarters

Often called in-law apartments, accessory dwelling units (ADUs), mother-daughter homes, accessory apartments, or granny apartments, these are separate apartments within or attached to a home, or built over a garage. An accessory apartment usually consists of a bedroom, bathroom, sitting area or small living room, and kitchenette, often with a separate entrance. It can be created by renovating a basement or garage, or by attaching a wing to a house.

Parents get to live near their children, but everyone also gets a little space and privacy.

Some communities allow these apartments to be occupied by people who are not related. This means that your parent could move into an accessory apartment attached to someone else's house, allowing her to stay in her community in a smaller and less expensive dwelling, where she has a close "neighbor" who might provide a little oversight and help.

Or, if your parent wants to stay in her own home but it's too big for her, or the expenses are too high, she might create an accessory apartment and then live in either the apartment or the house, and rent the other section to a tenant.

Some elderly owners make special arrangements, such as keeping the rent low in exchange for help with chores or other assistance. (Be sure your parent understands that taking in renters requires some work on her part and that there can be problems if, say, a renter fails to pay the rent.)

ECHO Housing

Elder Cottage Housing Opportunity (ECHO) homes are modular homes, separate from the main house, that are temporarily placed on the property of a single-family house, usually in the backyard.

These units, sometimes called "granny pods," are about the size of a large garage, and include a bedroom, bathroom, living area, kitchen, and eating area. Most are designed specifically for older people; they are single level, wheelchair accessible, equipped with ramps and grab bars, and well lighted. They should also have details such as lever faucets, raised electrical outlets, a kitchen countertop that allows for a wheelchair, antiscald controls on the faucets, and the like.

More expensive units come with high-tech monitoring devices and safety features—for example, small lights leading to the bathroom that go on as soon as you climb out of bed; a rubber floor that reduces injuries from falls; a lift that can be attached to tracks on the ceiling; a video system that alerts the family if there's trouble; and a medical home monitor that tracks oxygen, glucose, blood pressure, and heart rate, as well as distributing medications.

An ECHO home does not have to look like Mom drove up in a mobile home, although some do. Most can be designed to match an existing house, with the same windows, siding, roofing, and roof pitch, or they can be adapted to look like a guesthouse on the property.

A typical ECHO home is usually between 500 and 700 square feet, although a two-bedroom cottage will be bigger. They cost anywhere from $30,000 to $90,000 (and up, if you use a local builder and can't find a prefab unit). Some can be rented, which is great if you don't think you'll need it for more than a year or two. Most can be returned, for some money back, when they are no longer needed.

Check with the local zoning board to see if ECHO homes are allowed in the neighborhood. Sometimes, even if accessory apartments are not allowed, you can get a short-term variance for an ECHO unit, with the provision that it will be removed when it is no longer needed and that the property will be restored to a single-family residence.

Find out whether local regulations require a minimum of yard space, include requirements for access and parking, and allow utility hookups. Ask how such a structure will affect property taxes. Also, find out how difficult it will be to remove the unit when it is no longer needed.

Unfortunately, these units aren't easy to find. When searching the web, try "Elder Cottage" or "ECHO modular units" or "accessory dwelling unit" followed by the state name. The area agency on aging or housing department might be able to give you information about local manufacturers of ECHO homes. Anyone selling modular homes might also have some ideas about how you can find smaller units, or a contractor can build one to your specifications.

Before You Build

CALL THE LOCAL ZONING BOARD or buildings department. Accessory apartments are not allowed in some communities zoned for single-family residences, and if they are permitted, certain restrictions and regulations may apply. If you are told that accessory apartments are not allowed, ask about getting a variance or a special-use permit.

CALL THE LOCAL HOUSING AUTHORITY AND AREA AGENCY ON AGING. Some communities offer low-interest construction loans, tax deductions, and other financial assistance to help people build accessory apartments for the elderly.

CONSIDER THE FINANCES. Get an estimate on what it will cost to create a separate apartment. Adding a few small kitchen appliances to an existing studio or guest suite won't be that expensive, but building a bathroom, kitchenette, and separate entrance onto a second floor might be prohibitive.

Be aware that property taxes might be higher because of the addition. If your parent takes in renters, the rent will change his income level, which could affect his eligibility for Medicaid or Supplementary Security Income.

THINK ABOUT THE FUTURE. Before you shell out $25,000 for a renovation, be sure this is an asset that you can use in the future, or something that can be changed back. If your parent lives there for only a year or a few months, will that be a serious problem? Does zoning allow it to be rented to nonfamily members? The future is uncertain, so be sure this is something you can do, regardless of how long it is used.

TALK WITH A REAL ESTATE AGENT if you want to know the value of adding an accessory apartment or need someone to find renters and draw up lease agreements. (You can find generic lease agreements in most stationery stores and on the web.)

" My mother has lived with me for six years now. I feel unappreciated. This is not an easy thing to do.

Deep down, I think that she understands that what we're doing is great for her. But day to day, she doesn't get it.

She gets tired of her friends saying, 'You're so lucky.' She doesn't feel so lucky, because she doesn't have her own house, because she's not independent.

When she's upset, she says, 'Well, I never wanted to be here in the first place.'"

—Maggie B.

Chapter 20

An Array of Housing Options

Roommates and Shared Housing • Congregate Housing • Retirement Communities • Senior Apartments • Foster Homes • Assisted Living • Continuing Care Retirement Communities

Fortunately, your home and a nursing home are not the only alternatives. An expanding array of possibilities exists, ranging from villages to shared housing to full-service life care centers.

Check out the options and start talking about this early, as planning a move (and persuading your parent to even consider one) takes time. Also, some facilities have waiting lists. Postponing will mean fewer options and a frantic scramble down the road when your parent is frailer and the situation more dire.

As you look, try to be open-minded. Remember, you are not looking for a glamorous setting; you are looking for a safe and supportive environment where your parent will get physical care, mental stimulation, and companionship.

Be sure any housing arrangement will meet the day-to-day needs of your parent—today and for some time to come. This move may be extraordinarily difficult; it's best not to have to do it twice.

The previous chapter dealt with the decision to move, and the ins and outs of sharing a house with your parent. This one considers other housing options; the next looks specifically at the hunt for a good nursing home (but much of that information, such as what to look for in a facility, should be helpful when looking at any senior housing).

Roommates and Shared Housing

Shared housing has become popular in recent years, and understandably so. It's a great option that allows people to stay at home, cut costs, have help and companionship, and maintain their autonomy—a precious asset.

By definition, shared housing is a situation in which two or more unrelated people live together, somewhat like a family. The specific arrangements, however, vary from house to house.

Your parent can find a person to move in with him who will pay rent or help out and do chores in lieu of rent (or some combination of the two). Or, he can move into someone else's house and pay the homeowner extra to provide some care and supervision.

Sometimes friends get together, find a house, and share tasks and expenses. They can hire a housekeeper and/or aide and get the care they need at a fraction of the price.

Your parent needs to think about what she wants out of this and whether it would work for her. Does she get along well with others? If she has friends in a similar situation, are these people with whom she could live in close quarters?

WANTED: HOUSEMATES

Some communities have services that link people with potential roommates or find group housing for them. Most provide this service free, although some charge a fee. To find out if such a program exists in your parent's community, and to get more information about shared housing, contact the National Shared Housing Resource Center (nationalsharedhousing.org).

For help finding a roommate, writing an ad, interviewing, and writing up a contract go to sharinghousing.com.

FINDING HOUSING

Be leery of websites and companies that offer advice about housing, even large, established sites. Yes, it's free, but most take a generous commission on referrals, and refer only to a handful of facilities with which they have contracts.

To find out about housing options in your parent's community, talk to friends and contact the area agency on aging (eldercare.gov) and the long-term care ombudsman (ltcombudsman.org). The Family Caregiver Alliance has a Family Care Navigator that is useful (caregiver .org). The Alzheimer's Association also has a website that provides leads (communityresourcefinder.org).

CARF International (once the Commission on Accreditation of Rehabilitation Facilities, thus the acronym) inspects and accredits a variety of facilities and services. Their website (carf.org) has a list of assisted living homes, CCRCs (Continuing Care Retirement Communities), and other facilities that are accredited.

Keep in mind, however, that accreditation is a helpful, but far from perfect, yardstick. Application is voluntary, and the CCRCs pay a fee to be evaluated. Those that are not accredited may still have high standards.

If she is finding a roommate through the want ads or a roommate-matching program, she needs to decide what she wants in a housemate—a regular companion (in other words, someone who is not away at work all day) or simply someone who is available some part of the day or at night in case she needs help? Does she need someone who can do household chores and/or someone who can provide personal care?

When your parent (or you) interviews potential roommates, ask about pets, smoking, noise levels, visitors, laundry, sleep habits, and arrangements for shared meals and chores, as well as personal and financial references.

Once a match is made, be clear about the details of the arrangement from the start. Prepare a list of the house rules and each person's rights and responsibilities. If a roommate has agreed to

" I really like the Homeshare program because it means that Mum can be in her own house. She doesn't want to live with any of us, and the alternative is a nursing home. The roommate pays $150 a week for room and board and gives us 10 hours of labor. She has a baby monitor in her room. If Mum has a rough night, I pay her something.

We had to get rid of the first one after we found out she was medicating Mum so she'd go to sleep earlier. But we love her new roommate. She's a pistol. She has so much personality, and the change in Mum is noticeable. She participating in conversations and laughing more. She is sleeping better, taking shorter naps, and staying up later at night.

It was a long slog to get this in place, but well worth the interviews and effort."

—Diana R.

GROUP LIVING? NOT FOR ME!

Small group living arrangements like home-sharing and congregate housing can be fantastic, but alas, they are not for everyone. They are economical and provide companionship, stimulation, and other support. However, if they require that people eat together and take part in community life, and if your parent has been a loner all his life, he's not likely to adapt well to this experience.

Is your parent ready to share a living space, or does he need a good deal of privacy? Can he get along with others and enjoy their company, or does he find most people a nuisance? Can he compromise, adjust his schedule and habits, and be sensitive to other people's needs?

If you doubt his capacity to be flexible, he should look for a situation that allows for a great deal of privacy. Even then, he might want to spend some time there before signing a long-term contract.

help around the house instead of paying rent, be specific about the chores and how often they need to be done. Put in writing how and when rent, utilities, groceries, repairs, and other bills will be paid.

Housemates should also agree in advance how bills and responsibilities will be handled if one person can't hold up his or her side of the bargain. If, say, your mother has a young person move in who will help in exchange for rent, what happens if that person is ill?

Likewise, if things don't work out and your parent wants this person out of her house, how much notice will she give?

Be aware that two or three people sharing a house usually goes unnoticed, but once four or more unrelated people are under one roof, local zoning officials may be alerted. Check the zoning codes, because the situation may be considered "group or multifamily housing," which might be prohibited.

Congregate Housing

Congregate housing is shared housing, but it is typically a more formal arrangement that includes more residents, and staff who provide meals and housekeeping, and in many cases, recreation, transportation, and personal care. (Some states refer to assisted living facilities as "congregate housing," so the terminology can be confusing.)

Residents have bedrooms within a large house or a multifamily home, or they have small apartments within a building, often supervised by a house manager. All or most meals are shared in a central dining room, and residents might share a common living area.

Many communities are leery of congregate housing because of the challenges it has posed to local zoning ordinances, but resistance is fading in many areas. Government, nonprofit, for-profit, religious, and community groups have all gotten into the act, building, organizing, and sponsoring such homes.

The local housing department, senior center, or area agency on aging should be able to give you information about congregate housing opportunities in your parent's neighborhood.

Retirement Communities

Retirement communities are also known as "independent living communities" for good reason; people need to be largely independent to live there.

While the number of variations on this theme is growing—and even the classifications listed here overlap (congregate housing and CCRCs (Continuing Care Retirement Communities) are

IT TAKES A VILLAGE. REALLY.

Most communities have a menu of services that help seniors stay in their own homes, but some have gone further and formed cooperatives of people helping people. Residents can opt in, pay a fee, and receive help from other members— help with errands, shopping, gardening, social visits, dog walking—whatever they need. For more information, contact the Village to Village Network (vtvnetwork.org or 617-299-9638).

In a similar vein, naturally occurring retirement communities, or NORCs, offer a plethora of services for the elderly, but these usually stem from institutions (such as universities and hospitals) and are run by public money.

The area agency on aging (eldercare .gov) might know of NORCs in your parent's state, or you can find a list of communities at norc.org.

sometimes considered retirement communities)—typically these are gated communities set up specifically for retired seniors. Some, however, are open to other generations.

Retirement communities generally have apartments of various sizes, and sometimes small houses, on the property.

Residents can often get meals at a central location, although the apartments have full kitchens. They also offer social events and group outings and activities.

Most retirement communities are in warmer climates and cater to wealthier people who are active.

Senior Apartments

Some apartment buildings specialize in the needs of the elderly. Not only are all of the tenants older, but the buildings are constructed for seniors—no steps, ample pathways for wheelchairs, sturdy and stable furniture, handrails, good lighting, tight security.

From small buildings with a few units, to massive high-rises, these apartments are usually near shops and public transportation, and they often provide meals, activities, and other services.

Many senior apartments are government subsidized, through the U.S. Department of Housing and Urban Development. However, these often have waiting lists of three or four years, and they are available only to people with low incomes.

If your parent is frail and contemplating a move into a senior apartment, find out exactly what services are provided, including whether there are emergency provisions, such as a call button in the bedroom and round-the-clock staff. Also, find out in advance what would happen if your parent were to become ill, confused, or immobile. Some senior apartments evict residents who become infirm, even if they can afford to hire personal health aides or companions.

....

"My mother made the decision herself, without discussing it with anyone. She moved out of her apartment in New York and into an elderly housing complex.

I was upset because, you know, this is the thing you dread, your mom moving into an old-age home. I feared she would be miserable.

But she seemed happy there, and looking back, I remembered that she had talked about going into an old-age home with my father before he died. She said to him more than once, 'Wouldn't it be nice to be in a place where they do everything for us?'"

—Barbara F.

....

Foster Homes

Some families will take in an older person for a fee (anywhere from $500 to $3,000 a month) and provide the care and support that you might provide if you could. Most elderly people who live in foster homes have some physical and/or mental limitations and need help with daily tasks. The foster family cooks meals, does laundry, provides transportation, and generally helps the person through the day.

Before you gasp and shake your head, know that there are hundreds of wonderful foster home stories and, although it's not well tracked, there seem to be few disasters. Doing your research in advance, getting to know the foster family, and keeping an eye on things should help you avoid major problems.

If a foster family embraces and nurtures your parent, this can be an ideal solution—certainly better than the isolation of home or the confines of an institution. You might feel considerable relief, and even develop your own relationship with the foster family.

States have their own rules on foster care, specifying how many adults can live in one foster home, regulating costs, and defining eligibility requirements to become a foster family. The area agency on aging (eldercare.gov) should know about any adult foster care programs in your parent's state. Usually the older person (or his children) shoulders the cost, although most states offer Medicaid and SSI coverage to people with low incomes.

Despite all its benefits, foster care can elicit unexpected reactions. You may worry—rightfully—about whether a foster family is treating your parent well. And you might be visited in the late hours of the night by your old companion Guilt, who tells you that strangers are doing what you should be doing. Or you might grow jealous of the relationship that is developing between your parent and her foster family. *Mom wants to spend the holidays with them instead of us. I can't believe it.*

In the clear light of morning, the fact that your parent has found a good home should calm your anxieties and concerns. Just be sure to visit frequently and establish a rapport with the foster family.

> One day when she called and sounded particularly low, I said, 'Oh, Mum, I think I really missed the boat. I should have helped get you into a retirement home where you could have been with other people, because you love people so much.' I made it sound like a compliment.
>
> I left it so that if she was interested, she could bring the subject up later, as though it were her own idea, not something that I was pushing on her. It takes some time for this sort of thing to settle in her mind. She needs to mull it over, without any pressure from me. If I had suggested straight out that she move, she would have gotten all indignant and resistant."
>
> —Betty H.

HOUSING OPTIONS AT A GLANCE

TYPE	DESCRIPTION	COSTS
Accessory Apartments	An apartment within, or attached to, a single-family house	Renovations to create an accessory apartment vary
ECHO Housing	Modular units placed temporarily on the property of a family home	$30,000 and up
Shared and Congregate Housing	Anything from two roommates to a group of people who receive an array of services	Varies widely
Retirement Communities	Gated communities catering to active retirees	Varied, but usually moderately to fairly expensive
Senior Apartments	Apartments for independent elderly people; often for people with low incomes	Subsidized apartments accept only low-income residents; rents vary by area
Assisted Living	Facilities that provide a range of services for people who need some supervision and daily help	$3,500 a month on average; could be higher or lower, depending on the area and services provided
Foster Homes	A family takes in an elderly person and provides meals, housekeeping, laundry, and some other services	From $300 to $3,000 a month, but might be covered by SSI and other benefit programs
Continuing Care Retirement Communities	Large complexes that offer a full spectrum of care, from houses to nursing home care	Usually, a hefty entrance fee plus monthly fees (although the entrance fee may be refundable)

ADVANTAGES	DISADVANTAGES
Proximity while preserving privacy	Not allowed in some towns and can be expensive to set up
Independence and proximity to family, with independence	Not allowed in some neighborhoods
Companionship, shared expenses, and, in some cases, meals, transportation, and housekeeping	Less privacy; people might not get along
Activities, social life, and some services	Often not appropriate for someone who is frail or confused
Independence, without home maintenance. Most offer meals, laundry, housekeeping, transportation, and recreational and social activities	Typically there are long waiting lists for subsidized apartments, and they can be poorly maintained
Meals, housekeeping, supervision, activities, and custodial care; some accept residents with dementia	Your parent might not be able to remain if her health worsens
With the right family: loving care, emotional and physical support	With the wrong family: a disaster
Peace of mind that all future care is covered and no further moves will be needed	The cost makes this an option only for people with ample assets or cash available after selling a home.

Assisted Living

Assisted living facilities are an intermediate step, serving people who need help getting through the day but don't require the supervision and medical services of a nursing home.

Be sure you are clear on that last point. Most assisted living facilities offer supervision, *but not nursing care* and not full-time aides. If your parent needs hands-on help through much of her day, an assisted living facility might not be enough.

The services offered vary widely. Most offer on-call help, two or three meals a day, transportation, recreation, and exercise programs, housekeeping and laundry services, social services, and at least some help with bathing, dressing, toileting, and other personal tasks.

Some can handle incontinence. Others are set up to care for people with dementia.

Be sure a facility can truly provide the level of care they advertise. Many have gotten in over their heads, accepting frail residents they can't care for adequately. Tour the facility; ask about staffing levels.

Because residents generally have quite a bit of privacy, remain largely independent, and are surrounded by others who are still fairly able, they tend to remain healthier and more active than people who enter nursing homes prematurely. Furthermore, assisted living is, on average, about half the cost of nursing home care.

However, unlike nursing homes, assisted living facilities are not regulated by the federal government. Every state has its own rules and these are typically fairly lax. It is up to you, the consumer, to be on your toes when examining the options. Make sure any facility on your list is licensed by the state. Check with the state ombudsman's office to see if complaints have been filed again the facility.

Facilities range from large houses with a few rooms to tall buildings with more than 200 units. Most range from 25 to 125 units. In some residences,

A QUALITY CHECK

When you research housing options, ask the local area agency on aging or the long-term care ombudsman about licensing or any "quality assurance" program within the state. Also, check with the Department of Consumer Affairs or the Better Business Bureau to see if any complaints have been filed against a particular residence. Most important, talk with people who reside in the facilities and their families. Find out what they like and don't like about it.

HOW LONG WILL THIS LAST?

Whatever housing option you choose, find out what happens as your parent needs more care—because she will. If your mother needs help now getting meals, vacuuming, and doing her laundry, what happens when she needs help with toileting and dressing? What happens when your father becomes confused?

How long can he stay in this facility? Who decides when he must leave, and how do they decide that? How much warning will you receive? Do they help in finding a nursing home or other living situation for him? What happens if he is hospitalized and then in rehab for a period of time? Be sure you have a plan for what comes next.

people share bedrooms; in others, they have private apartments.

Smaller facilities, often called "board and care homes," usually offer fewer services and less medical care, and are only loosely monitored, if at all.

Assisted living can cost anywhere from $2,000 to $8,000 a month, with the national average falling around $3,500 a month, or $40,000 a year. But this is a base price and does not include all services.

Which brings us to this essential point: Find out exactly what is included in the price and what is extra. Get a detailed list of what is provided. All meals or just some? Full laundry services or only sheets and towels? Housekeeping in your parent's room or only in the common areas?

If needed, is custodial care (bathing, dressing, grooming, toileting) included or charged by the hour? Is it available around the clock or just during certain hours? Is there any nursing care at all? Also, find out how much the rates might increase each year. Is there some cap on increases?

Medicare and most private insurance plans do not cover the costs; however, if your parent has long-term care insurance, it should pay for room and board and perhaps a little more, assuming your parent meets eligibility requirements. Some states have arrangements to provide some coverage under Medicaid, and the VA has a program providing coverage in some cases.

Also of critical importance: Find out what happens when your parent becomes more frail and/or confused. Will she be able to stay? How will this additional care be provided, and what will it cost? Will they arrange for a move? If she is

> ❝ I spent an afternoon trying to convince my mother that I was her daughter, not a servant, and when I went to bed that night, I thought, 'We have to make another arrangement.' I'd put up with this for too long. I'd had it.
>
> The next morning I started making phone calls, and we found her an assisted living home within a few weeks."
>
> —Jane D.

hospitalized, does she lose her room? If she needs hospice care, can they provide it, or do they work with a particular hospice organization?

It's very difficult to move someone repeatedly, so assume your parent's skills will decline, and plan accordingly. Read contracts carefully, and be sure to review all details concerning cost, services, and discharge.

For more information about the regulations and residences in your parent's state, contact the area agency on aging (eldercare.gov), the National Consumer Voice for Quality Long-Term Care (theconsumervoice.org), or the Assisted Living Consumer Alliance (assistedlivingconsumers.org).

> " Dad wasn't all that frail, but he was lonely. He would come up with a hundred reasons to ask one of us to come over. A lightbulb was out, or a gutter was full, or he couldn't get the television to work. There was always something, and I was always running over there or worrying about him and feeling bad that I wasn't with him. I turned to my sister one day and said, 'This has got to stop.'
>
> I have three kids at home and a job, and I couldn't keep doing it. I couldn't handle the work and I couldn't handle the worry. That's when we started looking into other housing possibilities."
>
> —Skip M.

Continuing Care Retirement Communities

Continuing care retirement communities (CCRCs), also known as life care centers, are the prix-fixe meal on the menu of housing options. They offer it all—from independent living to nursing home care—usually for a fairly hefty price.

Many communities accept only people who can get around and live independently. Once a resident has been admitted, however, he has access to a spectrum of care for life.

These centers usually include houses and apartments for those who are living independently, and offer these residents a variety of activities, such as golf, swimming, tennis, a gym, lectures, movies, and trips.

They also have an assisted living floor or complex, which provides care and services for people who need help with daily tasks such as bathing, dressing, and eating. And there is a nursing home unit or wing for residents who are very frail or ill.

Consequently, there is a mix of residents, many of them healthy and active, so the atmosphere is less dreary than it is in some other institutions.

Most important, these communities offer companionship, physical and mental stimulation, full care, and enormous peace of mind. Your parent doesn't have to worry about nursing home care, where he will go, and how he will pay for it. Everything he will ever need is paid for (depending upon the type of contract signed), and he will never need to move again (except within the facility). When he needs more care, he doesn't leave his familiar stomping grounds.

Entrance fees vary greatly, ranging anywhere from $30,000 to more than $500,000. The entrance fee is often the cost of a house or apartment. Sometimes this fee, or some portion of it, is refunded when the resident dies or moves. There are also monthly fees, ranging from $1,000 to more than $5,000. The monthly fees cover meal plans, utilities, maintenance, transportation, housekeeping, and recreation.

For some people, the sale of a home will cover the entrance fee, and when they calculate what they save in home maintenance, taxes, utilities, and potential care, and what they gain by moving, the math makes sense.

CCRCs offer various and usually pretty complicated financial contracts, making it difficult to compare apples with apples. Generally, residents are asked to choose from among three types of arrangements:

- **Extended,** or life care, contracts (Plan A) cover everything. The entry fee and monthly fees cover all health care that is needed, including unlimited nursing care, without an increase in those fees while the person is receiving that care. This involves higher monthly fees.

- **Modified** contracts (Plan B) cover only a limited number of days of assisted living or nursing care each year. After that, the resident pays a fee that is usually about 80 percent of the full rate. However, the entry fee and monthly fees are lower.

- **Fee-for-service,** or pay-as-you-go, contracts (Plan C) provide residents with independent living, but require that they pay the full cost of any assisted living or nursing care needed. The entry fee and monthly fees are lower.

THE SEARCH

After you make a list of possibilities, call facilities to see which ones might be right for your parent. Once you've narrowed down your list, take a tour. Is the place clean and well kept? Do the residents seem occupied and content? Does the staff seem caring and respectful? Can the facility meet the particular needs of your parent? Ask a lot of questions—of administration, staff, residents, and their families. What services are offered? How much freedom do residents have? What is the total cost? How might this change? For a detailed list of issues to consider, see page 422.

Because this is a long-term commitment and a major financial investment, your parent should do a lot of research and have a lawyer experienced in such matters examine the contract. He (or you) should check the financial stability of the residence, the refund policy, Medicare and Medicaid certification, any costs not included in the monthly fees, health insurance requirements, possible increases in fees, and the availability of skilled-care beds.

Also, find out how decisions are made to move residents from one level of care to the next, how often residents need to supplement services with paid care, and what happens if your parent runs out of money.

Keep in mind that if your parent is moving into a life care center, long-term care insurance may be redundant. Talk to the financial administrators to see how such insurance would affect costs.

Tour a CCRC as you would any other facility. Go on an official tour and then return unannounced. Have a meal, talk to residents and staff, watch people interact, visit an activity, see if anyone is using the weight room or pool and what kind of supervision they have, and ask about staff-to-patient ratio in the nursing home. See page 422 for a list of things to consider when choosing any long-term care facility.

....

“ About three years ago, my parents moved into a life care center in the neighboring town. My sisters and I were shocked. They were healthy and active. It seemed as if they were giving up.

Now I am grateful. They love being there. They don't have the responsibility of caring for a house, and they do what they want to do. It's not gloomy or depressing. In fact, it's nice—much more like a country club than an old folks' home. Best of all, we don't worry about the future. It's all taken care of. It's really a blessing."

—Elizabeth J.

....

Chapter 21

A Good Nursing Home

The Decision • Starting the Hunt • What to Look For
in Any Facility • Getting In • Admission • Who Pays?

You hoped it would never happen. Maybe you even promised yourself or your parent it would never happen. But at some
point—often after great effort to avoid it, and agonizing days of
sadness and guilt—it becomes clear that the time has come. You need to
move your parent into a nursing home.

It is a devastating decision. But in many cases, it's the best option.
Yes, there are horror stories, but there are also plenty of success stories.
A good nursing home can provide a level of medical care, supervision,
companionship, and activity that is often not possible at home. And
if you are barely making it through each day, it's best to arrange this
move before you crash.

About 40 percent of people over the age of 65 will spend at least
some time in a nursing home. Most stay for just a few months, recuperating after an injury or illness. Some are long-term residents.

You are in no way abandoning your parent. In fact, even though
a move to a nursing home should relieve you of the daily demands of

her care, your job is far from over. Your involvement, and the involvement of other family members and friends, is vital to the success of
this move.

Your parent needs someone to monitor her care and to act on
her behalf. She needs someone who will talk with staff members regularly and speak up when things aren't right. And of course, she needs
your support, your love, and your warm touch now more than ever.

Sorrow may be unavoidable, but shake off any guilt. You are
doing your best and will continue to do your best, and that is an
amazing gift.

SOONER? OR LATER?

On the one hand, you should keep your parent out of a nursing home for as long as possible, because, well it's an institution, and people sometimes go downhill after such a move. There are many ways to do this—by being aware of issues that often send people into nursing homes (such as medications, hearing loss, incontinence, and falls), using community programs, renovating a home, and coordinating in-home services.

On the other hand, if a nursing home is clearly on the horizon, delaying, denying, and dodging it is a bad approach, for all sorts of reasons.

Many of the best nursing homes have waiting lists, so if a nursing home is even in the realm of possibilities, study the options and get your parent's name on any list, as it could be months before there is room. You can always decline when her name comes up.

Also, if your parent is even remotely near Medicaid eligibility, it's best to get into a facility that accepts Medicaid

before he runs out of money. If your parent can cover even six months of nursing home care, he may have a better chance of being accepted by the home of his choice. And then, when he switches over to Medicaid, he should be able to stay put (ask about this to be sure).

If your parent has dementia, it's best to start this process while she can still be part of the deliberations. Also, she might adjust more easily if she makes a move while she is somewhat lucid and can get used to new surroundings and make some friends.

Although her own home is usually better than an institution, it isn't always. Home can be isolating. Help can be unreliable. Neglect and abuse can happen anywhere.

And finally, despite what you might tell yourself, caregivers actually do have limits. Do not wait until you are hospitalized or severely depressed to make a change. Learn the options early, even if you believe you won't use them.

The Decision

The mere thought of a nursing home may conjure up images of muttering old people warehoused in stench and isolation, of abusive orderlies, indifferent nurses, and helpless patients strapped to chairs.

It happens, yes, but less than it used to. Public lobbying, consumer advocacy, litigation, and federal reforms have all forced nursing homes to rethink their mission and responsibilities. As a result, many have hired more staff and improved their training, stopped or cut back on the use of physical restraints and sedating medications, eased rigid schedules, renovated rooms, and developed a range of activities to keep residents engaged and stimulated.

Inspections still discover negligent and abusive situations, but there are more and more examples of good care—nursing homes where residents make friends, become involved, exercise, eat decent food, and are well tended to.

If you start early, do some legwork, and get your parent into a good nursing home, and then visit her regularly and advocate on her behalf, her move to a nursing home could be a boon for her and a great relief for you.

Nursing homes are invaluable if your parent needs more care, therapy, or supervision than is practical or possible at home; when family members cannot handle the physical and emotional demands of caring for an infirm person;

PROMISES MADE . . .

Whatever promises you made in the past, to yourself or to your parent, they were made when you didn't know the facts, when you weren't standing where you are today. It's okay to move forward with whatever the best choice is, given the current circumstances.

Most people in a nursing home have a spouse or child who swore he or she would never, ever put this person in a nursing home. Forgive yourself utterly and completely, from head to toe.

---

and when living in any other type of residence is not an option because of the severity of your parent's disabilities or behaviors.

Most nursing homes offer basic medical care and round-the-clock nursing supervision in addition to meals, laundry services, personal care, counseling, recreation, social services, rehabilitative

---

" I worked in a nursing home for 22 years. I was exceedingly knowledgeable about the process. But when it was my mother, when I was personally involved, well, part of me didn't want to know. I couldn't deal with it.

But eventually, the choice is taken away. They are in the hospital, and they have to go. My mother's house wasn't set up for this. We couldn't lift her. In the end, we had no choice."

—Laurette H.

programs, and pharmacy and laboratory services. Some have "memory care" units for people with dementia, and others provide "subacute medical care"—special

wings or floors that provide hospital-level care. Facilities are usually privately owned, publicly supported, or run by a nonprofit religious or civic group.

Starting the Hunt

Ideally, you'll have time to do some research, tour a number of facilities, revisit one or two that look promising, and ask a lot of questions. Ideally, your parent will have time to live with this idea and begin to accept it.

In reality, however, time might not be on your side, and your search might be frantic.

Unless this is a temporary move (for respite or recuperation), try to buy yourself a little time. If your parent is about

to be discharged from the hospital, you can usually get a reprieve of a day or two by appealing your parent's discharge. If your parent is at home, see if you can't hire temporary help while you review the options.

Moving is disruptive and stressful. If you "try out" a nursing home with the thought of moving your parent to a better one later, you will throw her life into chaos twice, create more work for yourself, and possibly hurt her chances

KEEP YOUR PARENT AT THE HELM (EVEN IF YOU'RE CHARTING THE COURSE)

No matter what your parent's physical and mental limitations may be—even if she isn't fully aware of what is happening around her—try to keep her involved in all stages of this decision, talking about the options, touring homes, choosing one, and signing up. Keeping her involved and informed should make the transition easier.

If your parent can't tour nursing homes, then collect brochures, menus, and activity schedules for her; take photos

or a video; and describe what you saw and the people you met. The facility's website might include a virtual tour (which, of course, isn't quite the same as a real tour but is still revealing).

While reviewing the options, focus on what matters to *her* and what would be best for *her*. A beautifully renovated building and lush gardens might wow you, but your parent might feel more at home in a smaller, less fancy facility with a warm and caring staff.

COMMON REACTIONS TO PUTTING A PARENT INTO A NURSING HOME

- Guilt that you are not doing enough for your parent
- Anxiety that the nursing staff won't do enough for your parent
- Guilt that your parent isn't in a nicer, more expensive home
- Anxiety over the high cost of the nursing home he is in
- Guilt that you don't visit more often

- Anxiety about having to visit so often
- Guilt because you are so relieved that your parent is in a nursing home
- Anxiety that it won't work and you'll have to devise another plan
- Guilt because you promised you would never put him in a nursing home
- Anxiety that you, too, will end up in a nursing home one day

of getting into another residence, as her placement may seem less urgent. It's best to get it right the first time.

Making a List
Start your search by putting together a list of local nursing homes. If you're not sure whether your parent should stay in his community or move closer to you or one of your siblings, find out about residences in all of those places. Certainly, it's best for him to be near family who can visit and monitor his care, but it's also important to find a good residence.

A few resources to use as you make your list:

HOSPITAL DISCHARGE PLANNER. If your parent is in the hospital, the discharge planner can guide you. Discharge planners should know quite a bit about local nursing homes, and they often have relationships with administrators, so they may be able to expedite your parent's admission. They also know

something about your parent's medical situation, so they can advise you on which homes are best suited for her. Sometimes nursing home administrators give priority to a hospital patient whose care will be covered, at least in the beginning, by Medicare.

Contact the discharge planner early in your parent's hospitalization. Be aware, however, that a discharge planner's main objective is to get your parent out of the hospital, so she may pressure your family to make a hasty decision. A hospital may also have a tie to a particular facility, biasing the planner's recommendations. (But if you ask, he or she should tell you about any such connections.)

MEDICARE'S "NURSING HOME COMPARE." On the Medicare website (medicare.gov), you can learn about nursing homes in the area and get information about staffing levels, certain quality measures, and any problems that have been reported.

A CULTURE CHANGE

Boomers have revised much along their path, and now they are changing nursing homes. The goal? No more long, sterile corridors, beeping call buttons, shift changes, or restraints. No more schedules and rules. No more gray meat patties. No more top-down institutions where life revolves around the nursing station.

No, now there is a growing interest in smaller homes, with maybe 10 to 30 residents, homey living spaces and open kitchens, wide gardens, sunlight, and, most important, a whole new philosophy of care.

In these homes, whatever size they might be, the focus is not solely on what residents *need* (drugs, rehab, medical care), but what they *want* (companionship, independence, purpose).

People wake up when they want, eat when they want, and do what they want, almost as if they were, well, people. Everyone who is able pitches in, setting the table, stirring the sauce, and arranging the flowers. The staff is more like family than overseers.

This movement, known widely as "culture change" or "person-directed care," gives people more say in their care and recognizes that people's needs are highly personal.

For example, while it might be convenient for a nurse to walk from room to room at the beginning of a shift, taking blood pressures and temperatures, most people do not want to be woken up at 5 a.m. The new approach: Take vitals when people get up, whenever that might be.

In addition to monitoring your parent's health, the staff might get your mother access to a piano if that's what she loves, or ask your father, who used to run a large business, to research the feasibility of building a pool at the home.

Culture change also includes something known in the field as "consistent assignment." Rather than rotating nurses and assistants, caregivers are assigned to residents so they develop relationships and are more apt to notice subtle changes that might indicate trouble.

When looking at nursing homes, or any residence for that matter, ask about the philosophy of care. Find out if your parent can sleep in, eat ice cream for breakfast, or help with the cooking, for example. You might get a bewildered look, or, with any luck, you might hear, "If that's what he likes to do, then of course he can."

For more information, contact the Green House Project (thegreenhouseproject.org), Eden Alternative (edenalt.org), or Pioneer Network (pioneernetwork.net).

Any nursing homes that is not certified by Medicare will not be included in this list, but that's a limited number, so this is still a good starting point for your hunt.

The website focuses on a five-star rating system, five being the best and one, well, it's generally best to avoid any homes with one star. (As always, though, there are exceptions, so if that's all that's near, don't despair. Go take a look.)

The stars are based primarily on three sources of information:

The first is the state health inspection report. Nursing homes that receive Medicare or Medicaid funding are inspected, on average, about once a year. The inspection report examines nearly 200 issues, ranging from the temperature of the tap water and whether the stew meat is fresh, to signs of abuse and neglect. You can look at the actual report and get specific information about any violations.

Most nursing homes have violations, so look beyond the numbers. Clearly, failing to file a medical report correctly is less serious than failing to prevent bedsores. See what the problem is and if the home has made efforts to remedy it. Repeated offenses should raise a red flag.

Be aware that states all have different rules and processes for inspections, so if you are comparing a facility in Arkansas with one in Tennessee, you might be comparing bananas with pineapples.

If you are interested in a facility, but there are violations that concern you, call and ask an administrator what has been done to correct the problem. The way the staff answers your questions— whether they are direct and apologetic, or indifferent—will tell you a great deal about how they regard their mission.

The second factor in the Nursing Home Compare section is staffing. The Centers for Medicare & Medicaid Services uses information provided by a nursing home to estimate the number of nursing hours per resident per day. The important number to look at is the number of CNA (certified nursing assistant) hours, as these are the folks who do the bulk of patient care. Four hours is optimal (although few nursing homes have this), and less than two hours of CNA time is actually dangerous.

Finally, the stars are based on several quality measures, such as whether residents have bedsores, whether they have

been delirious (which is often caused by inappropriate care), and whether they are gaining or losing skills, such as the ability to dress or feed themselves. These quality measures are compared with both statewide and national averages, and perhaps most helpful, you can compare ratings between facilities.

OTHER WEBSITES. Be very cautious about using websites to find a nursing home, as many are commercial and extremely biased ("advisers" are simply salespeople who get commissions if they get you to sign up with one of the homes on their lists). A few, however, are quite good. Check out the Informed Patient Institute (informedpatientinstitute.org), which rates such websites and can tell you about the better ones in your parent's state.

....

66 We looked for a nursing home, but we didn't like any of the facilities. One was in a basement. People were sitting in wheelchairs in the hallway. They weren't well groomed. They had food on their clothes.

I couldn't imagine my mother in a place like that. I probably looked at five, and they were all really depressing.

We put her in an assisted living facility, as a stopgap, until we could find something. Then I heard about a place run by the Lutheran church. It was really nice—clean, there were a lot of caregivers on the floor, and it had a nice feeling to it. There was enough oversight, and I could easily get there from my apartment.

She lived there for three and a half years. It was great for all of us."

—Angela S.

....

FRIENDS, FAMILY, CLERGY. Friends and relatives might have insight into local facilities if they have had a family member in a nursing home. Members of the clergy, who visit people in nursing homes, might also have recommendations.

AREA AGENCY ON AGING OR LONG-TERM CARE OMBUDSMAN. Each state (and some communities) has an ombudsman who is an advocate for nursing home residents and their families. They can provide information about nursing homes and help you sort through the facts, ratings, and inspections reports. The best ombudsmen visit nursing homes routinely and will know what each offers and the quality of care available.

If they can't help you, someone from the agency on aging should be able to. They all work together, but sometimes one person is simply more helpful than another.

Be aware, however, that an ombudsman can't tell you which facility to choose or provide personal opinions about facilities. However, he or she might subtly try to redirect you if you are headed in the wrong direction. *Why would you select Serene Acres? I think you should look at Barton's Landing. Are you sure Cedar Hollow is right for your parent?* Listen for those cues.

You can find the local long-term care ombudsman and the area agency on aging by going to eldercare.gov or calling 800-677-1116.

CITIZEN ADVOCACY GROUPS. Many states have nursing home advocacy groups that keep tabs on nursing homes, guide residents and their families, and advocate for better regulations and policies. They might be helpful in your search for a good residence. To find an advocacy group, visit the website of the National Consumer Voice for Quality Long-Term Care (theconsumervoice.org).

Note: Don't pass over nursing homes sponsored by religious organizations just because your parent is not affiliated with that religion. Nursing homes affiliated with a religious group are often among the best ones.

What to Look For in Any Facility

In a rural area, the choices might be slim. But in a populated area, there should be some decent options within a 30-mile radius, and thus, decisions to make.

Once you have a list of "maybes," go have a look. Go on a formal tour, and then, if a facility seems promising, return during the evening or on a weekend, when staffing levels tend to be lower.

When you tour, don't be blinded by fancy interior decorating, a glamorous lobby, or lush entrance gardens. Walk the corridors and observe how the residents are cared for, because that's what matters. Visit the common areas where residents spend time. Ask to look at several bedrooms, the kitchen, the infirmary, and any dementia wing or other special unit. If possible, meet the manager of the residence, financial director, head nurse, activity director, social worker, and/or medical director.

Talk with residents, their families, and staff. If you don't understand something or if a situation seems amiss, ask. This will tell you far more about the home than you will learn on any guided tour.

When making a decision about nursing homes, or any senior housing for that matter, here are some things to consider:

LOCATION, LOCATION, LOCATION. Being near family or friends who will visit regularly and keep tabs on care should be a primary criterion when selecting any housing. If your parent is mobile, find out whether the facility is near shops and restaurants and/or if a van or other transportation is readily available.

CERTIFICATION AND LICENSING. All nursing homes must be licensed by the state. A nursing home can choose to also seek certification from the federal government, which then enables it to receive Medicare and/or Medicaid payments.

It's generally best to find a nursing home that is fully Medicare and Medicaid certified because this means that, one, it meets federal guidelines; two, skilled nursing care that falls under Medicare will be covered, and three, if your parent becomes eligible for Medicaid he cannot be discharged solely because of finances.

Other kinds of facilities (such as assisted living) have far fewer and less stringent regulations.

GUT INSTINCTS. Your first instinct is often a pretty good one. What turned you off? What surprised you? What did you like?

THE NOSE TEST. That first waft is one indicator of the quality of a home. Is it fresh, airy, and odor-free? A facility shouldn't smell musty or rancid, nor should it reek of perfumes or cleaning agents.

WELL SCRUBBED AND MAINTAINED. Does it appear clean and well maintained, not just in the lobby and public rooms, but elsewhere as well? Are the buildings and furnishings in good repair, or is there plaster cracking off the walls?

YOUR PARENT'S NEEDS. Can this residence meet your parent's specific needs? What sort of care is offered to residents with dementia or to those who are deaf? Are residents who are incontinent helped to the toilet immediately (or, better yet, before the need arises)? Are people on hand to help residents eat? Can they handle your father if he's a curmudgeon or your mother if she has anxiety?

MONEY. Of course, this should be high up on your list, as it's a major issue. What are the entry fees, monthly fees, and additional costs? Find out exactly what is included and what is extra, such as laundry, haircuts, special meals, outings, physical therapy, dental visits, lab work, medical equipment, and prescription drugs.

Unless your parent is quite wealthy, be sure a nursing home accepts Medicaid, as many people end up needing it.

A FRIENDLY TAGALONG

If you are touring without your parent or a sibling, ask a friend to come with you, preferably someone who has been through this experience. It's not easy looking at nursing homes and imagining your parent living in one of them, and it's physically tiring to do so much walking and interviewing. A friend can help you think more clearly and less emotionally, and give you the moral support you need on such a difficult trip.

How much have monthly fees increased over the past three years? What sort of increases are expected in the coming years?

Can contracts be terminated? If so, under what conditions? What is the refund policy? If a resident is discharged, how many days' notice does he get? Who receives such notice?

How stable is this residence financially? (What happens to your parent if the home becomes part of another facility or goes out of business?)

MEDICAL CARE. What are the arrangements for medical care, dentistry, psychiatric services, foot care, eye care, preventive care, and other health-related needs? Does the facility arrange for residents to receive regular checkups by a doctor or nurse at the facility? Can they continue to use their personal doctors. (By law, they can as long as the resident can see the doctor, at the facility or at the doctor's office, often enough to meet nursing home regulations.)

Are nurses available around the clock? Is there a doctor on call? (This is required at nursing homes.) Is the facility close to a hospital?

Are residents often restrained, either physically or with medications? (See page 446 for more on restraints.)

What percentage of the residents are incontinent, and how is incontinence handled? (If a large number of patients are incontinent—half or more—it may be because the staff uses diapers and catheters in place of good toileting habits.)

A PLAN OF CARE. In a nursing home, each resident should have a "plan of care" that outlines any therapies, treatments, meal requirements, special activities, and so forth. How is this plan determined? How much input does the resident and/or family have? How often is it reassessed, and how closely is it followed?

THE HOMINESS FACTOR. Is the residence well lighted, attractive, and cheery? Would this be a comfortable place to live? Are the lounges cozy and the rooms adequate?

THE GREAT OUTDOORS. Are there gardens or grounds where residents are free to roam? Are there benches and wide paths? Are residents actually enjoying the outdoors? Sitting in a dark room is not healthy.

THE FOLKS WHO LIVE THERE. Do the residents look well cared for and content? Are they groomed and neat? Are they alert, or do they look sedated? Are they restrained physically?

What is their level of functioning, physically and mentally? Will your parent find people at his general level of functioning?

Talk with residents and their family members out of earshot of staff so they can be candid. Are they happy with the care they are receiving?

ENOUGH STAFF. Do staff members seem harried and overworked? Are residents neglected and chores left undone?

Nursing homes are required to have at least one registered nurse on duty eight hours a day, seven days a week, and an RN, LPN, or LVN (registered nurse, licensed practical nurse, or licensed vocational nurse) on duty 24 hours a day. Some states require additional staffing.

But this bar is exceedingly low. The National Consumer Voice for Quality Long-Term Care recommends that nursing homes have at least one "direct care" staff member for every five residents during the day. (These are people who directly care for patients, as opposed to those in administrative roles.) The ratio in the evening should be at least 1 to 10, and at night, 1 to 15. Staffing should be higher if people have acute needs and in special wings, such as a dementia unit.

Staffing levels are posted within each facility; ask to see this. Most nursing homes fail to meet these criteria, but a residence that you are considering should not fail by much.

An assisted living home that takes severely ill or dementia clients also should be amply staffed and have 24/7 emergency provisions.

CARING STAFF. Is the staff pleasant and helpful, or is everyone on edge? Do they interact easily and cheerfully with the residents? Do they treat residents with respect and kindness? Do they seem to enjoy their work?

Are they open and direct in answering your questions? Do they seem knowledgeable? Is there a high rate of turnover (which suggests trouble)?

Find out if the facility rotates staff or if one staff member on each shift will be assigned to your parent, so there is some consistency in her care.

" I visited two homes with wonderful reputations and found that while the grounds and buildings were beautiful, the staff were nasty to the residents and clearly unhappy in their work. Others I visited were better, but I still wasn't satisfied. I kept calling friends and friends of friends, trying to get more leads. Then someone mentioned a place that she said had been a wonderful nursing home years ago, but now was in a bad neighborhood.

I went out to see it anyway—the neighborhood was poor, but not dangerous—and while it didn't compare aesthetically with the other places, it was immaculately clean and the staff was cheerful. They seemed truly fond of the residents, and never seemed exasperated, even when patients were difficult.

My mother was very weak and confused, but she seemed content there and I felt good about it."

—Sara B.

PERSONAL FREEDOM. Are residents encouraged to be independent, to care for themselves and make decisions for themselves as much as possible? Can your parent eat when he wants, sleep in if he likes, leave his window open at night, and sit where he wants in the dining room? Can he have a pet? Can he skip breakfast if it's not a meal he's ever enjoyed? Can he watch television until 1 a.m. and have a snack at midnight, if that's his habit? What if he's a smoker?

He probably won't get everything he likes, but is the facility flexible? If he's not supposed to have salt in his diet, but he feels that he's 92 and will have salt if he damn well pleases, how stringent will they be?

> " Getting my father into a good nursing home was like getting someone with very poor grades into college. He was on Medicaid because we'd spent all of my parents' money during my mother's illness. He had advanced dementia, and he had become angry and disruptive. A social worker said that nursing homes in the area would not consider taking such a patient and suggested that we get him admitted to a hospital and let the hospital staff pull some strings.
>
> We represented my father as being cooperative and agreeable, as he had been before the dementia set in, and finally found a nursing home that we liked that was willing to admit him. We whizzed through the application process because we were afraid they would refuse him once they understood how difficult he could be. They took him, thank goodness, but it was quite an experience."
>
> —Sara B.

A VOICE FOR RESIDENTS AND FAMILIES. Is there a resident council that has some say in the operations of the home? Likewise, is there a council that provides a platform for families? How often do they meet? What kinds of issues do they discuss? How receptive is the home to suggestions and criticisms? When was the last time the council recommended a change that was adopted?

A ROOM TO CALL HOME. Are bedrooms private or shared? Are bathrooms private or shared? How are roommates matched? What if they don't get along or have different lifestyles? Can they change rooms?

Are the rooms large enough? Are there windows that open?

Are the rooms furnished nicely? Can your parent bring furniture and other items from home? Do the rooms reflect their individual inhabitants?

Is there privacy? Are there curtains around the beds in shared rooms? Is there a locked place to store valuables?

WHAT'S IN A DAY? What are residents doing when you visit? Are they staring at a television screen or sitting alone in their rooms? Or are they engaged in projects and activities?

Is there a monthly activity calendar, and does it offer a wide range of choices? Are there frequent movies, lectures, classes, outings, games, and meetings that your parent might enjoy, given her interests and abilities? How many people actually participate in a given activity? Is the activities director willing to offer new classes or organize new events based on a resident's interests?

Do residents get exercise? Is there a workout room? A pool?

SPECIAL CARE FOR DEMENTIA

If a nursing home claims to have special programs and services for people with dementia, find out exactly what that means. A "memory care unit" may be a few rooms with a locked door, or it may be a carefully designed unit with a highly trained staff. The only way to know what's really offered is to see for yourself.

A program doesn't have to be solely for people with dementia; many of the best facilities have a mix of residents.

A good unit should be quiet and calm, but also provide plenty of physical and mental stimulation. Residents should be encouraged to do simple exercises, engage in easy and entertaining projects, and receive lots of encouragement to do all that they can for themselves. They might be able to help with meals, fold laundry, set tables, and otherwise stay involved and feel useful.

The floor plan should allow them to find their way around easily and to wander safely. Doors, hallways, bathrooms, kitchens, and hazards should be clearly marked to avoid confusion.

The staff-to-patient ratio should be high, and schedules should be flexible to meet the diverse needs of residents, including those who are awake during the night or want to eat at odd hours.

The number of patients on sedatives or other psychotropic (mind-altering) medications should be low, and the use of physical restraints, such as straps or body vests, should be virtually nonexistent. Find out how the facility addresses behavioral symptoms; they should have a whole litany of approaches they try before considering any sort of physical restraint or antipsychotic drug.

Once your parent is in a residence, be sure she receives a thorough assessment. Plans for her care should take into account her special needs and unusual quirks—what she can and cannot do, what she enjoys and what makes her anxious, what gives her comfort, what medications she's on, what she eats, and the best way for the staff to help her.

Stay abreast of whether the staff is actually following the plan and whether changes are necessary. People with dementia can change quickly, going from critical and jumpy to calm and withdrawn in a matter of months.

Is there a library? Lounge? Card room? Can residents do paid or volunteer work?

Is the nursing home involved with the community? For example, are there school groups that visit? Cultural activities from the community? Volunteer visitors?

What are the rules about leaving the grounds? Are there planned outings? How are residents monitored if they leave the building? What sort of transportation is available to residents?

Do residents who are confined to their rooms because of illness or disability receive any kind of physical and social stimulation? Does someone help get them to activities?

THE CHOW. When you visit, arrange to have a meal. Does it look appetizing? Does it taste good? Is it nutritious

LGBT

To get help obtaining support, services, information, equal rights, and respect for lesbian, gay, bisexual, or transgender people, visit the National Resource Center on LGBT Aging at lgbtagingcenter.org, or SAGE (Services and Advocacy for GLBT Elders) at sageusa.org.

and well balanced? Does the daily menu change often? Are there ample choices? Can the kitchen accommodate special dietary needs?

Are meal hours flexible? Is food available around the clock? Can residents keep food of their own?

Is the dining room attractive, neat, quiet, and intimate? How is seating decided? Can residents choose their own dining companions?

Are staff members available to help people who have trouble eating on their own? Do patients confined to bed have help or company at meals?

THE HEAD HONCHOS. Get a feel for the philosophy of the institution, as well. An administration that is genuinely concerned about residents will see to it that your parent gets good, continuous care. If an administrator/director is willing to meet with you and is open to your questions and concerns, that's a promising first step.

THE VISITOR'S ROLE. Are visits encouraged and visitors made to feel welcome? Can visitors come for meals? Are young children allowed? Can residents have private time in their rooms with mates or spouses? Are there private places where you can be alone with your parent?

ROOM CHANGES AND DISCHARGE. You don't want your parent moved from room to room or, for heaven's sake, evicted. State and federal regulations cover these issues in nursing homes, but ask for specifics. Find out under what circumstances the home would move your parent to a new room or evict her.

How long will your parent's bed be reserved in the event that she needs to be hospitalized or is temporarily absent for some other reason? What happens if she exceeds that limit? (This is particularly important if your parent is on Medicaid, as the facility's time limit may be quite short or it may not hold a bed at all. If your parent loses her place, the residence must give her the first Medicaid bed available)

Find out if your parent might be moved to another section of the nursing home once he is on Medicaid. It is disruptive for an older person to switch rooms, especially if he has made friends on a certain floor or wing and developed relationships with staff members. Furthermore, some nursing homes put all Medicaid patients onto a floor or unit that is not renovated, more crowded, and poorly staffed. If there is a separate section of the nursing home for those on Medicaid, tour this section as well.

CULTURE AND RELIGION. Is the home sensitive to the ethnic and cultural norms of your parent? Are there other residents in the home who follow your parent's religion or are ethnically similar? Do they serve appropriate foods? Are there plenty of people who speak the same language as your parent? How will medical and other information be provided if there is a language issue?

What provisions are there for religious worship? Are there services in-house? Can residents go to churches or synagogues in the community? Is transportation provided? Do clergy visit frequently?

GENERAL SAFETY AND ACCESSIBILITY. Is the facility set up to prevent accidents, and to be manageable for those with canes, walkers, or wheelchairs? Are there grab bars by the toilets and beds and handrails along the hallways? Are pathways kept clear of clutter? Are there ramps, wide hallways, and elevators? (This should be true of all nursing homes.)

Is there ample security? Are there clearly marked fire exits, smoke alarms, fire doors, and alarms? Is an evacuation plan clearly displayed? Are there emergency call buttons that can be easily reached from both the bed and the toilet? Will your parent receive an emergency help button to wear?

And what about the neighborhood? Is it relatively safe?

HOSPICE CARE. If hospice care is of interest to your family, ask if the nursing home has any arrangement with a nearby hospice (and if so, which one) or dedicated beds for hospice care. Find out how often hospice has been used at the facility, and how much the staff understands and accepts the philosophy of hospice.

If your parent is in an assisted living facility, be sure they can accommodate hospice services. Find out what help the staff will provide under these circumstances and how they coordinate care with hospice.

IS A BED AVAILABLE? If not, how long will your parent have to wait? If you and your parent like a particular home, and a bed is not available, talk with the director of admissions at the nursing home about short-term possibilities. Could she be cared for at another facility until a bed is available?

Getting In

Finding a good nursing home is only half the battle. The other half is getting your parent accepted. In some places, where there are more beds than patients, getting in isn't a problem. But in many areas, popular nursing homes will have plenty of candidates vying for admission, and administrators pick and choose freely when accepting residents. The person with the most money or the

> " They said they had a certain number of Medicaid beds, with a long waiting list. I was desperate, so I put my mother on it. But I thought we'd never get in.
>
> They came and did an evaluation. The woman is there asking Mom questions and I'm answering because Mom is out of it. What do you weigh, what kinds of medications do you take, etc.
>
> I sensed she scored well. She didn't have any complicated diagnosis, just dementia. No other illness. She's light to pick up. She was pleasant, not a difficult patient.
>
> Then I got a phone call and they said, 'We have space,' and I hightailed it over there. I thought, 'This is too good to be true.' I never asked how or why. I just sensed she scored well."
>
> —Sara H.

fewest problems or the easiest personality (and family) will be given priority.

When you meet with an administrator, be honest, but also be discreet in what you say about your parent's angry outbursts or demanding personality. You need to know that the staff can meet his needs, but don't overemphasize any problems. If he's calm and easygoing, make that clear. Likewise, although you shouldn't hesitate to ask questions, be kind and polite. A family perceived as unreasonably demanding may be turned away in favor of one who understands the pressures of nursing home work.

You can't hide your parent's financial problems, because the nursing home will look through his records. Homes prefer self-paying residents and those who qualify for Medicare coverage. The longer someone can foot the bills privately, the better. If your parent is already on Medicaid, he may have fewer choices and may face lengthy waiting lists. It's always better to enter a nursing home when your parent can pay out-of-pocket for six to nine months.

If he has trouble being admitted, talk to the long-term care ombudsman, a local citizens' coalition, and, if possible, a savvy eldercare attorney.

Build a rapport with the nursing home's administration, and if your parent is put on a waiting list, call often and be persistent (but polite!) about making sure that he gets the first bed available.

Admission

The admissions process can be lengthy and exhausting, and it requires that you submit a variety of your parent's personal, medical, financial, and legal records. The nursing home's admissions or financial officer will tell you what is needed. Ask for all the paperwork in advance so you have time to review it and gather what you need before actually going through the admission process.

A nursing home might ask for a large deposit before admission. Find out what this covers and whether it will be refunded if your parent leaves early. Get any agreement in writing. If your parent's care is to be covered by Medicare or Medicaid, the home cannot require a deposit in advance.

Any nursing home contract should include detailed information about costs, payment schedules, services to be provided, penalties for failure to pay, the discharge policy, the rules of the house, the responsibilities and rights of residents, and the facility's refund and bed-holding policy should your parent be hospitalized or temporarily absent for some other reason.

Read the contract carefully or have an experienced lawyer read it. Ask the nursing home's director or the state's long-term care ombudsman to clarify any provision that confuses or concerns you or your parent. Beware of clauses in the contract that free an institution from liability for injury or lost possessions. It's best not to sign any pre-dispute arbitration agreement (which gives the facility control over any arbitration process and limits your ability to seek justice or compensation if there is neglect or abuse).

Who Pays?

What shocks most families is not just the exorbitant cost of nursing home care, but also the fact that Medicare and private health insurance cover so little of it.

Nationally, the average cost of a semiprivate room in a nursing home is more than $80,000 a year (and more than $90,000 for a private room). That's only an average; in many parts of the country, the rates are higher.

Furthermore, the daily or monthly rate quoted by a facility is usually just a base rate. Often, medications, doctor visits, wheelchairs, walkers, and other such services are extra (unless Medicare or Medicaid is footing the bill, in which case most services are included). In some homes, doing laundry, monitoring catheters, and preventing bedsores are considered extras. A survey by *Consumer Reports* found that nursing

> " I know my limitations as a person. I knew what I could do for her and what I couldn't. My mother lived with us for almost five years, and at the beginning we were able to manage. But she became too sick, too demanding. Moving her into a nursing home was the only choice. It was time. I don't have any guilt about it."
> —Nancy S.

> " I refused to put my mother in a nursing home. My sister and brothers kept telling me that we had to do it, that she was too difficult to manage, but I wouldn't listen. I cut back my hours at work and used up pretty much all of her savings to pay for aides and nurses at home. I stuck to my resolve.
>
> Then a friend of mine told me that I had created a home for my mother that was worse than any nursing home. And she was right. My mother didn't do anything or see anyone. She never got out or had any stimulation. And in the meantime, I was ruining my own life.
>
> I finally gave in, but I was mortified any time I had to tell people where she lived. The staff at the nursing home was reassuring and I gradually felt better, but it took time."
>
> —Alex B.

homes sometimes charge up to $1,000 a month for such extras.

Medicare pays for nursing home care only when "skilled" nursing care is needed within 30 days of a hospital stay that lasts at least three full days (and it must be directly related to that hospitalization). A doctor must authorize the need for care, and it must require the oversight of nurses and/or rehabilitation therapists.

If your parent meets all of these requirements, Medicare will pay for 20 days in the nursing home, and then it will pay a portion of the tab for the next 80 days. After that, you're on your own. Many supplemental insurance policies will cover the extra cost between days 21 and 100, but that's it.

Private long-term care insurance will cover some of the cost of a nursing home (usually for some limited period of time), but most people don't have such insurance. As a result, the majority of people who need extended nurising home care tap into their savings and when that is used up, they apply for Medicaid.

All of this comes as a great surprise to people who thought that they had a sufficient nest egg and then suddenly find that it is completely gone. Even a fairly hefty savings account can be depleted quickly.

Before your parent runs out of money, learn about Medicaid eligibility in her state and ways that your family might protect at least some assets. (See page 352.)

Unlike most other health insurance, Medicaid does cover nursing home care. In fact, Medicaid covers nearly half of all nursing home care in this country.

Most nursing homes accept Medicaid patients, but they favor self-paying and Medicare patients, and may limit the number of Medicaid patients they admit. For example, a nursing home with 200 beds might have only 20 beds earmarked for Medicaid patients.

If there is any chance your parent will end up on Medicaid, be sure that any facility you consider accepts Medicaid, and find out exactly what will happen if and when she switches to Medicaid.

If a nursing home is fully certified to take Medicare and Medicaid, it cannot legally discharge your parent for switching to Medicaid. Your parent should simply be able to stay put, without any changes at all.

But many nursing homes are not fully certified; they have just one wing or unit that is Medicaid certified. In this case, a home can evict a patient who is newly on Medicaid if the designated Medicaid beds are all taken. However—nothing is simple on the nursing home front—states have their own rules regarding Medicaid, and some states require that nursing homes guarantee a bed if a resident goes on Medicaid.

The bottom line: Know the policies and get everything in writing before your parent enters any nursing home.

As for the sort of care your parent will receive, it's true that most plush nursing homes do not accept people on Medicaid, but it is a myth that anyone on Medicaid will end up in a dreadful place. Some very good nursing homes accept Medicaid.

Remember, an expensive nursing home is not a guarantee that your parent will get loving, devoted care, just as a run-down exterior doesn't always mean shabby care. Appearance is an important clue to what kind of service is provided, but the quality of care comes from the people who work in the facility. The philosophy of the administrators and the devotion of the staff is what matters most.

Chapter 22

Making the Move Work

Moving Day • A Plan of Care • Visiting • Being an
Advocate • Long-Distance Caregiving • When Trouble
Brews • Is This Move Working?

You've found a nursing home, or perhaps an assisted living
residence or other housing, which should relieve some of the stress
in your life and provide your parent with much-needed supervision, care, and company. But, as you well know, your job is far from over.

You and others in the family need to help your parent prepare
for a big move that he might be dreading, help him adjust to his new
life, and then stay connected and be sure that he gets adequate care.

Unfortunately, nursing homes and other facilities are not without
their problems. Your involvement will help keep his spirits up, but just
as important, it will help you develop relationships with staff members
and be sure that your parent is being cared for properly.

While this chapter is geared toward those who have a parent moving into a nursing home, most of this information is relevant to any
group or institutional housing situation.

Moving Day

Moving day (as well as the weeks leading up to it) can be wrenching for everyone. You are likely to feel anxious (and relieved, guilty, worried, sad), and your parent may be downright terrified (and anxious, angry, worried, depressed). Put your own emotions aside as best you can, and focus on reassuring your parent.

Depression, withdrawal, and even some hostility are all normal responses. This is a big move. It's scary. It feels final. Your parent is leaving a lot behind and facing a great unknown at a very fragile time of life. Even though he knows on some level that this is not your fault, he may very well blame you.

It's not easy—not at all—but let him express these things. Don't take anything personally. Listen calmly and acknowledge what he's saying. Let him know that you hear him, understand, and will not desert him. His reaction is part of a process of letting go and moving on.

....

❝ I was prepared to be uncomfortable, to hate my aunt's nursing home. But I was surprised. It was attractive, and, more than that, many of the people living there were much healthier than I expected. One older gentleman even flirted with my aunt in the elevator. Her cheeks turned bright pink.

We both liked the home more than we expected, which came as a great relief.**❞**
—Fran M.

....

Avoid the urge to change plans at the eleventh hour, just as you're closing the car trunk. *I can't do this. I'll figure something else out.* You've given this a lot of thought. You've both come this far. Now give it a chance.

The Days Before the Move

If you have some time before the move—that is, if your parent is not going unexpectedly into a nursing home—find ways to make the transition easier. A few suggestions:

• In the weeks before the move, take your parent to visit her new home, several times if possible. Even if she's been there before, she will now see it through the eyes of a future resident, which will give her a different perspective. If she knows any of the residents, let them know when she will be arriving so they can greet her.

• Ask friends and family to offer encouragement and support. They might tour the home as well.

• Hold a party for your parent a few days before the move. (Have it around her hospital bed, if necessary.) Guests should bring gifts for her new life—framed photos, silk flowers, a bathrobe, a calendar with lots of visits already written in, soft new sheets, a grandchild's drawing for the wall, and if she doesn't already have one (and if she can operate one), a very simple laptop or tablet so she can video chat with family.

LOST IN TRANSITION

Medical errors and care disasters often occur when the baton is passed from one situation to the next—from home to hospital, from hospital to rehab facility, from rehab to nursing home, and so on.

Medical instructions, therapies, directives, and medications all need to travel with your parent without anything being forgotten or misinterpreted along the way.

Electronic medical records and accountable care organizations—groups of hospitals, doctors, and nursing homes that share information—have helped but not eliminated the problem, so you have to be on your toes.

Before your parent leaves home or the hospital, be sure you have a list of all her medications, medical instructions, therapy needs, dietary restrictions, allergies, and directives. Then review these with the nurse in charge and be sure nothing's been lost in transition.

- Before packing the car, find out exactly what your parent is permitted to bring, and what is not allowed, so you don't arrive only to be sent home with half of her belongings. Leave valuables behind unless they are absolutely necessary (things get lost and stolen in any institution), but include objects of comfort, such as a special chair, a favorite afghan, or family photos. Clearly label all of your parent's clothes and belongings, down to each book and pair of socks.

On Moving Day

- Get others to lend a hand. They might help you arrange your parent's room and then stay and have a meal with her. Or someone might stay home with your children so you aren't hurried while getting your mother adjusted. It's best not to move her in and then race out.

- If your parent has fixed habits and routines (and who doesn't?), ask the staff if they can be accommodated. After years of doing something a certain way—having a cup of coffee first thing in the morning, staying up every evening to watch *The Late Show*—it's hard to change the pattern. Being able to maintain old routines and habits will make this move easier. (Actually, nursing homes are required to provide "reasonable accommodation of needs and preferences," so if your first few polite requests are denied, it's okay to become a bit insistent.)

Likewise, if your parent gets magazine subscriptions or likes certain newspapers, see if they can be delivered. Or if there are special foods she enjoys—her oatmeal every morning, her tea at 4—perhaps that too can be arranged.

- If a group of people helps with this move, space your departures so that your parent doesn't have to deal with one enormous good-bye. Later that day, the group might meet back at your house to give you some support at the end of what is bound to be a draining time.

• Be sure plans are made for follow-up visits and that your parent knows you will return soon.

A Plan of Care

Once your parent is admitted, a nursing home must conduct a full assessment of his physical, functional, social, mental, and emotional condition. Staff will examine his overall health, hearing, and vision, and his ability to perform "activities of daily living" (bathing, toileting, grooming, eating, walking), as well as his ability to communicate, understand, and remember. They should take note of his past, lifestyle, habits, hobbies, and relationships.

Ideally this assessment is done on the first or second day; by law, it must occur within 14 days of a resident's admission, or within the first 8 days if Medicare covers this stay. (Because Medicare covers only short-term, intensive nursing care, these residents are usually in more serious shape than others.)

The staff then has a week to put together a "plan of care" that outlines your parent's medical treatments; describes the therapy and nursing care he will receive; recommends activities he should or shouldn't do; and specifies his diet, exercise regimen, and general daily schedule.

The plan should be devised in a way that keeps your parent as active and independent as possible. It should be drafted by an interdisciplinary team that includes nurses, dietitians, social workers, rehabilitation and occupational therapists, members from the activities staff, and any others who play a role in your parent's daily care.

You, other family members, and, if possible, your parent should all be integrally involved in designing the plan of care. Ask that the conference take place when you can attend. Find out how much time has been scheduled for it. (It might last an hour or more.) Be sure ample time is set aside so that discussions are not hurried.

....

" One of her friends called me and said, 'She's just not thriving there. They are like cattle in stalls there.'

I thought, 'I'm doing the best I can. You haven't seen what I've seen.' Mom had been in so many different assisted living homes, rehab centers, hospitals, and nursing homes.

Those comments were hard for me. Her friends would not see her for months, and then they'd go and immediately be critical."

—Maggie B.

....

If your parent can't speak for him- self, be sure the staff understands his schedule, what gives him pleasure, what upsets him, what calms him down, what times and tasks are most confusing for him, and anything else that seems pertinent.

Get a written copy of the plan, and be sure it is specific and reflects your par- ent's needs and any of your concerns. When you visit, check to see that the plan is being followed.

A plan of care must be updated every three months or any time there is a change in your parent's physical or mental health.

Visiting

Visiting can be stressful and time- consuming, but remember, even if a visit is brief, even if your parent com- plains the whole time or forgets that you came or who you are, your presence is invaluable. It lets her know that you care and that she is not alone. It helps you keep tabs on how she is doing and any problems that exist. And it sends a message to the staff that you are moni- toring her care.

Here are a few visiting tips:

- Although nurses and aides can be helpful in letting you know when your parent needs a visit, don't routinely schedule your trips via the staff. By dropping in unexpectedly, you will be better able to monitor her care.

- Nursing homes often have posted vis- iting hours, but these do not apply to immediate family. The nursing home might want you to think that they do, but by law, relatives can visit whenever the resident wants them to. You might have to go someplace where you won't bother other residents or keep your parent's roommate awake. Visiting at unusual times lets you see what is happening when staffing is lean. Be respectful of any particular reasons for limiting visiting hours, but know your rights.

- Plan your visits around your parent's schedule. If you can avoid it, don't interrupt her naptime, a therapy ses- sion, or her favorite class.

- Visits can be short; in fact, short is often better. Your parent may tire easily. Thirty minutes may be plenty.

- If your visits are tense or uncomfort- able, do something new. Take your parent to lunch, help her write emails, take her for a drive, look through a photo album, or read a book aloud to her. If your parent has dementia, tour the home together (it will always be fairly new to her or she might forget that she showed you the place yesterday). You can also defuse tension

WHEN COMMUNICATION FAILS

When your parent cannot communicate, visits can become awkward. She is sitting hunched over in her wheelchair, staring blankly. You are trying vainly to make conversation, to find something to say. If you're squeezing this into a tight schedule, you may wonder why you bother.

Even if she seems oblivious, your parent is probably more aware of these visits than you think. She may not know it is you, but she will sense the presence of someone kind and familiar. She will hear your voice, smell your familiar scent, and feel your hand stroking hers. Your visits are probably very reassuring and calming, even though it may not seem so at times.

Come prepared with stories to tell—about your day, what's happening with friends and family members, goings-on about the town, memories and tales from the past—or bring a book or magazine article to read aloud. You might also bring some favorite music.

If she likes physical attention, brush her hair or put lotion on her. Speak slowly, explaining what you are doing, so you don't startle her. Touch her, but also let her touch things—your hands, your face, or perhaps a cat or new scarf. And if possible, get her outdoors to smell the fresh air and feel the sunshine.

Don't worry. She knows, on some level, that you are there.

by talking to other residents. That will help your parent make friends and allow her to show you off as well.

- Pamper her. If you are used to having a hand in your parent's physical care, don't hesitate to continue in that role. Fix her hair, help her put on makeup, rub her back, give her a manicure or a foot massage. Looking good always makes people feel better.

- Hugs are potent medicine, and nursing home residents are woefully lacking in warm physical contact. Unless your parent is uncomfortable with touch, go ahead and be close.

- Silence is okay. Sometimes just sitting with her, being in the room, is reassuring. Bring some work, a book, or some knitting and sit quietly with her.

- If your parent has trouble eating, visit during mealtimes and ask others to do the same. You can help her eat, and if you are eating too, she might eat more than she would otherwise.

- Bring the children, unless your parent specifically asks you not to. Children can be noisy, but they also radiate joy, spirit, and energy—things in short supply at a senior home.

> **"** She's forgetful and she doesn't have much to say, so conversations can get pretty boring. Now we read a book. After she's eaten, I read aloud for a while, which gives us something to talk about."
>
> —Carol P.

- Obviously, if you have a cold or the flu or some other contagious illness, postpone your visit until you are better, not simply to protect your parent, but to protect all of the residents.

- Try not to say you will visit at a certain time unless you are sure you can do so. Visits trigger a lot of excitement, and a canceled visit is a huge letdown. If you have to cancel, let her know as soon as possible, and reschedule. You might let the staff know of your parent's disappointment.

- Keep your parent up to date on what is happening with friends and family. News from the home front is gold. Photos and home videos are wonderful.

- Take a few minutes during a visit to review your parent's wardrobe. Does she need new clothing or shoes? If she's become less mobile or is confused (which makes dressing difficult), ask an aide who regularly cares for her if there is something that might

> " I was there every day and was very involved. I was demanding, but I tried to be diplomatic.
>
> It's hard because if you lose your temper, they might not directly take it out on your parent, but they are aware of it.
>
> One time one of the caregivers cut my mother's chin very badly. It was an accident, but it was upsetting. and it wasn't handled well. I felt they should have called the doctor, and I told them so.
>
> All in all they were good about taking care of her, but I think it's because I was a presence. In addition to visiting, I went to all the monthly meetings and talked to everyone."
>
> —Angela S.

make getting dressed easier, such as sneakers, slippers, a new robe, or elastic-waist pants.

- Use your visits to establish a rapport with the staff. Get to know them and let them know how much you appreciate their efforts.

Being an Advocate

You are your parent's number one advocate. You know her the best. You care the most. So don't be afraid to speak up.

Build a rapport with the people who care for your parent. Get to know them, and talk to them about who your parent was, her daily routines, her likes and

dislikes, and any tips that might make their job easier.

Obviously, you need to be alert to any signs of possible abuse or neglect: bruises or wounds, bedsores, soiled bedsheets, incontinence, poor hygiene, weight loss, excessive fear, delirium, diminished self-esteem.

AN EYE ON DEMENTIA

A failing memory is a cruel foe. Your parent may not remember that you visited and insist that you never come see him. He might yell at you when you arrive and argue that you should leave. Do not be dissuaded. It is more important than ever that you advocate for him now.

He might not be able to tell you what's wrong, so be aware of mood shifts and changes in behavior that might signal trouble. Look out for anxiety and distress, sores and bruises, weight loss, poor hygiene and grooming, and other signs of poor care or even abuse.

New approaches to dementia have shown a variety of ways—ways that do not involve restraints or sedation—to ease anxiety, agitation, outbursts, and hostility. (See Chapter 23 for more on dementia.)

When you visit, understand how hard this is for the staff, show your appreciation of anything done well, and help them find ways to assist him. Tell them what he once enjoyed, and remind them of particular needs, quirks, and preferences. What is the best way to calm him? What schedule works best for him? What triggers anger and agitation?

As for his forgetting your visits, you can mark a calendar with your visits, but don't push your parent to remember something that he can't. What difference does it make, really, if he knows when he last saw you? Live in the present with him. And ignore any urge to visit less. Your advocacy is absolutely critical now that he can't fend for himself, and your presence is reassuring, whether he lets you know that or not.

Be alert to dangers if your parent is at any risk of falling (which most elderly people are). Check his room for such things as a slippery floor, lack of grab bars, anything that might trip him up or leave him unsupported.

Stay abreast of those ailments that are often overlooked or not adequately treated in nursing homes, such as vision and hearing problems, bedsores, incontinence, malnutrition, dehydration, insomnia, and overmedication.

Be aware of depression, as it is very common in nursing home residents and often ignored. A brief grieving period after this move is normal, but if it goes on for more than a few weeks, talk to your parent's doctor. Feeling hopeless and lethargic, losing weight, and a change in sleep habits are *not* normal parts of aging. They require attention and treatment.

Ask the staff to notify you immediately if your parent falls, becomes ill, seems depressed, or requires a change in treatment or medications.

Let them know when you have other, perhaps less urgent, concerns, as well. If your father's roommate keeps him up at night, if he doesn't like the food, if he isn't getting outdoors, talk to the staff.

Even if your parent is very frail, immobile, and suffering from severe dementia, he should get fresh air, proper nutrition, stimulation, and some exercise. Talk to the activities director about options. Your parent should not be alone, staring at a television screen all day.

If your mother used to have a particular interest, say, in gardening, talk with the activities director about how she might become engaged in some relevant task. Even if she is simply moving dirt around from pot to pot and replanting plants, it might make her feel useful. If your father is lucid but his days are meaningless, ask if he can visit people in the infirmary, read to residents whose eyesight is poor, help in the gift shop, or deliver flowers or mail to others. It's amazing how a little giving can lift the spirits.

Also, be sure that your parent is treated with respect and that he has some privacy, as these are vital to self-esteem yet are so often lacking in communal living situations. If your mother is uncomfortable about having strangers help her dress or bathe, see if the job might be limited to one or two regular attendants whom she likes. They might drape towels in such a way that she retains her dignity. If your father would prefer to be called Mr. Austin rather than Honey, let them know.

Two Golden Rules

1. As an advocate, you have to strike a balance between advocating assertively and supporting those who care for your parent—no easy task.

Certainly you should expect, and demand, reasonable care, and you should be outspoken when care is lacking. If you run into barriers, take an issue to the next step on the hierarchy.

But keep in mind, many people working in nursing homes have almost no training, receive low wages, and have far more work than they can handle. And it is no small task caring for elderly people who have complicated emotional, physical, and medical needs.

It can work in your favor to develop a rapport with those who care for your parent. Ask them about their own families and lives, and let them know that you are sympathetic to the pressures they face. They will usually show your parent the same kindness, understanding, and respect that you show them.

When someone makes a special effort or is especially kind, be sure to thank him or her. If you want to go a

CLARITY WHEN IT'S CRUCIAL

Be sure any essential instructions are very, very clear. You'll want to do this in any case, but when you can't visit often, it is especially important to do whatever you can to avoid mix-ups. Regulations protecting patient privacy might prohibit posting some signs in a clearly visible place, but usually a family can get permission to leave important reminders somewhere in the room. ("Mr. Potter is lactose intolerant" might be okay where people walking past his room can see it, but "Mrs. Miller is incontinent and needs to be taken to the bathroom every two hours" probably needs to be kept discreet.)

step further, give the person a small gift and send a letter of praise to a supervisor. Typically, tipping is not allowed, but the family council might pool contributions for staff gifts.

When you have a concern, rather than barking orders, work together with the staff to find solutions or resolve problems. Staff members can often make adjustments once they are made aware of a problem, but they will do so more readily, and care about your parent and your family more genuinely, if you show them respect. Have patience and a sense of humor about any minor mishaps.

It's difficult to let go of a parent's care. It's hard not to constantly correct and criticize those who now care for your parent, because of course they are not doing it as you would. But you aren't taking care of your parent day in and day out. They are. Try not to take out your grief and pain on an overworked aide.

2. Choose one person from your family to act as a spokesperson. You don't want a

> " There were a couple of very bad months at first. I spoke to the social worker at the home, and she asked me if I could hire a part-time aide to help my father adjust. Because he was on Medicaid, this wasn't really aboveboard— he would have been cut off if they knew we were paying for private care—but we did it anyway. And it succeeded beyond our expectations. The place became a home for him. He joked with the aides and nurses, and they treated him with affection."
>
> —Lillian R.

phone call from your brother to jeopardize an understanding you have carefully developed with an aide, or a comment from your sister to wreck a special menu you have worked out with the dietitian. Talk among yourselves and agree on a plan. Then have one spokesperson. This is easier for nurses and aides, and it reduces the possibility of mix-ups.

Long-Distance Caregiving

If you cannot visit your parent regularly, find someone who can. Talk with relatives and friends, and find out about any local volunteer visitors. A social worker from the nursing home, the state long-term care ombudsman, or a local consumer advocacy group should be able to tell you about volunteers and groups that visit the facility.

If you cannot find volunteers, consider hiring someone to visit on a regular basis and keep tabs on your parent's care. This is expensive, but if you can afford it, it's a worthwhile investment.

Ask a nurse supervisor how to stay in touch with the staff and find out the best times to call to get regular updates on your parent's care and condition. Try to create a relationship with one or two nurses or aides who see your parent regularly. You want to find someone whom you trust and who is sympathetic to your situation.

You might also contact the nursing home's family and/or resident council, which represents the needs and concerns of residents and their families. An active council should keep you abreast of what's happening in the home and might be able to find families who are willing to check in with your parent when they are visiting.

Lots of calls, even short ones, can fend off the loneliness your parent may

be feeling now. Send her a video of you and others in the family. If she can use the Internet, email notes and photos of yourself and grandchildren regularly. If possible, get her to video chat. Even if you connect while you're cooking dinner or doing chores, it will give her a sense of being with you, to some degree.

Send pictures drawn by grandchildren, care packages of special foods, or small gifts. Send jokes or cartoons, short articles you enjoyed, recipes you just made—anything so that there is a constant flow of communication. Even if she can't remember people, she will know someone cares.

Granny Cams

Sometimes families who are far away or busy at work want to install webcams—also known, in this case, as "granny cams"—in their parent's room. This way, a view of the room is available to you, at any time, on the Internet.

States have various laws about the cameras, and nursing homes have their own policies. Generally, you cannot install a granny cam without the permission of your parent and any roommates.

Of course, you have to consider your parent's right to privacy—is this something she agrees to, or would agree to if she were competent? Also, consider the practical value of a granny cam: Your parent is not always going to be within the camera's view. And it might create some animosity between you and the staff.

Use your best judgment and, if possible, discuss it with your parent, any roommate, and the staff.

> " When my mother stopped recognizing me, I visited less often, not because I thought she didn't know the difference, but because it was so hard for me. To have her turn and look blankly at me, to have her ask, 'Who is this woman in my room?' was very painful. I used to shout, 'Mom, it's Nancy!' and then be depressed for days after the visit.
>
> Then I discovered something that helps. When I visit, we look through an old photo album together. It is filled with pictures of her and her brothers when they were little. She doesn't have any idea who I am, but she knows who they are, and I see how it comforts her to tell me about them.
>
> For that one hour, she is a child again, living in a brown house in Richmond, Indiana, with a great big slide in the yard and two fun-loving brothers, and I think she is happy."
>
> —Nancy S.

When Trouble Brews

When you notice a problem, bring it to the attention of the staff as soon as possible. First, talk with the person directly involved—the aide who has repeatedly left your parent sitting unattended or who fails to change his wet sheets.

Once again, when raising a problem with a member of the staff, be patient and understanding of the demands on his or her time. Try to be helpful rather than reproachful at this stage. The worker may not even know that the problem existed.

Be specific about your concerns. Explain what you've noticed and when the problem occurred. Then listen to the staff member's thoughts on why this is happening and what might be done to resolve the matter.

If the problem is not resolved, talk to an immediate supervisor, again, being as specific as you can. If you still hit a roadblock, move on up the ladder, from the aide to the nursing supervisor or medical director, to an administrator, until you get results.

Be calm and respectful when you deal with each person, but remain firm in your resolve. Being rude, critical, or otherwise difficult might adversely affect your parent's care and future rapport with the staff, but reasonable complaints that are thoughtfully registered should not. In fact, once the staff realizes that you are not turning your back on the situation, your parent should receive better care.

Throughout the process, document everything. Keep notes on what happened and when, with whom you spoke, when you spoke with them, and what their responses were. Follow up phone calls with letters or emails, and request a written response. This assures that any agreement is clear, and it gives you backing in case the problem is repeated or becomes more serious.

If there is no resolution from the staff and administration, look into

> " After her stroke, my mother was moved from assisted living to the nursing home wing, which was hard for her, especially because she had to eat in a different dining room and most of the people in there had dementia. They were totally gone, being spoon-fed.
>
> I asked the head of the dining services if Mom could eat in the main dining room, with her pals, and she said no because they had to watch her, they had to be sure she ate certain things, drank enough fluids, that she didn't choke.
>
> I was trying really hard to remain calm, but I was going crazy. Mom wasn't eating; she was losing weight and getting depressed. But this woman wouldn't back down.
>
> So, I went to the vice president of the facility. I was armed for a fight. But within two minutes, he said, 'Of course she can eat wherever she likes.' And that was all it took."
>
> —Gina R.

the facility's grievance procedure and file a formal complaint. By law, all nursing homes are required to have such a procedure.

Also, talk with members of any resident or family council. Some are more helpful than others, but they should be alerted to complaints or problems. Most will at least advise you on how to proceed, and if several residents are affected, they should take action to address the problem.

Outside Help

If the problem is not resolved from within the nursing home, or if a problem is dire, go outside for help.

LONG-TERM CARE OMBUDSMEN are required by law to investigate all complaints, and if they can't resolve a problem, they will find an agency that can. Sometimes they will file lawsuits on behalf of residents.

The ombudsman can also explain laws and your family's rights, and can advise you on how to proceed with a particular problem. (To find the local ombudsman, go to ltcombudsman.org.)

THE STATE SURVEY AGENCY, which licenses and certifies nursing homes and conducts regular inspections, must, by federal law, investigate any dire situation (one in which a resident is in immediate danger) within two working days. (The long-term care ombudsman has contact information for the state survey agency.)

Unfortunately, less pressing complaints might not be investigated until the next time the residence is inspected, which could be months away. If the problem is recurring or affecting a number of

residents, be persistent. Get other families to file a complaint as well. There is power in numbers.

THE NATIONAL CONSUMER VOICE FOR QUALITY LONG-TERM CARE (theconsumervoice.org) has a lot of good information about residents' rights and laws. They also have a list of local advocacy groups.

CITIZEN ADVOCACY GROUPS monitor nursing homes within certain areas or states, and can provide families with some guidance about how to proceed when there is trouble. You can find one at theconsumervoice.org/advocate/cag.

See page 448 for information on what to do when you suspect abuse, neglect, or exploitation.

Restraining Restraints

Can you imagine being strapped down to a bed, your arms lashed to the rails, unable to move? Or how about being fed drugs that make you so dopey that you can't have a lucid thought, never mind that they are likely to kill you?

Nursing homes have been ordered by Congress, alerted by doctors, and warned by the Centers for Medicare and Medicaid Services to stop using restraints—physical and chemical means of controlling patients—except in the most unusual circumstances. Nevertheless, many facilities continue the practice. Know what to look for and how to keep your parent free from restraints.

Restraints are generally used on people with dementia who are considered difficult—hostile, aggressive, anxious, agitated—or are apt to wander.

They are also used on residents who have fallen or are deemed to be at risk of falling (falling down, sliding out of a chair, or rolling out of bed).

Physical restraints include everything from full-body vests to straps (used to tie someone's arms down) to innocuous-looking wheelchair trays that basically prevent a person from sliding down or getting up. Chemical restraints include tranquilizers, anti-anxiety drugs, antidepressants, sedatives, and hypnotics.

Any restraint is dehumanizing and dangerous. The drugs not only throw a person into limbo, but often worsen any behavioral problems and cause confusion, agitation, delirium, insomnia, hypertension, loss of appetite, and even death.

As you might imagine, physical restraints cause anxiety, depression, agitation, and isolation, but they also cause bedsores, constipation, poor circulation, incontinence, infections, and loss of appetite, among other things. Ironically, although they are used to prevent injuries, these restraints can lead to injuries, sometimes very serious injuries, when a person, in a state of panic, tries to escape or simply tries to get up in the middle of the night.

Indeed, restraining a person is usually more dangerous than leaving him be. And although restraints are largely intended to make life easier for the staff, people who are restrained often require more time, not less, from nurses, when compared with similar residents who are not restrained.

Residents of nursing homes generally do better in terms of falls, agitation, and unruly behavior when:

- their basic needs are met

- any pain or discomfort is treated

- they are allowed to operate on their own schedules

- they have friends and companionship

- they are involved in activities they enjoy

- they get outdoors regularly

- they get plenty of exercise

- they have ample opportunities to use the toilet

- they live in a safe environment

With a little training, ingenuity, and common sense, risks can be reduced so that falls don't happen or, if they do, they are not terribly harmful. Accidents can be prevented through exercise (which improves balance and strength, and relieves agitation and insomnia), the use of supportive shoes, lower beds and chairs, better lighting, clear pathways, handrails, sensors and alarms (that let the staff know when someone is trying to get up), and walkers.

Simply anticipating residents' needs can prevent accidents. For example, if your father always has to go to the bathroom right after lunch, then an aide should have that on the schedule so your father isn't trying to get up on his own.

Chemical restraints (antipsychotics and other medications) are more difficult to monitor because there can be many reasons for prescribing various medications. Know what medications your parent is on and why. If he seems unusually groggy or inattentive, find out if there has been any change in medications and why he might be acting this way.

Talk to the staff about the true risks of any behavior (is his pacing or hooting actually endangering anyone?) and what nondrug interventions have been tried. Brainstorm with them about what more can be done that doesn't include medicating your parent. If a drug is necessary to treat an ailment, be sure it is the lowest dose possible and that it is used for the shortest amount of time possible. But continue to try other approaches as well.

On the rare occasion when falls or serious behavioral problems cannot be avoided without restraints (and this is highly unusual), weigh the risks and benefits of the situation. Your instinct may be to protect your parent at all costs, but remember that it is usually better to risk a minor fall than to have your parent restrained and risk more serious injuries and complications.

If your parent is threatening the safety of others, talk with the doctor about any medical issues that might be triggering the behavior, and talk to a nurse or social worker about any unmet

" One of the aides, whom my mother loved, had heard a rumor that I had complained about her. I hadn't, but it took over a year to break down this barrier. I said to one of the home's social workers, 'Look, if she wants to be angry with me, fine. I can take it. I just don't want her to be angry with my mother.'

I tried very hard to mend the fences because I knew that much of the quality of my mother's care depended on what they thought of me."

—Barbara F.

need your parent might be trying to communicate (he's hungry or tired or in pain and doesn't know how to relay this information, so he becomes angry or aggressive). There may be ways to make him feel more comfortable and less threatened.

Restraints can be used only under a doctor's order, and your parent, or you, can refuse them even if a doctor recommends them.

Neglect, Abuse, and Exploitation

Physical and emotional abuse and neglect, financial exploitation, and theft occur with shocking frequency, especially when residents are too sick or confused to fend for themselves and families are not able to visit regularly. Be alert to signs of trouble and act immediately. Don't ignore subtle warning signs.

Again, visit often or have others check in, and do so unexpectedly. Lock up valuables and hide cash. Be sure that no one has (or can get) access to a checkbook or banking PINs or passwords. Anyone named as your parent's power of attorney should review bank statements occasionally to make sure nothing unusual is happening.

Ask about any unusual marks or bruises. (If your parent has fallen or otherwise been injured, you should have been notified immediately.)

If your parent has dementia, note changes in his behavior—accusations, fear, agitation, or outbursts, for example. Try to ascertain whether there might be a reason for his distrust and anxiety.

Obviously, any sort of hitting, shoving, pinching, slapping, or other such attacks are unacceptable, but a person doesn't have to touch your parent to be abusive. Saying things that make him feel threatened, demeaned, or afraid also constitutes abuse. Exploiting him financially is abuse as well.

Isolating a person, ignoring his physical or emotional needs, or failing to keep him safe, clean, fed, and toileted all constitute neglect. It is neglectful to repeatedly ignore a resident's call bell, to fail to reposition her to avoid bedsores, to fail to help her eat and drink, or to leave her to walk unassisted when she needs help.

However, unlike abuse, neglect may not be intentional. Staff might not have time to help or know how to help. Sometimes the problem can be remedied simply by talking to these caregivers.

Abuse, on the other hand, requires immediate and aggressive action. If there is any question at all of danger, get your parent out of the situation right away or ask that the person or people responsible be removed from your parent's care immediately.

Document any problems in writing and be specific about when, where, and what happened and who was involved. Alert the staff supervisor, the director of the home, and the doctor. Contact the local ombudsman, the local adult protective services agency, the nursing home licensing agency, and the citizens' advocacy group. If any physical assault, theft, or other crime has occurred, call the police.

Unwanted Room Changes and Discharges

Could your father suddenly be evicted or transferred out of his nursing home? It shouldn't happen, but it does.

Nursing homes can legally discharge or transfer residents who, after reasonable notice, fail to pay their bills. They can also discharge residents who go on Medicaid if the home is not fully certified and has no specially earmarked "Medicaid beds" available. (However, if the home is fully certified, it cannot evict residents who become Medicaid eligible.)

Nursing homes can also discharge residents or transfer them to another facility if the resident no longer needs nursing home care, if the nursing home closes, if the facility cannot meet the resident's needs, or if the resident presents a danger to himself or others.

These last two reasons really should not be an issue, as nursing homes, by nature, provide complex care and should be able to adjust that care and implement plans to meet the needs of almost any resident.

Unfortunately, nursing homes occasionally use these reasons to get rid of residents who are difficult, who have families who are seen as difficult, or who are switching to Medicaid, which means less income for the nursing home.

Before notifying a family and resident of any plans for discharge, the nursing home must make some real effort to meet the needs of the resident or alleviate any troubling behavioral symptoms through a plan of care. If, after this effort has been made, a resident is to be transferred to another nursing home or simply discharged, the nursing home must give 30 days' notice (except in some unusual circumstances). It must explain, in writing, why the resident is being transferred, where the resident will go, and when the move will occur.

This written notification must also include information about how to appeal the decision. States have different rules about discharge and transfer; contact the long-term care ombudsman if you need guidance.

Is This Move Working?

Your mother's belongings are in place, her room is relatively comfortable, the staff is reasonably good, and you have both settled into a new routine. But she seems unhappy. Her health has deteriorated. She is more confused than before, and she complains endlessly. Was this the right thing to do?

Give it time. People (elderly or not) usually need at least six months, and often longer, to adjust to a new environment, a new routine, and new relationships. There are often setbacks early on, but your parent is likely to adapt with time.

If your parent's complaints are vague, help him be specific. Is there something he needs or wants, or does he simply need to air his fears and worries? Once you've discussed his complaints and addressed any concrete problems, ask your parent to think of three things he likes about this new home. Redirecting his attention to the positive aspects of this move might take his mind off the less desirable factors, at least temporarily.

If you are not sure whether or not your parent is okay, keep these realities in mind:

- Nursing home residents sometimes complain bitterly and appear depressed when visitors are around and then, as soon as the guests are gone, return to activities, friends, and a more pleasant mood. If there is a staff member who has a good rapport with your parent, ask how your parent's mood changes with your visits. If your father simply needs to complain and you are an easy target, let him. Just be aware that you are getting all the bad news and none of the

ⓘ FOR MORE HELP

National Long-Term Care Ombudsman Resource Center
ltcombudsman.org
202-332-2275

....

The National Consumer Voice for Quality Long-Term Care
theconsumervoice.org
202-332-2275

....

The National Center on Elder Abuse
ncea.aoa.gov
855-500-3537

good. Take his complaints with a grain of salt.

- If your mother appears worse each time you visit, it may not be that her condition is rapidly deteriorating, but simply that you are more aware of her decline because you are seeing her less often than you used to.

- Adult children often project their own emotions onto parents they have placed in nursing homes. Who is really unhappy, your parent or you? You may not like seeing her in a nursing home, but given her age and infirmities, she may be doing just fine.

If, after you've given it some time, things are not working, ask for a team meeting with a nurse, a social worker, the activities director, and anyone else necessary. See if you can come up with a game plan. Talk with the long-term care ombudsman and see if he or she has some suggestions.

If nothing works, then it is time to explore other options. While a second move isn't ideal, sometimes it's necessary.

❝ At first my father didn't want to stay, and he kept trying to leave. The staff was kind and understanding about it, but we were really afraid that they would decide that he couldn't stay. He was angry and demanding a lot of the time, he was notoriously picky about what he ate, and he complained about everything. The staff told me not to worry, that he would adjust, but I couldn't believe it. I was sure he would wear them out, and then what would we do? I also felt like a monster for leaving him there, because he seemed so miserable.

About two months after his move, I went to see him and arrived to find him all smiling and happy. I have never been so grateful to anyone in my life as I was to the nurses who were so patient and good to him. They never suggested medicating him or made me feel that he was in any way a burden. It's odd. You love these people, these strangers, who care so tenderly for your parent, who do what you wish you could do. They become your friends, and you want to do good things for them.❞

—Brenda S.

When They
Forget

Chapter 23

The Aging Brain

What Is Normal? • Mild Cognitive Impairment • Dementia •
Getting Tested • Alzheimer's Disease • Vascular Dementia •
Lewy Body Dementia • Dealing with the Diagnosis •
Treating Dementia

A pile of unopened bills sits on your mother's desk, which is odd because she's always been extremely organized about paying bills. Now that you think about it, you've noticed a number of unusual things about her recently. She missed a lunch date with you. There was that silly incident over the dog that got her so upset. And last week she called and asked you to come over right away, but when you got there, she couldn't remember what was so urgent. In fact, she couldn't even remember calling you.

A cold wave passes through you. *Could it be . . . ?*

When memory fades, the possibility of Alzheimer's disease looms ominously, and for good reason—it's a road no one wants to walk. But don't immediately assume that your parent's waning retention is because of irreversible brain disease. Mild forgetfulness and confusion may be benign side effects of old age and mental inactivity, or they may be the by-product of grief, hearing loss, overmedication, infection, or some other treatable problem.

So before you drop off your parent at the nearest nursing home, get her to a doctor who is well versed in such matters. Find out what's wrong, what's treatable, and how to proceed.

Even if the symptoms are caused by Alzheimer's or some other type of dementia, life is not over. It has taken a dramatic turn, yes, but it's not over. It's time to make plans, learn new approaches, and address any issues that are compounding your parent's problems. If you can take a deep breath and remain calm, you can help both yourself and your parent through this journey.

What Is Normal?

The human brain, a chunk of firm jelly weighing about three pounds, is made up of a hundred billion nerve cells, all interconnected to form an elaborate communications web. But just as skin sags and bellies protrude, this fabulous control center reflects its age.

Up to half of people over 65 say they have more trouble remembering things than they used to. (And plenty of people over 50 say exactly the same thing.) But a little forgetfulness is nothing to worry about. Given enough time, healthy people in their 70s can do just as well as young people on memory tests.

Although the effects of time on the brain might be unsettling and inconvenient (as you search, once again, for your glasses only to find they are on top of your head), they are generally inconsequential. People might need an extra few minutes to remember a person's name or what it is they came into the kitchen to get; they might have a little trouble balancing a checkbook or following a long story. Despite these minor hiccups, most people remain sharp, imaginative, and productive.

> " Mom would forget something on the stove, or forget what she just did, and I'd think, 'Well, she's getting older. Maybe I'm just looking for problems.' But finally I said, 'No, something is not right.'
>
> She would wear the same clothes over and over and not care if she took a shower or washed her hair, which is really out of character, because she used to be immaculate. She would say, 'No, I didn't wear this yesterday,' or 'I washed them,' when I knew she hadn't."
>
> —Linda K.

MEDICATION WARNING

Overmedication can cause confusion and memory loss, and will certainly worsen any dementia, so be sure that any medications your parent takes are absolutely necessary.

In particular, some commonly used drugs, known as anticholinergics, interfere with an important chemical in the brain, acetylcholine, which is involved in thinking and memory. These drugs, which have been linked to cognitive impairment and memory loss, include ones frequently used to treat pain, colds, depression, asthma, insomnia, motion sickness, and incontinence.

Talk with your parent's doctor about her medications, and keep all medications to a minimum, even over-the-counter drugs.

After 80, almost everyone experiences some decline in memory (primarily forgetting names and words), as well as a dip in mathematical, verbal, and spatial skills. They might have trouble multitasking or returning to a task after an interruption. They process information more slowly, and their reactions are delayed (which explains some fender benders). This is what doctors often refer to as "age-associated memory impairment" (or "age-related memory impairment").

Although the passage of time is largely to blame, other issues that are common in old age certainly play a role—the use of certain medications, hearing loss, and grief, to name a few.

Sometimes brains shift into low gear simply because they are less active. If a vibrant, brilliant man loses his job and has little to do all day but stare at a television, his mental engine is bound to slip into idle.

Ironically, overstimulation can have the same effect. If your son tells you something while the TV is on, your phone is buzzing, and you are wondering if there is anything in the fridge that can be turned into dinner, you may very well look at him blankly when he later says, "I told you all of this already!" The younger generation has become adept at juggling the sensory overload of the technology age, but for our parents (and for many of us), it's a cerebral nightmare.

The bottom line: A little brain slippage is nothing to fret about.

Mild Cognitive Impairment

Somewhere on the scale between normal aging and dementia is what's known as mild cognitive impairment, or MCI. A person with mild cognitive impairment isn't simply forgetting the occasional name or where she put her keys; she is forgetting more substantial information, the stuff she would normally remember—appointments, conversations, an anniversary, a favorite recipe, an address. She might show poor judgment, get lost in a familiar place, and have trouble with complex situations, such as multitasking, understanding a complex plot, or following lengthy instructions.

Despite these problems, a person with MCI can get along just fine on her own, and usually only those in her inner circle will notice the gaffes.

Unfortunately, people with mild cognitive impairment have a higher risk of developing full-blown dementia. (Estimates suggest that 50 to 60 percent of people with MCI will go on to develop dementia eventually.) But don't panic. First of all, that means that nearly half of this group will *not* develop dementia. Also, many people who think they have MCI are just struggling with normal aging issues and worrying needlessly. Some are mistakenly given a diagnosis of MCI.

Keep an eye on what's happening with your parent, and talk with her doctor about any issues that might be causing or exacerbating any memory loss and confusion, such as the following:

- poor vision

- hearing loss (he can't remember what he didn't hear)

- medications (including many over-the-counter drugs)

- isolation and boredom

- illness and infection

- high blood pressure and/or cholesterol

- vitamin deficiencies, particularly B12

- thyroid problems

- dehydration

- use of alcohol or tobacco

- depression

- stress and anxiety

- insomnia or sleep apnea

Coping with MCI

Be patient. Although it may be hard to avoid, berating or embarrassing your parent for his lapses is not helpful. Try to remember that it's not his fault; he cannot try harder or think differently.

What he can do is use calendars, alarms, labels, notes, lists, and reminders. Get your parent a calendar or day planner that he can take with him everywhere. If he uses a smartphone, he should sync his calendars and set it up to give him reminders.

Stow important information—key addresses and phone numbers—in his wallet. Or, if possible, plug them into his smartphone, so he has the information he needs at his fingertips all the time.

Being organized and systematic will help as well. Store often-lost items such as keys, the remote, glasses, or a wallet in one, fixed location. Have a routine.

At this early stage, most people can learn ways to effectively use the memory that remains. For example, sometimes simply saying important things aloud and then repeating them—really focusing on the information—helps. So when you say, "I'll pick you up at 11," your parent should not just nod, but instead should look at you and say, "Yes, you will pick me up at 11." You can help with this by asking your parent to repeat information, several times if necessary.

> ❝ I'd come to visit and see that her bills were still in envelopes and they were written on. For example, it would say, 'electric bill.' I could see she had tried to file it, but she was having trouble. And she'd always been good with her bills."
>
> —Angela S.

Likewise, when your parent gets up to get a sweater, he might actually say it aloud—"I'm going upstairs to get my sweater." (Then he'll be less apt to forget what he's doing halfway down the hall.)

Help your parent find some humor in his slipups. Ignore some mistakes. And assure him that mild forgetfulness is nothing to be overly concerned about. Worrying excessively about memory loss, and becoming despondent because your loved ones are annoyed with you, will only exacerbate the problem.

Stay calm and hope for the best. But, as always, plan ahead. Think about what will happen if his mind slides further, and be prepared just in case.

Dementia

The word *dementia* comes from the Latin *de*, meaning "without," and *mens*, which means "mind." Dementia is not a specific illness, but rather a group of symptoms that have many causes, in the same way a fever and chills may be caused by the flu, meningitis, or malaria.

The hallmark of dementia is severe memory loss (especially short-term, or recent, memory); people forget what you've told them, what they did yesterday, or where they are going, for example. Other symptoms include confusion, poor judgment, disorientation, personality changes, and difficulty with language and math. People get lost, words get jumbled, and bills go unpaid. Higher function, also known as frontal lobe or executive function, may also decline, making it harder for a person to plan, self-regulate, or filter stimuli.

Dementia is not an inevitable part of aging; it is the result of a disease or injury. It is, however, common in the elderly, especially in the very old. It's estimated that 12 to 15 percent of people over 70 have dementia. The rates increase with age, approaching almost 40 percent for people over 90.

Causes

About 70 percent of all cases of dementia are the result of Alzheimer's disease. About 20 to 30 percent are caused by small, imperceptible strokes or other conditions that affect blood flow to the brain—something known as vascular dementia. Another 10 to 25 percent of cases (depending upon which studies you read) involve something known as Lewy body dementia.

Other types and causes of dementia include frontotemporal dementia, which causes personality changes and is often diagnosed in younger people (ages 40 to 70); normal pressure hydrocephalus, an often treatable illness in which spinal fluid builds up in the brain, causing memory loss, incontinence, and an unusual, shuffling gait; alcoholism; HIV infection; and Creutzfeldt-Jakob, Huntington's, and Parkinson's disease.

The numbers don't add up because medicine, particularly geriatrics, is rarely neat and tidy. In the case of dementia, there's often more than one villain mucking about in the brain. Alzheimer's and vascular disease frequently occur in combination, and Lewy body dementia often coexists with other illness, making it unclear exactly what is causing what or where the trouble began.

And noted in the previous section, a host of other issues cause confusion (sometimes referred to as pseudodementia) and will compound any existing dementia.

Symptoms of Dementia

Although short-term memory loss and confusion are the trademark symptoms of dementia, any changes in a person's normal habits and behaviors are suspect. Typically, symptoms are persistent and grow steadily worse. A change in environment and routine often compounds the problems.

Here are some of the most common symptoms:

MEMORY LOSS. Dates, events, and conversations, especially recent ones, are forgotten. People insist you never told them something and ask for the same information over and over.

CONFUSION. Everyday tasks, such as cleaning the kitchen, following a recipe, or paying the bills, are suddenly challenging.

DISORIENTATION. People get lost in familiar places, or forget where they are and how they got there.

LOSING THINGS. People not only lose things, but can't retrace their steps to find them. They have no clue where the lost item might be or when they last saw it. Because items seem to vanish, they sometimes accuse others of stealing.

POOR GROOMING. Personal hygiene is neglected, and clothing may be soiled or inappropriate for an event or the weather.

PERSONALITY CHANGES. People are "not themselves." They become uncharacteristically angry, agitated, fearful, rude, or worried. As the world becomes more challenging and losses become more evident, depression and anxiety are common.

LANGUAGE DIFFICULTY. Words are forgotten, misused, or garbled. Instead of saying "car keys," a person might say, "the thing you use to start up the car," or he might say "car kreys."

MATH AND MONEY TROUBLES. Counting, calculating a tip, or balancing a checkbook is a challenge.

POOR JUDGMENT. People often make unsafe, unwise, or unusual decisions.

TIME CONFUSION. People often get confused about the day, month, year, or season. They have trouble grasping how long ago something occurred or the idea of something happening in the future (such as a visit that won't happen for several weeks).

REPETITION. A person says or does the same thing over and over.

VISUAL AND SPATIAL CHALLENGES. People may have difficulty judging distances or seeing contrasts clearly.

TROUBLE CONCENTRATING. A person might have trouble following a conversation or get lost while telling a story.

WITHDRAWAL. For all of the above reasons, a person with dementia will often decline invitations and avoid social situations.

LESS COMMON SYMPTOMS

People with dementia sometimes lose their sense of etiquette and social norms, their inhibitions, and sometimes, their compassion and empathy. As a result, they might suddenly tell off-color jokes or make lewd or bigoted comments. They might become rude or mean. They sometimes embarrass others and don't understand why the person is embarrassed, or they do something and feel no embarrassment themselves.

A parent who has always been intensely honest might suddenly start telling lies because he actually doesn't remember the facts, because he is covering up for his forgetfulness, or because his moral compass and sense of empathy are askew.

A few more unusual clues that dementia might be at play:

- Your parent tries to eat things that aren't food, such as wax fruit or napkin rings that are on the dinner table. (*I know I sat down here to eat something.*)

- He's falling, stumbling, and tripping a lot. (This is caused by something known as progressive supranuclear palsy.)

- He doesn't get jokes or sarcasm anymore.

- He starts hoarding or shopping compulsively or becomes obsessive in other ways. This might be because he forgot that he just bought jam yesterday (and the day before that), or he might be trying to gain control over a world that is increasing illogical.

- He stares off or looks sort of glassy-eyed. People in the early stages of dementia sometimes lose the ability to move their eyes easily, something called "reduced gaze."

Dementia or Old Age?

In the early stages, it is difficult to distinguish between dementia and benign memory loss. The symptoms of dementia can be fairly innocuous at first, and most people compensate for minor mental slipups with reminders and notes, or find excuses for their errors. *Oh, I'm sorry about our date. I was sure we said Tuesday.*

Social skills are sometimes the last to go, so during short visits a person with early dementia may seem perfectly fine. He may chat about old times and remember who's who and what's happening. Family members and friends, who don't like to think that anything is wrong, are happy to dismiss a disheveled appearance or a few memory lapses.

At some point, however, the problems become hard to ignore. The dementia begins to interfere with relationships and the details of daily life, such as shopping, paying bills, making meals, or selecting clothing.

Your parent might get lost, make poor financial decisions, or lose a particular skill—an avid crossword puzzle fan may have trouble filling in the blanks, or a lifetime golfer may fumble about while selecting the proper club.

NOT JUST FORGETFUL

In dementia, memories aren't simply forgotten; they are lost. Normal memory lapses *(Where did I put my keys?)* become gaping memory voids. People don't forget something, rack their brains, and then—*Aha!*—remember it. Instead, they have no sense that something was forgotten; the information is gone, along with any recollection that it once existed.

For example, you might come out of the mall and think, *Hmm, where did I put the car?* and after a moment have some vague recollection of parking near the Macy's entrance, but someone with dementia might walk out and have absolutely no sense of how she got to the mall. Having no memory of driving herself, she is apt to become frightened

(How did I get here? How do I get home?) or angry *(I know I didn't drive here, so Marty must have dropped me off. Why isn't he here to pick me up?).*

A person doesn't just forget what you said; she forgets speaking to you at all. She doesn't simply miss an appointment; she insists she never had one. She doesn't simply forget the name of the movie she saw; she forgets that she went to a movie.

Because someone with early dementia still retains long-term memories, he might tell vivid stories from his youth or recount things in detail that happened two years ago. He simply cannot remember recent events—what he had for breakfast (or that he ate breakfast), what he did yesterday, whom he spoke with on the phone, what you told him last week or even an hour ago.

As a result, a person might ask the same question over and over again, making you irate, *Mom, I've told you this four times already! We are leaving for lunch at 11:30!*

When you try to jog your parent's memory—*Remember, I came over yesterday and we talked about going to Aunt Carol's today?*—it doesn't trigger anything. (She might pretend she remembers, however.)

As memories and abilities slip away, your parent might, understandably, become anxious. The world makes no sense anymore. He feels lost. People are angry with him. He's failing on several fronts, but he's not sure why. And it's terrifying.

Your parent might also become accusatory. *If I left my glasses by the bed and they aren't there now, then somebody must have stolen them. If I have no recollection that we were supposed to get together, it's because you forgot to tell me.*

> " At first Dad forgot the obvious stuff. He'd lose his reading glasses or forget something you told him.
>
> Then one day, he was driving and completely forgot why he was in the car and where he was going.
>
> He'd dropped some papers off for a client and had no recollection of doing it."
>
> —Sam K.

Getting Tested

If you suspect dementia, urge your parent to consult her doctor. A knowledgeable doctor should identify the cause or causes, address any treatable issues, and give you some sense of what to expect.

Ideally, a doctor will also connect you with a social worker who can counsel your family, teach you about lifestyle changes that will make everyone's life easier, and lead you to appropriate community programs.

A diagnosis will help your parent understand what is happening to him. It should prompt him to attend to important business and perhaps do things that he has put off. And it allows your family to plan for the future while your parent can still be part of that planning.

Learning the biological reasons for your parent's behavior should also give you a little more patience, empathy, and tolerance—things you will need in spades now.

Making the Suggestion

Persuading your parent to talk with his doctor about memory loss will be easier

> " I was planning my wedding and we were having lunch and discussing whether to have a nighttime party or something in the afternoon, followed by cocktails. I said, 'Which do you think is better?' and she said, 'I don't really understand the difference.' That was a significant moment."
>
> —Angela S.

if he has noticed the problems and wants to know what is happening to him. But if your parent is like most people and denies that there are problems, insists that it's just old age, and resents any suggestion that something is wrong, then you have a challenge before you.

Wait for the right moment, when your parent is calm and at his most lucid. Start by asking him if he's noticed any changes or has concerns. Or, next time he has forgotten or missed something, casually ask if he has noticed more of these slips than before, and if it bothers him. Ask what he thinks it might be and if he has mentioned it to the doctor.

If he draws a blank, then delicately mention some of the changes you have noticed, without criticizing or alarming him. Assure him that such memory lapses may be caused by simple things, such as medications or a vitamin deficiency, that can be fixed. If he resists, try the do-it-for-me approach: *It would really put my mind at ease if you had this checked out.* Or call your parent's doctor and alert him or her to your concerns. The doctor can raise the subject during your parent's next appointment.

If you get nowhere, make an appointment for yourself to see a social worker or someone from the local Alzheimer's Association to discuss your parent's symptoms, issues that worry you, and how to proceed.

An Evaluation

Doctors take different approaches in an evaluation. Some immediately order

" My mother was stung by a bee and she's very allergic, so my aunt took her to the hospital. She was on prednisone, and you have to start with more and then reduce it, and you can't screw around with it. You have to do it right.

But my mother couldn't figure it out. My aunt called and said, 'I don't think your mother is going to be able to handle this.' So I went down for a couple of days, and I could see that she couldn't focus on what she was doing.

My aunt was with her, and my mother said, 'I'm glad you called my daughters, because I just can't fake it anymore.'

She knew something was wrong. She knew she couldn't do things. She said, 'I get in the car and I can't remember where I am going. I feel insecure and so I just come home.' She tried hard to keep it together for a long time, and so it was a relief to have her say it. She said, 'I just can't do it anymore. I think I have Alzheimer's.'"

—Carrie L.

tests and set up appointments with specialists, while others focus on complaints, symptoms, and immediate needs. Sometimes the diagnosis is obvious on the first visit, but often a doctor needs to follow the patient over time to be sure.

Bring any information related to your parent's health, including a list of medications (both prescribed and over-the-counter), illnesses, treatments, family history, and symptoms. Also, bring a list of questions and take notes, because you'll be getting a lot of information and it's easy to forget it (no irony intended).

Alzheimer's is usually diagnosed through a process of elimination— a crude, but surprisingly accurate approach. In general, an evaluation will include some or all of the following:

A PATIENT HISTORY. The doctor will talk to your parent, as well as to you and other family members, about your parent's health, past medical problems, medications used now and in the past,

WHEN OTHERS REFUSE TO SEE IT

You see Mom regularly and her addled mind has become hard to ignore. She forgets to feed her cat. She leaves pots on the stove. She misses church. However, during your sibling's occasional visits, Mom pulls herself together and appears pretty lucid.

You know there's a problem; your sibling says you are imagining it. You want to prepare, perhaps even persuade Mom to move; your sibling says you're overreacting.

Trust your instincts. Don't let a sibling or other family member deter you from plans that need to be made.

If possible, get your sibling to spend more time with your mom. Or get him to speak with your mother's doctor, and/or get a nurse, social worker, or geriatric care manager involved. Your sibling might be more willing to hear this from a professional.

> ❝ My parents were married for 50 years, and about 5 years ago my mother started to be really horrible to my father. She went through these wild ups and downs when she would yell at him or become terribly depressed and not want to go out or do anything. I think she finally exhausted him, because he died two years ago.
>
> We all blamed her, and for a time I would have as little as possible to do with her. I was so angry with her for being so cruel. Then, last year, while visiting my brother in Florida she became so depressed that he took her to the hospital. They said she had been having ministrokes.
>
> Oh boy, did I feel bad. I mean, she didn't know what she had been doing. She couldn't control her rage or depression or paranoia. I'm just glad that I know now so that I can take care of her and stop resenting her so much. She really has no idea what she is doing."
>
> —Marge W.

memory problems, any difficulty he might have in carrying out daily tasks, changes in behavior, and other such matters.

A PHYSICAL EXAM. The doctor will check your parent's overall health and look for signs of illness or injury.

A NEUROLOGICAL EXAM. The doctor will test your parent's reflexes, senses, balance, gait, and coordination.

A PSYCHIATRIC EXAM. The doctor (or a psychologist or psychiatrist) will take note of your parent's appearance and speech and ask about his moods and any psychiatric problems he might have, such as hallucinations, obsessions, depression, anxiety, or phobias.

A MENTAL STATUS TEST. In a preliminary evaluation, most doctors will conduct some sort of test to evaluate mental function. This 15-minute test assesses your parent's ability to perform simple tasks, recall new information, think abstractly, calculate, and communicate.

He might be asked, for example, to count backward from 100 by sevens, state the date and his location, follow a simple instruction (hold this piece of paper in your right hand, fold it, and put it on that table), recall information given moments ago, and perhaps draw some familiar object.

Incorrect answers do not mean that a person has dementia, and doctors take into account the patient's education, age, nervousness, and previous abilities in judging the results.

During these questions, your parent may be frightened or embarrassed if she has trouble answering them. If you are present, don't give clues or advice, but do offer quiet reassurance and comfort.

If your parent does poorly on this test, the doctor will try to determine when the problems began and how they have progressed over time, and may order a more comprehensive mental exam, which can take several hours to complete.

LABORATORY TESTS. Blood and urine samples will be examined for the presence of a variety of disorders that cause or contribute to confusion, such as infections, anemia, kidney and liver disease, thyroid abnormalities, vitamin B12 deficiency, syphilis, and AIDS.

SCANS. If a doctor feels that the information isn't adding up or something seems amiss, a scan can clarify what's happening. Imaging technology (CT, MRI, and other scans) is used to take pictures of the brain to detect damage from strokes, blood clots, tumors, bleeding, or a buildup of spinal fluid.

Positron emission tomography (a PET scan) can detect the buildup of amyloid proteins, the hallmark of Alzheimer's. But the test is expensive and if your parent has Alzheimer's, there's really no effective treatment. More important, about 20 percent of cognitively healthy older people have amyloid buildup in their brains, so the value of such scans is questionable.

Alzheimer's Disease

Although dozens of diseases cause dementia, by far the most common cause is Alzheimer's disease, affecting more than five million people in the United States.

> " When the doctor told me it was probably Alzheimer's, I just kept saying, 'It's got to be something else. This can't be right.' My mother was such an active person. She raised eight of us by herself. She was completely independent. I just couldn't believe that her mind could be affected like that.
>
> I was very frightened. You read and hear so much about Alzheimer's. My first thought was, she's going to become like a baby, like a vegetable.
>
> So far, I've been managing. It's a challenge, that's for sure. We have good days and bad days, but somehow we get through them all."
>
> —Linda K.

In Alzheimer's disease, brain cells degenerate and the brain becomes littered with telltale debris, known as plaques and tangles. Amyloid plaques are clumps of an abnormal protein surrounded by dead or damaged tissue. Neurofibrillary tangles are twisted bundles of fibers (made up of a protein called tau) that build up within brain cells.

What causes this destruction is unknown. In fact, scientists are not even sure if Alzheimer's is a single disease with a single cause, or a number of related diseases caused by a variety of factors. In other words, different paths may lead to the same brain damage and symptoms.

Risk Factors

Growing old is clearly the greatest risk factor for Alzheimer's disease. After age 65, the rate of disease doubles with every five years of age.

Genetics also plays a role, which means that anyone with a parent or

THE STAGES OF ALZHEIMER'S DISEASE

Although people with Alzheimer's react uniquely to the illness and follow an unpredictable course, experts have tracked a few of the more common symptoms of the illness. The stages described below are only a rough outline of what may occur over the course of a person's illness, which can go on for more than a decade but typically lasts four to six years.

Stage I: *A person at this point is usually still alert and social, and may be very much enjoying life, although something is not quite right. Frustrated by the forgetfulness and afraid of what is happening, some people become anxious and/or depressed, which only exacerbates the memory loss and confusion.*

- Short-term memory wanes. A person has trouble remembering recent events, learning new things, retaining information, and concentrating.

- Speech is slightly impaired. A person confuses one word with another, or can't remember the right word or a name.

- Hygiene is not what it once was. Clothing may be soiled or disheveled, and bathing and grooming may sometimes be forgotten.

- Judgment is poor, and thinking abstractly is difficult.

- Emotional responses are erratic and exaggerated. A person may become easily upset, anxious, angry, or depressed, often in response to the changes taking place.

- Daily tasks, such as tying a shoe, balancing a checkbook, or putting dishes in the dishwasher, can be challenging and may take longer to do.

- A person at this stage might get disoriented in familiar places and on often-used roads.

Stage II: *The signs become obvious, and daily life is difficult.*

- Short-term memory is worse, or largely gone. A person might be unable to learn new information or skills, and may forget the names and identities of friends and family. He may also have trouble dealing with new or unexpected situations.

- Coordination is poor, creating a risk for falls and accidents.

- Confusion and poor coordination combine to make daily tasks even more difficult. People often require some assistance with bathing, eating, and dressing.

sibling with the disease is at greater risk. But don't become overly alarmed. In the majority of cases, the genetic link is not an overwhelming one. Genetic mutations are responsible for only about 5 percent of the cases of AD and usually happen at a very early age (in one's 50s).

- Making decisions or doing a task that involves a series of steps is overwhelming.

- Disorientation is pronounced. A person might not be sure how to get to the kitchen in his own home.

- People wander. Often they are looking for a place that is less confusing, a place that feels more "right," so this happens most often if they are in an unfamiliar place.

- Agitation and pacing are common.

- Moods are more exaggerated. A person might be uncooperative, hostile, or aggressive, although some people become serene and peaceful. (They may be less frustrated by the illness because they don't remember what they used to be able to do.)

- Many people become paranoid and have hallucinations and/or delusions.

- People often have trouble controlling impulses, so they might be rude or vulgar. They might undress in public or make sexual comments or advances.

- Language and speech troubles worsen.

- Ability to add, subtract, or do other calculations is virtually lost. (The checkbook may be overdrawn or bills left unpaid.)

- Sleep cycles fall out of sync, so a person may sleep at odd hours.

- Stories or actions are repeated monotonously.

Stage III: *At this point, people are totally dependent and require constant care.*

- Confusion is acute. All short-term memory and most long-term memory are gone.

- Communication skills, as well as the ability to walk, are also usually gone.

- People are incontinent.

- People often lose a good deal of weight.

- Physical rigidity and seizures may occur.

- Hallucinations (seeing or hearing things that don't exist), delusions (irrational or unfounded beliefs), and paranoia (in particular, a belief that others are trying to kill the person or that a spouse is cheating) are all common.

- Eventually, people are unable to speak, get out of bed, or feed themselves. They become susceptible to malnutrition, infections, dehydration, pneumonia, and other illnesses.

One genetic factor—apolipopprotein e4, or APOE-e4—has shown the strongest link in these cases of early-onset. Less is known about other genes. However, the disease may require that you inherit a faulty gene from both parents. Or you may inherit only a propensity for the illness, and some second assault, such as an injury or exposure to a particular environmental toxin, may be necessary for the disease to develop.

There is also mounting evidence that high blood pressure, high cholesterol, and diabetes increase the risk of Alzheimer's. So exercise, eat well, and keep the extra weight off.

Beyond these causes, researchers are looking at a number of other possible causes for Alzheimer's, including prior brain injury, toxins in the environment, the role of the immune system, viruses, or simply worn-out brain cells that run amok.

No link has been shown between Alzheimer's and aluminum, aspartame, silver fillings, or flu shots.

Vascular Dementia

At least 20 to 30 percent of all cases of dementia are thought to be wholly or partially caused by diminished blood flow to the brain. Usually this is caused by a series of strokes so small they go unnoticed—something known as multi-infarct dementia, or MID. (An infarct is an area of tissue that is dead or dying.) With each successive stroke, the brain loses more and more ability. Blood flow can also be hindered because of other damage to blood vessels and conditions that reduce circulation.

Diabetes, high blood pressure, high cholesterol, smoking, and abnormal heart rhythms, as well as plain old aging, all damage blood vessels. Doctors can often determine that vascular dementia is involved based on a patient's history, symptoms, and tests.

Although the symptoms are similar to those for Alzheimer's (and as noted, the two can occur together), the specifics depend upon what part of the brain is damaged. Sometimes the disease affects physical abilities before it affects thinking and memory, so a person might become weak, lose some vision, or become incontinent before he becomes forgetful or confused.

The symptoms typically grow worse in spurts, more like walking down stairs than the slow slide that occurs in Alzheimer's disease.

If diagnosed early, the progression of multi-infarct dementia can sometimes be slowed by improving circulation through diet and exercise; improving the management of diabetes; and with medications that treat high blood pressure, high cholesterol, or other causes of vascular disease.

> " Every time my husband enters the room his mother says, 'Well now. Where have you been?'
>
> For a while, he was hurt by it. But we actually find it kind of amusing now."
>
> —Kim R.

Lewy Body Dementia

Lewy body dementia is not as well known as other types of dementia, but it's the third most common form of dementia.

Lewy bodies are clumps of protein that develop in the part of the brain that controls movement and thought. LBD, as it's known, shares many of the same symptoms as Alzheimer's—confusion, memory loss, language difficulty, and so on—so it can be hard to differentiate from Alzheimer's. It also sometimes occurs in tandem with Alzheimer's and Parkinson's disease.

People suffering from LBD typically flip-flop between confusion and lucidity, and often suffer from recurrent, vivid hallucinations. They also tend to have the tremors and slow, rigid movements found in people with Parkinson's. Some people with Lewy body dementia also have a sleep disorder, which causes them to kick, thrash, and get visibly upset during dreams.

For more information, contact the Lewy Body Dementia Association (lbda .org or 800-539-9767).

Dealing with the Diagnosis

Under normal conditions, doctors meet privately with patients to discuss a diagnosis and then let the patients decide how much, if anything, they want to tell their families. But dementia derails everything in life, including the doctor-patient relationship.

Typically, with a diagnosis of dementia, doctors confer with the entire family, both because patients might have trouble understanding the ramifications and because every family member is profoundly affected by this illness. But that should be done only with your parent's consent. Ask him whether he wants to

talk with the doctor alone or wants one or more family members present.

A doctor should not discuss the diagnosis *only* with the family, bypassing your parent completely, unless your parent has specifically requested such a thing or there are some extenuating circumstances.

People with dementia often take the news far more calmly than their families expect. Of course it is upsetting—terribly upsetting—but they already know something is wrong, even if they don't readily admit it. They are worried and have suspicions about what is happening. A

FORGIVE YOURSELF

If you have been snapping impatiently at your father or criticizing him for being disruptive, forgetful, or rude, you may feel guilty once you realize that his behavior is caused by an illness. Forgive yourself. You reacted perfectly normally under the circumstances and have nothing to feel guilty about. In fact, even now that you know the diagnosis, you are sure to have a few angry outbursts. It would be almost impossible not to, given the nature of this disease. Give your parent as much love as you can, forget about what happened yesterday, and focus your energy on today.

diagnosis lets them know why their world is so askew. It also gives them the opportunity to begin to deal, both practically and emotionally, with what is to come.

Breaking the News

When you or the doctor talks with your parent about a diagnosis of dementia, try to understand what she may be experiencing. In addition to obvious feelings of devastation, she is, most likely, afraid of losing dignity and respect, and of becoming a burden to the family, among other things.

Listen to her concerns, offer warmth and support, and reassure her that she will not be alone. Tell her that you all, as a family, are going to get through this together. Without dismissing her fears, focus on all she can still do and on the good times she and her family can still have together.

Of course, you will have your own turbulent emotions to contend with as well. You may have suspected Alzheimer's and now realize you were totally unprepared for the truth. You may feel shock, horror, anger, grief, and helplessness. You may feel even more sorry for yourself than for your parent and deeply afraid of the work that lies ahead. You may secretly hope that the disease runs its course quickly. You are surely going to experience some grief over what you have already lost and what you are going to lose.

These are all normal reactions. Don't be ashamed of them. You have a great deal to comprehend and to come to terms with. Be kind to yourself. Take time to digest all this. Spend time with family and friends, or carve out some time to be alone. Let the grief and tears come. And know that there is a lot of good support out there.

Now What?

Okay, deep breath. The world might be spinning the wrong way, but help is available.

The doctor or a member of his or her staff should talk with your family about the future and set you up with a social worker who can provide referrals and counseling. If no help is offered, do some research on your own, because a diagnosis by itself is of little use.

Whether your parent has Alzheimer's disease or vascular dementia or some other cognitive impairment, contact the Alzheimer's Association (alz.org or 800-272-3900), which has local chapters throughout the country that run

ON THE LOOKOUT FOR COMPLICATING FACTORS

If your parent has dementia, be aware of other problems that can exacerbate the symptoms and make it harder for him to compensate. (These issues can also cause confusion on their own.)

DEPRESSION. Depression can mimic early Alzheimer's or can coincide with dementia, especially in the early stages. Frustrated and saddened by the memory loss, people often become depressed. But that will only worsen the symptoms. Treating depression can alleviate some confusion and memory loss.

DELIRIUM. Although delirium typically comes on suddenly—in a matter of days or even hours—it is sometimes confused with dementia or may coexist with it. Symptoms vary widely but often include disorientation, inattentiveness, and changes in personality. Delirium is reversible, but it must be treated immediately. (See page 268.)

MEDICATION. Antidepressants, heart medications, anti-inflammatory drugs, sleeping pills, ulcer medications, insulin, and cold medications can all cause confusion, agitation, and other symptoms. Your parent's doctor should be aware of all drugs that he takes, including nonprescription ones.

ALCOHOL. Prolonged, heavy use of alcohol can cause permanent brain damage and dementia, but even moderate drinking can worsen confusion. Urge your parent to stop, or at least cut back.

VISION AND HEARING IMPAIRMENT. Make sure that your parent gets his eyes and ears checked regularly, as poor hearing or blurred vision will make his world that much more confusing.

VITAMIN B12 DEFICIENCY. Medications or age can impede a body's absorption of vitamin B12, causing fatigue, depression, anxiety, memory loss, and other problems typical of dementia. The deficiency is treated with injections of the vitamin.

---

support groups and provide referrals to local services, from housing and legal aid to financial and medical assistance. Call other local senior service organizations as well if you need further guidance and information on specific topics.

While this diagnosis forces one to think about the future, it can also magnify the value of the present. Talk with your parent about her priorities. If she is still relatively lucid, find out if there is anything that she wants to do while she still can. Does she need to resolve an old conflict or visit a distant friend? Has she always wanted to take a trip to San Francisco? Try Vietnamese food? Return to a childhood home? See the ballet? Remember, even though it may be hard to believe right now, life is not over, for you or your parent.

Planning for the Future

Because your parent is going to need extensive care, and at some point will be unable to make decisions for herself, your family needs to plan now for

> " My mother had Alzheimer's for 12 years. The most painful part was when we were just realizing what it was. I cried on the flight home. That is when I really grieved, because I thought, *The mother I knew is over.* I thought, *This is it.*
>
> This might seem cold, but in all the years after that, I didn't feel sad. I felt happy to be helping her. I knew I was making her life better. And there were moments that were a lot of fun with her. She couldn't communicate, but we would play music and she would laugh. We'd take her in the wheelchair and roll her around town. And she loved sitting in the sun with us. I felt a joy in knowing I was giving her a happy ending to her life."
>
> —Karen S.

the future. It's not easy; no one wants to think about such things. But you will be so glad you did.

If she has not already done so, your parent should name a durable power of attorney and a health care proxy, have a will drafted, and sign and fully discuss advance directives. Also, she, or you, should gather other important documents, such as tax returns and insurance information (all listed on page 12), or know where these documents are kept.

Your family also needs to start planning your parent's future care and living situation. Learn about community services and home care.

Furthermore, as discussed in Chapter 3, it is essential—*essential*—that you take care of yourself now. Pace yourself. Take breaks. Get support. You'll be a better caregiver if you do.

Even if you think you would never, ever put your parent in any sort of senior facility, you might want to at least see what options exist. This disease takes a toll on all involved, and most families cannot take it on for years on end. Also, some of these facilities are actually very good at caring for people with dementia. (And the best ones will have waiting lists.)

Finally, think about who would care for your parent if something were to happen to you or another primary caregiver. Choose a family member, close friend, or trusted adviser who can take over as surrogate.

Treating Dementia

The best medicine for your parent will come from you, not the pharmacist. Right now, more than anything else, your parent needs a safe and organized environment, a simple and calm routine that can be adjusted to meet her changing needs, easy stimulation, a lot of reminders and cues, a good diet, exercise, social activities, and a hefty dose of love and patience.

Even difficult behavioral problems—the kind that land people in nursing homes (and sometimes get them tossed out of nursing homes), such as agitation, aggression, and delusions—can often be improved with changes in your parent's environment, her routines, and your approach.

To give your parent what she needs now, you need to learn about this disease and master some tricks for coping. You also need to find some way to deal with stress, and dig deep to muster up the strength, flexibility, and patience for all that lies ahead.

The next two chapters offer ideas for your parent's care, and yours, as the two go hand in hand.

Medications

Unfortunately, no magic bullets exist for dementia. Not even pretty good bullets.

Treating any heart condition or vascular disease to prevent further damage to the brain can sometimes slow the cognitive decline caused by vascular dementia. That means exercise and a healthful diet, of course, along with drugs that thin the blood, prevent clotting, lower cholesterol, and reduce blood pressure.

Other than that, scientists have not found a way to change the ultimate course of Alzheimer's and other forms of dementia. A few drugs seem to ease memory loss and confusion, but only a little, only in some patients (fewer than half),

and only for about 6 to 12 months. As a result, there is some debate over the value of such medical treatments. It's worth seeing if they help and making your own decision.

Currently, two types of drugs are approved for the treatment of dementia. The first, cholinesterase inhibitors, slow the breakdown of acetylcholine, a chemical involved in thinking and memory that is undermined by disease. The three in use are donepezil (Aricept), rivastigmine (Exelon), and galantamine

THE BRAIN GYM

Not surprisingly, people who travel, read, socialize, and debate current events score better on mental function tests. They also weather the dementia storm better, apparently because they have more reserves to call on. When damage occurs, other brain regions and connections, strengthened by years of activity, seem to pick up the slack.

However, once disease has set in, suddenly pushing your parent to learn bridge and tackle brainteasers will be a futile and frustrating enterprise for all involved. He cannot now restore what's lost.

What he can do, at least in the early stages, is learn new strategies for coping and remembering things, which are discussed in the next chapter.

Remember, your parent can't "try harder." He can't work his way out of this illness through mental gymnastics. His brain cells are not functioning the way they once did.

Encourage him to do what he can and what he enjoys, and help him find ways to cope in his new world. But you both need to try to accept what he can no longer do.

DRUGS USED TO TREAT SYMPTOMS OF DEMENTIA

Nondrug approaches should always be tried first; many of these drugs are dangerous.

PROBLEM	DRUGS COMMONLY PRESCRIBED (generic/brand name)	POSSIBLE SIDE EFFECTS
Depression Hopelessness, sadness, weight loss, social withdrawal, irritability	Citalopram/Celexa, sertraline/Zoloft, mirtazapine/Remeron, fluoxetine/Prozac	Drowsiness, constipation, anxiety, dry mouth, increased risk of falls
Apathy Lack of enthusiasm, motivation, interest	Antidepressants (above) Methylphenidate/Ritalin	(Same as above)
Anxiety Excessive fear or worry, agitation, restlessness, combative behavior	Lorazepam/Ativan, clonazepam/Klonopin Some antidepressants are used to treat agitation and anxiety.	Drowsiness, falls, confusion, loss of inhibition, agitation, anger (and increasing tolerance to the drug). *Caution:* These should not be used on a regular basis.
Psychosis Hallucinations, delusions, paranoia	Olanzapine/Zyprexa, quetiapine/Seroquel, Risperidone/Risperdal (some of these drugs are also used to treat nonpsychotic symptoms, such as aggression and agitation)	Drowsiness, rigidity, tremors, jerking, twitching, confusion, dry mouth, constipation, infections, increased risk of falls, stroke, and death. *Caution:* These should be used only as a last resort.
Aggression	Carbamazepine/Tegretol, oxcarbazepine/Trileptal, divalproex sodium/ Depakote (also sometimes used to treat depression, agitation, and anxiety)	Drowsiness, confusion, lack of coordination
Insomnia	Zolpidem/Ambien, eszopiclone/Lunesta, zaleplon/Sonata	*Caution:* These can cause falls and confusion and should not be used often.

(Razadyne). They must be taken early in the course of the disease, and can cause side effects, including nausea, diarrhea, and cramping.

The second type of drug, memantine (Namenda), works on a different chemical in the brain, glutamate, and is used for patients with moderate to severe Alzheimer's. It is sometimes given in combination with one of the cholinesterase inhibitors. Memantine may help certain behavioral symptoms, but in some people it actually makes behavior worse. It can also cause constipation, confusion (who needs more confusion?), dizziness, and headaches.

TREATING SYMPTOMS

Several medications are often given to alleviate specific symptoms, such as anxiety, agitation, depression, insomnia, and hallucinations, but be careful. Although it's tempting to reach for a pill—and doctors prescribe them readily—most of these medications can actually worsen some symptoms, cause new ones, and increase the risks. Drugs should be used only when other approaches (discussed in the next two chapters) have failed.

As we've noted, anticholinergic medications (used to treat pain, incontinence, anxiety, asthma, insomnia, and depression, among other things) can worsen confusion and memory loss. Antidepressants have been linked to a higher incidence of falls in people with dementia.

Antipsychotic medications are also worrisome. Although they are commonly used to treat delusions, paranoia, and aggression, these drugs have been shown to worsen confusion and language

skills, and increase the risk of falls. They are also associated with higher death rates.

Antipsychotic medications can also cause tremors, jerks, and other involuntary motions. An extreme form of these movements, called tardive dyskinesia, may not improve even after the medication is stopped.

Although people with Lewy body dementia frequently have visual hallucinations, they are at particular risk of serious side effects from antipsychotic medications.

Despite all this, these drugs are sometimes necessary—particularly when someone is violent, combative, or dangerous and cannot be calmed or controlled by other means. Ultimately, your ability to care for your parent, and to keep him in a less restrictive environment, may come down to the ability to control certain behaviors.

Before turning to medications, however, look for possible causes (infections, other medications, or illness) or triggers (a person, a place, or an activity). Try behavioral approaches. Then, determine the severity of the behavior. Is he a danger to himself or others? Often, these behaviors don't last long and improve more quickly without medications, so if a behavior is simply annoying, but not dangerous, consider giving it time to see if it resolves on its own.

When you must resort to drugs, remember the rule "low and slow"—start with a very low dose and then slowly increase it as necessary. Once a drug has had the desired effect, ask the doctor when your parent might be weaned off it, to see if it is still needed. People with Alzheimer's change quickly—a jumping bean who needs something to calm her down can turn into a couch potato as the disease progresses, making a drug unnecessary and dangerous.

Be careful about mixing drugs. Drugs that act on the brain to reduce hallucinations or paranoia, for example, do not mix well with alcohol or a number of other drugs, including over-the-counter pills found in most household medicine cabinets. The combined effect on the brain may cause greater confusion, agitation, and disorientation.

Consult your parent's doctor before she takes any new medicine, even if it seems benign. Some drugs, such as over-the-counter sleeping pills, act by lowering levels of acetylcholine, the very chemical that is already in dire shortage in the brains of people with Alzheimer's disease. These will only worsen confusion and other symptoms.

If your parent is not under your care, be keenly aware of her medications. Nursing home patients, in particular, are often given sedatives and antipsychotics simply because it's easier, and it's the way they've always done things. Nonmedical approaches are almost always more effective.

A Note on Other "Treatments"

Although the Internet is loaded with treatments for dementia (and everything else), most of them have been found ineffective.

Omega-3 fatty acids, found in fish oil, might help protect the heart and blood vessels, thus slowing vascular dementia. Other than that, high doses of vitamins, ginkgo, ibuprofen, and Chinese moss

(Huperzine A, which was touted for a time) don't seem to help.

Some doctors prescribe hefty doses of vitamin E, an antioxidant, to slow memory loss, but studies on its value have shown mixed results and suggest a slight increase in death rates. It's especially worrisome in people who are on blood thinners or cholesterol-lowering medications, as vitamin E increases the risk of bleeding.

Your parent should talk with her doctor before taking any dietary supplements, herbal extracts, hormones, or drugs.

To find out about current studies and possible participation in clinical trials, contact the Alzheimer's Disease Education and Referral Center (alzheimers.org or 800-438-4380) or the National Institute of Neurological Disorders and Stroke (ninds.nih.gov or 800-352-9424).

ⓘ FOR MORE HELP

Alzheimer's Association
alz.org
800-272-3900 (available 24/7)

Alzheimer's Disease Education and Referral Center
alzheimers.org
800-438-4380

National Institute of Neurological Disorders and Stroke
ninds.nih.gov
800-352-9424

Lewy Body Dementia Association
lbda.org
800-539-9767

Chapter 24

Living with Dementia

Helping Your Parent • Helping Yourself

If marriage, work, and children test a person's patience, then caring for a loved one with dementia is the final exam.

You are called upon to help your parent in ways you never fathomed—sometimes against his wishes or without his understanding. At the same time, you are losing him, the parent you once knew, bit by bit, and finding in his place someone you might not know or even like. And in the midst of all this grief and aggravation, you must muster up superhuman amounts of flexibility and patience. It's a ridiculously tall order, but truly, these are the keys to your parent's day and your survival.

Right now, you have to take care of yourself, in a big way, because your care and your parent's care are inseparable. His mental state will reflect yours. If you are on the verge of exploding, he will become anxious and unsettled. If you nag and criticize, he will feel inadequate and angry. But if you are rested and calm (as rested and calm as possible), if you are flexible and patient, your parent will be more composed.

The heartbreak of this disease can't be avoided, but honestly, if you take care of yourself, try to understand how your parent sees the world, and learn a few new approaches to daily life, you can alleviate the symptoms, defuse the stress, and even have moments of joy.

This chapter offers tips on how to help your parent now, and how to help yourself. The next chapter suggests ways of tackling specific daily tasks, such as bathing and dressing, and difficult behaviors, such as agitation and aggression.

Helping Your Parent

Making daily life easier for your parent will make life more manageable for both of you. Keep her environment simple and predictable, and learn what makes her anxious, what helps her relax, what distracts her, and what reassures her.

Simplify His World

The simpler your parent's world is—his house, his tasks, his conversations, his visits—the better life will be for everyone.

The problem is, your parent might not realize that the volume is too loud or the lighting too bright or the room too crowded for him. He just knows that he is unhappy, and so he becomes agitated or angry. It is up to you to be alert to his surroundings. A few general guidelines:

- Get rid of knickknacks, small rugs, mirrors, piles of papers, and clutter, especially in the room where your parent lives (unless all this chaos is familiar and oddly calming for him).

- Furniture should be simple and placed so that it can be easily used. Pathways should be clear. Once you clean up and arrange the furniture, don't rearrange it.

- Keep the noise level down. You might not notice that the television is blaring, the dog is barking, the vacuum is humming, and several people are talking at once, but any one of those things might completely confound your father.

- Use clear signs and labels—on the bathroom door, in bedrooms, on cabinets, on bureau drawers ("shirts," "pants," and so on), on toiletries ("shampoo," "conditioner," "lotion"). Sticky notes can be useful too ("Turn Off the Stove," "Feed the Dog," "Lock the Door"). If

➕ MEDICAL ALERT

Your parent might not be able to tell you what she's feeling or even comprehend herself what she is experiencing, so you or some other caregiver needs to be on the lookout for signs of trouble. Your mother might not be able to let you know when her head aches, or if she has abdominal pain, or if it hurts when she urinates. Instead, she might become agitated, critical, or whiny. She might moan, become angry, or resist using the toilet or (if she has dental problems) eating a meal. Be aware of shifts in behavior and mood, and if you suspect a physical ailment, alert the doctor.

your parent might not know which item in the refrigerator he should eat, write "lunch" across his sandwich bag. Use drawings and symbols if written words don't work (for example, a picture of a sock on the sock drawer).

- Get phones with large push buttons, which are easier to read and easier to use. Put photographs on all speed-dial buttons. (So rather than speed dial 1 and 2, there is a picture of you on one and your sister on the other; likewise emergency photos or symbols on fire and ambulance numbers.)

- Keep items that are often needed, and frequently lost, in the same place all the time. The remote is always on the coffee table. The house key is always hung by the door. His glasses are hanging from his neck.

- When you have questions, keep them simple. Don't ask what he wants for dinner (baffling); ask, "Do you want chicken or hamburger tonight?"

- When giving instructions, eliminate unnecessary steps and provide directions one step at a time. Each should require only a single action. For example, instead of asking your father to bathe, go through each step with him: "Take the shirt off. Step into the shower." And so forth.

- Minimize change. Simply going to the doctor's office may trigger a frenzy of fear and frustration. Certainly, a change in a living situation, or even a room change within the house, can cause pandemonium. The more life stays the same, the better. New people, new foods, new activities, and new schedules might throw him off.

Let Him Do What He Can

In the early stages, your parent should be encouraged to do whatever he still can (without your pushing him to do things that he can't). Day to day, it might be easier to do things for him, but it is important for your parent to remain active.

Think of tasks that he can manage on his own or with minimal help. Have him polish the silver, get the mail, cut coupons, or water the flowers. Ask him to hand you ingredients while you cook dinner.

Of course, letting your parent help might require more work from you and others (the laundry may need to be

> ❝ My father is losing his filter, but sometimes we laugh. We dance. We never did that before. So there's a little joy in this horrible disease."
> —Julie H.

refolded, the spilled juice wiped up). But people with dementia who are encouraged to stay active, remain social, and otherwise have some sort of a life are less depressed, less aggressive and agitated, and generally less dependent.

Use your imagination. If your mother was a pianist, running her fingers over an electric keyboard (even one that isn't plugged in) might give her hours of enjoyment. If she was a cook, stirring flour and water or "pretend" cooking might give her solace. If your father was a carpenter, gluing bits of wood together or tinkering with a few tools might feel familiar and make him happy.

Look for the Message

Your parent cannot fully understand the world around her or clearly communicate her needs, so you need to decipher her signals as best you can.

If your parent is agitated and anxious, maybe the radio is too loud or her sweater is too hot. If your parent strikes at a visitor, maybe that person came at

> " Over the years we tried to convince my father to use a cane when he became unsteady on his feet, but he always refused. He'd say he got around much better than any of us, or he'd get angry and change the subject.
>
> When his dementia got worse, he became much frailer, and one day I took out the cane we'd gotten for him and tried to slip it into his hand. Before I could do it, he looked at me with a concerned expression and said, 'Eric! I didn't know you used a cane!'"
>
> —Eric S.

her unexpectedly and frightened her or resembles someone she feared. If your parent is screaming obscenities or throwing things, maybe it's because her leg aches, or she has an infection, or she has to go to the bathroom. She cannot remember what this feeling means or how to say, "I need to go to the bathroom." She is simply reacting to her discomfort and wanting something to change.

When she's upset, think about possible causes. You might keep a log and watch for patterns. If she is more anxious at a certain time of day or in a certain place, perhaps there is something about that time or place that reminds her of something she should be doing.

Also, think about how she used to be and what she used to enjoy. If she has always loved reading, and now she can't, perhaps that is causing her agitation. Perhaps an audiobook will calm her.

Again, your mother is not trying to annoy you. She simply doesn't understand her surroundings and doesn't know how to communicate her feelings, get what she needs, or remedy what she doesn't like. Your task is to play sleuth and see if there isn't some message behind her actions.

Put Yourself in Her Shoes

Imagine being given a colossal assignment, one that you simply cannot do. You are overwhelmed by the challenge and humiliated by your lack of ability. You know, on some level, it's not difficult. In fact, you think perhaps you've been able to do it in the past. But today it feels like you are trying to scale the Empire State Building.

WHITE LIES

You grew up knowing that lies were wrong, but with dementia you'll need to skim over the truth routinely, and when that doesn't work, you might have to tell a few white lies (sometimes known as "therapeutic fibbing").

Before telling any lies, try some diversions. That is, instead of telling your father, again, that he doesn't work anymore and doesn't need to go to the office, let him wear his suit or ask him what he liked about his job. Or say, *Before you go to work, you need to have breakfast first.*

If he remains firm in his conviction that it's time for work and is getting upset, go ahead and tell him that it's Saturday even if it's Tuesday.

If your mother insists on staying up until her husband gets home even though your parents divorced 20 years ago, you might ask her about him—how they met, what she liked about him, and so on. See if she wouldn't like to wait up for him in bed. If nothing diverts her, then tell her that he's away and will surely check on her when he returns.

When your parent insists that you are bringing her to a bedroom that isn't hers, ask her if it wouldn't be okay to stay in this room for now. Or confirm any emotions that might be behind her comment. *I know you miss your home, Mom. But I'm here for you, just down the hallway, so you're not alone.* If she is still agitated, then tell her that her house is being painted right now.

It might not be comfortable for you, but remember, your parent is not living in the here and now. And you need to use whatever tools you can to ease her mind.

Making matters worse, someone is standing over you growing increasingly impatient and annoyed as you struggle and fail. The pressure and embarrassment make it harder for you to think, so you fumble even more.

For your parent, getting dressed or eating a meal, especially one that involves several foods and an assortment of utensils, are formidable tasks. She can't remember what to do next or why she is doing this at all. If you criticize her, hurry her, or grow annoyed, she will become more anxious and confused, and less able to perform.

If, on the other hand, you can lower your expectations, muster a good dose of patience and compassion, and give her ample time, she might actually be more successful with the task at hand. Or at least she might not get as upset about it.

Forget Logic

Anyone knows that bananas should not be put in the oven and hair should not be combed with a toothbrush. But if you attempt to explain the reasons to your parent, you will be wasting your breath. He is living in a world where everything is changing. Nothing is familiar, and nothing makes sense.

You can't reason with him, so stop trying. You are raising your blood pressure needlessly. Instead, give him a hug and hand him a comb.

Remain Patient and Calm

Staying calm will help you cope, but it will also help your parent get through the day (which will, in turn, help you maintain your serenity).

It's no small order, but your frustration and criticism (even if you think you're hiding it well) will only send your parent into more turmoil and deeper confusion. If she's made a mistake (another one), remain patient. If she's agitated, remain calm. If she's criticizing you and embarrassing you in public, remain steadfast. Of course, you won't always be able to do it, but do your best.

Treat Her with Respect

When dementia strikes, treating your parent with the respect deserving of an adult will be challenging, especially when she is acting like a two-year-old. But whether you are cutting her food or helping her bathe, remember that your parent is not a child and shouldn't be treated like one. She has lived a long life and has well-formed opinions, dreams, likes, and dislikes—even if she

can't remember what they are anymore. Help her maintain a sense of dignity. Address her with the same respect that you always have.

Make sure that your tone of voice is not condescending. Try not to scold or nag. Refrain from talking about her as if she were not in the room or unable to comprehend your words.

> " A few weeks before my mother died, I had everybody over for Easter. I thought, *What did I get myself into?* because I couldn't give my attention to anything else. She needed all my time.
>
> But she really enjoyed herself. My niece is a psychologist and she was trying to trigger my mother's memory, asking her questions, mentioning her favorite composers and songs. Mom loved music.
>
> I asked her that night if she had enjoyed her company. And the way she smiled at me I knew that it was a very, very successful day."
>
> —Sally T.

SUPPORT FOR YOU AND FOR YOUR PARENT

There are hundreds of support groups for the families of people with Alzheimer's and other forms of dementia, which is great, but know that there are also support groups for the patients themselves.

Patients, at least those in the early stages of the illness or those with mild cognitive impairment, are often relieved to talk about their fears, losses, aggravations, and other feelings, as well as how they and their families plan to cope in the future.

You, your family, and/or your parent can join an online support group (try alzconnected.org), or find out if there is a local support group, through the Alzheimer's Association (alz.org or 800-272-3900).

Instead, protect her self-esteem, dignity, and modesty, and ask others who care for her to do the same.

Stick to a Routine

Create a schedule that works for your parent, and then stick to it. If she is most lucid in the morning, schedule complex activities, such as bathing, for that time. If she gets restless and fidgety in the middle of the day, create a calm environment at that time.

You might also plan visits for the same time and day every week. Or if your parent goes to day care every weekday, then try to follow the same routine on the weekend by getting her up and dressed and then giving her some activity to do that is similar to what she does in day care. She won't remember the schedule, but she shouldn't be terribly surprised by it either.

Divert His Attention

Diversion is one of your best friends now. For some people, it's magic. Basically, the idea is to use all that forgetfulness to your advantage. When your parent is about to do something that you don't want him to do, divert his attention.

When your father starts into a tantrum or begins to tell a repetitive story, don't tell him to stop. Gently change the subject or suggest a new activity. Have him look at a photo album, sip a cup of tea, go for a walk, listen to music, sing a song, or flip through magazines. He might just forget what was upsetting him in the first place.

IN NEED OF SUPERVISION

Your parent might be able to live alone for some time after receiving a diagnosis of dementia, but not for long. If she becomes confused easily, has trouble using a telephone, wanders, leaves the stove on, or presents some other risk to herself or others, she needs supervision. Don't wait for a disaster to realize she needs coverage—plan in advance.

Find out about adult day care programs, companions, volunteers, roommates, aides, or other ways she might be supervised during the day.

If he gets riled up in the middle of a task that has to be finished, like getting out of the tub, divert him by pausing for a moment and singing a familiar song or telling an old family story. It should calm him, and when you return to the task, he might have forgotten that this is something he didn't want to do. A short break might calm you as well.

> " I've learned that I have to think ahead and make it look like I really don't want my mother to do something, and then she'll do it.
>
> I came home one afternoon to find her physically wrestling with Mildred, the aide who takes care of her while I'm at work. It was raining, and Mildred wanted her to go inside, but she wouldn't do it. I suggested that Mildred tell Mom to sit outside, that she didn't want her to go in the house. Then Mom wanted to come inside. You learn to do whatever works."
>
> —Carol G.

> **"** My mother had dementia, and I cared for her for nine years. But she was an easy person, and the fact that she didn't have other ailments made her care easier. I didn't have to worry about wounds or respiratory issues or heart ailments. I was caring for her as you would a child."
>
> —Angela S.

Ignore It

No one likes to be corrected all the time, so do it as little as possible. It is demeaning and confusing for your parent (and he probably won't understand what it is he is doing wrong), and exhausting for you. Instead, ignore some things—a lot of things—as long as they aren't dangerous or harmful.

Does it really matter if your parent remembers the cat's name or if he talks about his late sister as though she were still alive? Who is it hurting if he wears mismatched clothes or if he wants to eat cereal for dinner and turkey for breakfast? Ignore his mistakes, don't correct him, and agree with him, even when he's wrong. You might even join him in his mixed-up world and have turkey for breakfast, too.

When you must correct him, say something that will get him back on track without being critical. *You probably did take your medication, but let's check your pillbox just to be sure.*

When you have to correct him in public, do so gently and/or with humor. Rather than saying, "No, Dad, it's not Thursday. Today is Tuesday," either ignore the error or try something like, "This week's been moving so fast that it feels like Thursday, doesn't it?"

It's natural that you want your parent to remember, to get it right. It's a knee-jerk reaction to correct his mistakes. But a louder voice, confrontation, shame, or annoyance will not bring back old skills or memories; it will only make him feel more inadequate and confused. So let some things go.

Beware the Witching Hour

People with dementia often suffer what is known as "sundowning." That is, as the sun goes down, disruptive behaviors become worse. Agitation, in particular, becomes heightened.

It's not clear why this happens, whether it is the change in lighting or simply that the day has been tiring and exhaustion is kicking in. Certainly, children are less well behaved in the evening, and it's the time of day many of us reach for a cocktail, so maybe it's not limited to dementia.

If your mother is more confused and agitated in the evening, schedule complicated activities for an earlier part of the day, and keep the evening calm and soothing. Sometimes turning the lights on in the afternoon, before the sun starts to set, can help.

Be aware of it, schedule life accordingly, and repeat your mantra: *I am calm. I am calm. I am calm.*

Get Him to Exercise

Exercise? With all that you are dealing with? Why bother?

Even if your parent is very confused, some fresh air and sunshine, a walk around the neighborhood, or some modest stretching and/or lifting light weights will help her get through the rest of the day. If she's chair-bound or bedbound, she can still do some simple exercises.

When someone has dementia, exercise usually reduces agitation, improves sleep habits, reduces falls, helps people perform daily tasks, alleviates depression, boosts mood and self-esteem, and, best of all, improves people's interactions with their caregivers.

Pets, Imagery, Music, and Art Therapy

A pet can calm people when they're agitated, alleviate depression, and boost self-esteem. Your parent probably can't care for a pet now, but if someone else is around to do that, she might enjoy having a gentle companion to talk to, stroke, and hold. Find a pet that is a bit of a couch potato. You don't need two agitated souls in the house.

Music can also be soothing and relaxing. Sometimes soft "white" noise, such as the sound of ocean waves or other continuous sounds from nature, can decrease nervous chatter and calm a person with dementia. Music from her youth will transport her to better times.

She might sing along or even dance a little (good exercise). Children's songs can also be calming, as they often have simplistic, repetitive melodies.

Art is also a helpful outlet. A few colored pencils or a soft chunk of clay might tap her creative side (and keep her busy and distracted for a while).

Imagery can be very effective in calming the soul. Get your parent to close her eyes and then talk slowly and gently, describing a place or time she loved. Walk her through it, describing, for example, a walk on the beach, or the smell of the pine trees and sound of water lapping the rocks at a lake. Help her to relax in this place, to savor it.

Reassurance and Hugs

Warmth and love are strong elixirs. When your father gets riled, discombobulated, or anxious, gently stroke his hand or cheek. Tell him that you understand, that he's doing a good job. A gentle touch and a kind, soft word will help both of you get through the next few minutes—and a few minutes of peace can be a saving grace at this time.

Helping Yourself

Dementia calls for a stronger-than-usual arsenal of self-preservation measures. This illness takes such an enormous toll on caregivers that most families eventually find themselves at the door of the nearest nursing home.

Now more than ever, you have to—really, absolutely have to—take care of yourself. People caring for dementia patients are at extremely high risk of illness, depression, and, in the throes of frustration, aggression. You'll be no

SOCIALIZING WITH YOUR PARENT

Social isolation is one of the more serious side effects of this job. If your parent lives with you, the problem can become dire. You must find ways to meet your need for companionship.

Try to get out on your own regularly. When you have to include your parent, bear in mind the following tips:

• Keep gatherings small. One or two people will be more manageable than a large party.

• Whenever possible, socialize around a regular daily activity. Invite people over for a meal during your parent's usual mealtime, or have friends join you on your parent's daily walk.

• Although you need to get out and away, your parent might do better if people come to him. This way he will be more settled and can choose to go to his room when he gets tired or overwhelmed.

• If your parent has odd habits or troubling behaviors, warn guests in advance. Everyone will be more comfortable, and most people will understand and be supportive if they know what to expect. Don't forget your sense of humor. It will get you through some dark patches.

good to your parent if you're in a hospital bed or you're drinking away the blues or, most definitely, if you are abusive. This is an enormous undertaking. Do not minimize what is happening.

And remember, your parent's mood will, to some extent, mirror yours. If you are relaxed and patient, he will be calmer and more cooperative.

So take a deep, slow, calming breath, and then make your triage list, because you simply cannot do it all. What absolutely *has* to get done that only you can

do? What on your to-do list can go on your some-other-day list, or your not-that-critical-so-I'll-forget-it list? Who can help you with other tasks or give you some respite? What community services are available? (Use them.)

Exercise, eat well (sure, you know it, but you really have to do it), join a support group, schedule breaks, get plenty of help, and find ways to relieve stress and anger. Review Chapter 3 for more ideas on caring for yourself, and try the suggestions outlined below.

> " Sometimes it's as if the woman who raised me, the one that I used to go to for comfort, were dead. I don't have my mother anymore, and I miss her terribly."
> —Francine R.

Acknowledge the Situation

Early in this disease, it's natural to believe, on some level, that your parent will wake up one day and be the person she used to be. Or at least that she won't get much worse. That kind of hopefulness gets people through the day. But it also leads to frustration and despair when, instead, your parent wakes up each day less able than she was before.

If your parent has irreversible dementia, she will not get better. She will not be able to do things today that she couldn't do yesterday. She will probably be even less capable tomorrow. You cannot teach her new things or remind her how to do old things.

Acknowledging the situation, changing your expectations, and accepting these harsh realities is extraordinarily painful, but it is the only way to reduce the frustration, find new ways to deal with her, prepare for what lies ahead, and appreciate whatever you still have.

Remember, It Is a Disease

With dementia, there is no cast, there are no bandages, and there's not even a temperature for you to check. In the early stages, your mother looks much as she always did, so it's natural to expect her to be the same. But she is sick. She cannot control her behavior. She is not repeating the same questions over and over to exasperate you. She is not fidgeting frantically to annoy you. She cannot force herself to remember the answers any more than someone with a broken leg can force himself to walk.

Because of severe damage to her brain, your mother has lost not only her memory, but her ability to interpret the world or express her needs. She paces frantically and fidgets because her bladder is full and she doesn't remember what she is supposed to do about it. She wanders because she feels lost. She smacks the nurse who is putting on a blood pressure cuff because she is certain the nurse is trying to take her arm off.

Your mother may seem as if she has reverted to childhood, but she has not. A child can learn and take instructions. A child remembers that the stove was hot and doesn't touch it again. A child feels safe in your arms and knows that you are not trying to kill her with your embrace.

Your mother's world is not just fading; it is topsy-turvy, illogical, and scary. She is lost, out of control, and unable to understand her own fear.

This is not her; it is a disease. Keep this in the forefront of your mind: *This is a disease; she can't help it.* It might alleviate some of the frustration and help you keep some perspective.

See the Full Half

Okay, maybe this glass isn't half full. But if you can change your perspective, even a little, you might find that it's not empty either.

> ❝ When my mother was in the nursing home, I used to visit her at lunchtime and feed her. After she had eaten, I would hold her hand and talk about the past, and she would lie there and listen. She never really said anything, or at least anything that made sense.
>
> One time I was flipping through old photos, and she reached out and touched my cheek, and there was a warm and connected look in her eye when she stared up at me. She said, 'They're all gone, aren't they?' I said, 'Yes, they are. But I'm still here and Polly is still here.' And that was it. She was gone again. But I don't think I'll ever forget that moment."
>
> —Jim C.

The point is, looking for what is still good is better than staring down what is horrendous. So rather than being constantly and endlessly frustrated that your parent isn't who he used to be, try to appreciate who he is today. A tall order, no doubt, but give it a try.

People with dementia cannot remember, cannot do the math, cannot follow the story, cannot, cannot, cannot. So many *cannots*. But often, if we are open to it, we find there are still some *cans*—that they can create, laugh, have fun, hug, dance, share, and love.

Focusing on what still is, the *cans*, the good moments you still have with your parent, will certainly help him, and it might help you, too.

Time to Grieve

Whether you adored your parent, battled with her daily, or resented her silently, you are losing her now, one small piece at a time. And losing a parent, regardless of the past, is painful.

This particular good-bye is not only agonizingly prolonged, but it is complicated by the very nature of the illness. Dementia doesn't just take away a person's ability to remember or calculate; it steals his personality, his endearing quirks, and his beloved memories. You are left to care for a hauntingly familiar stranger, someone whose physical features and occasional glances may be heartwarming, but whose behavior and personality, more and more, seem to belong to someone else—someone you might not particularly like.

Witnessing such a transformation is unnerving. Your parent, the person who made vital decisions, is increasingly dependent, incompetent, and childlike.

Your father may throw tantrums, have trouble feeding himself, or forget his way home. Your mother may become slovenly and self-centered.

Although you might hold dear the person you knew, you might also feel some disdain or even, at times, disgust for the person your parent has become. You are losing her, but in many ways, she is already gone.

You are busy facing each day's new challenge, trying to get through each minute, and anticipating the future, but take time to acknowledge these complex emotions and to grieve, because that is largely what this is about. Grieving means allowing the pain and tears, it means recognizing a loss, and it means being kind to yourself.

Be Alert to Depression

No surprise, depression is common among people caring for someone with dementia. Be alert to the signs—for yourself and for anyone else caring for your parent. If you just can't face another day, can't stop crying or yelling at people, can't eat or can't stop eating, can't sleep or can't wake up, can't stop feeling miserable and worthless, and question the reasons for being alive, get help immediately. Call your doctor, a therapist, or a psychiatrist. This is a tough job, but depression doesn't need to be part of it.

Deflating Stress and Finding Patience

This bears repeating: Your mission is to stay calm in a situation that evokes every emotion but calm. When your parent pees on the couch, accuses you of trying to kill him, or stores the car keys in the

> ❝ I have said things that I would never have dreamed I could say to my mother. I've yelled and screamed at her. I've cursed her. Sometimes I hate her.
>
> I was brought up to know that you don't do those kinds of things. But you get to a point where you just don't know what else to do. I'm usually a pretty controlled person, but with this, you don't have any control.
>
> I don't like what's happening to me. Every day I pray for patience."
>
> —Martha S.

freezer, you are going to feel anything but calm. But it is the one emotion that will get you through the moment.

Find ways to relieve the pressure, to think clearly, and to draw out the patient caregiver that resides deep within you—yoga, tai chi, deep breathing exercises, support groups, walking around the block a few times. Of course, going into your room and yelling, punching pillows, swearing furiously, and falling into a puddle of tears has its benefits as well.

In addition to some long-term approaches, like a regular lunch date with a friend and a stint at the gym each morning, you need some emergency techniques that will take you to that serene, superhuman place in a pinch.

When your parent pours a whole bottle of shampoo on your rug because she saw a dirt spot, or throws dinner in the garbage because she saw bugs crawling on it (they were black pepper flakes), pause before responding. Just pause. Don't say anything. Look away. Look at the ceiling. And then look quietly at

the situation and decide if it has truly ruined your life. Take a few slow breaths. Roll your neck from side to side several times. Repeat your mantra: *I am calm. I am calm. I am calm.* Breathe deeply a few more times. And then, ever so softly, tell your mother that she's probably right about the bugs. When she's not looking, pull the roast chicken out of the garbage and rinse it off, or make some peanut butter sandwiches.

Then, give yourself a hug. You need a big one right about now.

Vent Your Anger— Someplace Else

Your worst anger may erupt during the early stages of the disease, when you are still fighting what is happening, trying to hold on to the person your parent was, and struggling unsuccessfully for a logical explanation.

Before seeing your parent, you promise yourself that today you will be patient. But within minutes of walking in the door, you find yourself snapping at her. *Mom!! What have you done? How many times have I told you not to rip up the mail? Why do you do this to me?* Minutes later, you hate yourself for getting irate, and you hate her, or this disease, for turning you into a shrew.

Welcome to dementia. It distorts the personalities of not only patients, but their caregivers as well. People who never used to swear suddenly know every four-letter word in the book. People who were kind become crabby. People who love their parents dearly suddenly want them to disappear.

The problem is that while dementia breeds anger, it also feeds off it. Yelling at your parent or yanking his shirt

BEWARE OF ABUSE

When a parent has dementia, the stress can be overwhelming, and you may find yourself lashing out, shaking, pushing, or even striking your parent. If this happens, get away from him immediately. Drop whatever you are doing and walk away. Call a neighbor, a relative, or a friend to take over for you. You need support and you need a break, and you need it right now.

Contact the Alzheimer's Association (alz.org or 800-272-3900). Many chapters have help lines that can get you through a moment of crisis and arrange emergency respite care. Also contact the area agency on aging (eldercare.gov or 800-677-1116) to find out about community services and support.

Focus on the Good Times

Embrace any passing moments of intimacy or apparent awareness. You may not get them toward the end, but early on there may be breaks in this storm when your parent returns to you. Suddenly, there is a moment of intimacy, a comment, a familiar look, a hug, some laughter, or, with any luck, a "thank you." Savor it. Remember it. Make a note of it and pin it to your wall. This is a shot of strength and pleasure that you may not get again.

Don't Assume She's Miserable

Early on, when your parent is still aware of what her abilities used to be, she will be upset about what she can no longer do. But as the disease progresses, she might become content in her mixed-up, timeless world. She might not realize that life used to be different. No matter how involved she used to be, she might be happy just sitting, stroking a pet, watching the birds at the feeder, or listening to a favorite song. So while it saddens you, she might not be as unhappy as you think.

Remember Your Sense of Humor

If your mother thinks you stole her stockings so that you could wear them over your head and rob her, it's sad, but it's also amusing. Help her look for her stockings and assure her that you are not going to rob her. Then, when you repeat the story to your sister, go ahead, pull

off because you can't stand to wait while he fumbles with each button can trigger a wild tirade. If you can back off and cool down, things will go more smoothly, and you may actually get him dressed and fed faster.

When you can't cool off, vent your anger elsewhere. Make sure your parent is safe, and then leave the room. Yell out loud, kick a wall, or punch a pillow. Be sure to have a list of friends you can call when you need to release some steam.

Forgive Yourself

When you do slip and lose your temper with your parent, which you are bound to do, forgive yourself. You acted naturally. If there is anything positive about this disease, it's that your parent will forget that you ever even raised your voice.

> " Sometimes, she says something—
> a little joke or a comment—that
> shows me she is still there. Buried under
> that disease, a piece of my mother still
> survives. It's that little piece that remains,
> the memories of who she was and those
> soft, familiar hands that keep me going."
> —Marge W.

the stockings over your head, and have a good laugh about it. *What was I going to steal, her dentures?*

You need to grieve, of course. You are losing your parent in a very painful way. Yet despite the gravity of the situation—and because of it—give yourself permission to laugh. Indeed, seek out friends, movies, or books that will make you laugh. It's potent medicine.

Give Yourself a Lot of Credit

On one level you know you are doing a good job. On another, you feel like a failure. Some days, it just feels that you aren't giving your parent the time or attention that he needs. You aren't kind or patient enough. At times, you may wish that he would die.

You would have to be a saint to do otherwise.

Give yourself a lot of credit. If it helps, write a list of all that you are doing for your parent and put it someplace where you will see it regularly. Then stand in front of the mirror and tell yourself that you are an amazing daughter or son. You are. In fact, anyone caring for someone with dementia is an unsung hero.

Remember, if you are in a support group or know people who are in a similar situation, don't compare yourself with them. They are handling different symptoms, they have different relationships with their parents, different supports, entirely different pressures in their lives. No comparisons, please.

Use Help and Respite

To preserve your sanity and health, get help early, early, early in the game, and take regular breaks, even if you think you don't need them.

Before your parent is accustomed to a routine that includes only you, get her used to other caregivers—people in the family, companions, or a day care program.

- Don't ask your parent if she wants to go to day care or if she wants to have a particular person care for her. Gently tell her what is going to happen. Don't make it a choice. To give her some sense of control, ask if she wants to wear this outfit or that one, or if she wants to have something to eat before leaving, but don't question whether or not she wants to go.

- If possible, ease into the arrangement gradually. If your parent fears strangers and you are having a companion or aide come to the house, have him or her come very briefly the first time, and then build up. Or, if you are taking your parent to day care and your parent clings to you, stay with her for the first day. Then leave her for an hour, working up to half a day, and so on.

- Schedule the changing of the guard for a time of day when your parent tends to be calm.

- Provide detailed instructions about your parent's daily routines and habits, and suggest ways of dealing with difficult behaviors. If possible, have the aide watch you in action once or twice, so she can follow your lead.

- Make it clear when you will return. Put a calendar or clock on the wall, marking the day or indicating the time that you will be back. An aide can draw an X through each day or cross off each hour as it passes.

- Keep a regular schedule. Your parent should go to day care or the aide should arrive at the same time each day, if possible.

- If your parent says you are abandoning her, accuses the aide of stealing, or refuses to go to day care, consider any underlying reasons she might have for behaving this way. Maybe she is afraid you are leaving her for good, or worried that this other person is going to hurt her. Logic might not work, but you might, for example, leave a large picture of yourself and a note saying that you love her and will return soon.

- Be committed to this arrangement. Give yourself a month or so to put up with the fussing that may accompany it. Don't give in. The longer the new arrangement is sustained, the easier it will become for your parent to accept it. Determination is key.

"I tried to leave my mother at a day care program, and the next thing I knew she was running after me.

I'd spent a lot of time finding a situation that would be right for her, and I was very upset that she refused to cooperate. Several months later I tried again, at a new place. But this time I got my mother there early, before anyone else. It was like starting somebody off in kindergarten. We began with one day a week until we had worked up to four days. It was all very gradual. When my mother got anxious, the staff put a sign up: 'Sally will be here to pick you up at four.'

She came to love the place. That's the funny part. She looked forward to it. Of course, as soon as she got off the van, she couldn't tell me where she had been or what she had done. But while she was there, she was happy. And that's all I cared about."

—Sally T.

Chapter 25

Managing Day to Day

Hygiene and Dressing • Incontinence • Eating • Communication • A Sense of Time • Other Challenges • Problem Behaviors • Psychotic Symptoms • Late-Stage Dementia

---

I t's been a long day already. Now the mail has disappeared, your mother is insisting that you are her sister Margaret (whom she never liked), she's refusing to eat dinner, and you've just discovered that she put her clothes in the oven instead of the washing machine. Tonight, of all nights, is bath night. It's enough to make someone consider a one-way ticket to Bora Bora.

Before you head for the airport, try some of the approaches in this chapter and see if you can't protect your mail, the house, and your sanity. Unfortunately, there are no uniform rules or answers. What helps one person may be of little use to another. Try different tactics and see what works. (Of course, what helps this week might not be of any use next month, so you might have to switch your methods over time.) A little ingenuity, perseverance, and compassion will make this journey smoother for both of you.

Chapter 7 suggests general tips for managing every day when a parent is elderly, many of which should be helpful to you now. This chapter offers additional ideas on handling those same daily tasks when someone has dementia, as well as tips on handling particularly challenging behaviors.

Good luck.

Hygiene and Dressing

When the smallest tasks become Herculean battles, it's tempting to let things go. But your parent's hygiene affects not only her risk of infection, but also her self-esteem and the well-being of others who spend time with her.

Bathing

The conflict sometimes begins at the mere suggestion that you or someone else help your mother with a bath. She might insist she just had one. Or insist that she can do it herself. Goodness knows, she's done it herself forever. The trouble is that while she recognizes that it's something she used to do for herself, and something that is private and done alone, when she gets into the bathroom, she can't remember how to do it.

If you think about it, hygiene requires a lot of steps. For an addled mind, it's complicated and demeaning. A few tips for making it bearable:

- Daily baths are not necessary; your parent needs to bathe only two or three times a week. Sponge baths are fine when proper bathing isn't possible.

- If sponge baths are an ordeal, try splitting them up; the lower half can be done in one day and the upper half, the next.

- If she can get out and can afford it, have her hair washed by a professional once a week, which might be a treat and will take that part of the job off your hands.

- If possible, do this when she is most lucid and has the most energy. If your parent is more confused in the evening (a phenomenon called "sundowning"), then obviously, that's not a good time for baths.

- Stick to a routine. If bathing is done after breakfast, try to do it at that time on every bath day.

- Give her simple choices—enough so that she has some sense of control, but not enough to derail the activity. "Do

REMEMBER THE BASICS

SIMPLICITY. Simple tasks. Simple instructions. Simple choices.

PATIENCE. Everything will take longer now. That's a given. Ironically, any impatience on your part will only drag things out. *Dad, come on. Just get your pants on! Hurry up. We have to go.* Patience is the key to moving things forward and getting them done. *It's okay, Dad. Take your time. Just put your right leg through this hole.*

COMPASSION. He is not trying to be difficult; he is ill. Remembering how hard this is for him, and what he's up against, will help both of you.

ROUTINES. Adhering to some sort of routine should help both of you get

through the day. Find one that works and, as often as possible, stick to it.

FLEXIBILITY. You had a plan for the day. A schedule. But he's wet the bed (and the floor), and now all your plans are dashed. Time to breathe slowly, respond calmly, and rethink the day.

Hope for a plan, prepare for chaos, and forget all the rules. No, your dad can't wander out unattended, but let him wear socks that don't match, eat ice cream for breakfast, or watch TV at 2 a.m., if that's what works for him.

HUMOR. When life gives you lemons, find the humor in it. Sometimes, in all the craziness, there is nothing left to do but laugh.

---

you want to take your bath before or after you have your tea?" Or "Do you want a shower or a bath?"

- Give her, and yourself, plenty of time for demanding tasks like this. Schedule them when you aren't hurried.

- Take a moment beforehand to gather your patience. Don't walk into this braced for a fight and ready to erupt at the first protest. Get your Zen on. Remember how terrifying and difficult this is for her. Your calm reactions will make her feel secure.

- If your tone suggests that you are happy about this and you act as though this is something she loves—a special

treat, something wonderful and relaxing—she might just believe you.

- Be prepared. Draw the bath, have towels nearby, open the shampoo bottle, have clothes laid out in the order that they go on, and so forth.

- Create a safe and easy environment. Make sure the water is a comfortable temperature. Warm up the bathroom. Install grab bars on bathroom walls and safety handles on the tub. If she showers and has trouble standing, put a small, sturdy seat in the shower stall. If you help her wash her hair, buy a handheld attachment for the faucet. Use a no-slip bath mat.

A SAFETY CHECKLIST

❑ Lock (or install childproof latches on) any cabinets that contain household cleaners, solvents, medicines, matches, lighters, liquor, knives, laundry detergents and bleach, scissors, or other dangerous items. Check for hazards outside the house as well, such as paints, clippers, saws, grills, and lighter fluid.

❑ Turn the temperature on the water heater down to 120°F and label all hot water faucets clearly (with large red letters or by painting the handle red). A person with dementia might not test the water temperature, and if it's too hot, he may not realize immediately that he is being burned or react quickly enough to escape serious injury.

❑ Don't wait to find out that your parent wanders. Assume she will either wander out or get lost at some point. Get her a medical alert bracelet (or necklace) that identifies her as having dementia and provides contact information. Have a recent photo of her on hand. And sign up with the Alzheimer's Association's Safe Return Program, a national program that helps locate people with dementia who get lost.

❑ Get an ID tag of some sort for yourself as well (or any primary caregiver), so that if you are injured, emergency crews will know that your parent needs help.

❑ If exterior door locks could be a problem in an emergency, consider putting alarms or bells on exterior doors to prevent wandering.

❑ Post clearly written instructions for calling 911 by every phone. Include the street address, as your parent is likely to forget his address in an emergency.

❑ Install handrails and grab bars throughout the house, as dementia (and the medications used for it) affects coordination and balance. Remove loose rugs and clutter on the floor. Check that chairs are sturdy and have

• Be sure that hidden areas, folds of skin (under the breasts, between tummy rolls), and genitals are cleaned. Just getting in a tub and swooshing some soap around is not enough.

• Be flexible. You know how a bath or shower should go, but you're in Wonderland now. If she wants to put the shampoo in her hair and then get in the shower, or get in with her clothes on and then take them off, go

for it. Using a clothes dryer is easy; an upset parent with dementia is not.

• You may need only a few inches of water in a bath. A full tub might worry her or make the bath more complicated.

• Respect your parent's modesty as much as possible. If it makes her more comfortable, give her a towel to hold in front of herself, or stand behind the shower curtain while aiding her.

strong armrests. Buy a cane or walker if necessary.

❑ Remove bedroom and bathroom door locks that are operated from the inside so your parent can't lock himself in.

❑ Hide a spare key outside your house in case your parent locks himself (or you) out.

❑ Even in the early stages, your parent should not smoke when unattended. He might forget a burning cigarette or drop a smoldering butt in the wrong place.

❑ If your parent might leave the stove on, lock the stove, remove the fuse, turn the gas off, or (if you still need to use it) use knob covers or get an electrician to install a remote on/off switch.

❑ You can buy a small fire extinguisher that attaches under the stove vent and goes off automatically in case of a small stove fire.

❑ Remove artificial fruit, food-shaped magnets, or anything else that might be confused for food. Sometimes even items stored in a bowl in the kitchen, such as tacks, erasers, corks, and paper clips, can be mistaken for food.

❑ Place decals at eye level on any glass doors or large windows so your parent doesn't accidentally walk into the glass.

❑ Use contrasting colors to make steps clearly visible.

❑ Install automatic lights that go on when someone moves or enters a room so that your parent isn't fumbling around in the dark looking for a light switch.

❑ Buy an automated pill dispenser that locks pills in and dispenses them on a timer.

❑ Clean out the fridge occasionally and get rid of old food. Someone with dementia might not realize that milk is sour or cheese is moldy.

If possible, have someone of the same sex bathe your parent.

• Give simple instructions. Instead of saying, "Wash your hair now," say, "Tip your head back. Now close your eyes."

• Describe what you are doing as you do it so she knows what's coming. *I'm going to put a little shampoo in your hair now.*

• Let her do what she can for herself, even if it's not done perfectly.

• Show her what you want her to do. Mime pouring shampoo or wiping with a washcloth so she can follow your lead.

• Limit the conversation to basic instructions and reassuring comments. This is not a good time to start talking about tomorrow's schedule or your problems at work.

PHYSICAL AID

When you are lifting or moving your parent, helping to bathe or dress him, or assisting in some other way, keep these tips in mind:

• Approach from the front, so as not to startle him. Make eye contact and try to keep it.

• Take it slow. Whatever else is going on, try not to hurry; it will only add more time to the task.

• Speak gently, letting him know what is going to happen before it happens.

• Reassure him that he is doing fine, that everything is going well.

• Keep instructions short and simple, going one small step at a time.

• Support him along his larger muscles and bones. Rather than holding a hand, hold a shoulder. Rather than turning him over by pulling an arm and leg, pull the hip and thigh.

• Lift with your legs, not your back. Bend your knees and push up using your leg muscles, not your back.

• If you can't lift or maneuver your parent, don't. Call for help from a neighbor, friend, or if necessary, the police.

• You can buy a "transfer belt," which helps lift people to a standing position, at any medical supply store or on the Internet; or consider buying chair lifts, straps for cars, and other devices aimed at lifting and maneuvering people.

• When things get rough, try a new tactic. Do it at a different time of day. See if a bath, rather than a shower, is easier.

• Buy her something special—lavender bath soap or a soft new towel—and see if it doesn't pique her interest in bathing.

> " I cannot leave him alone for even a few minutes. Yesterday he went and laid a nice fire—newspaper, fatwood, firewood, etc. It would have been great if he'd put it in the fireplace, but it was in the kitchen, under the sink. I caught him with the matches."
> —Todd F.

• Speak calmly and soothingly, encouraging her all the way. Remind her that you are there, helping her, and that she's doing it just right.

• As she grows more frail, her skin will become thinner and more susceptible to damage. Don't scrub. Blot gently. Use gentle soaps and moisturizer. A little talcum powder between folds of skin will reduce friction. Bath time is a good time to check for rashes and sores.

Oral Hygiene

Keep up with oral hygiene as well, even if it's tempting to let this task go. It's still important to prevent infections and tooth decay.

As always, your attitude will help. Remain calm and act as if this is a good thing the two of you are doing, not a horrible chore that you dread. Keep instructions simple.

- Try different things to find what works—a toothbrush with a longer handle, a softer brush, a smaller brush. An electric toothbrush is easier for some people because it requires little hand or wrist movement; however, it terrifies and confuses others.

- It's still important to floss, if at all possible. Most drugstores sell a variety of floss and flossers. See what works.

- Be sure dentures are kept clean.

- Talk with your parent's dentist about other ways to keep up with oral hygiene.

- At some point, you might have to switch to disposable dental swabs and just do a quick wipe.

Grooming

Although you should keep to your parent's usual and familiar routines, you also need to simplify. Ease your mother toward a simpler hairdo and away from any rollers or dyes. If she wears makeup, gradually get her to use less of it. She might still want to put something on, but a quick swipe of blush and lipstick might be enough to satisfy her.

As soon as possible, move your father to an electric razor, as regular razors will become increasingly difficult for him and dangerous. Once you have to shave for him, he might want to put his hand over yours so at least he feels as if he is doing it himself.

" He was getting into dementia and showing very poor judgment. He wanted to buy a motorcycle. Adopt children. Start golfing. He'd never golfed in his life.

I said, 'If he wants to adopt children, go ahead and let him try. They'll never let him, so I'm not going to argue with him.'"
—Maggie B.

Let your parent do whatever she still can herself (as long as it's not hazardous). Simply brushing her own hair repeatedly might soothe her.

Dressing

Find some balance between what's easy and manageable (the same pair of sweatpants every day) and what might boost your parent's self-esteem (a bright dress or silky blouse). Where you draw this line depends on who your parent was, who she is, and how far this disease has progressed.

Once again, take a deep breath and gather your patience. Allow plenty of time, plan ahead, and keep instructions very, very simple.

- Find easy-to-wear clothing, such as elastic-waist pants or sweatpants; shirts without buttons (either pullovers or ones that snap up the front); clothing with Velcro, which is easier than buttons, zippers, or snaps; tube socks, which don't have a front or back; and slip-on shoes or sneakers (or buy elastic laces that never need tying).

- Clearly label dresser drawers ("Shirts," "Pants," "Socks"), and if necessary, mark the front and back of clothing.

LOST AND FOUND

Losing and hiding things is par for the course with dementia. Be prepared.

• Keep two sets of anything that's important—eyeglasses, keys, dentures, hearing aids.

• Attach small items to large key chains so they can be found more easily.

• Get in the habit of checking wastebaskets before emptying them.

• Keep important things in the same place, always. The house keys hang next to the door, the dentures go in the glass by the sink, and so on.

• Attach house keys or glasses to a strap that hangs around your parent's neck.

• Check all pockets carefully before clothing is laundered or dry-cleaned.

• Limit hiding places by locking cabinets and closets.

• Keep a neat house if at all possible, so there are fewer places to lose items.

• You can buy a gadget that allows you to connect a pager to items that are frequently lost—TV remote controls, cell phones, house keys, and so forth.

• If your parent is still dressing independently, lay out his clothes in the order in which they go on.

• Minimize choices. Keep only a few outfits in the closet, and stow away any clothing that is inappropriate for the weather.

• If your parent is prone to undressing at inappropriate times, get him clothes that are not so easily shed.

Incontinence

Incontinence might be caused not by a problem in your parent's urinary tract, but by a disruption in the brain's messaging system—the bladder's cry for relief is not registering. Or your parent might not remember how he's supposed to respond to this urgent feeling or be able to get his clothes off fast enough. Or perhaps he's forgotten where the toilet is or how to use it.

First, talk to his doctor to rule out infections, medication problems, weakness of the pelvic muscles, or other medical causes. Try the incontinence remedies offered on page 243, and also consider these ideas:

- Make it easy to find the bathroom. If possible, leave the door open and the light on. If the door is closed, mark it clearly with large letters or a picture. Create a trail of night-lights.

- Clear a path to the toilet.

- Draw attention to the toilet by using contrasting colors. Hang brightly colored fabric behind it. And be sure there's ample lighting.

- Be sure he wears clothing that is easy to remove quickly.

- Make the toilet easy to use, with a raised toilet seat and grab bars.

- Remind your parent to use the bathroom, or set a timer for established intervals. Monitor his habits and schedule bathroom visits accordingly. Have him go just before he normally does, even if he insists he doesn't need to.

- Once you help your parent to the bathroom, you might have trouble getting him to actually use the toilet. If possible, leave the room to give him privacy, or at least look the other way. Encourage his urination by turning on the tap water. Remind him gently why he is there and what he needs to do. Then give him time to empty his bladder and bowels.

- If your parent confuses other objects—such as buckets, wastebaskets, and flowerpots—with toilets, put lids on them, put them out of sight (or at least out of the bathroom), or label them.

- Look for cues that your parent has to go to the bathroom. He might play with his fly, suddenly become fidgety, or look toward the bathroom without actually getting up and going. If he has speech trouble, he might say, "I have to key." Or he might revert to childish words, such as *doo-doo* or *poopie*. Listen for any such hints that he needs to go to the toilet.

- Try not to show anger when there is an accident (yet another saintly feat). He cannot help it. Reassure him that it's not a big deal, that it's okay.

- Put plastic liners and other protection on furniture and his bed (being sure it's either under a fabric layer or textured so he doesn't slide off it).

- Use a portable commode or urinal when getting to the bathroom becomes too difficult or confusing.

- When nothing else works, he might need to use diapers or a catheter, but only as a last resort. Talk with his doctor.

Eating

Sometimes people with dementia fail to eat because shopping and cooking are too confusing. Sometimes they have trouble getting the food from the kitchen to the plate, or from the plate into their mouths. Some people think they have eaten when they haven't, or forget they've just eaten and insist on having another meal. Some forget what to eat and have a box of chocolates for lunch (worse things could happen).

In addition, medications can interfere with the absorption of certain nutrients, alter appetite and sense of taste, and upset the stomach. (Ask the doctor about this.)

Below are some strategies for making sure your parent eats healthfully. (See page 88 for other tips on meals and diet.)

- Simple, simple, simple. No long spaghetti to spin on a fork, shells to crack, meat to cut up.

- Keep the place setting and choices simple, too. Place only a napkin and fork at his plate—no confusing extras. It will be easier for him to distinguish food on a white plate than on a decorative one. When possible, serve only one or two foods at a time.

- Be sure food is the proper temperature, as your parent might not realize something's too hot and burn his mouth.

- When utensils present an obstacle, serve finger foods, such as chicken nuggets, cut-up fruits and vegetables, tiny egg rolls, stuffed mushrooms, cheese and crackers, and sandwiches. If your parent likes to pace, he can take such foods with him as he strolls.

- Try cups with handles on both sides, cups with straws, and utensils with thicker, weighted handles. Use unbreakable dinnerware in case something is dropped or thrown.

- If you are dealing with a constant eater, use a timer or place a mark on a clock showing what time the next meal will be served. Or simply keep some low-calorie snacks in the house—carrots, celery, cucumber, raisins, low-salt crackers, or butterless popcorn. Instead of arguing with your parent about whether he did or didn't just eat, give him a healthful snack.

- The snack approach is also helpful for a reluctant eater. Instead of forcing your father to the dinner table, leave a plate of healthful snacks in front of him at all times—fruit, smoothies, cheese, vegetables with a hearty dip, peanut butter on crackers, or a diet-supplement drink.

- Keep distractions to a minimum during mealtime.

- Give him time to eat. If the rest of you must go, then start your father early

> ❝ My mother will eat with each member of the family as they come and go. Sometimes on Sunday mornings, my daughter's boyfriend will get her coffee and an egg sandwich before he leaves, and she won't say anything to anyone about it. Then she'll eat breakfast again with my husband and me an hour later. It's not a big deal, I guess, but how much can one person eat?
>
> She got four boxes of candy for Mother's Day and ate all of them single-handedly. I keep imploring people, 'Please don't give her candy,' but they don't listen. Now I hide the candy or even throw it away. She doesn't remember it existed.❞
> —Carol G.

WHEN HOME COOKING ISN'T POSSIBLE

At some point, your parent will likely have to have all her meals provided for her. You will have to sign her up for a meal delivery program or make other provisions, such as adult day care or a companion. Learn about the options sooner rather than later. Check with the area agency on aging (eldercare.gov), the Meals on Wheels Association of America (mowaa.org), and/or the National Adult Day Services Association (nadsa.org) to find out about local programs.

on a course before everyone else sits down, or allow him to continue eating while you clean up. It's not ideal, but it's often necessary.

- When you're not around, be sure your parent has food that is ready to eat (sandwiches, salads, stews, soups).

- Put leftover or loose food in see-through containers and mark them clearly. If you are leaving something for lunch, mark it: "Mom's Lunch."

- Check that dentures fit properly. Sometimes, someone with dementia doesn't realize what the problem is; he simply knows that eating is difficult.

Cooking

If your parent is still cooking for herself, make sure the kitchen is safe. You'll have to judge her abilities and determine when it's time to remove the knives, switch from glass to plastic, and get her to stop using the stove. Just don't wait until the kitchen is ablaze to do so.

Although you might want to make the kitchen off limits right away (*Mom, just sit here while I make dinner*), cooking, or helping someone else cook, will make

your parent feel useful and relieve some stress and anxiety. In the end, giving her a job or two might actually make your life easier. She could just stir something, wash the lettuce, or break the ends off the string beans. (Sometimes, you might need to invent a job for her.)

If cooking is part of her daily habit, quitting might be difficult. If so, make this transition slowly. Get meals delivered occasionally or persuade her to eat meals that require minimal cooking from time to time, so she begins to adjust to the idea. Plan other activities for the time when she always cooked. And be supportive. Maybe she always hated cooking, but this is yet one more loss for her, and that alone can be painful.

A few tips:

- As with everything else, simplify. Throw out anything that clutters the kitchen shelves and adds to the confusion. (*What is this? Cranberry chutney? From 2008?*) Have only what's necessary in the cabinets. Get rid of any gadgets she won't be using.

- Put signs on all the cabinets and drawers. "Forks," "Soups," "Breads," "Bowls."

> **❝** I brought my mom home, and my dad opened the door and the whole side of his face was puffed up and red. It had been burned.
>
> My mother wasn't there to cook for him, so he put a can of beans directly on the electric burner and then picked it up and opened it. The beans shot out. They were all over the ceiling and the floor. He was burned all over.
>
> But all he was worried about was the mess and who was going to clean it up."
> —Maggie B.

- If your parent is still using the stove, post a clear reminder above it: "Turn off stove." Place a timer by the stove ("Set the timer"). Clearly mark the OFF position on each burner (red nail polish works).

- You can hook up a gadget that turns off the stove automatically if your parent leaves the room and doesn't return within a predetermined amount of time.

- Burner covers (for electric stoves) will reduce the heat. They are still hot enough to cook on, but less apt to cause a fire if your parent swipes a sleeve past them, sprays oil on them, or holds a newspaper over them.

- Get a teakettle with a very loud whistle (being sure your parent will know what this whistle means and won't just be terrified by it). A microwave might be better for simply heating up a mug of water for tea, as long as you have a good mug that doesn't get hot.

- Be sure her cookware is sturdy and has protective handle covers, and that her potholders are flame-resistant and not worn thin.

- When she can't use the stove safely, disable it, use knob covers, remove the knobs, hide the pots, cut off the gas, and/or get an electrician to install a remote on/off switch. Newer stoves have lock features that might deter her.

- Microwaves are somewhat safer than stoves, but not foolproof. Get rid of nonmicrowaveable bowls and cups. Put a sign on the door: NO METAL.

- Toasters and toaster/ovens can be just as dangerous. (Will she stick a fork in to get her toast or put the toast in for too much time?) Again, signs usually help. But at some point, get rid of it, unplug it, or hide it.

- People with dementia also forget to turn off the water. It's not so dangerous, but it's still a potential disaster if flooding damages the house or sends your parent into a fit (or makes you late for work again). Post a reminder to turn the water off, remove any plugs, or use an antiflood plug (available online). You can also get a faucet that allows about 20 seconds of water before you have to push down on it again.

- If your parent might cook when you can't observe her and isn't a safe lone ranger, unplug appliances during those times, remove appliances, or install a timer that shuts each unit down during certain hours.

Communication

Over time, dementia skews communication in a number of ways. People have trouble with grammar or finding the right word. They might talk fluidly, but the words have no meaning. Sometimes they can formulate and write words and sentences, but have difficulty pronouncing them. They lose their train of thought, drifting off in midsentence. They have trouble finding the right word for an object and say instead, "that thing that you play music on." Or they might jumble their words, so that *needle* becomes *beedle*, or *food* becomes *fide*.

Your parent will have trouble not only expressing herself, but understanding what others say. She might be able to read a sign, but have no idea what it means. She might understand what you say in person, but not what you say over

the phone. She might be able to repeat a message, but not interpret it, so she says, "Oh yes, I understand" and repeats your instructions beautifully, but then doesn't follow them.

When Communication Fades

- Have your parent's hearing checked.

- Be sure your parent has no dental problems that might be hindering her speech.

- When you talk with your parent, find a quiet place (turn the TV off); do it at a time when you won't be interrupted or distracted.

- Face her when you speak. Be sure she's looking at you.

- Use simple words and sentences. Speak slowly and deliberately. A deep voice is better than a high-pitched tone, which can be more difficult to understand and may suggest that you are upset.

- Supplement your words with nonverbal cues. Point to things. Use photographs, pantomime, and touch.

- If you are giving your parent instructions, don't assume she understands what you are saying, even if she assures you that she does. Double-check by asking her to repeat the instructions and explain what they mean. (Of course, if the instructions pertain to something in the future, she may not remember them, even if she understands them.)

> " Eventually, my mother couldn't express what she was feeling. I would say, 'What's wrong?' and she really didn't know. One time she said, 'I want to be free,' and I understood that she wanted to leave, to be free of the disease, to go back to some other part of her life. Later, she wanted to go home to her mother, who was waiting for her, she said. That made me very sad, because I figured she was preparing to die.
>
> But after a while I realized that she wasn't sad. In fact, I think she was quite ready to go. I was projecting my own sadness, my own sorrow, onto her."
> —Mary W.

- Listen carefully when your parent is trying to tell you something. Give her your complete attention. Look directly at her and try not to interrupt. If she hesitates, forgetting her thought, give her time to try to finish.

- When communicating becomes more difficult for her, listen for words that are repeated or seem meaningful, and respond to those. As you look for meaning in her words, be aware that common themes people with dementia try to express are loneliness and fear, concern about family, and a desire to be well again.

- Let your parent talk even if she is making no sense. She thinks she's making sense, and the sound of her own voice and feeling that someone is listening may be reassuring for her.

- Correcting her mistakes will only increase her frustration and confusion. Encourage your parent, even if you don't understand what she's saying.

When Communication Is Gone

It's hard to know which of the many losses of dementia is the most difficult or the most painful, but when the lines of communication fall silent, an enormous and critically important door shuts. Your parent, no longer able to relay his needs, his pain, his fears, or his wishes, becomes isolated. Caring for him becomes even more challenging and very lonely.

Monitor your parent's comfort and health carefully now, because he can no longer explain when something is amiss. Watch his body language carefully. Facial expressions, such as a smile, a grimace, or a frown, or body movements, such as a clenched fist or a turn of the head, can be revealing.

When he can't talk to you, keep talking to him. He may still understand what you are saying, but even if he doesn't, your presence and the sound of your voice will bring him comfort.

A Sense of Time

Your parent has lost (or is losing) any ability to track time. As a result, you may find that she is constantly worried about doing things at the wrong time. She may get nervous that she is late for an appointment that actually isn't scheduled until next week. Or she may be concerned about wearing out a welcome

and say it's time to go just minutes after she has arrived for a visit.

Try to understand her concerns. Imagine how confusing it would be to have no idea what day it is, what time of day it is, or how much time has passed.

If your parent needs to track the hours or days, keep clocks and calendars clearly in sight. Sometimes an analog clock is helpful because when you go out, you can put colored tape on the clock where the hands will be when you return, with the words "Janie will be home at this time." Or, if she has a doctor's appointment at two and is worried about missing it, put a small, bright note on the clock in the two position.

Various timers are available that can help remind your mother when to take her medications, when to eat, when to use the toilet, and so on.

If large clocks and notes don't help, reassure your parent (or post a note) that you or someone else will help her get to where she needs to go on time, and that you will keep track of when it's time to leave.

A Place in the Past

Your parent may have trouble remembering not only the day and the hour, but also the decade. Many people with dementia become lost in the past, talking about people who are long dead or a job they left many years ago.

This can be extremely upsetting, not only because it is a stark reminder of just how confused your parent is, but also because you may want to talk about today when your parent can talk only about yesterday. You may want to tell your father you love him, but he is lost in 1950, a time when you didn't exist.

As hard as this is on you, the past is probably a very comforting and safe place for your parent. It is a place he can remember and a time when he was fit and able. It might also be that he needs to deal with some unfinished business from the past. Either way, forcing him into the present could disorient and upset him.

If your father is happy in 1950, let him stay there. In fact, encourage him to talk more about that ride he took at Coney Island or the days he spent at his grandparents' farm.

When he says that he is going to visit Wayne, a friend who died 10 years ago, don't try to convince him that Wayne is gone. Instead, try something like, "Wouldn't it be nice for you to see your friend Wayne? Tell me about how you met him, Dad."

Other Challenges

It may feel that the list of challenges never ends. Here are a few more issues that might arise and that often require a different approach when someone has dementia:

Sleep (or Lack Thereof)

Restlessness, confusion, and a disrupted internal clock all make getting a good night's rest difficult. If your parent is wandering the halls at 2 a.m., tossing and turning at 3 a.m., and getting a snack at 4 a.m., he'll be tired, and perhaps more important, so will you. Trouble sleeping, and its effect on the whole household, is one of the top reasons why people with dementia eventually end up in nursing homes.

Whatever the causes, sleep problems eventually subside in most cases. In the meantime, here are some tips for helping your parent get his Zs (more sleeping tips are listed on page 216):

- Make sure your parent gets outside in the fresh air and gets some exercise most every day.

- Cut out caffeine and other stimulants.

- His internal clock is irregular or absent, so your parent has to rely on external clocks. Schedule naps and bedtime and then stick to the schedule. Don't let him doze off at 7 p.m. (even if that seems like a gift at the moment) or he'll want to start his day at 3 a.m. Try to keep him awake until other people in the household retire.

- Guide him to activities that are calming before bedtime, such as listening to music or an audiobook. If undressing is a nightmare, help your parent get into his nightclothes half an hour before bedtime so he can calm down from the effort before going to sleep.

- Make sure your parent has gone to the bathroom before going to bed.

- Don't lay out clothing the night before. Your parent might wake up in the middle of the night and think it's time to get dressed.

- Make sure your parent feels safe in bed. Keep familiar furnishings and photographs near the bed. Also be sure the room is at a comfortable temperature and that he has appropriate covers.

- Be sure there's a night-light or other dim lighting in your parent's bedroom, and put night-lights in the hallway so she doesn't become disoriented on the way to the bathroom.

When your parent's restlessness keeps you awake and nothing seems to work, get help. Although medicating your parent is not a good idea, it might be the only way to get through the week. Talk to the doctor.

Driving

The question of when to give up the car keys is a sensitive subject with any older person, but it can be explosive when a parent has dementia. When you express your concern, your parent may have no idea what you are talking about despite several recent dents. Or when you steer him away from the ignition, he may accuse you of holding him hostage.

" My father's license expired and he couldn't get a new one because he couldn't pass the test. But he was happy to take the car out anytime, even without a license. He took the keys out of my mother's drawer, where she hid them, and had copies made.

His doctor told him he shouldn't drive. Everyone told him he shouldn't drive. We tried to reason with him. But he said, 'No, that's my independence.'

My husband and I finally had to disable the car."

—Maggie B.

SCAM ALERT

Be extremely alert to fraud. All elderly people are vulnerable, but those in the early stages of dementia—when they still control their finances, yet have questionable judgment—are at the highest risk.

This is not something that happens to someone else. Scams and fraud are rampant, and come in all shapes and sizes, from massive telemarketers to a new best friend (who happens to need a loan). See page 326 for more.

Talk with your parent about driving early in this disease, *before* he needs to quit. (He should quit pretty early on, though, because disorientation and confusion can easily lead to a serious accident.) If he is already a danger and needs to be stopped immediately, take action regardless of his response (kindly, of course, but firmly).

If possible, get rid of the car so there is no threat of his driving. If the car is needed, get an auto mechanic to show you how to remove the distributor cap so it won't start. When you need to use the car, you can put the cap back on. There are also gadgets you can buy that will temporarily disable a car.

Medications

Very early on, your parent might be able to take his medications on his own. An automatic pill dispenser or phone reminder system might help (see page 144). But eventually, pills, like everything else, will become a problem.

- If your parent resists taking a pill, wait a few minutes and try again. Remind him why the pill is important.

- Ask the doctor if it's okay to crush a pill and mix it with food.

- Lock up or hide medications so they aren't taken accidentally.

- Don't just hand your parent a pill and walk away. People with dementia sometimes hide pills, toss them, or tuck them in their cheeks out of fear and confusion. Watch that a pill is actually swallowed.

- If your parent can't swallow a tablet, talk to the doctor about liquid or melt-away versions.

Money

Your parent's ability to manage his money will decline. Early in the game, bills will be forgotten, calculations confused, and money may become meaningless. If your parent used to be thrifty, he might start spending money recklessly. He might invest in obvious scams. Or he might make smaller mistakes, like handing over $20 for a candy that costs 70¢ and walking away without any change.

As soon as possible, start shifting financial oversight or control to yourself or someone else (with ample safeguards in place). If it makes your parent feel better, let him carry small amounts of cash and a few expired credit cards in his wallet.

GADGETS TO MAKE LIFE EASIER

A vast array of products exists to make life simpler and safer for people with dementia—reminders, alerts, motion detectors, easy-to-use phones, medication dispensers, stove-top fire fighters, automatic faucet controls, and so on.

This Caring Home (thiscaringhome .org), created by Weill Cornell Medical College, provides detailed, room-by-room safety tips and reviews of products. The Alzheimer's Store (alzstore.com or 800-752-3238) sells products for people with dementia. Even if you don't buy anything, scanning these websites should give you ideas for things you can do yourself.

It's a tough subject, but deal with it early, because people can suddenly find themselves in dire financial straits.

Telephones and Mail

If your parent lives with you and you aren't getting your bills or are wondering why there are never any messages on your answering machine, it is time to make some changes.

Of course, getting your bills online and telling important callers to use your cell phone should solve the problem. But if you are dependent upon a home phone, ask the phone company for a call-forwarding service so your calls can follow you, keep the answering machine in a locked drawer (so your parent can't turn it off), or turn the ringer on the phone and the volume on the answering machine off.

You can buy a phone that allows incoming calls even when the phone is left off the hook (look for phones with an "auto on-hook" feature).

For your parent, phones with large numbers and speed dial with identifying photos will be easiest to use. Some literally have nothing else on them but four or six buttons with a place on each one for a photo.

Regarding the mail, get a post office box or put a latch on your mailbox that is a little difficult to undo. If you live in a suburban or rural area, you might be able to work out a plan with your mail carrier to leave the mail on a shelf in the garage or in the neighbor's box.

If your parent lives alone and is having trouble handling the mail, arrange with creditors to have her bills sent to your address, or arrange to have them paid automatically from a bank account.

> " Last week Mom raced me to the mailbox and I actually had to wrestle the mail away from her. She had it all stuffed under her sweatshirt, and I knew I would never see it again. Finally I put a bungee cord on the box. She can't figure out how to get it off. The mailman has a little trouble with it, too, but he's getting better at it."
>
> —Carol G.

Problem Behaviors

No matter what your parent is doing now that is making your life challenging, it will change. Maybe not tomorrow, but usually in a matter of weeks or months. A person who is hitting people and having tantrums often becomes calmer and quieter with time. A person who is always poised on the edge of danger, hiding scissors under couch cushions, will eventually lose interest in such things.

A barrel of patience, a list of strategies, and the knowledge that this too shall pass will help you cope.

When a particular behavior is causing trouble, keep a record for several days or weeks (or make a mental note) of when the trouble began, anything that might have set it off, what approach was tried to resolve the problem (distraction, reassurance, medications, and so on), and when it stopped. You might begin to see a pattern and thus, find ways to head off problems before they start.

Sometimes it helps to simply ignore a behavior, as long as what your parent is doing isn't dangerous. Everyone has to agree to simply look the other way. When an action doesn't trigger a reaction, it can become boring. It's worth a try, anyway.

Hiding and Hoarding

If your parent is hoarding food, money, or other items, and her actions are not harmful, let her do it. People with dementia sometimes stockpile things because they are afraid that they will have to care for themselves in the future, that they will be abandoned, that people are stealing from them, or that people are trying to harm them. It may give your parent some peace of mind to squirrel things away.

In fact, if you can, help your parent stash some items. Provide a tin for food or a safe hiding place for small change. You will be less apt to find moldy cookies,

DEPRESSION AND DELIRIUM

As we've noted, people with dementia often become depressed, especially in the early stages of the disease. Depression is treatable and not an acceptable part of this illness. Don't ignore it or think it's to be expected. Talk to your parent's doctor.

Delirium, the sudden onset of acute confusion and inattention, is common in elderly people, especially if they are moved to a new location, undergo surgery, get dehydrated, or become sick. Again, know the symptoms and alert the doctor immediately, as delirium is a medical emergency. (See page 268 for more on delirium.)

> ❝ For somebody whose mind is deteriorating, she does really well. She's fast. She'll snatch things off the table and put them in her pockets faster than you can see her.
>
> I made hot-cross buns for Easter, and by the end of the meal, her pockets were filled with them. I think she's saving in case of a flood—I mean, we have more than enough to eat. Nobody goes hungry around here, and she certainly eats well. She's always putting food away as though she might not get another meal. I keep asking her, 'What are you doing that for?' But I'll never get an answer."
>
> —Carol G.

spoiled cheese, and piles of coins in drawers and closets.

Also, keep an eye out for new hiding places and check them occasionally, without letting your parent know that you're on to him.

Agitation

Your parent picks up a magazine. Puts it down. Goes into the bathroom. Comes back. Sits down. Stands up. Walks into the kitchen. Comes back into the living room. Rocks in her chair. Asks you what she should do. Goes into the kitchen again. Comes back. Asks you what she should do.

Tranquilizers start to look awfully tempting about now. Although medications are sometimes necessary, they are not the best solution. First, try some of the tips offered earlier in this chapter and, as always, remember your mantra: *I am calm. I am calm. I am calm.* It will help tremendously if you can keep your cool and use a steady, reassuring voice. Also:

- Make sure your parent isn't consuming any drinks, food, or drugs that contain caffeine or other stimulants.

- Try to figure out what triggers the agitation—a particular activity, a certain room or place, or a time of day. Then be prepared next time you head into that zone, or avoid it altogether. If, for example, she gets agitated every time you vacuum, try to do the vacuuming when she isn't around or at a time when she is less upset.

- Be aware of any personal need or discomfort that might cause agitation, such as hunger, a full bladder, fatigue, or thirst.

- Sometimes agitation is prompted by some unspoken concern. Your mother may be wringing her hands or nervously bouncing her leg up and down because she is worried about being late for an appointment or about getting home safely from a visit. If you can figure out what's worrying her, you might be able to calm her fears.

- Reduce stimulating noise, bright glare, and commotion. Turn off the TV (you can buy headsets for the television so she doesn't have to listen to it). Move guests into a different room. Turn down the music or radio.

- Encourage your parent to exercise daily, even a little bit, so she'll use up some of the nervous energy. If she wants to pace, let her do it (it's exercise). Get someone to go for a regular walk with her, get her to a gym or pool, or, if she can handle it, buy simple exercise videos that might keep her occupied for a while and use up some energy.

MY FATHER DOESN'T KNOW IT'S ME

As dementia weaves its way through your parent's brain, destroying his abilities and his memories, it will eventually get around to that cherished pocket that holds his memories of you. He might know who you are at one moment but not another. He might know your name but forget that you are his daughter. This is the heartbreaking nature of dementia.

At this point, the magnetic forces that drew you to care for your parent, and kept you at it when things got rough, can wane. Your father doesn't look at you with a familiar gaze, full of knowledge and memories, but with the blank look of a stranger or the angry glare of a victim.

With all that you are losing, this is a debilitating blow. But as you well know, your parent needs you now more than ever. Not only does he need you to protect him because he can no longer fend for himself, but your warmth, your gaze, and your touch are powerfully reassuring for him, even if he can't say so, even if he doesn't know why.

He has little to give you, and needs everything from you. It is a lot to ask. Love him with all you have left, for even though he doesn't remember your name or the past, you are his entire world now.

- See if there isn't something that might soothe her, like a cat or special pillow or sweater or photo album.

- Give her something to do, such as shelling peas, stuffing envelopes, folding laundry, or polishing silver. Or make up a task. *Mom, I need all these pages folded in half. Could you help me?*

- Distract her. When she starts to pace, get her doing or thinking about something else—a song, a photo album, a memory, a story she loves to tell.

- Try relaxation techniques, such as massage or therapeutic touch, imagery, and soothing music.

Wandering

A person with dementia may start out on an errand and forget where she is going and where she started. Or she might just amble aimlessly out the door and into the night.

Even if your parent has never wandered before, be sure she wears an identification bracelet or necklace, at the very least. If wandering is a concern or becomes a regular problem, talk with your parent's doctor because certain medications can make it worse.

Follow some of the guidelines for dealing with agitation, as the two are related. And don't forget, exercise and cutting out caffeine will help reduce any nervousness or pent-up energy.

A few more tips:

- If your parent simply needs to roam, take her for walks and give her ample space to pace at home. Clear pathways. Make sure she has slippers, socks, or shoes that provide adequate traction. Use nonskid strips, if necessary.

GRANDPA IS SCARING ME

A beloved grandfather says bizarre things. He wets his pants or makes a mess of his food. He's crass or mean. It's hard for an adult to bear; for a child, it can be terrifying. It can also leave them with unhappy memories of someone who is dear to you.

Explain it as well as you can—that Grandpa's brain is injured, that he doesn't mean what he says and can't remember what's just happened.

Your reaction will determine your child's reaction, to some extent; if you stay calm and kind, it sends the message that this is nothing to worry about. If possible, find some humor in odd behaviors, excusing Grandpa for that loud belch or racy statement and giving him a supportive hug.

Assure children that Grandpa still loves them, even though he may not be able to show it now (or remember their names). And encourage them to discuss their feelings about this with you.

If you ache for your children to know your parent as he was, offer them a glimpse into the past with stories of your childhood and his life, and old photos.

Once they accept what is happening, children can be wonderful company for an older person with dementia, and a big help to you. They are often more forgiving than adults and might be able to interact and play at the same level as your parent. A child might like to sing songs, watch a cartoon, or play games that are manageable for a grandparent with dementia.

For help explaining dementia to a young child, several books are available, including *The Memory Box* by Mary Bahr and David Cunningham, *Grandpa Doesn't Know It's Me* by Donna Guthrie, *Always My Grandpa* by Linda Scacco, *The Sunsets of Miss Olivia Wiggins* by Lester Laminack, *What's Happening to Grandpa?* by Maria Shriver, and *Still My Grandma* by Veronique Van Den Abeele.

- Put a sign on the door: "Jack, Do Not Leave," or simply, "STOP." (This might work only for a short time and only in the early stages.)

- Disguise exits with posters, wallpaper, curtains, or other decorations.

- Lock doors with latches placed high or low on the door, or use plastic child-proof knobs. Better yet, , install alarms on doors, or attach a bell so others are alerted when the door is opened. You can also buy monitors that alert you when your parent opens the door

Some allow you to record your own voice: *Dad, please stay in the house.*

- Alert neighbors and the local police to the situation. Have photographs of your parent on hand so that if he does get lost, you can hand them out. Ask neighbors to let you or your parent's caregiver know if they see your parent strolling by.

- Get a GPS tracking device, which will let you know where your parent is. You can put it on his cell phone or, better yet (as he's likely to head out the door without a phone), put a device on a wrist strap that he keeps on all the time.

- Sign up with the Alzheimer's Association's Safe Return Program (alz.org or 888-572-8566). Your parent will receive identification cards and jewelry, and be entered into a national database, so that anyone who finds her knows whom to call. Local police departments also have access to photos and information from the database that will help them locate your parent.

- Along with an ID card, put a note in your father's pocket with instructions for him: "Dad, stay calm. I'll be there soon. Call this number."

- Consider buying motion sensors or pressure-sensitive alarms that alert you when your parent gets out of bed, leaves his chair, or approaches the door.

- Install a sturdy fence around the property.

- If your parent disappears, do not wait to get help. Do a quick search, and then alert the police that someone with dementia is missing.

Repetition

Repetition is the Chinese water torture of dementia. The first few drops land on the head with little impact, but as the minutes and hours pass, each drop, each repeated tale or tic, echoes more irritatingly and painfully than the last. Other people can't understand why you are getting so angry, and neither can you. But you are certain that if your parent

asks you whose shirt he's wearing one more time, you will scream.

Sometimes, like nudging the needle on a skipping record (for those of us who had LPs instead of iTunes), you can prod your parent out of a repetitious behavior by changing the topic or the activity. Divert her attention.

If your parent asks the same question over and over, either stop answering it or reply in a different way. When she asks for the 18th time, "When's dinner?" instead of telling her one more time that it's at 7, say, "We'll have dinner after Charlie comes home" or "when the table is set."

If the problem is a repeated motion, touch often works better than words. For example, if your parent is nervously stroking one elbow, rub her other arm or a leg for a moment. (Or give her a dollop of moisturizer and ask her to rub it onto her leg.)

When nothing works, focus your own attention on something else. Take some deep breaths. Tune her out. Try to ignore her motions. Don't respond to her questions. In other words, when you can't divert her attention, divert your own.

Accusations and Insults

Dementia doesn't simply obliterate personalities; it rearranges them. Certain traits become more pronounced, others fade away, and oddly enough, brand new traits can appear.

It's not uncommon for people with dementia to become mean and insulting. Your father might complain that you never visit, that you don't feed him enough, that his wife is cheating on him, or that you've hidden things from him (which you may have, and for good reason). He might call people names or be rude to strangers, leaving you to apologize for him.

Given all that you are doing for him, such attacks can shatter the patience and control you are trying so hard to sustain. No matter how confused he might be, a parent's criticism hits a very sensitive nerve, and the insults may be impossible to shrug off. But shrug you must.

Whenever your parent makes a biting remark, remember that he doesn't know what he is saying or mean what he says. Try hard not to take such comments personally. Think of yourself as one of those blow-up clowns that you punch and they pop right back up—the blow was meaningless and did no harm.

Consider what might be behind your parent's comments, especially if the same criticism is made repeatedly. For example, people with dementia often accuse others of stealing things because that explains why they can't find things. Your parent might claim that someone is keeping him prisoner because he is aware that he is losing his independence and that other people are now in control. He might accuse a spouse of infidelity because he feels inadequate as a mate. He might insist that you are mean because he knows that he is increasingly dependent on you and is angry about it. Not knowing where else to fire that anger, he fires it at you.

Next time your father accuses you of taking his clock, rather than yelling back, "I did NOT take your clock," simply accept the blame. *Maybe I did take it. Let's see if we can't find it together.* Rather than arguing, "I am not cruel to you," console your parent and address his real fears. *I know the world feels cruel right now. I don't like this either. But we have each other, and we will get through it together.*

You are going to waste a lot of energy—energy you sorely need now—if you continually try to reason with your parent. It's not likely to help. Simply do what you can to reassure him that people love him and that he is safe.

Your father might not stop making the comments, but if you understand why he makes them, or at least accept that there is no reason or logic to them, you will be better equipped to put up with them.

Talk to others who care for him, as well, and explain all this. You might have to make up for your parent's anger and criticism by apologizing for him and then being especially appreciative and complimentary.

Inappropriate Sexual Behavior

Inappropriate public behavior is common when people have dementia; inappropriate sexual behavior is not. When either one occurs, first decide whether the behavior is worth your attention. Sometimes what is construed as sexual behavior, such as sitting outdoors naked or rubbing one's crotch, may simply be an effort to get comfortable. It might be hot outdoors, and the crotch might itch.

If your parent's behavior is not hurting anyone—if your father is masturbating alone in the living room—ignore it, if you can. It will undoubtedly be painful and bewildering for you. But you cannot force him to adhere to social norms that have disappeared from his mind. Ignoring the behavior might

APPROPRIATE SEXUAL BEHAVIOR

In the early stages of dementia, romance, intimacy, and even sex can be quite appropriate. As long as your parent can still make somewhat reasonable decisions, is not upsetting or abusing another person, and is not the target of fraud or abuse himself, love and passion are perfectly normal.

Unfortunately, your befuddled parent might make poor relationship decisions. He might call his new love by your mother's name (or call your mother by someone else's name). He might insist that some woman he just met is married to him, or that they are siblings, or that they have been together for years.

As jarring as all this might be, let it be if it makes him happy and no one is harmed. If you are concerned, talk with his doctor or someone from the nursing home.

If your parent has a spouse, sexual and intimacy problems might arise, not surprisingly. Most people do not talk about these issues but struggle silently. Urge your "well" parent to talk with a counselor. A support group might also help her.

reduce it, and learning to look the other way should save you a lot of aggravation.

Sometimes people with dementia mistake one of their adult children for a spouse. Again, if possible, ignore it or just go along with it. If it's too much to bear, find a new approach. When your mother is making romantic advances on your brother and insisting he is her husband, rather than repeatedly correcting her verbally, get your brother to change his look slightly (does he wear his hair like Dad or have the same glasses?). Or you might go with a white lie. *Yes, he looks like Dad, but Dad isn't home yet. He'll be back later.*

When a certain behavior has to be curbed, head it off before it starts. If your father is apt to play with his genitals in public, be sure that his hands are busy with something else. If he urinates in unusual places, buy him a belt or pants with a button-up fly rather than a zipper—anything that is slightly difficult to open. Then as soon as you see him struggling with his belt or waistband, steer him toward the men's room.

Stay one step ahead of your parent. If you know that a long line or a wait at a restaurant will set your father off, tell the waiter in advance that you need to be served quickly. As soon as your mother starts being lewd or unbuttoning her dress on the street, suggest a diversion—one that she enjoys, like having ice cream or calling a grandchild.

Don't make a fuss when your parent embarrasses you in public, as that will only draw more attention. Instead, gently convey the message that your parent is ill. Rather than criticizing him, get him back on course, console him and calm him, apologize to anyone he offended, and exit quickly, if possible.

When your parent's sex drive is out of control, talk with the doctor.

Psychotic Symptoms

Certain issues—violence, delusions, and hallucinations—can immediately become too much for a caregiver. Try the tips outlined throughout this chapter and the preceding one. If nothing helps, and you simply cannot handle it, know that you have a lot of company. It may well be time to find other housing and care for your parent.

Aggression and Violence

Some of your parent's anger and aggression is understandable; life has taken a terrible turn, and each day is a series of failures, losses, and frightening experiences.

Some of it is caused by damage to the part of the brain that regulates and reins in emotion. This can abolish

> " My mother went through a violent stage, which was the scariest part of her dementia for me. She was a different person. It was horrible. She would yell, scream, and swear—at me, at the rest of the family, at the doctor. She would come right up to my face and threaten to hit me.
>
> When we were in public, she would get frustrated and there was no controlling her. I would take her to church, and if somebody moved their head in front of her or talked, she would say, 'When is he going to shut up?' very loudly.
>
> She would never have done that before, never be rude. It was horrible for all of us."
>
> —Linda K.

inhibitions and disable normal filters. As a result, your parent might not only behave badly, but not realize that there is anything wrong with what he is doing. Family members who no longer like this angry imposter, but who still have to care for him, face an agonizing conflict.

Be sure your parent is getting exercise and that his needs are met and ailments addressed. Avoid and derail his outbursts as best you can. Look for cues that set off the rage, and be ready to jump in and divert his attention. Remain as calm as you can, because yelling back will only escalate the anger.

Although it's unusual for a person with dementia to become physically violent, it happens. Remove or lock up potential weapons (knives, guns, baseball bats, umbrellas, scissors, and so on), and post emergency numbers by the telephones.

If an outburst is physical but not dangerous—if your parent is storming around the room cursing violently, or banging his fists on the bed—let it happen. Provide a safe environment where he can explode, such as a room in which there are no sharp edges, glass, or other dangerous items. Hopefully, he'll tire himself out quickly.

If your parent attacks you, get away from him as quickly as possible. If necessary, call the police.

When your parent can't be calmed down in any other way, aggression can be treated with medications. It's not ideal but it's sometimes unavoidable. Talk with the doctor. Be sure to start at

THE BEST MEDICINE: A LEVEL HEAD

The best medicine for your parent now will be the most difficult one for you to find: a calm response. If you can stay composed during an outburst or tirade, it will help your parent immensely (and thus, help you immensely).

When he is throwing his food against the wall, screaming about charging herds, or pacing in agitation, find your Zen. Speak slowly and calmly, using as normal a voice as you can muster. Don't argue with him or scold him or threaten him. Accept what he says as fact, and then redirect him to a new activity or location.

a low dose and check regularly to see if other, nonmedical approaches would be more effective.

Delusions and Hallucinations

Your mother insists that the neighbor is trying to poison her. Your father tells you that he just spoke to Vanna White. As if you didn't have enough to worry about.

Delusions—believing things that are not true—are common with dementia largely because people tend to misinterpret what is happening around them. Your father might not understand the difference between a person on television and a person in real life. Your mother believes she is being starved because she can't remember her last meal.

Hallucinations—seeing things or hearing things that don't exist—are less common. Your father tells you that there is a pig in the corner of his room or that elves speak to him. You can no more convince your parent that these things aren't true than someone could convince you that what you see is not there.

Talk with the doctor about possible causes, such as medications, infections, pain, or vision or hearing problems.

Look for other causes or underlying meaning. When your mom says that her bed is on fire, find out if the electric blanket is on too high. If your dad says that a home care worker is trying to kill him, ask how the worker is going to do that. Maybe your parent feels that the aide is trying to suffocate

" My mother would wake up in the middle of the night screaming, 'Get them out of here! Get them out of here!' She would say she saw people, little children, at her bedside. I didn't know what was going on. At one point I had a minister come and talk to her. I didn't know what else to do. I thought maybe he could help get rid of any demons or spirits in her life, but it didn't help. Then one day it just stopped on its own. She stopped crying out. I asked her later about the little children, if she had seen them lately, and she didn't know what I was talking about. She told me I was nuts."

—Mary W.

him because she keeps all the windows closed and smokes all day. Sometimes patterns in a carpet or on wallpaper can trigger hallucinations in an addled brain.

Don't argue with your parent. In fact, do just the opposite. If the hallucination is not frightening—and some are actually amusing or pleasant—let your parent tell you about it and accept her word as true. Likewise, if a delusion is not causing any trouble, go along with it or ignore it.

If the beliefs or visions are upsetting your parent, assure him that he is safe, that the goblins are friendly ones, or that you will shoo the pig away. Take a bite of any "poisoned" food first or let your parent keep her own box of snacks if she feels she is being starved.

As always, distractions can help. Hallucinations sometimes go away if the person simply moves to another part of the room or house, or starts a new activity.

Increase lighting. Get rid of any excess noise that might be contributing to hallucinations. Cover mirrors, paintings, or other props that might be prompting a vision or belief. (She doesn't want to get undressed because people— in the photographs—are watching.)

Also, be sure your parent isn't watching upsetting or violent television shows as she might have a hard time separating television from life.

Late-Stage Dementia

Toward the end of this disease, your parent will need constant help and supervision. He might not remember who you are or be able to have a conversation. He will need intensive help with all daily tasks—bathing, dressing, eating, and using the toilet.

As the muscles become more rigid and the brain's ability to direct the muscles wanes, he will probably be in a wheelchair or bed, unable to hold his head up for more than a few seconds. Swallowing will be impaired, and eating anything that isn't soft will be impossible.

Although it might not seem so, your parent is still in there, to some extent. That is, even though he won't call you by name, he will most likely be comforted by your presence, your voice, and your touch.

Your parent's senses still work, for the most part, so even if he is hunched over in a wheelchair and mute, he might enjoy listening to music, eating a favorite food, or looking at family photographs. Rubbing in lotion, brushing your mother's hair, or sitting in the sun should also be soothing.

Be alert to any signs of discomfort. Your parent can't relay information about pain except by groaning, fidgeting, or grimacing. Agitation, pulling, and shouting or mumbling can also be signs. Be aware of physical signs of injury too, such as sores, swelling, fevers, and the like. If you suspect abuse or neglect, get help immediately.

People with dementia die from various causes—pneumonia, choking, heart disease, dehydration, and malnutrition. Essentially, as nerve cells die, the body simply can't function anymore. People can't eat or drink, they can't digest, and eventually their organs stop functioning.

With any luck, your parent has talked to you in the past about his wishes concerning medical care, and specifically how aggressively he wants to be treated at this point.

Know that much of the care that is routinely given at the end of life only worsens the pain and symptoms. This is particularly true in the case of dementia. A respirator, for example, is extremely uncomfortable and can cause infections and injury (and require that a person be tied down), but for someone with dementia, it is also likely to be terrifying because he won't have any idea what is happening to him.

Chapter 26 discusses end-of-life care. Although denial is comforting and completely natural, try to face what's to come and plan how you might protect your parent from unhelpful medical intrusions.

The Last Good-bye

Nearing the End

Well in Advance • Making Decisions • Your Parent's Perspective • Communicating • Caring for Your Parent Now • Taking Care of Yourself • Care at Home • Hospice Care • In the Hospital • What Death Looks Like • The Moment After

At some point, it becomes clear that your parent is neither invincible nor immortal, that despite your labor and love, the best efforts of doctors, and the prayers of friends, she will not be around much longer. If you have been giving ceaselessly and worrying constantly, or if your parent has suffered miserably through illness and infirmity, this may not be a completely unwelcome thought. At the same time, it is an agonizing one. Inconceivable, in a way. How can this person who has been with you from the start, cared for you, guided you, and fought with you ever be gone? No matter how sick your parent is, no matter how much or how little she can say or do now, she is still there and still your parent. How could it ever be otherwise?

The looming death of a parent is painful to think about and even more difficult to talk about. In fact, you might be tempted to deny it or ignore it. But as your parent nears the end of her life, keep in mind that this time and, ultimately, your parent's death, belongs not to hospitals and doctors, but to your parent, to you, and to other people in the innermost circle of her life.

Your family may have more control than you think over this death. You can usually choose which medical treatments will be used and which refused, where your parent will be, how she will spend this time, who will be with her, what will be said, what comfort will be given, and, when it's over, what sort of memorial will honor her life.

Death is a process, a final passage of life, that demands both practical and emotional involvement from everyone. Do not turn away. You and other family members are facing a great loss, but you can still cherish this time with your parent and help her find some comfort and peace in this passage.

Death is not simply a grim and heartbreaking betrayal. When we are willing to face it, to be involved in it, death is also a potent reminder that despite all the aggravations in a day, life is precious—very, very precious. To whatever extent you are able, be part of this process and, in doing so, celebrate life.

Well in Advance

Perhaps your parent has signed papers explaining his wishes to avoid futile, aggressive medical care at the end. Maybe you have promised that you won't ever "let it be dragged out." You know what he wants. You know what to do.

But do you really? Are you sure?

If those broad parameters are all you've discussed, then the odds are good that he will die in a hospital, receiving brutal treatments and suffering needlessly. To avoid this nightmare and make your parent's death as peaceful as it can be, it is essential that you do more.

Before your parent is facing end-of-life decisions, ideally before any specific decisions are on the table, prepare. Talk about his wishes. Don't wait, because it can become too late quite suddenly. (For more on talking about late-life medical care, see page 653.)

" One afternoon I was wiping my father's face with a damp wash-cloth. I was exhausted, and he was barely conscious. He was very thin and pale, but I could still see my father there, the young, strong man that I knew. I stroked his forehead, his cheekbones, the hollows and curves of his neck.

He was still there, but he wasn't going to be there much longer. I knew that. I could still love him and touch him and hug him, but just for now. Maybe not again. And at that moment I loved him more than I have ever loved anyone in my life."

—Mack C.

Find Those Directives

By now, your parent should have a living will outlining her wishes regarding medical care at the end of life, and a power of attorney for health care, authorizing someone to make medical decisions on her behalf. Find them. Be sure that you have a copy on hand, and that her doctor has one as well. If she hasn't signed them already, get them signed now.

Communicate

Although you may know on some level that your parent's time is limited, talking about that means exposing both of you to a set of razor-sharp emotions. Because of that, most people avoid such conversations. Indeed, you may find yourself saying, "Everything is going to be fine," when you know full well that it won't be. It's as if by saying the words we make it happen, and by dodging them, we cling to hope.

Whether anyone says it openly or not, your parent most likely knows that his life is drawing to a close—maybe not this week or this month, but soon. But he may be doing exactly what you are doing—avoiding the subject because it's scary and he doesn't want to upset those around him. Talk early on, at least a little, about the decisions that lie ahead.

START WITH THE DOCTOR. Although no doctor has a crystal ball, he or she should discuss the prognosis, the issues, and the decisions that your parent faces now, as well as those that likely lie ahead, and the various paths your parent might take.

This isn't particularly comfortable territory for anyone, even doctors, so you will have to push to have an open conversation, and to get realistic information and a complete menu of options.

A CALL TO HOSPICE. Yes, hospice. It's a scary word, and a seemingly inappropriate one if your parent doesn't seem ready for such a thing. But remember, you are simply gathering information and learning the options. Doctors often don't discuss, or even know much about, palliative care. Talk with a palliative care specialist or hospice nurse early in the process, long before you think your parent would ever need such care.

Hospice care is focused on comfort and meeting a patient's goals (such as lucidity, mobility, seeing a particular loved one, or getting to some event). Typically, hospice care is provided in the home, although some hospices have inpatient facilities or arrangements with local hospitals and nursing homes.

Hospice staff will review the situation and explain what services they provide. This will not only help you understand the options, but also give you a contact so that if things become complicated, if tough decisions have to be made quickly, you have someone to consult.

If your parent is in an assisted living facility, nursing home, or other group home, find out if they work with a particular hospice, and how services might be coordinated.

A FAMILY POWWOW. Your parent, if he is still able and willing, will be front and center in such discussions, but how do you even start such a conversation?

If it's too difficult to raise these issues outright, ask questions and let your parent steer the conversation. Ask what the doctor has said and/or what your parent thinks lies ahead. If that doesn't get you anywhere, be more specific. *Dad, remember those conversations we had when you signed your living will? Do you still feel that way? If for some reason you stopped breathing now, would you want to be put on a machine? The doctor mentioned dialysis. Do you understand what that involves? Is that something you would want to do?*

If your parent can't understand the choices or communicate his wishes, or if he simply does not want to have such

> I asked her about dying. I said, 'Do you think about dying much?' And she said, 'No, I really don't.' And that was it. That was the end of the conversation.
>
> I was blunter than I usually am, but I wanted to give her a chance to talk about it. I didn't get anything, but I know it didn't offend her, either. We're just different. I enjoy introspection, thinking about life, and she doesn't. She's always been that way."
>
> —Betty H.

conversations, you and other family members should discuss the situation at length. Review possible scenarios, options, and likely outcomes. Think about who he is and what he would want. Even though it will be difficult for everyone, try to be realistic about the choices that might arise, how he might fare, and what you will do.

DNR and POLST

Your parent's legal directives—his living will and medical power of attorney—state his wishes, but they are not medical orders. People who have signed these documents can end up on life support, regardless of their directives.

To avoid specific procedures, your parent needs a doctor's orders written into her medical chart. Talk about these options early—very early—because it is incredibly hard to make decisions in a crisis, and people routinely end up with treatments they don't want.

The most familiar of such orders is a DNR, or Do Not Resuscitate order. A DNR alerts medical staff that if a patient stops breathing or goes into cardiac arrest, there is to be no attempt to restart his heart or lungs. DNR orders are usually written when resuscitation efforts are likely to be unsuccessful or, at best, likely to leave a person severely and permanently incapacitated.

Frail, elderly people have little chance of surviving resuscitation and leaving the hospital. Cardiopulmonary resuscitation, or CPR, is not just some oxygen and chest compressions; it is a pretty violent effort to force air into the lungs and jolt a lifeless heart, and it often results in broken ribs and torn airways, neurological damage, and death.

Medical orders can protect your parent from other unwanted treatments as well. The specifics vary by region, but in most places, you can get orders to prevent intubation, artificial nutrition and/or hydration, and hospitalization. Sometimes an order simply says, "Comfort Only."

Many states and regions have POLST (or MOLST) forms—Physician (or Medical) Orders for Life Sustaining Treatment—that allow for a range of instructions concerning medical care. For example, a patient might want to avoid resuscitation attempts and hospitalization but still want to receive

....

66 I had a general idea that my dad didn't want to be on machines— no extraordinary medical procedures— but as far as specifics go, we hadn't discussed it. He was a sick man. I knew that he would die of his breathing problems. But I didn't know that, given his situation, life support was likely to be in his future. I was never told that in an emergency situation, a respirator would be indicated.

He was on a respirator and hooked to all sorts of tubes for 20 days. I watched him being tortured in front of me. I could hardly touch him because there were tubes everywhere.

One day a doctor came in and saw me stroke his calves and said, 'Oh, he's getting a massage.' But I was touching him there because that was the only place where I could reach him. I couldn't even touch his face.

Those are my memories. That's what I'm left with."

—Katherine D.

....

antibiotics in case of an infection and IV fluids in case of dehydration.

(*Note:* If your parent is at home, be sure such orders are clearly visible. Put them on the refrigerator, behind the front door, or above your parent's bed, and make sure they are noticeable and that everyone involved in your parent's care knows about them and understands them.)

Once again, these orders and your efforts do not mean that your parent will die sooner; it simply protects him from needless pain and suffering.

Spread the Word

Make sure that your parent's doctor, any aides or caregivers, and other family members are aware of these discussions and plans, are clear about your parent's wishes, and are ready to abide by them. If even one sibling disagrees with a decision to forgo a procedure, it will complicate matters at a time that is already difficult.

Be persistent in ensuring that your parent's wishes will be honored. If he is in a hospital or nursing home, be sure that his advance directives and any medical orders are on file, and speak with nurses or aides involved in his care. Make sure they understand his wishes or the family's decision and will abide by them. Find out exactly what they will or will not do in specific situations.

Likewise, if your parent is at home, be sure anyone involved in his care understands the plan. Will they call 911? If not, what will they do? How will they keep your parent comfortable? Whom will they call? Basic instincts to call 911 often kick in at these moments if someone hasn't thought out how to respond.

Brace Yourself

Now for the big step. Talking is one thing, but you and others also need to be ready to act. Maybe you are all in agreement that your dad, who has acute lung disease, will not be intubated because he would never get off a ventilator. But are you actually prepared to refuse such a thing? Does he have orders in his medical chart?

We think we are ready, but the reality is always more difficult than anyone anticipates, largely because the choices we expected are often not the ones we ultimately face. Using the above example, what do you do when an impacted bowel or broken hip requires surgery, and that surgery requires a ventilator?

You can't anticipate all the possibilities, but you can prepare yourself to make some very tough decisions. Honest

> " My mother would say, 'I'm tired. I've had enough. If anything else happens, I don't want any more.' But I think she was thinking in terms of an operation. She was thinking of her brain surgery. I'm not sure. She didn't ever spell it out.
>
> When she had a heart attack, we just weren't ready for that. She went to the emergency room and was put on life support.
>
> We assumed we were pretty savvy, that we knew what was going on. But we were stunned. I look back and wonder, *What were we thinking? What happened?* But the whole thing just snowballed."
>
> —Joann C.

information, discussions, and planning, along with a little soul-searching, will help.

Making Decisions

You talked and planned, and you thought you knew what to do, but standing at the bedside, with the clock ticking and your heart breaking into a zillion pieces, it all looks completely different from what you expected.

"Extraordinary treatment," "futile," "no reasonable chance of recovery." These are the things you discussed. But none of it seems relevant now.

Now there are chances, albeit slim ones. Now it's not clear whether a treatment just possibly might help.

What was meant by "futile"? What is a "reasonable chance"? How much "pain and suffering" is too much when the other option—refusing potentially life-sustaining treatment—feels very, very final?

Whether or not to jump-start the heart of an old and dying person with electric jolts when there is no chance of survival should be clear-cut. It's not only futile, but inhumane. But how does one know when radiation is no longer useful, when dialysis should be stopped, when surgery should proceed, when a transfusion would be useful, or when antibiotics no longer make sense?

There is no right answer. For one person, being in a wheelchair with an oxygen tank, half a mind, and an ostomy bag would be unthinkable. For another, a minuscule chance of survival is still a chance, regardless of what life might be like.

Get all the facts. Seek a second opinion if necessary, and talk with a hospice or palliative care expert. If you are uncertain or family members disagree, take your time if possible. If that means delaying a procedure a little or keeping your parent hooked to a machine for an extra day, then go ahead. You need time to make this decision and accept it.

A few things to consider while you deliberate:

GOALS AND PROGNOSIS. Consider the goals, benefits, side effects, and risks of any treatment. Is it meant to prolong life, to preserve independence, to keep her mobile, or to make her more comfortable? If the aim is to prolong her life, how much more time might it give her and what will that life look like? What are the odds of this treatment being successful? What does life look like on the other side? If the plan is to try an approach, how long will this trial last?

Once you are clear about the goal of a treatment and the chances of reaching that goal, decisions about specific procedures should be clearer.

WHAT WOULD SHE WANT? When patients can't speak for themselves, doctors often ask families, "What do you want to do?" But it's the wrong question.

> " The nurse called me at work and told me that my mother was vomiting and had diarrhea. The nursing home needed my permission to start an IV line for fluid and nutrition. I was about to say yes when I stopped myself. Was this really what she would want? No. I knew my mother wouldn't want it. So I said, 'No. Give her whatever she will take on her own.'
>
> It was a very, very long day, and I didn't sleep at all that night. I live far away, and I'd been back and forth twice that week already, so all I could do was wait by the phone. She died the next day.
>
> Do I regret my decision? Not at all. Could I do it again? I hope so."
>
> —Carl L.

The right question is, "What would she want?"

What *you* want about now is to go home and cry, and not make such enormous decisions. What you want is for your parent to be alive and well. Even if there's been a lot of forethought, you might find words pouring uncontrollably out of your mouth. *I want you to do something. Anything. Just don't let her die.*

But the question is, What would *your parent* want? What would she say to you right now if she were looking at this situation? Think about her, listen for her voice in your ear. What did she value in life? What did she think about aggressive treatment toward the end of life?

If you turn this question away from your own needs, if you think not about what *you* want, but about what *she* would want, you will make the right decision, whether that means ending treatment or continuing it.

WHERE IS "THERE"? When questions arise about the value of a treatment or the possibility of hospice care, families often insist that they are "not there yet." It's not time. Not now. Not yet.

It's a common approach and, indeed, a completely understandable one, but be careful. Waiting to be "there," people often find themselves standing in an intensive care unit staring at a person full of tubes, wondering where "there" went and how they got "here."

We wait for an obvious moment when we should shift gears, for a clear dividing line between living and dying, between useful treatments and futile ones. But that defining moment rarely comes. Instead, we face odds and possibilities and unknowns. For example, a procedure might give your parent a few additional months, but she will probably be quite dependent, and it's possible that she won't even survive the procedure. Not exactly the end-of-life choice we expected.

The point is, we are "there" all along this path. Every time we have a conversation, consider the options, and make a decision about medical care, we are "there," determining the course of both life and death.

THE NATURE OF HOPE. When someone is facing the possibility of death, loved ones and doctors tend to tone down or hide bad news, and inflate or invent the good. They do it in the name of hope, to give the patient hope. *We can't tell her this because she might lose hope.*

Hope is good. But lies and half-truths do not create hope; they create deception. And deception is isolating. Deception also makes it impossible for someone to make informed choices. The truth, if your parent can hear it, allows him to prepare and to make decisions about his care.

Certainly there is no reason to dump dreadful news on someone who is clearly not ready to hear it or force someone to accept a fact that he simply can't. That's not the point. But be aware of what's being said, and avoid blatant lies and misleading suggestions of hope.

If you're not sure how to proceed, ask your parent what he thinks the future

OUTSIDE HELP

If your family cannot agree on your parent's medical care, or if your wishes regarding treatment clash with those of the doctor and you have no power of attorney giving you the authority to make decisions about her health care, contact the hospital ombudsman, the social worker, or the hospital's medical ethics committee.

Compassion and Choices (compassion andchoices.org or 800-247-7421) works to expand options for dying patients and has counselors in every state who are versed in legal and medical end-of-life issues. The National Right to Life Committee (nrlc.org or 202-626-8800), has information on keeping a person on life support and securing aggressive medical interventions.

> **❝** I knew my father probably wouldn't make it through the year. But we didn't talk about it. We talked about his illness and treatments, but not about his dying.
>
> At one point, I mentioned his lack of appetite. He said, 'That's what happens in the terminal stage.' It was as if a window shattered. There was silence for several seconds. Finally I said, 'Are you afraid?' And he said, 'No. I want to be sure that your mother is going to be all right. But I'm not afraid.' And that was it. We didn't say anything else. I just wrapped my arms around him and we held each other.
>
> It was as if a veil was removed. After that, every look, every touch was so intense and so close because we both knew, and we knew the other knew."
>
> —Mack C.

holds, and how much he wants to know. Let him determine how much news he gets and how he wants to handle it. If he knows the facts and continues to talk about cures and a long future, let him. It's where he needs to be. Don't erase his fantasy, but don't confirm it either. (You might say, "That would be nice, wouldn't it?" instead of, "Yes, I think you're going to beat this thing.")

Keep in mind, hope has many faces, and hoping for a cure is only one of them. People can hope to live until a certain date, or hope to be free of pain, or hope that their life had value. They can hope for all sorts of things. Accepting that death is near, knowing the truth, does not mean hope is lost.

MISDIRECTED BLAME. We live in triumphant times, but medicine's victories have left us in this horrible position of making life-and-death decisions. It's a power none of us wants. And yet, these decisions are made every day in every hospital by people no better or wiser than you.

Because we hold this power, it sometimes feels like we are not simply allowing death, but *causing* it. We might want our parents to die peacefully, but we certainly don't want to be accomplices.

Whatever you do, whether your parent dies at home or in the hospital, whether you opt for more treatments or palliative care, you did not cause this death. You have to know this in your heart. Your parent is dying. He is going to exit this world one way or another. You are simply determining, based on the information on hand, whether further medical procedures are likely to be beneficial or detrimental. You are trying to make death, which is not optional and not caused by you, the best it can be.

WHITE COATS. Even the strongest among us can feel lost in the land of doctors. We don't know what they know; we don't speak their language. *Just tell us what we should do.* We want facts and answers. But the truth is, they don't have answers and often don't have many facts. Sadly, on this particular journey, most are not terribly good guides.

Doctors spend all their training and working days trying to avoid death. When that's not possible, most want to leave the room, and some actually do. Doctors, for the most part, know very little about palliative care or how to make death gentle or easy. That's not to say they aren't competent and caring.

It's just that this is not particularly comfortable turf.

So, it's up to you to push for answers, make your own decisions, and then fight for what you want.

THE MYTH OF HOSPICE. Hospice care is not about giving up, or waiting for death, or overmedicating someone to the point of causing death. Hospice and other palliative care is state-of-the-art medical care. The difference between this and more aggressive treatment is that the primary goal is to maximize comfort, mobility, and lucidity. In other words, the aim is to have good days, not just more days.

Interestingly, people receiving hospice care do not necessarily die sooner than those receiving aggressive medical care. In fact, people often live longer than they would otherwise. Once people are free of pain and symptoms, surrounded by those they love, and relieved of fear and anxiety, the desire to live is powerful.

YOUR FAMILY'S RIGHTS. By law, your parent has the right to refuse any and all medical treatment. If your parent is unable to speak for himself, his assigned health care proxy is in charge. If there is no proxy, a doctor will usually turn to family members to make a decision.

Not only can you legally refuse treatment, but you can also stop treatment that has been started. Although it's more difficult to stop treatment than to reject it in the first place, it is possible, legal, and done routinely.

NO ONE ELSE MATTERS. This is your family's decision. It does not belong to a doctor who laid out the choices. It does not belong to the nurse who raised her eyebrows or made a slicing comment. It does not belong to a friend or acquaintance who believes they understand where you stand. It is private. Do not be swayed. Hold on to your convictions.

A SENSE OF FAILURE. Some odd language has crept into our lexicon. People talk about patients "fighting bravely" or "beating a disease" when they continue aggressive treatments. They talk about people "letting go" when they opt for palliative care. And when traditional treatments hold little promise, doctors often say, "There's nothing more we can do."

If your parent or your family opts out of aggressive, painful treatments, it is not because anyone "gave up" or "stopped fighting." And when traditional treatments cannot keep a disease at bay, there is still much that can be done to keep your parent comfortable and make the most of these days.

Whatever decision is made—whether you opt for invasive treatments or hospice care—nobody failed. It's all horrendously complex and overwhelming. Your efforts, your deliberations, your compassion—all of this is heroic.

Understanding Some Issues

We think of end-of-life decisions in terms of "pulling the plug" and "stopping life support," but the fact is that critical decisions are made long before such choices are on the table.

For most people, the path to a peaceful death begins with decisions about routine medical care—surgery, transfusions, dialysis, hospitalization, and medications. Nevertheless, it's helpful

HASTENING DEATH

If your parent wants not only to skip aggressive treatment, but to speed up his dying, don't be alarmed. (You probably will be alarmed, but catch your breath and think calmly.) People often ask about suicide because they want to know the options and want some control in a situation that feels frighteningly out of their control. Once they have information and reassurance that their wishes will be followed and they will not be in pain, they often lose interest in suicide.

Be certain your parent is not suffering from dementia, depression, or another mental disorder. Be sure that he fully understands the course of his disease and the scope of pain relief and comfort care available.

Although physician-assisted suicide is illegal in most states, some doctors will help a patient hasten death if the patient is terminally and incurably ill, and deemed to be mentally competent. Some will supply ample doses of narcotics without comment, while others will provide directions for and even personal help in using them.

People sometimes hasten death by refusing to eat or drink, but most people who are dying have little interest in food or fluids anyway, so this will probably cause you more pain than it will him. (Those who are not so close to death will often forget their plan as soon as they get hungry and dinner is served.)

If your parent's desire to hasten death is based on complete information, then you have little recourse but to support him as best as you can. His plans may trouble and anger you. But even if you do not agree with his decision, stay with him. Your parent needs you, and you will surely regret it if you abandon him now.

to understand some of the hot issues that can arise. (*Note:* DNRs and other medical orders are discussed on page 527.)

LIFE SUPPORT. The phrase commonly refers to a ventilator, also known as a respirator, which is a large machine, about the size of a mini-refrigerator, that forces oxygen into the lungs through a tube that is inserted into the nose or mouth, or directly into the windpipe (trachea). Although younger people are often put on life support temporarily and then successfully weaned, a frail, elderly person often cannot get off the machine and resume breathing independently.

Patients on ventilators usually need catheters, tubes for hydration and nutrition, and links to various monitors. Mucus must be sucked up regularly and their lungs monitored for infection. Some patients must be sedated or tied to their beds to keep them from pulling out the tubes, which are irritating.

PULLING THE PLUG. When life support is withdrawn, doctors do not actually pull a plug. "Pulling the plug" is a coarse way of saying that treatment will be stopped and machines turned off, with the understanding that death will follow. It seems drastic, but this death does not have to be painful. In fact, it is likely to be less painful than if the treatment were continued.

A patient is often given sedatives and painkillers. Once the drugs have taken effect, the air is turned down and the ventilator is stopped. After the tube is removed, a patient might be given oxygen to keep him comfortable.

Family members can stay with him, talk with him, hold him, lie with him. Sometimes people die immediately; sometimes they continue to breathe on their own for hours or even days.

FOOD AND WATER. Food and water are the most basic forms of human care, so refusing treatments that provide nutrition and hydration can seem unthinkable. The fact is, artificial nutrition and hydration—pumping liquids and nutrients into a body—is an invasive medical treatment. It does not resemble a sip of water or bite of food. It is painful and involves complications and risk. For your parent, at this stage of life, it may be dangerous.

The human body, once it has finished its initial struggle to live, is remarkably adept at dying. People who are close to death lose their appetites and don't want more than to wet their dry mouths and lips. The organs are shutting down. The body does not need and can no longer process food and water.

Forcing nutrients and fluids into a body that can no longer digest, circulate, or dispose of them can lead to all sorts of complications, including shortness of breath, a backlog of water into the lungs, severe constipation or diarrhea, bloating, and infections.

Dying patients who grimace because of a wound do not show signs of hunger or thirst. In fact, the body often releases endorphins, natural pain relievers. Dehydration, which causes a patient to lapse into a coma, is sometimes called "nature's anesthetic."

DOUBLE EFFECT. Doctors sometimes talk about "double effect," the idea that medications used to treat pain and symptoms might also hasten death. As a result, they are often stingy with pain medications, even when someone is dying.

First of all, if your parent is in pain, it needs to be treated. There is no reason for her to suffer now.

Second, this effect is woefully overstated. If you suddenly gave someone a megadose of morphine, it would likely kill him. However, when a dose is increased gradually over time, as is typically done, patients adjust. Their bodies learn to tolerate it.

If a doctor withholds pain medications, find another doctor or a palliative care expert, quickly.

COMAS AND PERSISTENT VEGETATIVE STATES. The border between life and death becomes especially fuzzy when most of the brain, but not quite all of it, is damaged or destroyed, and a patient

> 66 My mother was in a coma for 10 days in the hospital. I knew we were finally saying good-bye because I saw her dying before me, little by little, and I just wanted her to go. I wanted it to be over. After all those years of watching her be strangled by this disease, I knew she was finally going to be free."
> —Sally T.

falls into the twilight zone of a coma or a persistent vegetative state. Families are left to wonder and wait.

In older patients, these states usually are caused by stroke, heart attack, or Alzheimer's disease. When a person is in a coma, most of the brain no longer functions. The comatose person behaves much like someone under heavy anesthesia. She does not respond consciously to stimuli, such as shouting or poking, although she may be able to breathe on her own and might react reflexively.

Once in a deep coma for more than a month or two, patients usually enter what is referred to as a persistent vegetative state. Few recover from this, and none recover fully. In the case of an older person, the chance of any recovery is virtually nil.

The situation is sheer hell for family and other loved ones. The person is there, soft and warm to touch and hold, and, in some sense, alive. She may even have normal sleep-wake patterns, and her muscles may react involuntarily. Her eyes may open and blink. She may cough or yawn. It's a horrifying trick played out by medicine and human biology.

The last stage of this continuum between life and death occurs when the brain completely stops working, a state that doctors sometimes refer to as "brain dead." Although the term seems to leave room for doubt or hope, there is no difference between it and death.

Your Parent's Perspective

To care for your parent now, it helps to understand some of what he is going through. Of course, everyone's experience is unique, but there are common themes.

WILL THIS HURT? People are often more afraid of dying than of death. In particular, people fear pain. Straightforward information about what is to come, what treatments will be avoided, and how pain will be controlled should alleviate much of this fear. If your parent is not in hospice, ask the doctor for a consultation with a palliative care specialist, who can discuss pain and symptom control.

WILL I BE ALONE? Unfortunately, we all have to do this one alone, but reassure your parent that she is safe and that you and others will be by her side. Let her know that she will not be abandoned.

AM I A BURDEN? People worry about overloading their loved ones with work (but then ask that more be done for them, alas). Let your parent know that you and other loved ones will gladly take care of her, and that she is not a burden (even if she is).

WHAT'S ON "THE OTHER SIDE"? Whether or not your parent ever believed in heaven and hell before, such possibilities might haunt him now. Many people become extremely frightened that they will be punished on "the other side" for some sin. Others simply fear the vast unknown. *What is it like being dead?*

This can cause enormous anxiety. Your parent might not discuss his distress, but if you sense that he harbors such fears, reassure him that all is forgiven and that he will be at peace.

Others might imagine a reunion with a loved one, or some other pleasant "beyond." If your parent talks about seeing her father or sister or some other deceased relative, go with it, regardless of your own beliefs.

Certainly, no matter what your parent's leanings in the past, he might want to talk with a member of the clergy now.

DID I LIVE A GOOD LIFE? People often want to know that their lives have been worthwhile, that they have accomplished certain things, and that they were loved.

If your parent is alert and able to talk, ask her about her life. What is she most proud of? What are her fondest memories? In any way you can, let her know that her life was well lived.

If your parent was neglectful or abusive, or she otherwise failed in her life or in her role as parent, this isn't the time to rub that in.

IS MY WORK WRAPPED UP? Those who are dying, especially those who have dependents, want to know that their affairs are in order, their family is cared for, and any conflicts with others are reconciled. They want to know that nothing crucial is left unsettled or unfinished.

If you sense that your parent is worried about something he's left undone,

help him bring it to a conclusion. Urge an estranged relative to speak to him, or help him dictate a note or find a needed file. Or, just let him know that all is okay. Honestly, even if he's left a mess in his wake, brush over it. Let him go without regrets. It's not an easy gift to give, but it is a generous one.

WILL I BE REMEMBERED? Your parent might want to know that he left some legacy behind. Talk about the lessons he taught you and the memories that will be passed on to future generations. Let him know that the grandchildren still talk about the time he took them to New York, that they value all he taught them, or that they repeat a story he used to tell. If your parent has gifts or possessions to pass on, help him accomplish that.

WILL YOU BE OKAY? This is not the time to tell your parent how miserable you will be without her. Let her know you will miss her, but that you and others will be okay. As the end draws near, let her know that it is all right for her to go; give her permission to leave.

Five Stages

Elisabeth Kübler-Ross defined five stages of dying. They may be less accurate for elderly people, but your parent might be going through some of these emotions. For the most part, you simply have to allow them.

The reactions noted here (somewhat modified) are by no means sequential; people bounce among them, moving, for example, through a period of denial, a few days of anger, and then back into denial. Some adopt several at one time, angry about some things and hopeful about others.

DENIAL AND FALSE HOPE. Sometimes the brain simply pulls down the shades and looks the other way, announcing to the world, "This cannot be happening." This response is completely normal, developed through years of evolution to protect a person from information that is just too painful to bear.

Denial often goes hand in hand with hope—hope that the news isn't true, that a treatment will work, that a miracle will occur.

Don't encourage your parent's denial or unrealistic hopes, but allow them, especially early on. Urge him, gently, to face decisions that he must, but don't force him to accept facts needlessly. If he insists that he is going to get well when the doctor has told him otherwise, simply say something like, "That would be nice," or "Either way, we're going to make the most of this time."

ANGER. Your parent may become angry—angry at himself for being ill, angry at others who are not ill, angry at doctors who bear bad news, and angry at family and friends for any reason or no reason at all. He may express his anger loudly, in fits of rage, or he may bottle it up. Again, allow your parent his reactions. Give him a place to vent. If you become his target, don't escalate things by arguing.

BARGAINING. People often go through a period of bargaining, usually with God or whatever higher power they believe in. *Let me get well, and I'll stop smoking, cheating, being unkind, etc.* Your parent might bargain for his health, or he might bargain for comfort, love, or time—perhaps he wants to be around for a specific event, such as an anniversary, a birthday, or a celebration.

WORRY AND GRIEF. Realizing that there is no escaping death, no bartering with God, people often begin to mourn. Your parent may mourn things he failed to do in the past and dreams he will not be able to fulfill in the future.

Some people worry about specific issues. *Will I need life support? How will we pay for these medical bills? Am I a burden?* Some of these concerns may be eased with reassurance, but if not, once again, allow these reactions.

Sadness and grief are normal, but clinical depression, even at the end of life, is not. If your parent sinks deep into depression, talk with his doctor.

....

66 My father had a wonderful death. That's a funny thing to say, but his whole countenance changed. He was a difficult and demanding man, and he made a lot of people angry during his life. But when he learned he had only a few months to live, he became very sweet and tender. The minister came frequently to see him, and prayed with him. It made him very genuine and real, and you could say anything to him. We were very close during those weeks. I spent a lot of time up in his room, sitting at a card table trying to write. It was a lovely, sort of profound relationship.

The minister told me much later that he'd never seen a person prepare himself for death as beautifully as my father had. I don't know where it came from, but I hope that I can do the same. It was a tremendous gift that he gave us all, at the end."

—Betty H.

....

ACCEPTANCE. At some point, most people become resigned, acknowledging what is happening and realizing that there is nothing they can do to change it. Some fully accept death, and this can be a calm, almost peaceful time. The struggle is finally over.

If he accepts death before you do, there might be discord. You want him to continue a treatment, and he is saying no. If his resignation is based on full information, then try to be with him, to accept what's happening, and be happy that he's at peace with it.

If you are on the same page, this can be an extraordinary time for your whole

> ❝ The best therapy for us was laughter. She and I loved to giggle together. Even toward the end, we were laughing. Those are the memories I treasure."
>
> —Kim D.

family. The loss is sad, yes, but these final days can be a time of intense love, humor, intimacy, and joyful memories. It can be almost "otherworldly" as you close the door on day-to-day life and enter a place that only a privileged few get to share.

Communicating

Maybe you've found a way to talk with your parent about his medical care. Maybe you've been honest with him about his prognosis. But how do you talk about anything else? How do you stop commenting nervously on the weather and the hospital décor?

Standing at the bedside of someone who is terminally ill is painful, but it's also just plain awkward. What do you say? *How are you feeling? Nice weather we're having. What about those Red Sox?* You may want desperately to tell him you love him, that you'll miss him, that you'll never forget him, but it's all too close, too stark, too massive.

It's fine to talk about the ugly blue vinyl hospital chairs and the cool day

outside, but if it all starts to feel a bit empty, go ahead, cross the border. You can jump in, or just dangle a toe. Conversations don't have to be long and heavy. At a time like this, a few words, a bit of reassurance, even a look, an embrace, or a touch can say a great deal. The important thing is that you allow communication if you and your parent want it.

Ask gentle, open questions that allow your parent to speak or not speak, to take the conversation wherever she needs it to be. Be ready to listen.

Quite often, important issues arise on their own, at unexpected times. Your parent might say out of the blue, "I'm going to miss you," or "I'm afraid." Or

PLEASE DON'T GO

You may find that you are not only having trouble talking openly about death, but when the subject comes up, you plead desperately with her not to die.

In your own way, you are telling your parent that you love her and that you will be sad when she is gone. But be aware that such denial can shut your parent out, leaving her unable to share (aloud or silently) her pain, love, or fears. And at a time when she has so much personal work to do, it puts her in the role of worrying about you.

If you want to tell your parent that you love her, that you wish things weren't this way, that you will miss her, do so. But if you find yourself telling her not to go, think about how your words are affecting her, and try to take a different approach.

who is dead, or she might make references to traveling—getting tickets, packing bags, going on a boat, or leaving someone behind.

Be ready for these moments, because you can easily be caught off guard and shut your parent off. *Oh Mom, don't talk like that.* Try to offer her a safe place to express her thoughts.

Even if your parent can't speak, try not to stand numbly by the door, staring at her. You won't be able to avoid doing some of this, but it sets a mood of "just waiting," which is depressing for everyone.

You might look through family photo albums, play her favorite music, talk about wonderful times you've had together. Even if she can't join in, hearing you and others reminisce and laugh will fill her heart. As your parent grows closer to death, keep lights low, noise down, and interaction to a minimum, it's as if someone were falling asleep; don't keep jerking her awake.

she might say something like, "I want you to know where my valuables are stored," or "I need to give you your birthday present early."

People sometimes broach the subject in more cryptic ways. Your parent may talk about a relative or a friend

Caring for Your Parent Now

Whether your parent is in a hospital, in a nursing home, or at home, there is a lot you and other caregivers can do to care for her and keep her comfortable now:

• Watch for pressure sores. She'll need to be moved and rearranged slightly, as any pressure and friction on bony spots—elbows, heels, buttocks, the back of the head—can cause painful sores.

- Make sure your parent's mouth is not dry. Give her ice chips or sips of water. Keep chapped lips lubricated. Wipe her teeth, gums, and tongue with a damp cloth, or use disposable mouth swabs.

- Several other symptoms, including breathing difficulty, nausea and vomiting, constipation, confusion, and infections, are common as death nears, but most can be treated. If you are aware of such symptoms, alert the doctor or nurse.

- Be aware of her mental and spiritual health. She should have the opportunity to talk to a counselor, social worker, psychiatrist, or clergyperson. (Even if she can't communicate, she might be consoled by his or her presence and words.)

- Think about what she might find comforting. Does she want to be left in silence? Would she like to listen to music? Would she like to hear stories

" I don't know where she ends and I begin, our lives are so intertwined. Part of me is very much looking forward to losing her and being free. But frankly, I think that when she goes, I'll feel like, Oh, my God, I'm going to die now, too."
— Sasha L.

about old times or have someone read aloud?

- Treat your parent with respect and dignity, and ask others to do the same. Respect her modesty, even if she seems unaware of such matters. Ask people around her to call her by the name or title she is used to. Even if she doesn't seem to hear you, talk to her as you (or others) move her or touch her. *I'm going to lift your right arm and put a pillow under it.*

- If your parent has always enjoyed physical interactions, then gentle touch might be welcome now. If she's in the hospital, touch might be

A NOTE ON PAIN

Pain is no simple matter. It radiates from, and is compounded by, disease, treatments, emotional anguish, fatigue, and, ironically, the fear of pain. The stress of knowing pain will come, in itself, creates and worsens pain.

Determine any treatable causes of your parent's discomfort and address them as best you can. And be adamant that your parent receive ample pain medication.

If your parent is in pain, he should receive medication at regular intervals, before the pain begins (alleviating pain is more difficult than keeping it at bay in the first place), and extra doses of medication as necessary.

If your parent's pain is not adequately treated, ask for a consultation with a palliative care specialist and/or be persistent. There is no reason for your parent to suffer now.

difficult, but don't be deterred. Hold her hand, stroke her arm, or even snuggle next to her.

- Even if your parent can't express her thoughts or she seems oblivious to what is happening, assume that she hears and understands what is going on around her. Hearing is the last sense to go, so take private conversations out of the room and don't talk about your parent as if she were not there.

Taking Care of Yourself

Whether you are with your parent or not, you are living this death almost every minute of the day. Sitting down the hall, you might hear your parent's raspy breathing, sense the health aide's presence, or smell the soiled bedsheets. Even when you leave the premises, you will worry about her. Your sleep may be disjointed and you might have little appetite.

If this is a prolonged process and the end is not in clear sight, get help early. Hire a home health aide or companion. Recruit other family members and close friends to take shifts, make meals, run errands, or do anything else that helps you. Then, when others are caring for your parent, get away. Go for a walk, see a friend, run errands, or go for a drive.

If your parent's care continues for more than a couple of months, look into respite care. Your parent can be moved into a nursing home, hospice, or hospital temporarily, or you might be able to get round-the-clock aides to care for your parent at home. Take a few days and get away. Tend to your own needs and to other important relationships.

Even when time is short, you still have to take care of yourself. Get food and sleep, take breaks, and try to talk, a little bit, about something else. Meet with a grief counselor or member of the clergy.

> **"** We felt we had to do it all ourselves, so we took shifts. I would stay with Mom until midnight, and then my daughter would sit with her. My sister would come during the day, and if she couldn't come, then one of my aunts would come. We were on this round-the-clock schedule, which was fine as long as everybody showed up for their time slot. It got to be, *Okay, we've made it through today. Now let's hope everybody's in place again tomorrow.*
>
> In the end, that last week before she died, I found that I couldn't deal with it. I hadn't had any sleep. I was exhausted. I totally broke down. I started crying and couldn't stop. I called the hospice, and they sent someone over right away.**"**
>
> —Susan V.

If you feel that you can't leave the house at all because your parent is close to death, at least get out of earshot occasionally and get your mind on something else. You don't have to be at his side every second. Really. Go have a cup of coffee, flip through a magazine, take a nap, soak in a hot bath. And be sure to have a good meal now and then. (Yes, junk food and liquor might seem to fill some emotional hole briefly, but it is really only wearing you down.)

Even during this grim time, don't be afraid to laugh. It may seem disrespectful, but it is not. Watch a comedy or read a funny book. Your emotional core needs strength, and laughing is a great recharger.

If your family opts to care for your parent at home and you run out of stamina, don't be ashamed. Talk to the doctor or nurse or hospice about possible solutions. Many terminally ill people who are cared for at home die in a hospital or nursing home because their care becomes too much for family members to bear. Give what you can, but don't be ashamed of your limits.

Care at Home

Your parent may be able to be at home, with the help of hospice or visiting nurses. She will be surrounded by the people she loves and have control over what she wants to do—sip sherry, watch television at 3 a.m., have quiet time alone, or sit with the grandchildren.

At home, you create an opportunity for intimacy, for treasured moments of warmth and humor. You will be able to grieve, love, hurt, and care for your parent freely, privately, and completely. It will be, without question, a life-changing experience.

All this intimacy comes at a price, however. Such an undertaking can mean turning a home temporarily into what feels like a hospital, and it can entail sleepless nights and challenging days of demanding physical care. Even if health aides and nurses are enlisted to help, the constant proximity to death can be draining. These are long hours spent watching your parent become sicker and weaker and closer to death.

Caring for a dying person at home can be rich and rewarding, but it is not for everyone. Think about whether you have the time and energy to give, and

> Would we do it again? Yes, she was my mother, and Michelle's grandmother. Those months were wearying, but it was a special time. There was an incredible closeness and tenderness among all of us. I worried about Michelle because she's just a teenager, but she developed a bond with her grandmother."
> —Terry C.

whether other family members might help. Think, too, about whether you will be able to handle such immersion in the dying process.

If you are interested in caring for your parent at home, call the local hospice. They can tell you what to expect, what help they can provide, and what your role will be. The sooner you call, the more help they can offer and the easier this will be.

Practical Details

If your parent is going to be cared for at home, you might have to do some rearranging. Where is the best place for her bed? Does she need a hospital bed? If there's no downstairs bedroom, then a living room or dining room might be turned, for a short time, into a bedroom with a few adjustments. Chapter 7 offers tips for caring for someone at home and modifying a house.

Hospice Care

Hospice, the philosophy and practice of caring for people who are approaching death, is based on the belief that death is a natural and inevitable part of life and that at some point, rather than battling illness and fighting death at any cost, all efforts should be focused on enhancing what life remains.

Care is usually provided in a person's home, but is sometimes offered in a hospice facility, a nursing home, or, in some cases, within a hospital.

Hospice nurses and doctors do not try to cure patients, and discourage the use of aggressive medical treatments. Instead, the focus of care is palliative, aimed at relieving pain and symptoms such as nausea, dizziness, and constipation. However, most hospices will arrange for invasive medical procedures if those procedures will ease pain or treat symptoms.

Hospice nurses, who often work with a patient's primary physician or hospice doctor, are extraordinarily adept at managing pain and symptoms without causing unnecessary grogginess.

As important as the physical care is the social, psychological, and spiritual support the hospice staff provides. Nurses, aides, and social workers guide families through the daily regimen, the dying process, grief, and other emotional and practical issues. They help resolve conflicts, and offer financial guidance, pastoral support, and bereavement counseling.

There are more than 5,000 hospice programs across the country. Most offer home care and respite services. They typically have a medical director, nurses, home health aides, social workers, psychiatrists, nutritionists, speech and physical therapists, clergy, and volunteers, all of whom work with the family and patient, as well as the patient's own doctor. Whatever a family's specific

DETACHING

As your parent grows closer to death, his world will shrink. He will lose interest in the wider world, and then the outer circle of friends and family, and finally, all but the most intimate inner circle.

At some point, he won't want many visitors. He might not even want to see people whom you consider "inner circle." It's not that he doesn't care for these people; it's simply that leaving this world is hard work. He is detaching, bit by bit.

As your parent loosens his grip on life, let him do so. He is moving on. Don't keep pulling him back. It's best not to get his old friends on the phone (unless he asks), bring in visitors, show him photos of grandchildren, or talk about people he has already left behind.

Once he is clearly on a path out of this world, drifting in and out of consciousness, dim the lights, and use soft voices and gentle touch. (Strong physical contact—lots of hugging, kissing, and firm touch—can also impede his journey, as it pulls him back into this physical world.) Although you might very much want to keep your parent in your world, it is time to let him go.

needs, staff members are usually available 24 hours a day to answer questions or visit if there is an emergency.

Some hospices will make arrangements for short-term care, either by moving a patient temporarily into a hospice facility or nursing home, or by arranging for nurses and aides to fill in at home while a family takes a break.

Medicare and other insurance cover hospice services.

Hooking Up with a Hospice

Contact the local hospice early in the game so you can learn the options, meet the staff, discuss options, and, if appropriate, start making arrangements. It's best to do this long before things get dire.

Before a patient is accepted for hospice care, Medicare and other insurance companies require that a doctor determine—as much as such a determination is possible—that the patient has less than six months to live.

To find a hospice, contact Caring Connections (caringinfo.org or 800-658-8898).

....

" When we chose hospice and brought my mother home from the hospital, a boatload of equipment had been delivered. There was a backup generator in case the electricity went out, tanks of oxygen, a commode, and a special bed. I thought, *What am I doing?*

But we saw an improvement in her almost right away. She perked up, being at home. She started her crocheting again. She could walk down the hall— she refused to use the walker—and sit in my room in the sun. She seemed so much happier. And I knew that what we were doing was right."

—Nelly O.

....

AVOIDING 911

If you are caring for your parent at home, decide what you will do in an emergency. If you call for an ambulance, it's going to be difficult to avoid certain interventions and hospitalization. If you're not going to call 911, how will you comfort him? Talk to the hospice staff and have a plan; prepare emotionally and practically for such an event.

If you are worried that someone in the household might, in a state of panic, call 911, get the doctor to write an at-home Comfort Only or Do Not Resuscitate order, a legal document that releases paramedics from their obligation to resuscitate. Post it in an obvious place (such as on the refrigerator or inside the front door) where it will be spotted immediately.

Hospice Outside the Home

If your parent is in a nursing home, hospital or other facility, talk to the staff early about the possibility of arranging for hospice care.

Even if they are willing to allow hospice services, be sure they understand what is involved. If the staff seems uncomfortable working with hospice or doesn't fully understand palliative care, ask a hospice nurse to talk with them.

Sometimes when hospice gets involved, the staff at a facility assumes your parent is now being cared for and their services are not needed, which is not the case at all. Communicate. Make a plan. Be sure everyone knows who is doing what.

> " The nurse at the hospital wasn't willing to give Mom the morphine the hospice had prescribed. I said, 'She's going to die either way. What can you live with?' She gave it to her."
> —Emma P.

Find out if appropriate medications will be allowed and who will administer them, and be clear about what will happen and what will *not happen* in a crisis.

When There Is No Hospice

If you are interested in caring for your parent at home, but there isn't an established hospice organization in the area, don't despair. Hospice is not just an institution and a group of people; it is a philosophy of care. You can still take care of your parent at home; you will just need to do a little more legwork and organize your own support system.

Call a home care agency and let them know that you are interested in hospice-type care. More and more home care agencies are offering this sort of care, whether or not they are certified as hospices. Talk to your parent's doctor and contact a social worker, member of the clergy, or psychotherapist who specializes in bereavement.

In the Hospital

In the hospital, the reality of death will be less stark than if your parent were with you at home, and you won't have to provide hands-on care.

But hospitals have enormous drawbacks. For starters, unless there is a palliative care unit or hospice wing, it's hard to buck the system, and the system is founded on keeping people alive—at any cost.

Also, hospitals are impersonal places that impose physical and emotional distance between patients and their loved ones. You might not be able to be there as often as you like, or at the times you like. If your parent is receiving aggressive treatment, the medical machinery and staff intrusions will get in the way of your having any private or intimate time together. You may be unable to hug your parent, hold her hand, or even find a body part that can be touched. Furthermore, you and your parent will have little control over her care and daily life.

But there are things you can do to regain some control, even in a hospital.

- Be sure that your parent's advance directives and any medical orders regarding end-of-life care are filed in her medical record, and that the nurses and doctors overseeing her care are aware of them and prepared to follow them. You might put a note by her bed stating clearly what is to be done (and *not* done) in an emergency. Include your phone number.

- Be there as often as possible, and when you can't be there, find others who can be. You need to monitor her care closely, and if she doesn't want certain procedures, you need to be sure they aren't performed.

- Unless you want all-out medical treatment for your parent, keep her out of the intensive care unit. The beeping monitors, bright lights, and bustle of personnel is unsettling, and it hinders the kind of communication and physical contact that is needed now. Many ICUs also have rigid rules about visiting, further impeding proximity and solace.

- While you need to be diligent in fending off certain treatments and tests, you need to be equally diligent in being sure your parent gets the care and attention she needs.

Dying patients (and their families) typically receive less attention

" I know they are short-staffed in hospitals, but my mother was not a demanding person. That was her big thing, not to bother anybody. But when she called for a bedpan or painkillers, the nurses responded very slowly. Then, one afternoon, I was there and she wanted to walk, and the nurse said she would have to wait until later. But 'later' never came.

That did it. I said, 'I've had it. Let's get her home.'"

—Jane P.

> " At the end, she stopped eating because she couldn't swallow, and then she couldn't drink. So we knew it was a matter of days.
>
> I stayed in her room. I slept on the bottom of her bed, curled up by her feet.
>
> That morning I went to make toast, and I came back and she was lying there, and all of a sudden she started breathing really hard, and I called hospice and they said, 'It's okay. Stay calm. We're on our way.'
>
> I just held her hand. She stopped breathing. Then she suddenly took in a big breath and she looked at me, wide-eyed, and our eyes met and there was this contact between us that we hadn't in a long time. Then she was gone."
>
> —Angela S.

than other patients in hospitals, as the staff is busy with urgent care and has little or no training in how to tend to the needs of dying patients and their families.

- Track down a hospital social worker or chaplain, or bring in one on your own, to address the emotional and spiritual needs of your parent and family now.

- Make sure your parent is getting all the pain relief she needs. There is no reason to limit medication if it makes her more comfortable.

- Ask the nurses if you or another family member can spend the night. Some hospitals have units where family members can sleep, and others may allow you to sleep in an extra bed or cot in your parent's room.

What Death Looks Like

How do you know when the end is near? What can you expect to see? What will your parent experience?

In wonderful old movies, a dying person is propped up on clean, downy pillows, her hair is in place, her face is tired but still attractive, and she gazes lovingly at someone before gracefully lowering her lashes and taking a final breath. In the real world, death is less picturesque. Usually, a lot less.

The scenario is different for each person. Some people die slowly, some go unexpectedly in their sleep, some lapse into a coma, and others are alert right up to the final hours. More often than not, death is not a single dramatic moment, but a slow process, a gradual departure.

As a person becomes sicker, he gets weaker. He becomes less mobile and, usually, incontinent. Many dying people have trouble swallowing, and all eventually lose their interest in food and drink. As the person eats less, he becomes thinner, until his face is quite sunken and sallow. (Remember, this disinterest in food and water is completely natural and helpful.)

Your parent will become less aware of what is happening—because of the illness and any pain medication—and he may drift in and out of consciousness. Sleep patterns are often disrupted. Communication will grow limited. At times your parent may stare off as though he is thinking about something, his eyes may look glassy, and you may not be able to draw his attention.

Some dying people see and chat with people who have died, or talk about being in some distant place. This may startle you, but usually these experiences are pleasant, or at least not unpleasant. Your parent may also twitch or jerk occasionally, but this is nothing to worry about. It is usually not a sign of pain, just a restless muscle.

In the last days or hours, your parent's fingers, toes, elbows, nose, lips, and other extremities may feel cold and turn a bluish gray. At the same time, his temperature may rise, and he may have bouts of sweating (be sure to sponge your parent off and keep the sheets clean and dry).

His breathing may be labored, and as secretions gather in his throat and the throat muscles relax, he may make a gurgling sound when he breathes, something known as a death rattle. It sounds a little like someone sucking up the last bits of a drink into a straw. This noise does not mean that your parent is having any discomfort, but it may be frightening for you. Drugs can dry the secretions, but this is only for your comfort, not his.

Eventually there may be gaps in his breathing—he will stop breathing for a few seconds (and so will you), then gasp for another breath and continue breathing normally for a while. Near the end, these pauses will become longer until the breathing stops altogether.

The final moment is often quiet and uneventful, though a few biological reactions can take place that will be less upsetting if you are prepared for them. Sometimes the bowels and bladder release. The eyes and jaw may remain open. Sometimes people let out a howl or yell. It's not a cry of pain or despair, but simply a last muscular spasm of the voice box.

....

66 During the last week, Dad couldn't talk or respond. The hospice nurses told us that he had only hours to live, but five days passed like this. The tension of thinking, 'This is it,' for such a long time got to be too much.

A hospice worker told us that we had been spending so much gratifying time with Dad—talking about what he meant to us, about experiences we'd shared and how much we loved him, and reading his favorite Robert Frost poems—that he was fighting to stay alive. She said, 'He's going to hang on as long as this stuff keeps coming. He's loving it. There is so much energy here. You have to leave him; only then will he be free to leave.'

She suggested that each of us go in and say good-bye. And rather than clutching him close to us, that we stroke him very lightly, moving down his arms, and out beyond his body into the space of the room. This was a very physical way of letting go. Each of us did this, and we went to bed around midnight, more calm ourselves. Around 2 a.m. he died very peacefully."

—Ruth S.

....

> " At about I a.m. my sister woke me and said, 'She's choking. Something is happening.' I ran in and found my mother dying. I held her for a moment and then she was gone.
>
> We pulled a blanket up, tucked her in, and then made some tea and sat in the living room. It hit us both at the same time and we just started to cry. The exhaustion, the reality of this death, looking around that familiar room. After all we had done, our mother was gone."
>
> —Susan V.

Sometimes people appear to make a last, energetic effort just before they die—sitting up, trying to stand, gasping for another breath—which is upsetting, but such activity is largely reflexive, and usually not a conscious effort.

If you are aware that your parent is dying, it's hard to know what to do during these last hours, minutes, and seconds. You may feel paralyzed, awkward, and intensely helpless. Focus your energies on making your parent feel loved and safe. By now he will have little, if any, ability to communicate, but it is likely that he can still sense your voice and your touch. Speak gently to him and let him know that he has nothing to fear, that he is safe, that he has had a good life, and that he is free to go.

Missing the Last Breath

If you had hoped to be with your parent when she died, and weren't—whether you were far away or just made a quick trip to the store—you may feel cheated out of something, or guilty that you didn't extend your last visit.

Don't berate yourself. People often die after loved ones, who have sat with them hour after long hour, leave for a moment. Perhaps they don't want their loved ones to watch. Or perhaps they can't let go as long as they are stimulated. Think of it like falling asleep; it's hard to do until people leave the room.

Your parent may have chosen, in some way, to die when you weren't present. This is something you will never know. But you did nothing wrong. You gave your parent love and care long before that final moment, and that is what matters.

The Moment After

Your parent has taken his last breath, and you are standing beside him. Whether you are weeping or numb with shock, you face the question of what to do next.

Actually, you don't have to do anything. If you are in the hospital, you don't need to call for a nurse. If you are at home, you don't have to contact anyone right away. There is no need to whisk the body away.

You can sit with your deceased parent, touch his hands and face, say good-bye, and weep. You may want to pray, take part in another religious ritual, or tend to your parent's body in some way. You can pick out clothing for his burial or, if you choose, dress him. Some people find that such a task is actually a healing and tender final gift. Do what feels right for you. This time and these acts belong solely to you and your family.

When you are ready, call the nurse or your parent's doctor to confirm the death. You may want to call a member of the clergy. Don't worry if it's the middle of the night. Most clergy would rather come when they are needed than the following morning when the crisis is over. Once death has been confirmed by a doctor, nurse, or coroner, call the funeral home so someone can pick up the body and begin the process of filing a death certificate and preparing the body for burial or cremation. (If it's late at night, they may not come until morning.)

As soon as you are able, call members of your parent's immediate family. Do not hesitate to "bother" someone who is on vacation or at work. Most people want to be told as soon as possible, and feel cheated or deprived if they are not notified of the death until days after it has happened. If your family is large, make a list of people to be called and ask other family members to share the task. Emails can go to those outside the inner

> "Death—being part of that passage—was a turning point for me. It gave me strength.
>
> I know a lot of people saw my mother's skeletal body and her discomfort, and left the room and didn't know anything else. Their only thought was, 'Oh, my God, I'm going to deteriorate and be in such discomfort.' But when you're there through the whole process, you see that as just a minor part. The rest of it is coming to terms and having your good-byes.
>
> At one point, just before she died, I was lying next to her, and with the last bit of energy, she turned on her side and gave me a huge hug. She hadn't moved in over a day. It was amazing how she got those long arms wrapped around me. I don't know how she did it, but that was my good-bye.
>
> She died that night. She was in her own bed. She had this peaceful expression. She looked absolutely beautiful."
>
> —Kim D.

circle, alerting them of what's happened and when any services will be.

Get a cup of tea, wrap yourself up, and be proud of all you've given. Take a little time now to take very good care of yourself.

Chapter 27

The Aftermath

A Funeral Director • The Obituary • Planning a Funeral • Taking Care of Business • Dividing Possessions

After a parent has died, in the midst of your grief or before you have had a chance to even absorb what's happened, there is work to be done—people to be called, services to be planned, obituaries to be written. While these tasks may seem overwhelming, they can also be therapeutic.

Funerals and memorial services are valuable rituals, allowing your family to deal with the reality of your parent's death, to share the tears and memories, and to see, in the midst of your emotional disarray, that life still has some order.

You do not need to follow any preconceived notion, or a funeral home's pitch, of what this entails, nor do you have to spend a fortune. Devise a plan that reflects your parent and suits your family, whether that is a religious service and lavish gathering, or an intimate graveside memorial and backyard barbecue.

Do what feels right to you. What's important is not how much you spend, but that you take part in this last farewell.

A Funeral Director

For most people, the first step in planning a funeral is to talk to a funeral director, who will deal with the body and guide you through the process. (Know that, in most states, a funeral director is not required; you can plan this on your own if you so choose.) Find a funeral director who has a good reputation because, although many are trustworthy, some are scoundrels who inflate prices and push people to spend way more than necessary. A mourning family is easy prey.

Ask friends or family for recommendations. If you want to go a step further, the Funeral Consumers Alliance (802-865-8300 or funerals.org), a nonprofit consumers' rights organization, may have a local chapter that knows of reputable funeral homes in the area. The local regulatory board will be able to tell you which funeral homes have complaints filed against them.

If you have choices, get a price list from each, because prices, even within the same area, vary dramatically. By law, funeral homes have to give you a price list. They should give you this list in person or over the phone or via email or fax.

Filing Complaints

Funeral homes are regulated by state licensing boards and by the Funeral Rule of the Federal Trade Commission. They must provide a price list; they must let you buy individual goods and services, and not just packages; they must give you an itemized list of the total cost of the funeral and a "good faith estimate" for any services not directly provided; they cannot charge for embalming or other "care of the body" if you have not requested it; they cannot charge a "casket handling fee" if you chose a casket elsewhere; and they cannot charge you for "supervising a service" if they are not involved in services.

If you have questions or feel that you have been misled or cheated in any way,

ACCEPT ALL HELP

If people ask if they can do anything to help now, by all means say yes. "I'm okay, thank you" might begin to slip out of your mouth, but hold it in. Give jobs, and be specific. Ask others to babysit, run errands, prepare a meal, pass on information, or put up out-of-town guests.

You might also ask those who were close to your parent to write down their memories of him, especially if they start reminiscing over the phone with you. You may be too raw and preoccupied to absorb or remember such stories, but you will want to hear them later.

contact the funeral home directly first. If that doesn't solve the problem, contact the Funeral Consumers Alliance (funerals.org or 802-865-8300). You can file a complaint with the state consumer protection agency, state funeral examining or licensing board, and/or the FTC (ftc.gov or 877-382-4357).

The Obituary

While you sort out funeral arrangements, someone needs to write an obituary or death notice. Send it to any local newspapers (for example, where your parent lives now and where she lived in her youth), alumni magazines, and association newsletters. You can also post it on an online site like legacy.com. This way, the news can travel through a wider social circle, it can include photos and videos, and friends can share their memories and sympathy in an online guest book.

You can simply provide basic information, or draft an extensive record of your parent's life. Some papers will give you a form to fill out. The funeral director can also help you. (Many newspapers will rewrite anything you send.)

An obituary should include the full name of your parent; any nickname; his date of birth; schooling; recent career (where he worked, in what positions, and during what years); memberships in organizations; military service; awards received; hobbies; the full names of his siblings, children, spouse, and other survivors; and the date and cause of death.

Include the time and place of any funeral or memorial service, and note any fund or charity where people should send donations in lieu of flowers. You may send a photo as well.

Some larger newspapers charge fees to print death notices. Local newspapers, association newsletters, and school alumni magazines will usually print longer, more personal obituaries, in which case you should provide information about your parent's past, personality, hobbies, and anything else that's relevant. Relay any anecdote or event that occurred in that town or at that school.

LOCK IT UP

If your parent's house is now empty, lock it up. Only the executor should have the key. Stow valuables in a safe place. Thieves search obituaries to find out which homes are vacant. You might also alert the police that the house is empty.

Planning a Funeral

As you mull over how to commemorate your parent's life, you'll have to decide how to handle the body, when and where to have any gathering, and what that gathering will look like. You'll have to decide whether your parent will be buried directly or cremated, whether to have a viewing, and whether to have a religious ceremony, a secular service, or just a social gathering.

People usually schedule some sort of memorial within a week or two of the death, but you can put it off several weeks or, if a body is cremated, even months. Or, you can have a small burial service soon after the death, and then hold a larger memorial service months later when you have the energy, and when friends and family can be present.

Decide on a day and place as soon as possible so people can start making travel plans and so you can book a location, if necessary.

If you are planning religious services, contact any member of the clergy or person who will officiate, and begin planning the program. If you do not have anyone in mind, the funeral director or head of a congregation can make recommendations.

A Note on Cost

Cost might seem like a crass subject at this time, but it's an important consideration. It's easy to spend an exorbitant amount of money and get talked into all sorts of extras you don't want, given your frame of mind. Funeral homes will pressure you to spend more and often try to make you feel bad for spending less, but remember, the cost of a funeral does not reflect a family's love.

While a direct cremation (bypassing the funeral home and going directly to the crematorium) and potluck gathering at your home could cost less than $1,500, more elaborate funerals can easily cost $10,000 and up. Indeed, the casket alone can cost more than $10,000. Add a service and reception with flowers, food, alcohol, and limousines, and you can spend more than $30,000.

Think about what you want to do and what you want to spend, and then compare prices. Don't hesitate to negotiate. Most funeral homes quote high prices, but faced with the prospect of losing a customer, they will usually come down.

Negotiating may be more than you can handle now, but know that people do it all the time and that it is perfectly acceptable, even in a time of mourning. In fact, if your parent was at all frugal, if he worked hard and saved, he would want you to shop around and get the best price. Do it in his spirit.

Whatever you do, do not go into debt over a funeral. A simple event is just as meaningful as a more expensive affair.

In addition to any obvious fees (casket, flowers, food, rentals, and so forth), you'll have to pay a funeral director's fee, which is a fixed charge for using that home. It can run from a few hundred dollars (which is what it should be) to several thousand dollars.

You will also be charged for transporting the body. However, the price

THE LAST GOOD-BYE

FINANCIAL HELP

Some states have programs to help cover funeral costs for low-income families. For information, contact the local human services, or social services, department. You can also find information about low-cost funerals through the Funeral Ethics Organization at funeralethics.org.

quoted might cover only the price of getting the body to the funeral home; most funeral homes charge an additional fee for transporting the body to the church, gravesite, or crematory, and for other transportation, such as picking up the death certificates or burial permit.

You will have to pay extra for additional services, such as a hearse, a limousine for the family, a flower car, or a motorcycle escort for the funeral procession.

Handling the Body

Your parent's body may be a candidate for autopsy or organ donation depending on where and how he died. And no matter what, you'll have to decide what should be done with the body long term. If your parent had specific wishes about how his body is to be handled, they should be honored, if possible. If not, what would make you and others in the family most comfortable?

AUTOPSY. An autopsy is an examination of the body performed by a coroner, medical examiner, or physician, usually when a death is regarded as suspicious or unnatural. However, such an examination

might also be useful for medical research or teaching purposes. You must give your permission before such an exam is performed.

ORGAN DONATION. Organs are needed for donation, and medical schools use bodies for research and education. If your parent dies at home, with hospice, you may have to make arrangements for donations in advance. For more information, contact the Coalition on Donation (shareyourlife.org or 804-377-3580).

INTERMENT. The body is placed in a casket and buried in the ground, usually in a cemetery.

ENTOMBMENT. The casket containing the body is put in a mausoleum, a structure usually made of marble, stone, or concrete, with rows of crypts or, in some cases, individual rooms for caskets.

CREMATION. The body is put in a crematory furnace where, over several hours, intense heat reduces it to a few pounds of bone fragments and ashes. The ashes, or "cremains," are returned to the family in a box. They can be placed in an urn or other container (known as inurnment) and then buried in the earth, put in a niche at a cemetery or church columbarium, kept by family or friends, or scattered in some meaningful place.

Cremation simply speeds up the natural process of decay (all bodies, even those that are buried in expensive caskets, decay). Most religions allow cremation, although some conservative and orthodox faiths oppose it.

You do not need a casket for

cremation. You can opt for a simple box—sometimes referred to as an "alternative container"—of wood, pressboard, cardboard, or canvas. (You can buy a cardboard casket over the Internet for about $20 and line it with a soft blanket, if you like.) If you choose to have a viewing before cremation, you can rent a casket with a removable liner from the funeral home (usually for about a third of the retail price).

Cremation costs about $2,000 through a funeral home, or about half that if you go directly to a crematory (although many work only through funeral homes).

EMBALMING. During an embalming, the body is washed and disinfected. Blood and other body fluids are drained out, and chemicals—formaldehyde, glycerin, and alcohol—are injected into the arteries to make the tissue gel and to prevent the growth of bacteria. The undertaker can repair any damaged areas—plump sunken skin, dye skin, and replace missing hair. (Find out what is to be done;

otherwise, your parent may be unrecognizable. *Mom never wore red lipstick a day in her life! And is that a wig?*)

Embalming is not required by law (although a few states require it when a body is transported across state lines). Funeral homes might insist on embalming if there is a viewing, but they must seek permission in advance.

Embalming is rarely necessary, adds tremendous expense to a funeral, and involves highly toxic chemicals. It does not prevent the body from decaying; it only delays the process.

Caskets and Urns

Walking through rows of caskets is unsettling and impersonal, to say the least, and it's easy to be pressured into something you don't want or need. If you decide what you want and how much you want to spend in advance, it will expedite the process.

Don't be swayed by eager salesmen. No casket will stop a body from decaying, and your love for your parent is not measured by the amount of mahogany

BENEFITS FOR VETERANS

Military veterans are entitled to a free burial (including opening and closing of the grave, care of the grounds, headstone, and grave marker) in a national cemetery.

If your parent is buried elsewhere, the Department of Veterans Affairs will provide a grave marker and a large American flag to drape over the casket. Families of eligible veterans can receive some reimbursement for funeral and burial expenses. (Be leery of any private cemeteries offering free burials to veterans. They often charge other fees that cancel out any savings.)

A funeral director or the regional VA office should be able to help you apply for these benefits. To reach the regional office, contact the VA (www.cem.va.gov or 800-827-1000).

> " It felt so distant looking at these caskets in the funeral parlor. It was like going to Kmart. There was no connection to my father. So we decided to build one ourselves.
>
> We bought beautiful pine boards and built the interior frame like a boat because my father was a boater. It had crown moldings, wood panels, hand-forged brass hinges, and rope handles for carrying it. We lined the interior with a thick soft blanket that had been given to my father years ago.
>
> All my brothers and sisters and the grandchildren helped. We worked straight through the night, sawing, sanding, polishing, and varnishing.
>
> It was a wonderful experience. I can't really explain it. We laughed and cried. We talked about Dad and things we'd done. It gave the funeral a whole different feeling, having a focus like that. It gave the family a connection to the process because everyone had a part in it."
>
> —Peter W.

or velvet you sink into the ground.

Caskets come in wood, metal, fiberglass, or plastic. The wooden ones are hardwood (mahogany, walnut, cherry, oak), softwood (pine), or plywood; they may be solid wood or veneer. The metals include stainless or rolled steel, or copper bronzes of varying thicknesses (the lower the "gauge," the thicker the steel). Caskets are usually lined with cloth—twill, crepe, velour, or velvet (although you can use your favorite cloth, quilt, or comforter). Some have padding or mattresses in them, and you can opt for a spring contraption that raises and lowers the body for viewing.

Funeral directors will offer to have a casket sealed, which is usually done with a rubber gasket, to prevent water from leaking in and rust from forming. As with embalming, sealing a casket—no matter how tightly or with what materials—does not prevent the body from decaying.

Prices vary widely. At the lower end, a cardboard container sells for less than $50, and a pine box might be $200. At the higher end, well, the sky's the limit.

Most consumers buy one of the first three models they see, usually the middle-priced model of the three. So, salesmen usually show people three higher-priced models right away. Lower-priced models may be stowed in a back room, or not on display at all.

Get a list of caskets with descriptions and prices in advance, and look at it carefully. Find out if there are lower priced models not on the list (which there often are). Then select three or four to look at, rather than marching dutifully behind and letting the funeral director lead the way.

You can buy a casket elsewhere, which is usually much cheaper than buying it from the funeral home, although it is also a bit more complicated. Numerous companies now sell caskets over the Internet. Scanning websites in the privacy of your home may be less stressful than walking through a funeral home showroom. You can buy one and have it shipped directly to the funeral home, or you might just scan websites so you have an idea of options and prices before heading to the local showroom. You can also make a casket or have a local carpenter make one to your specifications.

VAULTS AND LINERS

Some cemeteries require that you buy a grave liner or vault to prevent the ground from sinking as the casket deteriorates. You can buy these from the funeral director, the cemetery, or a third party.

A liner is a simple concrete box that costs several hundred dollars. Sealing or lining the concrete with asphalt adds several hundred dollars to the price. A vault of ungalvanized steel costs almost twice as much as concrete, and a vault of galvanized steel triples the price.

The funeral director may advise you to choose a steel vault or special sealants to preserve the body, but again, nothing prevents a body from decomposing; this is simply a way of jacking up the price.

URNS

The urn story is much like the casket story. The choices are extensive and expensive, but simple is fine.

You can buy solid bronze urns or urns shaped like cowboy boots, golf club bags, hunting trophies—you name it. You can buy clusters of urns so that each family member can have their own handful of ashes, or cremation jewelry, in case you want to carry a sprinkle around in a locket. You can pay to put the ashes in a mausoleum vault.

You can also find your own appropriate container (a cookie tin for a baker, a flowerpot for a gardener), or buy a simple box and then cover it with family photos.

Services and Gatherings

A burial and funeral usually follows the tradition of your parent's religion. You might personalize this by having family members and selected guests read poems, say prayers, reminisce, or play music that has special meaning.

The funeral can be whatever your family wants it to be. Some people have viewings and religious services followed by a sit-down dinner, while others have potluck lunches, memorial walks, or cocktails and dancing on a boat. It's completely individual.

A GREEN BURIAL

According to the Funeral Consumers Alliance, each year in the United States, burials use more than 800,000 gallons of embalming fluids, 100,000 tons of steel and copper, 30 million board feet of hardwood, and 1.6 million tons of reinforced concrete for caskets and vaults.

A green burial is one that considers these and other environmental factors. The body is not prepared with any embalming fluids or other toxic chemicals. It is simply wrapped in a shroud or put in a biodegradable container and placed into the earth. Dust to dust, if you will.

Green cemeteries, which are few and far between, are basically nature preserves. They are not mown or fertilized or manicured. Instead of headstones, graves are marked with GPS chips, plantings, or local stones.

For more information, contact the Green Burial Council (greenburialcouncil.org).

As you decide what the mood and the message will be, think about what you want out of this. Do you want a joyous gathering that celebrates your parent's life or a solemn service that helps people come to terms with death? Do you want something that reflects your parent's passions (a party in a bowling alley), or something that soothes your family (an intimate gathering at home)?

Memorials can last 10 minutes or several days. Ceremonies and receptions are often held at a funeral home, a private home, a hall, a church, or a synagogue, but they can be held at any favorite spot.

At some burials, each person takes a turn putting a scoop of earth on the coffin; each guest carries a flower and places it on the gravesite; or guests arrive with photos, markers, and pens and write notes and decorate a large poster or a white coffin.

Sometimes guests are asked to share a story or say what's on their mind or tell how they knew your parent. Each person might light a candle or place a flower in a central circle after speaking.

Following the Japanese Odon festival, people sometimes decorate or write messages on paper lanterns, which are lit and sent down a river. Another popular tradition is to hand each guest a stone (which you can buy at a gardening shop). They hold their stones during the service, thinking about your parent, and then lay them on the grave or in a garden.

The point is, do whatever will have meaning for your family.

A NOTE ON VIEWINGS

Although certainly not for everyone, an open-casket wake, or viewing, gives people an opportunity to accept the reality of death—to see, quite literally, that the person is gone. Be prepared, though, because this body, drained of warmth and life and fixed up by embalmers and cosmeticians, might not resemble your parent or give you the "closure" you hoped for.

Usually a family can have a "private viewing" of the body at the funeral home and no embalming or fancy caskets are needed. The body is laid out on a table and the family is left alone to grieve.

The Cemetery

Most communities have a municipal cemetery as well as several cemeteries owned by religious or private organizations. Veterans have the added option of being buried at a national cemetery.

CHILDREN AND FUNERALS

Although children are often excluded from funerals, wakes, and memorial services, they often want to be included in the ritual, and they stand to learn from it. If you are not sure whether to bring a child, describe what the event will be like and let him or her decide whether to attend.

If the service is going to be quite long—too long for a child to sit still or remain quiet—bring a supply of toys and snacks, or include the child for only part of the service and arrange for a sitter to be nearby.

DO-IT-YOURSELF FUNERAL

Some people find it therapeutic and meaningful to plan the funeral, build the casket, and in some cases, even bury the body themselves.

Most states allow you to arrange the funeral and burial or cremation without a funeral director, as long as you comply with public health codes. Home burials are described in the book *Caring for Your Own Dead* by Lisa Carlson, or you can get information from the Funeral Consumers Alliance (funerals.org).

Your parent may have made plans for his burial and chosen a cemetery. She may even already have a plot. If not, choose a cemetery that appeals to you. Although people are usually buried near home, you might pick a cemetery near family, so they can visit.

Within a cemetery, you can buy a single grave plot or a family plot. Some cemeteries also sell space in a mausoleum or a columbarium. Find out if the cemetery requires some sort of grave liner or vault, and if it has any restrictions on markers, monuments, or plantings.

Taking Care of Business

If you weren't taking care of your parent's business before he died, you can only hope that he was well organized, because there is a lot of paperwork to be done now. A funeral director should help you with the most pressing issues, such as sending out death certificates. If you are the executor, a lawyer will walk you through probate and estate administration.

Much of the work doesn't have to be done immediately. Take time to grieve, and then attend to these tasks when your head and heart are a little more stable.

Some steps that need to be taken by the executor or family members:

CONTACT RELEVANT PARTIES, such as your parent's lawyer, financial planner, or accountant. If your parent didn't have a lawyer, you may need to hire one now.

LOCATE THE WILL by checking the likely places—her safe-deposit box, files, and desk drawers—or by calling your parent's lawyer. If there is no will and no lawyer, then the estate will be handled according to state laws.

A FUNERAL CHECKLIST

- ❑ Make a list of people who should be notified in person or by phone. Split it up and have others do some of the calling.
- ❑ Choose a funeral director.
- ❑ Choose a date for any services, and book any reception halls or other locations.
- ❑ Decide who will officiate, and meet with him or her to plan services. (Some religious organizations require that their own representatives officiate or at least have some part in any service, so ask in advance.)
- ❑ Send an obituary or death notice to appropriate publications.
- ❑ Decide if you want a particular organization to receive memorial donations (instead of people sending flowers). This information should go at the end of the obituary.
- ❑ Decide whether the body will be cremated or buried, or embalmed for viewing.
- ❑ Find out if your parent owns a plot. If not, contact local cemeteries.
- ❑ Pick out a casket or urn.
- ❑ Determine who will speak at the memorial.
- ❑ Select music. Talk to any musicians or music director involved.
- ❑ Decide on flowers, candles, guest books, or other extras.
- ❑ Do you want photos, letters, or other reminders of your parent's life on display at the service? Should someone make a poster or slide show?

FIND YOUR PARENT'S SOCIAL SECURITY CARD. Contact the Social Security Administration if you have problems locating it.

CHECK WITH THE PROBATE CLERK'S OFFICE in your parent's town to get a list of deadlines. If your parent has property in more than one state, be sure to check with the probate clerk's office in each state.

GET 5 TO 10 COPIES OF THE DEATH CERTIFICATE from the funeral director or health department. You will need these when reporting your parent's death to insurance companies, banks, the Social Security office, the IRS, and so on.

CONTACT YOUR PARENT'S BANK to close accounts and to find out if there is a safe-deposit box. These boxes are closed at the time of death in some states, but you may be able to check the box for a will and list the contents for tax purposes.

FIND YOUR PARENT'S MARRIAGE CERTIFICATE if your parent's spouse is alive

❏ Ask people to serve as pallbearers and/or ushers at the service, if necessary.

❏ If your parent was a veteran, contact the VA about benefits. Notify the local American Legion if you want a military component at the funeral.

❏ If there is to be a graveside service, decide whether the casket or urn will be lowered into the grave while people are present, and if so, who will do this task (family members or people from the cemetery or funeral home).

❏ If there is a gathering after the service, will everyone be invited or just family and a few close friends?

❏ Will a meal be served? Do you need a caterer or bartender?

❏ Ask a neighbor who will not be attending the services, or the police, to keep an eye on your parent's home (and perhaps yours) during the services. Thieves often track obituaries to find unwatched homes.

❏ Write up any program and get it printed. (Sometimes funeral directors keep sample programs on hand. They should also be able to recommend printers.) Order extra copies for friends and family who cannot attend.

❏ Think about where visitors will stay and, if necessary, how they will get from the airport or train station to the services. You are not responsible for this, but it's helpful to make recommendations.

❏ Email directions and instructions.

❏ If you have chosen an earth burial, at some point you need to select a grave marker or headstone. (This can be done later, however.)

and will be applying for benefits. The town clerk in the town where your parents were married should be able to provide copies if you can't find them in your parent's files.

NOTIFY INSURANCE COMPANIES (life, health, mortgage, accident, auto, credit card, employer policies). File all claims, switch any policies over to a spouse's name, and/or change the names of beneficiaries. Do this early so beneficiaries can receive their money as soon as possible. (Some health insurance policies provided by an employer can be continued in a spouse's or in children's names.)

CONTACT THE SOCIAL SECURITY AND VETERANS AFFAIRS OFFICES. You may receive a death benefit to cover funeral costs and other benefits to help a surviving spouse. Contact the Social Security Administration (ssa.gov or 800-772-1213) for information, and if your parent served in the military, contact the local Veterans Affairs office (va.gov or 800-827-1000).

> " The hard part was cleaning out the house. We came across all these reminders, bits and pieces of our child-hoods and memories of Dad. That was upsetting.
>
> My sister and I took care of it at our own slow pace. We met at the house three or four times over the course of a month or more, taking one room at a time. Then we would always go out for a beer when we were done. There was a lot of crying and a lot of laughing. Dividing things up didn't divide us. If anything, it made us closer."
>
> —Alicia B.

CONTACT FORMER EMPLOYERS if you think your parent may be owed pension benefits, salary, or pay for unused vacation or sick leave.

MAKE A LIST OF ALL ASSETS. If you are your parent's executor, gather titles and deeds to any property, automobiles, or boats; ownerships or partnerships in businesses; stocks, bonds, savings accounts, and checking accounts; and profit-sharing plans, pension plans, and retirement accounts. You'll need to change the name on any titles and deeds if property is transferred to a surviving parent or child.

LIST ALL DEBTS from mortgages, unpaid bills, charge accounts, and so on. Cancel all credit cards and pay the balance out of the estate.

FIND A COPY OF YOUR PARENT'S MOST RECENT INCOME TAX RETURN. If your parent was required to file a tax return, you will have to file one for the year in which he died. You can get an extension, if necessary. Call the local IRS office for information. Federal taxes are also due on larger estates. There are usually state estate and inheritance taxes as well.

TALK TO THE SURVIVING SPOUSE ABOUT REVISING HIS OR HER WILL. The will of a surviving spouse may have to be changed if it lists your deceased parent as a beneficiary. The same goes for any insurance policies. A surviving parent will also need to update any-thing held under joint names, such as bank accounts, property, credit cards, and so on.

Dividing Possessions

While some parents divvy up pos-sessions in advance or leave explicit instructions, most wills note only that property should be "divided equally" among the children. This seems simple enough, but be forewarned: This division, if not done with extraordinary care, can damage or destroy even close family relationships.

Although a poorly written will or fractured family increases the odds of trouble, all families, under all circumstances, are at risk. It doesn't matter whether you are dividing valuable art or worthless junk, whether you are best friends or estranged.

At such a time, your father's torn high school sweater or a water pitcher from your childhood can become an invaluable icon that you can't live without. People fall into painfully familiar roles—someone's bossy, someone wants to please, someone's greedy, someone withdraws. Siblings often feel things are unfair, that a brother is getting more than his share, or that a sister who got something years ago doesn't deserve more. All sorts of feelings you never imagined crop up as these tokens of your parent and your childhood are divided.

Proceed with open communication, a detailed plan, kid gloves, and a big heart. A few suggestions:

- If possible, put this off several months, even a year. Put everything into storage. Wait until the grief has subsided, when emotions aren't so volatile and perceptions askew. Immediately after a parent's death, yellowed letters and moth-eaten scarves may be precious. Six months later, it all should look a bit different.

- Talk with your siblings and come up with a method of distribution that all, or most, can live with. (Of course, the executor has the final say.) Be specific about how *everything* will be split, even the stuff you don't think anyone will want (because people will suddenly want it). Discuss whether any items are exempt from the agreed upon plan. For example, does jewelry go to the women in the family and war memorabilia to the men? Also, will purely sentimental items be treated differently from those with monetary value?

- If the property has any real value, get an appraisal (which you'll have to do for probate anyway), and then be sure everyone walks away with roughly the same cash value (or cash in lieu of property).

- Create an inventory of your parent's personal belongings, and if people can't convene, attach photos.

- If relationships are particularly icy, get a mediator, member of the clergy, or trusted family friend to oversee the division.

- Many families choose to give something extra to a sibling who was a primary caregiver. Think about this in advance.

- In-laws will eagerly throw in their two cents (or, in some cases, much more), which can cause untold trouble. Keep them out, along with others not directly involved. Direct heirs only, please.

- Unless you are going to split things up informally, avoid discussions about who wants what before the distribution, because one person's interest in

> My sisters and I went around and around taking our pick, and the one thing everyone wanted was the sugar spoon. It was an unusual shape, and it was on the table all our lives and everybody was attached to it."
>
> —Charlie B.

a desk or painting might pique someone else's interest in it or make others feel the item is spoken for.

- Before you start, think about what is truly important (the water pitcher or your relationship with your brother), and how to do this with a generous spirit.

- Know in advance that squabbles are normal. Expect them, and they might not seem so awful.

- Once it's done, plan a family gathering if appropriate. Congratulate yourselves for a job well done.

Methods of Division

People divide estates many ways. Sometimes each sibling writes down a list of choices, in order of preference, and then an outsider goes through the lists, making sure everyone gets some of their top choices.

Some families have inter-family auctions, with siblings bidding on items, but this can be lopsided if one sibling is less affluent than another. In a version of this, siblings are given equal budgets, in essence Monopoly money, and when they are out of money, they are finished.

One of the most common and effective approaches is to draw straws or pick names out of a hat or go by birth order, and then walk through the house

> " With the money my mother got selling her house, my husband and I were able to put a down payment on a bigger house so she could move in with us.
>
> Later, when we sold our house, I thought, *Here we have all this money.* But my brother said right away, 'You keep it. You deserve it.'
>
> I felt like I should divide it up with my siblings, but I took care of her for nine years and they wanted me to have it."
>
> —Angela S.

selecting items in order. Turn the order around each time, so whoever picks first in the first round picks last in the second round. In other words, if there are three siblings, you would pick 1, 2, 3, 3, 2, 1 and back around again.

You can make a list of items with photos and do any division online. The plus is that people don't have to travel, they can do it at their leisure, and it's a little less emotionally fraught. The minus is that you can't see the items up close.

If beneficiaries are unable to agree, the executor can divide assets into "approximately equal shares." If there are irreconcilable differences, then the property can be sold and the heirs receive cash.

Chapter 28

Good Grief

Facets of Grief • Caregiver Grief • Growing from Grief •
The Surviving Parent • Children and Grief

Your parent is gone. No matter how expected this might have been, the loss is jarring. Your world has changed. A piece is missing.

Grief, in all its many forms—shock, sorrow, guilt, rage, regret—rolls in like waves. It can pulse evenly, or crash down on you when you least expect it. For a caregiver, these emotions will be colored by years of illness and duty and may be overshadowed by a profound sense of relief.

You can't control your grief, shake it off, or speed it up, nor should you try. Grief is a necessary and valuable process that allows you to accept this loss, say good-bye, and move on with your life and other relationships.

Whatever your relationship with your parent was like, whatever your duties entailed, your life has taken a sharp turn. Be exceptionally kind to yourself now. Allow yourself to grieve in your own way and at your own pace, and know that whatever you are feeling, however unusual it may seem, you are not alone.

Facets of Grief

Although each person's grief is unique, psychologists have mapped out a number of common reactions to loss. Less well documented, but no less real, is caregiver grief, which is often quite different from the grief experienced by other loved ones. We'll start by examining some of the more "traditional" routes of grief; the particulars of caregiver grief are discussed later in this chapter.

You may experience only a few of these reactions and do so in no particular sequence, bobbing from one emotion to another, feeling fine for a time and then returning to old feelings you thought had long disappeared. Quite often, the deepest grief isn't felt for many months or a year after a death.

Know that your reaction is "normal" and is not a measure of how much you loved your parent. Logic suggests that the more you loved your parent, the more deeply you will grieve her death, and conversely, that a troubled relationship means you will grieve less (and perhaps even welcome this departure). But in fact, often the opposite is true. Conflict, disappointment, and distance can all make a parent's death more difficult to process.

> " When my mother died, I felt total relief. I remember that morning, I felt lighter.
> Even though she was in a nursing home, I was going all the time. It's always there. You're always thinking about it, and you're always worried."
> —Angela S.

If your parent was sick for some time, you may have done much of your grieving over the years, long before this moment, while others face the reality of this loss for the first time. Other stresses, losses, supports, and worries will also affect your grief.

In other words, each person will respond in his or her own way, at his or her own speed. If you aren't responding as you think you should, or your sibling is responding in a way that seems unusual, let it go.

These descriptions should assure you that your reactions are natural, and should also give you some insight into the feelings of others who may be mourning your parent's death.

The Immediate Impact

In the days immediately after a death, some people sob endlessly, while others respond with cool detachment, and some just need to be alone. Some people become forgetful and inattentive, others become adept organizers. One family member might crawl under the covers, while another is scrubbing kitchen counters, cleaning out closets, and organizing events. There is no right way to grieve.

Numbness, disbelief, and shock are common first reactions. No matter how old or frail your parent might have been, there is often a sense that this didn't happen or couldn't have happened. The notion that he is actually gone seems impossible.

In the days and weeks after your parent's death, take time off from work and

> " After my father died, we went into the living room and collapsed on the couch, and to be perfectly honest, we started laughing. That sounds horrible, I know, but we were completely exhausted. We had worried so much and cried so hard that I don't think we had any other emotions left."
>
> —Tina L.

other responsibilities to care for yourself. Spend time with family and friends. The more support you have, the better you will cope. Be willing to ask for favors or a shoulder to cry on when you need it. Most people want to help and are complimented that you trust them enough to ask.

The Aftershocks

In the weeks after the funeral, family members return to their homes, friends no longer offer words of condolence, and employers run out of sympathy. Eventually, people may think it's time for you to be your old self again, but you will still be grieving and may not be able to carry on with business as usual. In fact, many people experience grief only after the formalities and commotion subside, or the initial pain gives way to deeper despair and depression. Some people become irritable, and others become anxious and restless.

Give yourself time. Ignore those who try to talk you out of your feelings. Make yourself and your own care a priority.

ANGER AND GUILT. As you digest the reality of your parent's death, you may feel angry at him for leaving you, angry at the medical system for failing you, angry at siblings who didn't do what you wanted, angry at people who still have their parents, angry for all sorts of reasons. Be careful. Things said now cannot be unsaid. Release your aggression, but not on innocent (or even not so innocent) friends and relations.

You might also feel guilty now for things you said or did or failed to do or say. You can rewind this tape over and over again and keep finding imperfections. You're only human. Forgive yourself.

SHEER PAIN. At some point—in fact, at many points along the way—grief is just painful. It might feel quite literally as if someone has stabbed you in the chest or kicked you in the gut. It hurts because you have indeed been injured.

Be aware that acute grief can weaken the immune system, tip hormones out of balance, upset an appetite, and disrupt sleep. Some people become physically sick in the early stages of mourning, and suffer from chronic headaches, the flu, or other illness.

OUT OF SYNC. Even though this meteor struck your family, the rest of the world is still walking their dogs and getting haircuts and buying groceries. Birds are still chirping. Planes are still flying. But you know that the world is no longer spinning on its proper axis. Everything is out of alignment. Why don't other people know this?

YEARNING. You may find yourself searching for your parent, visiting his grave or his favorite spots, looking at photographs, trying in some way to stay close to him. Some people adopt the habits and mannerisms of a deceased

> ❝ I have kept myself so busy since she died, perhaps because there has been so much to do, perhaps because I want to be distracted. But now I find myself crying sometimes when I'm driving home from work. During that quiet time alone the reality sets in that she's not here anymore. ❞
>
> —Nelly O.

parent and, in a few cases, even the symptoms of the person's final illness. (Such an obsession, along with its symptoms, will pass.)

For months after the death, you may think that you see your parent out of the corner of your eye, or sense for a moment that you hear her come into the house. You pick up the phone to call her and then remember that she is gone. It's not uncommon to have dreams about your parent, which can be upsetting or reassuring.

DRUGGING GRIEF

Think twice before using drugs or alcohol to dull your emotional pain. Grieving is a necessary and natural response to a loss, and dulling the pain may only prolong or postpone it. Sleeping pills in particular can cause dependency and severe reactions. If you are suffering from clinical depression or from sheer exhaustion because you can't sleep, medication may be necessary for a short time, but be sure to use it in low doses and only under the supervision of a doctor.

OTHER LOSSES. You might revisit other losses in your life—loved ones who died, friends who moved away, relationships that were severed. It's as though this death ripped off old scabs and all the losses of your life become one giant, unbelievable heartache. If losses weren't recognized and mourned when they happened, this may be an opportunity to grieve for them, too.

A SEARCH FOR MEANING. After a loved one dies, people often speculate about the phenomenon of death, the meaning of life, and their own spiritual or religious beliefs. It may help to talk with a member of the clergy even if you have no connection with a particular religious institution.

A Year Later

A full year later, when you think that you've moved forward, the true impact of this loss might suddenly hit you with a wallop.

Odd, but true. Many people find themselves suddenly, unexpectedly drowning in grief after many months of being completely fine. In fact, sometimes this grief is more profound than anything experienced in the immediate aftermath.

The anniversary of a death—not always the precise date, but the general time period—is powerful. It's in the air, the color of the leaves, the warmth or coolness of the breeze. Something resonates and draws you back into this loss.

This second wave of grief may be particularly acute when

WHEN GRIEF BECOMES DEPRESSION

Pain and sorrow are normal parts of grief, but when the hurt doesn't let up, when sadness turns into despair and stretches on for months, get help.

The border between grief and depression is fuzzy at best. Most people who experience a profound loss, cry. They retreat from normal life. They don't eat properly. They can't sleep. They don't want to get out of bed. Life isn't fun. But sometimes, rather than emerging slowly from this dark pond, people get sucked down and begin to drown in it.

Caregivers in particular are at risk of developing clinical depression, especially when losses and burdens pile up—a second parent needs help, money is short, a marriage is threatened by caregiving duties. If you think you need help, get it. If you think a sibling or surviving parent has been pulled under by grief, get help for him.

---

someone dies after a long period of decline and disease. It can take time, sometimes a year, for the memories of the parent you knew, the younger, stronger, healthy parent, to return. Now finally you can really recall, and grieve, the parent who protected and coddled you in childhood.

It can be healing to have some ritual with family or get together with friends around the first anniversary of your parent's death.

Life Review

After some time, crying bouts, sleeping and eating problems, and moments of despair start to abate. This tends to be a time of reflection and growth. With the acute pain gone, people often review their relationship with the parent they have lost and reminisce about time spent together. Friends and mates may try to get you to focus on the present or the future, but this review is an essential part of saying good-bye.

Recognizing your parent for who she was and reconciling, or at least accepting, your differences and unmet needs will help you detach. It may also help you sort through your own personality traits—the ways in which you are like or unlike your parent and how you might relish that or try to change it.

If the relationship was full of conflict, if your parent failed you or hurt you, you may be left with unresolved anger and dueling emotions of love and hate. Of course, the problem is that now there is no one to confront; you have to reconcile the relationship on your own. The good news is that sometimes when this figure is gone from your life, you finally can move on, grow up, let go.

If the turmoil persists, a support group or psychotherapy can be invaluable in resolving such a struggle. See if your local mental health center, hospices, or community center offers bereavement groups or counseling.

> ❝ My brother is dealing with extreme guilt because he rarely called or went to see our mom. He withdrew, while I drew closer to the flame.
>
> Later, I saw an envy in him because he didn't make the effort."
>
> —Julie H.

Moving On

Eventually, life begins to return to normal. If you have allowed yourself to grieve, accepted the loss, and adjusted to the changes in your life, you should be able to face each day with more energy and spirit. You won't think of your parent as often. In fact, you may go through many days and weeks without thinking of him at all.

Sorrow may come only at certain moments now—at a wedding, a celebration of a new job, the birth of a child, and other important events your parent cannot witness.

Although the hole is still there, and always will be, it does grow smaller and less painful.

Caregiver Grief

Little has been written about caregiver grief, but conversations with families suggest that caregivers can have different, and often unexpected, dimensions to their grief.

RELIEF. Given your parent's age, illness, and the caregiving duties involved, it's not surprising that your first reaction to death may not be sadness or shock, but relief—relief that it's over, both for your parent's sake and for your own. The pain and illness, the doctors' appointments, the pillboxes and walkers, the relentless worry—all gone.

You might actually feel a bit light, airy, even elated. It's not that you didn't love your parent. It's just that he was so sick and the job was wearing. It's as if you've been lugging around two overstuffed suitcases, and now that you've put them down, your arms rise up of their own volition, as if the earth's gravity has released its pull.

GUILT. Of course, if everyone around you is weeping and telling you how sorry they are and how sad you must be, any sense of liberation you're experiencing might seem a tad inappropriate.

Don't feel guilty for a lack of sorrow or feelings of relief. If your parent was suffering, slipping away, or lost to dementia, you have grieved plenty. You may feel a bit out of sync, but relief right now is perfectly normal.

REGRET. When a parent dies and there is no longer a chance to do more or do differently, people often feel regret or guilt.

SIBLING JEALOUSY

After all is done, siblings who were less involved may feel suddenly jealous of a sibling who was doing the daily caregiving. This parent is gone, and now you wish you had more time—time that the primary caregiver did have.

Try to remember that this was work, a lot of it. Don't romanticize what this caregiving was about. When you visited, things were, most likely, very different from how they were day to day.

Be careful not to aim your grief, and the hurt and anger that often accompany it, at a sibling who is exhausted. Now is the time to be grateful to any sibling who did the lion's share of the care.

Perhaps you got angry at a father who was confused, or fed up with a mother who needed a lot of care. Perhaps you didn't do as much as you think you could have.

Let it go. It was a lot of work, and you did your best.

Remember all you did for your parent, how much you gave, and what you shared. Think about the days of worry, the calls, the care, the unending love and support. Be proud.

ANGER. After the ceremonies are over, your siblings get to climb into their cars and return to their previous lives, but if you were on the frontlines, your life is totally changed. It might suddenly be apparent to you what you've given—and what you've given up.

You might feel angry that others didn't help more, that siblings don't have a clue what you've been through.

Talk with a friend or therapist, cry out your anger, but be very careful what you say to your siblings. Think long and hard before hitting the send button on that fiery email. It can't be recalled. If you want to tell them that you are processing some difficult emotions and you'd rather not talk with them for a time, fine. But proceed with caution if you need to rant.

CONFUSION. In those first months after a parent's death, there is often a disconnect between who your parent was—strong, competent, and healthy—and who she became. You are grieving, but the person you really miss has been gone for so long that you can barely remember her. The person fresh in your mind may be muddled, incontinent, and slightly smelly. These images, the sights and scents that linger, can make it difficult to grieve the mother you knew, the mother you miss and have not seen in so long.

....

66 After my father died, I found myself furious at my siblings. This was completely unexpected. I think it was because I realized just how much I'd done, all I'd given up, and how little they'd done. Maybe I was upset that they weren't aware of that—or appreciative."

—Sarah G.

....

MOURNING IN THE AGE OF TECHNOLOGY

The 21st century has brought a new aspect to mourning. Months after your parent's death you found you've "pocket called" her.

There it is. Her face on your cell phone smiling out at you, her phone number printed above. You emit a silent gasp.

The funeral is over, the tears have dried, and life is slowly returning to some shade of normal. But here is a curious facet of grief. When do you remove her from your speed dial? Do you delete her from your contacts list? Surely, you can never, ever unfriend her on Facebook.

Technology has given us a new, final stage to mourning, and of course there are no answers. You might want to stop the pocket calls, but the rest can, if you want, live on.

With time, these images will fade and others will return. It can help to find photos of your parent when she was younger.

LOSS. Your caregiver duties, whether you liked them or not, gave shape to your day and your life. So while you might be relieved they are finished, you might also feel a bit adrift now, unsure of what to do without all those pressing demands on your time.

The job might also have given your life a sense of purpose and, in a way, come to define you. No longer in the role of caregiver, people can feel unhinged and unsure of their priorities and their own value.

This role often defines relationships as well. If you were the center of family discussions about Mom, and Mom is now gone, all sorts of relationships and regular communications can slip away, and you find you are no longer central in the family.

Be careful now, because you might, without realizing it, grab a new project—a sick friend, a troubled family.

Take time for yourself before taking on new caregiving tasks.

DISORIENTATION. If a parent's care has consumed you for some time, you might have missed what was happening in the world, not only the news, but books, movies, the arts, and technology. The world kept going, the culture changed, and you might not have been part of that. After your parent's death, people talk about things that you simply know nothing about. Don't worry. With time, you'll catch up.

LONELINESS. It might be that you have lost not just a parent and a schedule, but a host of other relationships—relationships with aides, nurses, doctors, secretaries, and physical therapists. Connections that might have been oddly intimate or intense are gone, often without any farewells.

Don't hesitate to visit the people you felt closest to now or to write them. Usually, they appreciate it when family members reach out, as they lost someone, too.

UNAPPRECIATED. If your parent was hugely grateful and your siblings repeatedly thanked you for all you did, you may be able to bypass this particular reaction. But many caregivers talk about feeling unappreciated, even invisible, after a parent dies.

Sometimes a caregiver's ability to juggle things, to manage a parent's care, makes it all look easy. Things happen. Events are planned. A parent is cared for. There is no sense that a person actually did all this backstage work to make it happen. Ironically, siblings and others may have no understanding of all that was done because you did it so well.

But your parent knew and that's what matters. And with time, your siblings might slowly figure some of it out (although, without having gone through it, they will never fully understand it).

PTSD. In the months after a parent's death, caregivers sometimes have anxiety attacks, flashbacks, or nightmares as they reexperience the stress, worry, and pressures of being a caregiver. Some

> ❝ I took care of my parents for 20 years, dealing with their financial problems, their health problems, taking them to therapies. It was a part of who I am. Now I'm not teaching. My kids are gone. I don't have my parents. I was a caregiver my whole life. So who am I now? A whole part of me is gone."
>
> —Maggie B.

psychologists refer to this as a form of post-traumatic stress disorder. While it is upsetting, it does not usually get in the way of daily tasks, and it subsides with time.

SATISFACTION. Now this is where you need to focus your attention. You took care of your parent through good days and bad. You were there, at her side, when she needed you. You called the doctor and managed the meds and juggled the day and cleaned up the mess. You gave her an enormous gift. You made her life better. As these days pass, try to remember that and be proud.

Growing from Grief

L ife will never be the same. Whatever sort of relationship you had with your parent, your life is different now.

NEWFOUND INDEPENDENCE. Whether you are 17 or 75, when your only surviving parent dies, you become an orphan. That may leave you feeling, at least for a time, afloat, rootless, and profoundly alone. You may have lost a safety net or a confidant, and you've certainly lost a link to your childhood.

The awareness that you are truly on your own, that you are no longer someone's child, can be a crushing and unexpected aspect of grief, but with time

> " I had a very difficult relationship with my mother. I struggled in those last years to get close to her, to build some sort of loving mother-daughter connection, and nothing ever worked.
>
> Given how little we had together, I was amazed at how much I missed her. After she died, there was a big hole, this big, empty hole in my life that I couldn't seem to fill or escape. I am still trying to figure out what that is about. Do I miss her, or do I miss the relationship I never had with her?"
>
> —Jane M.

it can also be an impetus for new growth and bolder independence. If your father guided you financially or your mother fed your ego, you will have to learn to do these things for yourself now. If you had a stressful relationship with your parent—if your mother was domineering or your father made you feel inadequate—the loss can, with time, be liberating.

A CLEARER VIEW OF ONE'S SELF. A parent's death brings you face-to-face with your own mortality. You don't have a buffer against the future anymore. You are now the older generation, and therefore the next in line to go.

You may have already studied your own wrinkles and white hairs, pulled at the sides of your face, and pondered a face-lift. You may have settled into retirement and your "golden years." You may have contemplated your own death. After a parent dies, the ruminations become stark. *Will I be like she was? Will I have this disease? Will my children*

care for me? Without children, who will care for me?

This confrontation with mortality can depress you, but it can also serve as a clarion call to recognize how precious life is and to make the most of it—and perhaps to do better in old age than your parent did.

REDIRECTED ENERGY. If you have been a caregiver for some time, you may have distanced yourself from friends, cut back on your hours at work, stopped exercising, and become accustomed to a superhuman pace. Now there is a void and a great deal of adjustment to be done. Finding a new purpose in your life and reestablishing broken ties will take time. It requires patience and awareness. Go slowly, but find worthwhile tasks and new goals for yourself.

CHANGES IN FAMILY STRUCTURE. Certain family patterns and rituals may disappear with your parent. You no longer know what your sister is up to, because your mother isn't there to spread the news. Holiday plans are now open, because Thanksgiving was always spent at your father's house. Although the change is disorienting, getting together as a family is now a choice, and perhaps a chance to create your own traditions.

With time, old roles may disappear and family alliances shift. A sister who was closer to Dad may create a new, stronger relationship with Mom.

This is a time of testing and sampling. Let it happen and participate in it. It may be uncomfortable at first, but your family needs to establish new rituals and relationships.

REVIEWING YOUR RELATIONSHIP WITH YOUR PARENT

After the worst of the grief has subsided, people sometimes find it helpful to explore a parent's life and to consider any unresolved issues. Approach these projects only when you are ready, and only if doing so feels right for you.

WRITE. Set aside time when you won't be interrupted to write letters to your deceased parent. Say all the things you never had the nerve to say. Tell him how he angered you or what you appreciated about him. And when you are ready, tell him good-bye.

INTERVIEW. Talk with your parent's relatives and friends about his childhood, his work life, and his relationships. Pursue whatever interests you and delve into areas you may have avoided when your parent was alive.

COMMEMORATE. Create rituals to honor and remember your parent. Visit her grave, frame photos, return to a favorite spot, plant a memorial tree, or have a family gathering on the anniversary of her death.

JOIN. Find a local support group, join an online discussion, or attend seminars on grief (hospice organizations sometimes hold or know about such meetings).

EXPLORE. What was good about your relationship with your parent, and what was bad? How are you similar and how are you different? How can you affect that? Why might your parent have been the way she was? What values or traits live on in you that you might pass down to your children?

REVIEW OF OTHER RELATIONSHIPS. In the midst of all this sorting-through, your relationship with your spouse may come under review, and strains in the relationship may suddenly loom large. Remember, your spouse cannot fill the void that your parent has left, or know what you are feeling unless you tell him. Communicate. And again, give it some time.

Your relationship with your children may also come under scrutiny. You may worry about what kind of parent you are or have been, and compare yourself with the kind of parent your parent was. Are you repeating your parent's mistakes?

Are you a good role model? Do you give your children the things your parent gave you?

You do not have to become your parent or repeat his mistakes. Make this a time for growth and enrichment, not despair.

> " My mother died nine years ago and I still wonder, *Where is she? Where did she go?*
> I can't seem to let go of this feeling that she is still here, somewhere."
> —Barbara K.

The Surviving Parent

O ften, widows or widowers become extremely depressed and isolated in the months, and even years, after the death of a spouse, especially after the funeral is over and friends and family have resumed their own lives. They may have trouble sleeping and eating normally and may become physically ill.

They also may face overwhelming practical hurdles—how to manage finances, cook for one, do household repairs, or relate to friends. While you need time for your own grief, you also need to support your surviving parent.

STAY IN TOUCH. Call regularly and visit often. Share your grief and allow her to share hers. As you do this, remember that her relationship with her spouse and her role as caregiver was very different from yours. Let her deal with her grief and express her feelings in her own way, without comparison or reproach.

GET HER OUT. Although your parent may not have the energy or the will to go out, social contact is very important now. Encourage her to see friends, and include her in family gatherings.

FOSTER INDEPENDENCE. Control your impulse to provide more protection than your parent needs. You may have a lot of caregiving energy on your hands, or you may assume that your mother can't survive on her own. Be careful. She has to adjust, learn about her new life as a single person, and regain her confidence and independence. If you take over her affairs or deluge her with advice, it may offend or cripple her. Love and support her, but let her learn to live on her own.

LIMIT DECISIONS. In general, a surviving parent should not make any major decisions, such as moving or selling a home, immediately after a spouse's death. It's better to get through most of the grieving process (which can take a year or more), let things settle, and sort out finances first. In the confusion of mourning, people sometimes make decisions they later regret.

STAY HEALTHY. Encourage your parent to see her doctor regularly and to take care of her physical health. Poor health will make her more susceptible to depression and illness. If she is using antidepressants or sleeping pills, be sure that she understands their side effects and potential dangers.

BE MINDFUL DURING THE HOLIDAYS. The holidays can be particularly difficult. Try to make sure she is surrounded by family.

....

" In the spring after my mother's death, I was planting a tree when I realized that it was my mother's birthday. So I called it Mary's Tree. And I tended to it, and fed it and watered it with care and love.

When I'm in the backyard, I look up at this tree, which is quite tall now, and I say, 'Hi, Mary.' And it helps."

—Rita W.

....

Also, mark your calendar with your parents' wedding anniversary, your late parent's birthday, the anniversary of his death, and other special dates, and be in touch on these days.

SUPPORT GROUPS AND COUNSELING. When she is ready, a support group for widows can provide practical guidance, emotional support, and friendships. Senior centers, family counseling centers, and hospices often run or know of such groups. You can also find some online.

GET HER INVOLVED. As she starts to heal emotionally, urge your mother to take classes, work, travel, and get involved in whatever activities interest her. With time and encouragement, she will find in herself the will to enjoy living again.

ALLOW FOR CHANGE AND GROWTH. You may find that your parent undergoes a surprising personality change now that her spouse is gone. A mother who played second fiddle may prove to be quite capable and even assertive. One who was introverted may become extroverted. Any perceivable change is likely to be troubling for you—you may prefer the "old Mom"—but let your parent find out who she is as a single person, and let that person thrive.

Children and Grief

No matter how we try to shield them, children, even very young children, are profoundly affected by dying and death. They are affected by their own loss, and also (and often more intensely) by your distress. There are no magic words, no right way to address this issue. Let your children express and explore their feelings when they are ready, and then respond to their questions as honestly as you can.

While you should help a child to share his concerns and pain, don't make him feel that there's something he should be feeling, or that something is wrong with him if he is not grieving. Children often accept death far more readily than adults. And in this particular case, a child might feel relieved that your caregiving duties are done and you can go back to being a parent.

START THE CONVERSATION. Sometimes children don't ask questions because they don't know what questions to ask. They simply know that the household is astir and they are scared by it. Explain briefly what is happening—why Mommy is upset, why the child has been sent repeatedly to a friend's house—and ask if he has questions.

LEAVE THE DOOR OPEN. Once you've talked, don't assume that it's over. A few days later you might ask a child if there

BOOKS FOR THE KIDS

A number of books can help a child come to grips with old age, illness, and death.

FOR PRESCHOOL CHILDREN:

The Dead Bird by Margaret Wise Brown, illustrated by Remy Charlip

The Tenth Good Thing about Barney by Judith Viorst, illustrated by Erik Blegvad

FOR CHILDREN FIVE TO EIGHT:

Annie and the Old One by Miska Miles, illustrated by Peter Parnall

Nana Upstairs and Nana Downstairs by Tomie dePaola

My Grandpa Died Today by Joan Fassler

Something to Remember Me By by Susan V. Bosak, illustrated by Laurie McGaw

Love You Forever by Robert N. Munsch, illustrated by Sheila McGraw

FOR CHILDREN EIGHT AND UP:

A Taste of Blackberries by Doris Buchanan Smith

Charlotte's Web by E. B. White, illustrated by Garth Williams

The Birds' Christmas Carol by Kate Douglas Wiggin

Little Women by Louisa May Alcott

---

is anything more he wants to talk about. Be aware that children may ask the same questions over and over. Answer them

❝ In the beginning, I welcomed the pain I felt when I thought about my mother. I wanted to remember her, to think about her, and I thought that as long as I felt the pain, she was still with me, still alive in some way. I was afraid that when I stopped hurting, she would be gone. It seemed like a betrayal to stop mourning.

Now I realize that it's okay not to grieve. The memories have faded, but they never go away. She'll always be with me, a part of me. ❞

—Barbara K.

over and over. Sometimes it takes a few repetitions for the information to sink in.

BE HONEST. Avoid canned responses to death: *God took him away. She is asleep and won't ever wake up. He went on a long trip and will never come back.* Children take things literally. (You may end up with an atheist, insomniac, or homebody.) If you tell a child that a grandparent is in the clouds watching over the family, he may worry about practical matters, like where Grandpa is on clear days or whether an all-knowing Grandpa sees every private thing he does.

Explain that Grandpa was old, his body was very sick, and it stopped working. Use examples from the child's own experience, like the death of a pet. You might add that the deceased person lives on in everyone's memories, or find an explanation that reflects your religious beliefs.

Explain that Grandpa is in no pain, that, in fact, he is out of pain; that death is not a punishment, but a natural thing that happens to everyone; that death is not contagious; and that the child is in no way responsible for the grandparent's death. These are all frequent concerns of children.

LET THEM BE CHILDREN. Although it may be hard for you, allow your children to play and laugh at this time. They are not being disrespectful; they are only being children.

Let them find their own way to grieve. Young children sometimes use play to work through their feelings and questions. They may have a doll or stuffed animal that "dies," which they then bury. Or they may lie still, pretending they are dead, as they try to figure out what it means to be dead. They may also express their grief by misbehaving or withdrawing.

Early in adolescence, children learn to be cool, and believe that it is uncool to reveal one's fear or pain. If your child reacts in this way, don't corner or push him into admitting something he doesn't want to admit. Let him know that you are there for him, and then let him have some room. You might also, when the time feels right, talk about what you are feeling. Hearing about your emotions may help him deal with, and perhaps even talk about, his.

A Final Note

Chapter 29

You're Next

Talk About It • Paying for Old Age • A Question of Where •
Your Body • Your Mind • Your Life

Through all of this, a question looms. It trails silently behind
you, wakes you at 3 a.m., and whispers to you as you tend to your
parent: *What will happen when I grow old?*

Who will take care of you? How will you pay for care? How will
you protect your children from some of what you've been through?
(If you don't have children, then what?) How will you create for yourself an independent, even joyful, finale?

Whether you are 30 or 70, there is work to be done. (Certainly if
you are 70. For Pete's sake, get going!) There are documents to sign,
papers to find, issues to discuss, and moves to consider.

If you want to make your late years the best they can be and protect
your family from some of the trials of caregiving, then you have to
face, head-on, some difficult subjects. You have to think about growing old, and growing frail, and even dying. Don't be put off. And don't
put it off. Learn the options. Make decisions. Don't delay.

Of course, you also need to take good care of yourself, both physically and mentally. This is critical stuff that directly affects how you
age and, quite honestly, whether you get the chance to age.

But that's not all. In fact, if you walk away from this experience gleaning nothing more than retirement basics, you will have missed the point. For beyond the advance directives and IRAs, beyond the megavitamins and yoga classes, there is a life to be lived.

How we age, how we live our last years, what burdens or gifts we bestow on others, and finally, how we die, is not wholly dependent upon the size of a pension, the complexity of a will, or how many miles we jog. It is determined largely by how we live.

In the end, what really matters is what sort of people we have become, what we have done with our time on this earth, and, most important, whether we have loved fully, forgiven readily, and laughed every day.

Talk About It

We're ending this book right where we started it—by urging you to talk. Talk with your spouse or companion at length, and repeatedly over time, about all of this. As your kids become adults, talk with them as well.

It's so easy to put this off, to assume everything will work itself out, or figure that there's not much you can do about it. Or maybe you dodge it because it seems too depressing.

But there is much you can do, and it is *not* depressing. Just the opposite. It's about taking charge of your life, having choices, and actually enjoying what might be several decades of living.

Start the conversation today.

You and your spouse should discuss all the issues laid out in this chapter—where you want to grow old, how you will be cared for, and how you will pay for that care. You also need to talk in depth about your wishes concerning medical care near the end of life. (See page 525.)

Open communication—now and repeatedly over the years—will ease the worry, and help you get the most out of these years. It's also a tremendous gift to your children.

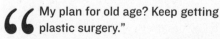 My plan for old age? Keep getting plastic surgery."
Chloe M.

Paying for Old Age

People are living longer than ever before. Indeed, 85 is the new 75, and more and more people will be seeing 100. Perhaps even you. That's great, but how are you going to pay for all those years? You don't want your children shouldering that bill, and you don't want to live in poverty. So what are you going to do?

Whether your finances are in good shape or virtually nonexistent, sit down (preferably with a good financial adviser) and review the situation. Dozens (maybe even hundreds) of books and websites can guide you through the details of pensions, Social Security, annuities, 401(k)s, and retirement planning.

The single most important thing you can do, however, can be summarized in one word:

Save!

Although you should get all the appropriate documents, investments, and accounts in place, the secret to paying for old age is pretty basic: Save money now.

You can't count on Medicare and Social Security, or even Medicaid, as they don't cover all the bills and, in all likelihood, will be cut back as the elderly population swells. You need your own nest egg.

Retirement pros will tell you that you need about 80 percent of your current annual budget (adjusted for inflation) when you retire, but retirees will tell you this is hogwash. Maybe you won't have a mortgage or college tuition to pay, but you'll have time on your hands

and you'll want to travel, eat out, and visit your grandkids. And eventually you will need heart pills, dentures, walkers, health aids, and possibly a nursing home.

Eighty percent of your current spending budget may be tight. Best to have the whole enchilada.

So how much do you need to cover that? A number of online retirement calculators can give you a personal estimate, but here's some quick and dirty math: For every $1,000 you (or you and your spouse) need a month, you need just under $200,000 in the bank (assuming 20 years of retirement and leaving nothing behind in the account, so this isn't generous). In other words, if you need $5,000 a month for 20 years, then you need $1 million in savings (more if you plan to have a lengthy retirement).

If this makes you a bit nauseated, hang in there. Don't close your eyes or look away. It's time to do something about it. You might not reach your goal, but you can get closer and then arrange your future accordingly.

....

❝ Caring for my mother was a great awakening, an enormous education. The experience opened our eyes big time to what we needed to do. Mostly, we needed insurance. We knew that one of us needed a job with a regular paycheck and employee benefits.

My husband said, 'I don't want you to end up in some dump,' like the kind of places we saw."

—Rachel M.
....

On a cheerier note, it isn't too late. You can save a surprising amount in fairly painless ways, one small step at a time. Sure, you should forgo all sorts of big, unnecessary expenses— new car, the latest laptop, and resort trips. But small savings add up. Skip the $4 lattes. Turn down your thermostat. Save eating out for special occasions. Quit smoking (double benefit). Shop around for gas, clothes, and groceries. Weatherize your house. Forgo the bottled water (double benefit). Avoid "dry clean only" clothes. Get movies and books from the library. Honestly, it's amazing what these little cutbacks will do for your monthly budget (and thus, leave for your savings account).

Let's say you buy lunch from a deli on most weekdays, spending $8 a day, or $160 a month. If you switch to making a bag lunch that costs only $2 (and may be more healthful), you'll save $120 a month. Over five years, that's $7,200 saved (more if you add interest). And that's just a little lunch money. It's hardly noticeable. But it adds up. Imagine if you saved in numerous other ways as well. Try it for a month and see what happens.

Since saving money is a bit like dieting—a good idea for a week or two, but it grows old quickly—take the decision out of your hands. Have a certain amount deducted automatically from your paycheck and deposited directly into a retirement or other savings account. Certainly put the maximum allowed into any company 401(k) or other matching pension plan. While you're at it, chuck your credit cards.

SIGN THOSE DOCUMENTS

You should absolutely, without a doubt, have an up-to-date will, durable power of attorney, living will, and power of attorney for health care, regardless of your assets, age, or plans.

Although generic forms and will-writing software are fine in some cases, in most situations it is worth it to spend a little money and get it done by a lawyer. One mistake can make an entire document invalid.

Retire Later

Another way to pay for retirement is to simply have less of it. That's right. Work longer. You might work fewer hours or even change jobs, but maintaining an income will help immensely.

Long-Term Care

As you probably know if you have cared for a parent, Medicare and private health insurance does not pay for much nursing care or the daily help most of us will need one day—help getting bathed and dressed and fed.

The vast majority of this care— 80 percent of it—comes from family members. Mom takes care of Dad, and then the children take care of Mom. Of course, we don't want our kids shouldering all of this duty, and we don't want our spouses drowning in it, either. But the other option—private care—is expensive, particularly if it is needed for any length of time.

Nursing home care costs about $80,000 a year on average (more for a private room). Care in an assisted living facility is about half that, at about

> " I know I shouldn't say this, but I don't think it's so horrible for kids to have some responsibility for their parents. I took care of my mother and it wasn't easy, but I wouldn't have it any other way. She's my mother. I wanted to care for her. So should my kids have to take care of me? I can say no, of course not, but some little voice in me thinks, why not? I mean, not a lot of care, but a little help. Isn't this what family is all about?"
> —Susan R.

$45,000 a year. Aides who come to your home charge about $20 an hour (which adds up quickly).

If you need a good deal of care for some time, and if your family is not going to provide that care, will you have enough savings to foot the bill? Would you become eligible for Medicaid, government insurance for people with very low incomes, which covers these costs? Could you get cash out of your home or trade in a life insurance policy? Or should you consider long-term care insurance, which will cover some (but certainly not all) of the cost?

LONG-TERM CARE INSURANCE

No one wants to think about this, but think you must. The longer you wait to buy insurance, the higher the premiums and the greater the chance of being denied coverage. You should ideally buy a policy between the ages of 55 and 65.

But don't buy in a panic, and don't be swayed by scare tactics. Learn the facts. Take time to decide if this is a worthwhile investment for you, because it is not for everyone.

As with all insurance, this is a gamble. If you end up needing years of care, then the insurance was a good buy; if you die without using much or any private care, then it was a bust. It's important to understand that you are not insuring yourself against the probable (a few months to a year of care), but against the catastrophic (many years of extensive care).

READY FOR MEDICAID

People sometimes give their assets away, usually to their children, so they can qualify for Medicaid and avoid paying for long-term care. Of course, letting taxpayers pick up one's tab raises all sorts of moral questions. Know that being on Medicaid also means that you will have less control and fewer options for nursing homes, home care, and medical care. And despite any promises made, if you give your assets away, you might never see them again.

If you are considering such a step, talk to a lawyer, as the details are tricky. Assets must be given away five years before care is needed (or you must pay enough to cover the amount transferred before getting Medicaid), and taxes may be owed on any transfer. See page 354 for more information.

REWIRING, NOT RETIRING

Despite longer life expectancies, most of us still see 65 as a magical border between long workdays and relaxation. But think about this carefully. If you retire at 65 or, heaven forbid, earlier, what are you going to do with all that time? If you live until 85 or 90 (or more), you could spend an awfully long time playing shuffleboard.

Forgetting for a moment how you'll pay for those years, what will you do with them? Play golf? Knit? Travel? Watch Netflix?

Examine your long-range view. When do you want to retire? Why do you want to retire then? What will you do? Might you launch a second career or continue working part time? Or, if you already are set financially, might you devote some time to community service?

It's a new world out there. The idea that you can work until 65, then kick back and enjoy life for 10 years, at which point you suddenly drop dead, just isn't realistic. We have to rethink when we retire, and look at it not as an ending, but perhaps simply a change of venue.

WHO SHOULD CONSIDER LTC INSURANCE?

PEOPLE WITH AMPLE—BUT NOT ENORMOUS—ASSETS. The reason to buy long-term care insurance is to protect your assets in case you need a lot of long-term care. If you don't have much in the way of assets, if you would be eligible for Medicaid within, say, a year or two of entering a nursing home, then a policy is not necessary.

As a general guideline (and there are exceptions), someone should have at least $200,000 in assets, not including a house and personal belongings, before buying long-term care insurance.

On the other end of this spectrum, people with ample savings, say more than two or three million dollars (other than their home), may not want to buy such insurance because, if need be, they could pay for this care out-of-pocket. They might rather save the money that would be spent on premiums, which, for a couple, could easily cost $100,000 if they buy a policy at 55 and don't need it for 30 years.

PEOPLE WITH ADEQUATE INCOME. Can you afford to pay the premiums? Does $200 a month fit into your budget? Can you continue to pay the premiums for years to come? Can you continue to pay them when the rates go up (and they do go up, sometimes considerably) or if your income dips?

If money is tight, retirement saving, health insurance, and, for those with

> " I am measuring out how much I need a year to live on, and I have a bucket list. I would like to sky dive, travel, spoil a grandchild. . . . Then, when there's no more money left—I don't want to be penniless or so old I can't enjoy life—do me in. I do not want to be old and decrepit."
>
> —Olivia R.

> " I'm looking at long-term care insurance for myself, because it's too late for my parents. But when I think about the expense, I wonder if it's really worth it. I'm only 53—too young to think about nursing homes. But then, that's what always happens with these things. You don't think about them until you really need them, and then it's too late."
>
> —Nelly O.

dependents, life and disability insurance should take precedence. Be sure you won't spend money on premiums only to drop the policy later.

PEOPLE WHO ARE LIKELY TO NEED EXTENSIVE LONG-TERM CARE. If you buy long-term care insurance, you don't get to simply decide that you are ready for some help. For a policy to pay out, you have to meet eligibility requirements—usually, you have to have severe cognitive impairment or need help with at least two basic daily tasks, such as dressing or bathing.

Furthermore, under most policies, you have to pay for such care for three months before the policy kicks in. (Note that you have to *pay for such care*. You cannot wait out this period, struggling alone or depending upon family members in the interim. You have to pay for services from approved providers during this "elimination period.")

Given that the premiums are likely to cost an individual well over $50,000, and the policy won't pay out for the first three months, and it won't cover the cost of all care needed, then a policy is worthwhile only if you end up being significantly disabled and dependent for some time (at least a year).

No one has a crystal ball, but certain factors sway your odds.

If your father and grandfather both died of sudden heart attacks, then you are less likely to need protracted care than, say, a person who has a family history of Alzheimer's disease or diabetes.

What about your lifestyle? Do you exercise, smoke, eat well, or drink heavily? If you love nothing better than a remote control and box of doughnuts, then you may need long-term care sooner than your peers.

Another factor to consider is the care that might be available to you. Do you live alone, have nary a relative and a strong independent streak? Are you adamant that no one in your family will ever take care of you? Or does your daughter, a doting, single nurse, live down the street?

Married people are less apt to need private care than single people (because a spouse will provide much of the care). And women, who live longer than men, are more apt to need paid long-term care.

What sorts of services exist in your community? Are there loads of programs for seniors and a full-service adult day care center? Or do you live in a rural community with little in the way of eldercare?

If you plan on entering a life care, or continuing care, retirement community, which provides (for a large fee) all levels of care, then long-term care insurance might be redundant.

Finally, if you become ill, confused, and immobile, are you going to want all that medicine can offer? Or would you be looking for an easy exit? If you are quite certain that you don't want things "dragged out," that you will call hospice when things look bleak, then your odds of needing extensive long-term care are lower.

THOSE WHO REFUSE TO SAVE. If you have ample income but simply can't get yourself to put money aside, then a policy might be a method of forced savings.

THOSE WHO WANT THE EXTRA PEACE OF MIND. Here's something the economists and financial experts can't measure. If you are an incessant worrier and the thought of long-term care bills has you pacing at 3 a.m., then by all means, buy insurance. And get some sleep.

SELECTING A POLICY

Do your research. This is a big investment, so take the time to do it right.

Buy from a strong, reputable company that has been selling these policies for many years (although none have track records of more than a few decades, as the policies appeared on the market in the 1980s). A number of companies have stopped offering the policies, others have gone out of business, and all have increased premiums significantly. You can check insurers' ratings at TheStreet.com (thestreet.com/insurers/index.html).

Find out what happens if a company shuts down. Ask how much rates have increased recently. (While they cannot raise rates on an individual because of, say, health problems or age, they can raise rates on whole groups of policyholders.)

Then, compare several policies. These policies vary in many ways— when they kick in, what they cover, how benefits are paid, and so on. Prices for a policy with basically the same provisions can vary dramatically between companies. Companies also have different standards for eligibility. That is, if you have diabetes, smoke, or have a bad back, one company might deny coverage, while another will accept you.

Talk to an insurance broker who is experienced and knowledgeable. Find one who can tell you about policies from numerous companies, not just one. Get an "outline of coverage" detailing a policy's benefits, costs, restrictions, and limitations. When reviewing policies, be sure that special features are worth the higher premiums. Any extras will add substantially to the cost.

Be aware that whatever your premium is the first year, it will probably be higher in future years. Plan for it.

Some issues to consider when looking at long-term care insurance:

THE AMOUNT OF COVERAGE. Most policies pay a fixed amount for each day of care, typically between $100 and $250 a day. (Most people opt for about $150 a day.) If you are unsure of how much

> **"** I've seen firsthand what an incredible responsibility it is to take care of my mother, and it is not anything I'd want for my daughter. Absolutely not. Never.
>
> What I want to do is create a facility for my friends and me to buy into, where we'd have all the services we'd need. I have to figure it out and put it together because I will never put my daughter through what I've been through."
>
> —Syd S.

coverage to buy, find out the average cost of care in your area (at longtermcare .gov) and compare this with what you might be able to pay out-of-pocket. (If you live in an area where care is less expensive, you might need a less generous policy.)

Some policies provide a daily maximum for a set period of time, maybe three to five years, while others cover expenses up to some maximum amount. In the latter case, if you buy a policy that covers $150 a day and you need only $100 a day in services, can you tap into the rest later, turning what was a three-year policy into a four-year policy?

Some policies have different benefits for different types of care (they might reimburse you $200 a day for nursing home care and only $100 a day for in-home care).

THE START DATE. As noted, almost all policies include an "elimination period," which is essentially a deductible. The policy doesn't kick in until you have paid for care for a certain number of days (90 is common). Any waiting period of fewer than 20 days will make a policy prohibitive. On the other hand, a waiting period of more than 90 days significantly reduces the chance that you will ever put the policy to use.

Some policies have different elimination periods for different types of care. You might have no waiting period for home care and 90 days for nursing care, for example.

Make sure you understand the details. Most companies start the clock on the first day you pay for services and then run on a calendar, but some count only the days on which services were needed. That is, if you need someone to come in three days a week, do all seven days of that week count toward the 90 days, or only three?

Also, see if they offer a once-in-a-lifetime elimination period. That is, if you need care for a few months, to recuperate from a fall, for instance, will those days count as your elimination period if you need care later?

THE SCOPE OF COVERAGE. Today's policies are broad, and most cover care in a nursing home or assisted living facility, as well as home care, adult day services, hospice care, and respite care. Some go a step further, providing coverage for the unknown—new services and technologies that have yet to be developed (like robotic aides). Most policies require that services come from a licensed or certified agency, but check these details.

THE CRITERIA FOR COVERAGE. When does a policy consider you eligible for benefits? Most policies kick in when you cannot handle two "activities of daily living"—bathing, dressing, eating, getting from a bed to a chair, and getting to the bathroom alone. Most policies today also kick in when cognitive impairment requires supervision. Find out who determines eligibility—your doctor or someone hired by the insurance company.

INFLATION PROTECTION. If you buy $150-a-day coverage today, but don't need it for 20 years, the price of nursing home care may have gone up so much that your policy won't cover meals. Inflation protection means significantly higher premiums (it can add 50 percent to the cost of the policy), so it may not

MEDICAID PARTNERSHIP

Most people land in a confounding middle place—too many assets to qualify for Medicaid and not enough assets to pay for long-term care or insurance. In an effort to get these folks to buy insurance, most states have established innovative partnerships between Medicaid and the insurance industry.

Although the details vary from state to state, these programs allow people who buy long-term care insurance to get Medicaid coverage when their insurance runs out, and still protect a chunk of their assets (within certain income limits).

For example, in some states, a person gets to keep the amount of money the insurance policy paid for care. So if a policy covered $150,000 of care, that person would be able to go on Medicaid and hang on to $150,000 (plus the $2,000 or so normally allowed).

The policy has to be approved by the state, and you might have to receive care in that state or in a state with a reciprocal agreement. Call the state insurance department to find out if such programs exist in your state, or visit the website of the Long Term Care Partnership Program (dehpg.net/ltcpartnership).

be worthwhile for someone who is older. But people younger than 70 should find a policy that allows for 3 to 5 percent inflation, compounded annually.

You might be able to skip the inflation protection (making the policy cheaper), and then, at a future date, increase the daily benefit without having to pass another physical; however, the new rate will be considerably more.

WAIVERS. Pretty much all policies now include a waiver that frees you from paying premiums while you are receiving long-term care. Check for any restrictions on this, such as the number of days or type of care that must be received before premiums are waived.

GUARANTEE OF RENEWAL AND PROTECTION FROM CANCELLATION. Virtually all long-term care policies are guaranteed renewable, but check,

because this is imperative. A company should not be allowed to cancel a policy unless the premiums are not paid or someone lied on the application.

RETURN CLAUSE. All companies should allow you to return a policy within 30 days of buying it and get your money back.

NONFORFEITURE PROTECTION. Nonforfeiture guarantees that you will receive some value from the policy if you decide you don't want it anymore. The value—either money back or partial long-term care coverage—is based on the premiums paid before cancellation. This provision can add significantly to the price of a policy.

Most companies offer "contingent nonforfeiture benefits," which kick in if premiums rise more than a specified amount. Say you buy a policy and five

ALL IN ONE PLACE

If you really want to be kind to your children, get your finances in order, your documents signed, and your plans laid out, then put all necessary paperwork and information neatly in one file or binder notebook. Be sure to update it regularly. Let them know where it is or, if they are young, let a sibling, close friend, or attorney know where to find it.

Your binder should include your will or instructions for finding your will; copies of your advance directives and power of attorney; a list of all assets and debts; names and numbers of attorneys, investors, accountants, and so on; information about accounts and credit cards; burial instructions; personal instructions about your home, pets, belongings, or other property; old tax forms or information on where they are located; insurance policies; company benefits; information about a business; military/veteran papers; deeds and titles; and so forth. (See page 12 for a complete list of important papers that your family might need.)

years later the premiums go up 25 percent. Rather than paying the higher premium, you could opt to stick with your old premium rate and reduce the amount of coverage.

MARITAL DISCOUNTS. Most plans offer discounts of 5 to 15 percent if both halves of a couple buy policies. Some

> After their father died, my daughters said, 'Think about what should go to whom, because everybody's been fighting over Dad's stuff.' They had me write it all out and sign it. And then they said, 'Think about what casket and what music you want.'
> It was hard. I thought, *Here I am, planning my demise.* I wasn't prepared for that thought. It pulls you up short and makes you think, *I'm going to die one day.*"
> —Mae H.

plans allow couples to split benefits, in which case they buy two policies, but if one person dies, the other gets the total coverage remaining. In other words, if each person buys a policy covering three years of nursing home care, and one dies without ever needing such care, the surviving spouse now has six years of coverage, or vice versa. A couple might also buy a single policy, providing a set amount of benefits, regardless of who uses them.

FEW RESTRICTIONS AND EXCLUSIONS. Once you know what a policy covers, consider what it doesn't cover. Most don't cover self-inflicted injuries, alcoholism, drug addiction, or mental illness. Some policies won't cover any illness that existed at the time the policy was purchased, or deny coverage for a certain amount of time. In this case, the restriction should last for no more than six months.

Also, look for restrictive clauses in a policy, such as "usual and customary costs," "prevailing costs," or "appropriate costs." Find out what this means and how coverage might be limited.

TAX QUALIFIED. Find out if the premiums are deductible as a medical expense and also whether a policy's benefits can be taxed (usually not).

COMBO PRODUCTS. Some companies offer a bundled package of an annuity or whole life insurance combined with long-term care insurance. (Sometimes the long-term care insurance can be added as a rider to existing life insurance.) Generally, whatever funds are used for long-term care are subtracted from the final benefit. This way, if the long-term care benefits are not needed, all is not lost. However, it requires buying a universal, or whole life, policy, which is far more expensive than a simple term policy and may be more than you need.

> " My mother talked all the time about how she didn't want to be a burden to us kids and how she would *never* move in with any of us. She would see other people depending on their kids and be very critical of them.
>
> But that's all she did. Talk. She never made a plan or took any action. Her emphysema got worse, and her diabetes got worse, and she just kept talking about how she didn't want us to have to care for her. But she never dealt with it in any practical way.
>
> So of course, we all had to take care of her, and it was a ton of work.
>
> My husband and I are very proactive about this. I'm a bit neurotic about it, to be honest. We have long-term care insurance and an account that we put money into every month for our old age. Whatever it takes, we do not, ever, want our girls taking care of us like that."
>
> —Betsy M.

A Question of Where

If you are over 60, it's time to start thinking about where you will live in your retirement and beyond. It's not too early. These things take years to iron out. Start now so you end up where you want to be.

Obviously, the first question is whether you are going to move to a new town. Do you want a different climate, a different cost of living, a place that's urban or rural? Do you want to be closer to your siblings or your children? (If so, be sure they aren't going to move soon after you do.)

As you consider where to live, think about what you might need beyond retirement, when you need help. Does any community you are considering provide ample services for elderly people? Are there adequate transportation

> **"** I don't ever want to be a burden on my kids. I am going to live with my sisters. I think our husbands will die before we will.
>
> If my sisters and I pool our resources, we can live together and afford help, as needed. Could be fun, or it could be a disaster."
>
> —Melissa T.

services, adult day services, meal services, and other programs?

Once you've got the geography sorted out, think about any house you are considering. Any home you buy, build, or renovate should have a bedroom on the first floor, wide hallways, at least one large bathroom (wheelchair accessible), an entrance that doesn't have steps or that would allow for a ramp, and so on.

As you look forward, be creative. Talk to friends about what they might do.

Perhaps they would be interested in moving somewhere as a group or setting up a creative arrangement—linked apartments, a large group home, or one-level homes on the same block.

Actually, It Does Take a Village

Once upon a time, extended family members lived in the same community, and women, for the most part, didn't work outside the home. Mom and Dad lived two blocks down and were regularly visited by an assortment of family and neighbors who brought over a pot pie, drove Mom to the doctor, and repaired the loose back step.

Then, of course, we moved apart, got jobs, and discovered our parents had no one nearby to help them in their old age.

Now, more and more communities are re-creating and even improving the old scenario with what are known

AGING WITHOUT CHILDREN

If you don't have kids or just don't want them involved in your old age, then create a circle of friends and trusted advisers who can serve as decision makers and care coordinators.

Talk to them about your goals and wishes—how long you want to remain at home, where you might live if you have to move, who would provide care, how your finances will be handled, and so on. Assign someone to oversee financial issues, someone to manage your care, and someone to make health care decisions. Assign proxies, and be

sure everyone knows about any legal documents.

Talk to them all at length in a group, and be sure everyone clearly understands what's to be done. Then write it up in detail and have everyone sign it. Depending on the duties assigned (and the depths of the friendships), there might be payments involved.

Choose people whom you trust (obviously), and who get along, can communicate readily, and are young enough to be counted on when you are old.

as "villages"—cooperatives that allow seniors to stay in their homes and be part of their communities.

Generally, it works like this: People who are over 50 pay an annual membership fee, ranging from $35 to $900 (some cooperatives offer discounts based on income). In exchange, they get help when they need it so they can stay in the community as they age.

A crew of volunteers is available to do most anything—transportation, errands, household help, home repairs, shopping, gardening, and social visits. Local merchants, handymen, dog walkers, caterers, home care agencies, and so on (all of whom have been vetted) offer discounts to members.

The cooperatives also organize social events for seniors—potluck suppers, walks, book groups, exercise programs, trips, and lectures. And, of course, members of a village do what any good neighbor would do: provide a sympathetic ear, friendly advice, and, when tragedy strikes, coffee, pastries, and hugs.

Funded by donations, grants, and membership fees, villages often have paid staff, but are manned largely by members of the village, most of whom volunteer as long as they are able.

NORCs

Sometimes, a neighborhood or high-rise unintentionally finds itself with a large concentration of elders. The next thing you know, you have a NORC—a Naturally Occurring Retirement Community (or, in rural areas, NORR, for Naturally Occurring Retirement Region).

The sheer number of elderly residents means power—power to create a

> ❝ I am doing a lot of planning and research because I've seen friends' parents die in ways that I never want to die, all alone in their houses, which is the booby prize.
>
> I want to live in a walkable community, where there is activity close by and I walk to the grocery store and wave to people. And I want to be surrounded by people who are active participants in life, who exercise and eat well, and want to take on meaningful projects. I also want to live in a net-positive-energy-and-water community, so I'm researching building models and cohousing.
>
> I'm excited about my future and all of this."
>
> —Dorothy R.

community that meets their needs. That might mean generous community services, innovative programs, social events, and a physical environment suited for seniors (ramped sidewalks, bright street lamps, and so on). Local merchants often offer discounts to seniors. Local universities or hospitals are often involved, providing leadership or volunteers.

So rather than having a patchwork of social services crop up somewhat randomly, the community itself designs, plans, and oversees the web of programs, as well as the physical layout (accessible parking, wide sidewalks, plenty of ramps, good lighting, and so forth).

As with villages, NORCs allow people to stay in their own homes as they age. Unlike "villages," which are completely self-run, NORCs are generally funded by federal or state monies, and have to adhere to specific guidelines.

Your Body

Although genetics plays a role in determining why one person lives to be 98 with their own teeth intact, and another is bedridden at 72, it is a smaller role than you might imagine. It turns out that the discrepancies in how we age are largely determined by luck and lifestyle.

People who age well—those who suffer the fewest ailments and infirmities and are vigorous and happy in their old age—are the ones who exercise, eat well, don't smoke, spend time with family and friends, and stay active and involved. It's that simple.

Most ailments that hinder people in old age, including diabetes, cancer, stroke, heart disease, arthritis, Alzheimer's, and osteoporosis, are associated with diet and exercise.

So, take care of yourself. You know how: Eat plenty of fresh vegetables and fruits, get lots of fiber and fluids. Stick to foods that are low in fat and salt. Avoid processed foods. And exercise. Stretch, flex, and lift. Take long walks. Try yoga, weight lifting, or basketball. Get outdoors. Get fresh air. Stretch your lungs and your muscles. This makes a tremendous, *tremendous* difference.

While you're at it, buckle your seat belt. Limit the booze. And definitely, toss the cigarettes.

ANTIAGING MIRACLES

Yes, you can down bottles of glutathione, picolinate, manganese, d-alpha tocopherol succinate, coenzyme Q10, HGH, and DHEA and hope it all merges to create the fountain of youth.

Or you can freeze your corpse in the hope that one day the cure to what killed you will be discovered, along with a safe way to defrost you. Some people sock away a set of their DNA in the hope of becoming rebuilt or cloned at a later date. And others believe that through "cybernetic immortality," they can download all their thoughts, memories, desires, impulses, biases, and everything else that makes them who they are onto a computer. Then, when their bodies are kaput, the cyber-them can go on, teaching their children, writing their books, and calling their friends.

Most antiaging approaches are less far-flung, but most of them are still a huge waste of time, energy, and money. Many are downright dangerous.

Stay healthy and active. Eat your greens. Work your muscles. Use your mind. Skip the cake. Spend time with friends. But don't be fooled. Don't waste these years buying into scams. And don't let dreams of immortality distract you from what really needs to be done—living your life, taking care of yourself, and planning for the inevitable.

You've heard all this before. Now try it. You won't believe what a difference it makes until you set yourself to the task. If you can alter your lifestyle, even in small ways, it will not only make for more and better years, health, and independence, but it will also make you feel younger, more energetic, and more optimistic right now, today.

While you're tending to your body, be sure to get good medical care. Don't put off that pelvic exam or prostate test. Find a good doctor, have regular check-ups, and be alert to signs of trouble. (And don't forget the dentist!)

Your Mind

O nce again, use it or lose it. Brains are not all that different from the rest of the body; they need exercise. People who study, travel, and explore are happier in life, more independent in old age, and generally live longer.

Plus, using your mind is fun and makes you a more interesting person. Oh sure, you use your mind while working and playing with your apps, and that's great. But use it for new things, as well.

Doing the same old thing every day—whether it's crunching numbers, editing manuscripts, or writing business reports—exercises only one part of your mind, a part that is already well defined. Fire up those neglected synapses. Learn Spanish, take oil painting, pick up chess, join a fencing club, make Thai meals, study Mayan culture, go to a lecture on Eastern philosophy.

Not only is it critical to keep your mind active, but it's important to remain productive, to feel that you contribute to society in some way. Volunteer in a school overseas, with an environmental group, at a hospital. Teach children, disabled people, or other adults. Get involved in politics or social causes.

Tapping into your creative juices is also beneficial. Even if you've never done anything creative in the past, take up sculpting, poetry, or dance.

Armed Against Dementia

Although brain gymnastics doesn't seem to ward off Alzheimer's and other forms of dementia, studying, learning, exploring, and otherwise exercising the brain will give you a reserve tank that should lessen the effect of disease.

You can also improve your odds by keeping healthy. High cholesterol, diabetes, and high blood pressure all increase the risk of cognitive impairment. Avoid saturated fats, stick to fish and small amounts of lean meat, and again, enjoy your fruits and vegetables.

Exercise has also been shown to keep dementia at bay, as have stress-relieving activities (meditation, deep breathing,

HALFZHEIMER'S

If you are convinced that you are halfway to dementia because you can't remember where you left the car (never mind the keys) or what you came up the stairs to get, don't sign up for a room in the Alzheimer's wing just yet.

A certain amount of forgetfulness is completely normal in middle age. When people are really cognitively impaired, they aren't forgetting a friend's name or messing up an entry in the checkbook. They forget important appointments and events. They get lost in familiar places and have trouble following a movie plot or conversation. They often have poor judgment and become impulsive.

If you are concerned, talk with your doctor. Many things—some of them reversible—cause cognitive decline. And sometimes forgetfulness goes away on its own. But don't stay up at night, because you are probably fine, and lack of sleep will only worsen your muddled mind.

imagery). These are the same things that will help fend off other ailments common in old age and make your life better all around.

Brain injuries clearly increase the risk of dementia, so wear a bike helmet.

Finally, certain medications, when taken for a long period of time, interfere with the workings of the brain. These drugs, known as anticholinergics, include common painkillers, antihistamines, and antidepressants. Even weaker anticholinergics can have a cumulative effect when people take multiple medications. You can see the anticholinergic strength of your medications on the Anticholinergic Burden Scale at indydiscoverynetwork.org/AnticholinergicCognitiveBurdenScale.html.

Your Life

Now that you've signed your will, stocked your fridge with kale, and signed up for yoga, it's time to get down to the really critical stuff. It's time to live life. Let go of any gripes and regrets, and get out there. Seize the day because you never know what's to come. Enjoy life and make the most of whatever remains.

The bonus of this is that friendships, an optimistic attitude, and a good hearty laugh can actually add years to your life. These factors may even be more important than things like cholesterol level or blood pressure.

To live long, it turns out that you need to live well.

Friends and Family

Your sister might make you angry. Your kids might drive you nuts. Your marriage might be boring. And you might not have time for your friends. Well, change your ways, because this is important stuff.

If you don't have time, make it. Call an old friend. Visit your brother. Take time out for your kids. And never be stingy with words like "I'm sorry," "I forgive you," and "I love you."

Foster your relationships. Nourish them. Water them and feed them. Work at them and enjoy them. Because when you're sitting in your wheelchair with little hair and no teeth and only a faint memory, the fact that you were promoted at work, or won a race, or made money, or cleaned out your basement won't mean a darn thing. But having loved ones around will. Ask anyone who's 85.

Find Your Soul

If you don't have the time or inclination for religious services, you might still spend a little time each week with your soul. Take a moment and get away from the noise, pressures, text messages, and distractions. Find a silent place, sit quietly, and listen. As the minutes pass, if you can clear your head of the commotion, you will begin to hear it, the voice of your soul.

If you do this routinely, just a few minutes each day, these moments alone with yourself will ease your stress and remind you of your priorities.

What does this have to do with growing old? Everything. It is this voice that guides us to where we need to be, and gets us through times of turbulence, pain, and loneliness. Any solace or spirituality you can find now will help later, when your knees hurt, your eyes don't work, and death is looking in your direction.

Laugh

Everything else—the friends, the forgiveness, and maybe even a certain form of spirituality—will happen more easily if you find the humor in life and have at least one good laugh every day.

Check Your Personality

Cantankerous. Curmudgeonly. Cranky. Surly. Grouchy. Grumpy. Crabby. These are the seven dwarfs at 90. If some of these adjectives already apply to you, imagine what words they'll be using when you arrive on the steps of Twin Oaks Memorial Home.

It's not just about being a nice person so your kids don't pull the plug too soon. It's about being the person you want to be. It's about being tolerant and kind, or creative and wild, or ambitious and bold. It's about knowing that people can change. It's about making choices about who you are and feeling good about yourself. (It turns out that you do not have to be your parent after all.)

Be Adaptable

If you talk with geriatricians and nursing home staff, they will tell you that the people who age best are flexible. They adapt easily to sickness, to bad news, and to changes in their housing or lifestyle. These adapters are less of a burden

BURIAL PLANS?

Although this isn't essential, and may seem a bit macabre, it is helpful to give your family a few general instructions on what to do when you are gone.

Do you want to be cremated? Do you want a religious service or a dance party? Or both? Do you want to donate your body for organ procurement or research? Do you want your ashes spread in some meaningful place? Or do you have a cemetery plot? Do you want someone in particular to officiate, or a certain song played?

You don't want to tie their hands (*I don't want any services or gatherings. Just throw me in the landfill*). After all, funeral and burial rituals are meant to soothe survivors. But some general thoughts can be helpful.

If this matters to you, put it in writing, especially if there might be any squabbling or confusion among family members. Some states recognize written wishes, and some allow you to legally name someone who will oversee funeral arrangements.

Unless there are extenuating circumstances (for example, you are "spending down" to become eligible for Medicaid), don't prepay for a funeral. As outlined on page 555, too many things can go wrong.

to their families. And studies show that they live longer, too.

With age, many people become entrenched in their ways, more stubborn and unbending with each passing year. But just as we can stretch our bodies and become more flexible, we can stretch our personalities and become more adaptable.

Work at letting go of things and going with the flow from time to time. Try it in small ways. Let go of the reins. Let others make plans, and don't fuss when plans are changed. Rearrange rigid routines from time to time. With time, you may find that you are more resilient, more agreeable, and better prepared to face the changes that certainly lie ahead.

Love Thyself

Sure, you should know your shortfalls, and even work to improve them, but know your pluses, too. Know all that is great about you. Forgive yourself. Like yourself. Give yourself credit. Know what is wonderful about you.

Change Your Ageist Attitude

It turns out that negative stereotypes about old age are actually bad for you. Whether you make cracks about old drivers and seniors in the checkout who can't manage their change, or you spend a bundle on hair dyes and wrinkle creams so you don't have to be one of them, you might be hurting yourself. People who view aging in a positive light seem to live longer than those who view it harshly.

People who accept old age as just another stage of life, who view themselves as wiser and richer as they age, and who still see themselves as valuable members of society when they are old, live longer. This seems to actually have a greater impact on longevity than blood pressure, cholesterol, weight loss, and exercise.

So rethink your views. Do it because it might extend your life, and, more important, because it might expand it. For all that is rotten about old age, most elderly people have amazing insights and joys. They have suffered and grown and accepted. And they have much to teach us. No matter how slowly they might drive, they have much to contribute to our lives and to our communities.

By changing our views, by respecting this older population and caring for them adequately, by recognizing our own aging process and seeing our gains as well as our losses, we will all be richer.

Be patient with your parents, polite to the old lady digging for change, and respectful to the elderly gentleman nodding off at the head of the table. Be nice, because whether you like it or not, you're next. And that might not be so bad.

Resources

Useful Organizations

Although you can find accurate and useful information on the Internet (along with plenty of pointless but oddly alluring distractions), be careful. The web has become an advertising whirlpool. Sites that appear reputable and unbiased are often the fruits of large corporations or trade associations and have one underlying message: *Buy a hearing aid! Get a reverse mortgage! You need more insurance!* Some cater to advertisers, swaying information to please a drug company or retirement community, and others have "free advisers," who get commissions for selling you something or signing your parent up for a housing facility, financial tool, or other product or service.

Know what you're dealing with. In the following pages we've provided some of the most useful and trusted sites.

TEN PARTICULARLY USEFUL WEBSITES

PROGRAM	CONTACT	DESCRIPTION
Eldercare Locator	eldercare.gov 800-677-1116	Start your hunt for local services here. The helpline and website will lead you to the area agency on aging that oversees services to the elderly in your parent's hometown.
National Long-Term Care Ombudsman Resource Center	ltcombudsman.org 202-332-2275	This website will direct you to a local ombudsman, who can help you find nursing homes, assisted living centers, and other long-term care facilities, apprise you of your rights, and help resolve conflicts within a facility.
AARP	aarp.org 888-687-2277	AARP provides all sorts of information on caregiving, financial and legal matters, and a variety of other issues facing the elderly and their families. It also has information on "universal design," ways to make a home safer and more accessible.
Family Caregiver Alliance	caregiver.org 800-445-8106	Started in California, the alliance runs a National Center on Caregiving and provides information on a wide variety of topics useful to anyone caring for an elderly person. It also has a Family Care Navigator to help you find programs in your area.
BenefitsCheckUp	benefitscheckup.org	This website searches for federal, state, and local private and public benefits and entitlement programs for people 55 and over. It also provides information about prescription drug programs that can save money.

PROGRAM	CONTACT	DESCRIPTION
Medicaid	medicaid.gov	This federal website has basic state-by-state Medicaid information, but most important, it will direct you to local Medicaid offices, which can help you navigate the system.
Medicare	medicare.gov 800-633-4227	This government website offers extensive information about Medicare, Medigap, and state insurance departments. It also provides information on choosing and paying for long-term care.
Alzheimer's Association	alz.org 800-272-3900	Although focused on Alzheimer's disease, the association provides an enormous amount of information on all forms of dementia—medical information, as well as support guidance, and referrals to local chapters and support groups.
National SHIP Resource Center	shiptalk.org	This national website will direct you to the State Health Insurance Assistance Program (SHIP), which provides one-on-one health insurance counseling to people on Medicare and their families.
Caring Connections	caringinfo.org 800-658-8898	Created by the National Hospice and Palliative Care Organization, this website provides information about advance planning and end-of-life care. You can download state-specific advance directives (legal forms that include a living will and a durable power of attorney for health care). Counselors are available through the helpline.

ACCESSIBILITY AND HOME MODIFICATION

AARP
aarp.org
888-687-2277

AARP has information on "universal design," ways to make a home safer and more accessible for an elderly person, and a checklist to be sure that a home meets a person's current needs.

ABLEDATA
abledata.com
800-227-0216

This federally funded program has a database of assistive technology and rehabilitation equipment, as well as information about the price and manufacturer or distributor. ABLEDATA's website also offers a resource center and "reading room," and has some reviews of products.

Disability.gov
disability.gov

This federal government website has information about civil rights, benefits, and options for people living with disabilities.

Fall Prevention Center of Excellence
homemods.org
stopfalls.org
213-740-1364

Based in California, this center sponsors two websites. Homemods.org will get you into a database of local organizations and contractors that do home repairs and modifications for the elderly and disabled. Stopfalls.org contains information on home safety and preventing falls.

National Rehabilitation Information Center
naric.com
800-346-2742

This federally funded resource provides information about accessibility and rehabilitation, facilities, funding, organizations, and other issues.

Paralyzed Veterans of America
pva.org
866-734-0857 (benefits helpline)
800-232-1782 (health care helpline)

This private, nonprofit advocacy group provides information on benefits, living with a disability, modifying a home, and other topics. It also makes referrals to local services.

This Caring Home
thiscaringhome.org

This Caring Home, set up by people at Weill Cornell Medical College for people with dementia, is actually useful when caring for any elderly person. It goes room by room, providing advice on how to make daily life safer and manageable, and reviews a variety of products.

ADULT DAY SERVICES

National Adult Day Services Association
nadsa.org
877-745-1440

The association's website will refer you to adult day centers in your parent's area.

AFRICAN AMERICAN SERVICES

National Caucus and Center on Black Aging
ncba-aged.org
202-637-8400

The center works to improve the quality of life for African American seniors and other minority or low-income seniors. The website can direct you to information about affordable housing, community service, and employment programs.

ALCOHOL AND DRUG ABUSE

Adult Children of Alcoholics
adultchildren.org

Using a 12-step, spiritually based, recovery program, like AA, ACA holds support groups around the country to help adults deal with issues connected to being raised by someone who was an alcoholic.

Al-Anon Family Groups
al-anon.org
888-425-2666

These groups help family members and friends of alcoholics cope. The website has information for families and referrals to local chapters.

Alcoholics Anonymous
aa.org

AA assists alcoholics in becoming and remaining sober through local self-help groups.

National Council on Alcoholism and Drug Dependence
ncadd.org
800-622-2255

The council has information on addiction and treatment, support for family members, and referrals to local services.

Rethinking Drinking
rethinkingdrinking.niaaa.nih.gov

This website, put out by the National Institute on Alcohol Abuse and Alcoholism, has a vast amount of information on drinking patterns, risks, and ways to cut back or stop.

ALZHEIMER'S AND OTHER FORMS OF DEMENTIA

Alzheimer's Association
alz.org
800-272-3900

Although focused on Alzheimer's disease, the association provides an enormous amount of information on all forms of dementia—medical information, as well as support, guidance, and referrals to local chapters and support groups. The phone line offers help 24/7.

Alzheimer's Disease Education and Referral Center
nia.nih.gov/alzheimers
800-438-4380

Run by the National Institute on Aging, this center has information on all aspects of Alzheimer's disease.

Alzheimer's Foundation of America
alzfdn.org
866-232-8484

The AFA works to raise awareness and educate the public about Alzheimer's disease. The website has information on the disease and caregiving, and social workers answer the hotline.

Alzheimers.gov
alzheimers.gov

This government website has a wealth of information on treatment options, paying for care, coping with daily challenges, and caregiver support.

Lewy Body Dementia Association
lbda.org
800-539-9767

The association offers information on Lewy body dementia.

National Institute of Neurological Disorders and Stroke
ninds.nih.gov
800-352-9424

Part of the National Institutes of Health, this center has information about a variety of brain diseases and disorders, and provides referrals to local clinical research centers.

This Caring Home
thiscaringhome.org

This Caring Home, set up by people at Weill Cornell Medical College for people with dementia, is useful for any elderly person. It goes room by room, providing clear advice on how to make daily life safer and more manageable, and reviews a variety of products.

ARTHRITIS AND OSTEOPOROSIS

Arthritis Foundation
arthritis.org
800-283-7800

The foundation provides information and makes referrals to local chapters, which sponsor support groups, events, and classes.

National Institute of Arthritis and Musculoskeletal and Skin Diseases
niams.nih.gov
877-226-4267

This federal clearinghouse is part of the National Institutes of Health and has information covering a host of disorders and diseases that affect bones, joints, and skin.

National Osteoporosis Foundation
nof.org
800-231-4222

This organization offers information on the causes, prevention, detection, and treatment of osteoporosis.

NIH Osteoporosis and Related Bone Diseases National Resource Center
www.osteo.org
800-624-2663

Part of the National Institutes of Health, this center has information on osteoporosis, as well as other bone diseases.

ASIAN SERVICES

National Asian Pacific Center on Aging
napca.org
800-336-2722

This national advocacy organization has several employment programs and provides helplines in numerous languages, assisting people with Medicare and benefit programs.

ASSISTED LIVING

(See "Nursing Homes and Assisted Living.")

CANCER

American Cancer Society
cancer.org
800-227-2345

Staff members can answer questions on a broad range of subjects, such as cancer detection, treatment, and the latest research. The website has information about diagnoses, treatments, and trials, as well as emotional support and local chapters, which can refer you to local services.

National Cancer Institute
nci.nih.gov
800-422-6237

The NCI helpline and website provide information on the detection and treatment of cancer, finances, and home care. It provides referrals to local organizations, cancer centers, and support groups.

National Coalition for Cancer Survivorship
canceradvocacy.org
877-622-7937

This private, nonprofit group is a survivor-led advocacy organization. It offers information on cancer treatments, costs, and insurance coverage, and refers people who have received a cancer diagnosis to support groups.

CAREGIVER COORDINATION

A number of websites provide ways for families and other caregivers—siblings, doctors, friends, neighbors, aides, and volunteers—to communicate and coordinate care. Although they can be a tremendous help to caregivers, you have to find the one that's right for your situation.

When looking at these sites, know that some charge a fee; others make money through advertisers (and target advertising based on your personal information); and some sell personal information. *Exception:* Caring Bridge is nonprofit and relies on donations.

Carepages
carepages.com

Carepages lets you create a personal website so friends and family can share information, post photos, and send messages.

CareZone, Saturing, and Tyze
carezone.com
saturing.com
tyze.com

CareZone, Saturing, and Tyze are all slightly different, but all of them help families and groups of caregivers organize care. Generally speaking, these services let you share information about your parent's care; coordinate tasks, appointments, and work shifts; send messages; and safely store information (such as medical records, legal documents, financial information, contact lists, prescriptions). All of this can be accessed from computers, smartphones, and tablets. Most also let you send out alerts to your group. Some charge fees, some have advertisers; some share some data, others do not.

Caring Bridge
caringbridge.org

Caring Bridge lets friends and family share news and photos, and send messages. It also provides SupportPlanner, a calendar that helps you coordinate care.

Lotsa Helping Hands
lotsahelpinghands.com

Lotsa Helping Hands lets you share updates and photos and has a calendar where people can sign up for tasks.

CAREGIVER SUPPORT AND SERVICES

AARP
aarp.org
888-687-2277

AARP provides all sorts of information on caregiving, financial and legal matters, and a variety of other issues facing the elderly and their families.

Caregiver Action Network
caregiveraction.org

Originally the National Family Caregivers Association, the Action Network is a nonprofit organization that provides information, support, and referrals to caregivers. CAN also helps members connect to local volunteers who provide education and support.

Eldercare Locator
eldercare.gov
800-677-1116

Run by the U.S. Administration on Aging, this is a good place to start looking for local services. The helpline and website will lead you to the area agency on aging that oversees services to the elderly in your parent's hometown.

Family Caregiver Alliance
caregiver.org
800-445-8106

Started in California, the alliance runs a National Center on Caregiving and provides information on a wide variety of topics useful to anyone caring for an elderly person. It also has a Family Care Navigator to help you find programs in your area.

National Association of Professional Geriatric Care Managers
caremanager.org
520-881-8008

Primarily a trade association for care managers, this group provides referrals to geriatric care managers who will, for a fee, help you navigate caregiving, find community services, and deal with family disagreements.

VA Caregiver Support
www.caregiver.va.gov
855-260-3274

This website and "careline" are meant to help caregivers of veterans find services and get support.

Well Spouse Foundation
wellspouse.org
800-838-0879

The foundation offers support to people caring for a sick or disabled spouse. Although your focus may be on your needier parent, your "well" parent needs help and support. Members are directed to support groups, can be assigned pen pals if desired, and receive a newsletter.

DEATH AND END-OF-LIFE PLANNING

(See also "Hospice Care.")

Aging with Dignity
agingwithdignity.org
888-594-7437

This organization sells "Five Wishes," a document designed to help people express how they want to be treated if they become seriously ill and are unable to speak for themselves.

Caring Connections
caringinfo.org
800-658-8898

Created by the National Hospice and Palliative Care Organization, this website provides information about advance planning and end-of-life care. You can download state-specific advance directives (legal forms that include a living will and durable power of attorney for health care). Counselors are available through the helpline.

Compassion & Choices
compassionandchoices.org
800-247-7421

Compassion & Choices provides one-on-one counseling and information on choices at the end of life, and ways to ensure that one's wishes are followed. It also has state-specific advance directives.

National Right to Life Committee
nrlc.org
202-626-8800

The committee, a grassroots organization that opposes abortion and euthanasia, has drafted a "Will to Live" form that states a person's wishes to be kept on life support regardless of the medical prognosis. The committee also provides help for people seeking treatment that a doctor or hospital refuses to provide.

DEMENTIA

(See "Alzheimer's and Other Forms of Dementia.")

DENTISTRY

American Dental Association
ada.org

The ADA's website helps you find a local dentist and provides a glossary of oral health. There's information available on dentures and oral changes caused by aging.

National Institute of Dental and Craniofacial Research
nidcr.nih.gov
866-232-4528

Part of the National Institutes of Health, this institute offers information on oral health.

DEPRESSION

(See "Mental Health.")

DIABETES

American Diabetes Association
diabetes.org
800-342-2383

The association provides information on diabetes, medical treatment, and related financial issues, and can direct you to state chapters for referrals to local doctors and support groups.

National Diabetes Information Clearinghouse
diabetes.niddk.nih.gov
800-860-8747

Sponsored by the National Institute of Diabetes and Digestive and Kidney Diseases, the clearinghouse has information on all aspects of diabetes.

DIGESTIVE DISEASES

National Digestive Diseases Information Clearinghouse
digestive.niddk.nih.gov
800-891-5389

This information service of the National Institute of Diabetes and Digestive and Kidney Diseases provides information on digestive diseases, from indigestion and gas to ulcers and gallstones.

DRIVING

AAA Senior Driving
seniordriving.aaa.com

This website, sponsored by the AAA, discusses driving skills, what family members should do when they feel an elderly person shouldn't be driving, and ways to improve driving skills. It also offers referrals to refresher courses and professional assessments. An interactive online tool, Roadwise Review, evaluates physical and mental abilities needed for driving.

EXERCISE AND PHYSICAL THERAPY

Arthritis Foundation
arthritis.org
800-283-7800

The foundation has information on exercise and rehabilitation (as well as arthritis), and makes referrals to local chapters, which often offer exercise classes.

Go4Life
go4life.nia.nih.gov

The website for the NIH's campaign to get older adults moving has information on getting started, safe exercises, and motivational tips.

Move Forward
moveforwardpt.com
800-999-2782

This site, by the American Physical Therapy Association, has information and makes referrals to local certified physical therapists.

National Senior Games Association
nsga.com
225-766-6800

The NSGA is a not-for-profit organization dedicated to promoting healthful lifestyles for active adults 50 and over through education, fitness, and sport. They organize the Senior Olympic Programs nationwide.

FINANCES

(See also "Medicare, Medicaid, and Other Insurance Issues" and "Fraud.")

BenefitsCheckUp
benefitscheckup.org

This website searches for federal, state, and local private and public benefits and entitlement programs for people 55 and over. It also provides information about prescription drug programs that can save money.

GovBenefits
govbenefits.gov

This website provides private, online screening to determine eligibility for government benefits. If you (or your parent) qualify for a program, the website provides necessary contact information.

Home Equity Advisor
homeequityadvisor.org

Created by the National Council on Aging, this website helps people examine their housing situation, expenses, and options.

Internal Revenue Service
irs.gov
800-829-1040

Tax information and forms are available online.

National Foundation for Counseling Credit
nfcc.org
800-388-2227

The foundation makes referrals to local Consumer Credit Counseling Service offices, which provide free or low-cost counseling on budgeting and debt management.

Pension Rights Center
pensionrights.org
202-296-3776

The center can lead you to a pension counseling office that provides workers, retirees, and their families with information and legal guidance.

Social Security Administration
ssa.gov
800-772-1213

Use this site to apply for benefits, estimate future benefits, arrange for direct deposit of checks, or to get general information on Social Security, SSI, or disability benefits.

FOOT CARE

American Podiatric Medical Association
apma.org
301-581-9200

The APMA offers information on foot care and disease, and referrals to podiatrists.

FRAUD

National Adult Protective Services Association
napsa-now.org
217-523-4431

NAPSA is a nonprofit organization with chapters around the country that advocates for vulnerable adults. Its website has information on abuse, reporting, and local services.

National Center of Elder Abuse
ncea.aoa.gov
855-500-3537

The center, part of the Administration on Aging, can direct you to the local offices of Adult Protective Services and hotlines, and provides basic information on abuse, neglect, and exploitation.

National Consumers League
fraud.org

This site has a variety of information on fraud and recent, popular scams to watch out for.

FUNERALS

Funeral Consumers Alliance
funerals.org

This group offers guidance on planning inexpensive and dignified funeral and memorial services. It can also direct you to a local consumers' funeral society in your area.

Funeral Ethics Organization
funeralethics.org
802-482-6021

Started by longtime consumer protection activist Lisa Carlson, this website lays out each state's laws on funerals, burials, and prepaying for funerals.

Green Burial Council
greenburialcouncil.org
888-966-3330

Visit the site for information on burials that are environmentally responsible.

National Funeral Directors Association
nfda.org
800-228-6332

This association offers guidance in locating a funeral director and planning memorial services and burials.

GAY, LESBIAN, BISEXUAL, AND TRANSGENDER ISSUES

HIV Over Fifty
hivoverfifty.org

Although this is actually the website of the New England Association of HIV Over Fifty, it has information for any elderly person dealing with HIV.

LGBT Aging Resources Clearinghouse
asaging.org/lgbt-search

The American Society on Aging has a list of resources for LGBT elderly adults and links to local service providers and organizations.

National Resource Center on LGBT Aging
lgbtagingcenter.org
212-741-2247

In partnership with several other organizations, SAGE (below) runs this resource center with information on housing, legal issues, caregiving, rights, and other matters for lesbian, gay, bisexual, and transgender older adults.

SAGE
sageusa.org
212-741-2247

SAGE is the nation's oldest and largest social service and advocacy organization for lesbian, gay, bisexual, and transgender seniors. SAGE (which was originally Senior Action in a Gay Environment, but is now Services & Advocacy for Gay, Lesbian, Bisexual & Transgender Elders) provides services, advocates for LGBT elders, and helps people find local programs.

GENERAL

AARP
aarp.org
888-687-2277

AARP is one of the largest and most powerful lobbying and educational organizations in the country. It has information on a wide range of topics such as housing options, home care, caregiver stress, and financial plights. There are money-saving programs for members, such as a travel service and a mail-order pharmacy, and volunteer programs and services. Call or visit the website to find out about local chapters, membership benefits, and publications.

Administration on Aging
aoa.gov

The AOA has information about federal programs and provides links to other programs and websites.

National Council on the Aging
ncoa.org
202-479-1200

This private, nonprofit organization advocates on behalf of the elderly. Although largely administrative, the NCOA makes referrals to local services and has information and special programs for seniors and their caregivers (housing, support groups, social services, legal and financial support, nutrition, and health).

National Institute on Aging
nia.nih.gov
800-222-2225

The NIA, a division of the National Institutes of Health, supports research on aging and health, and puts out loads of information on a variety of senior issues, including health topics.

USA.gov for Seniors
USA.gov/topics/seniors.shtml

USA.gov is the portal to an enormous information network, providing links to millions of websites on a vast array of topics. USA.gov's senior page will generally lead you to reputable websites with information on every caregiving and senior issue, ranging from legal and financial issues to health and travel.

HEALTH AND MEDICINE

American Geriatrics Society
healthinaging.org

Established by the AGS Foundation for Health in Aging, this consumer-oriented website has health information for seniors on virtually every topic.

HealthFinder
healthfinder.gov

This website, created by the Department of Health and Human Services, is a portal to all sorts of basic health information.

Informed Patient Institute
informedpatientinstitute.org

The institute is an independent, non-profit group that reviews websites that

rate doctors, hospitals, and nursing homes, state-by-state. Before using any of these rating websites, check with IPI first.

Mayo Clinic
mayoclinic.com

Run by the Mayo Clinic in Rochester, Minnesota, this website has trustworthy information on symptoms and treatments for a variety of ailments.

Medline Plus
nlm.nih.gov/medlineplus

Run by the National Library of Medicine and the National Institutes of Health, this consumer website has detailed information on diseases, disorders, treatments, and prevention. (Read the basic information, then go to "Learn More" for in-depth information.)

National Center for Complementary and Alternative Medicine
nccam.nih.gov
888-644-6226

This branch of the National Institutes of Health offers scientific information on alternative and complementary medicine, as well as alerts and advisories.

National Institute on Aging
nia.nih.gov
800-222-2225

The NIA, a division of the National Institutes of Health, supports research on aging and health, and puts out loads of information on a variety of senior issues, including health topics.

National Organization for Rare Disorders

rarediseases.org
800-999-6673

This nonprofit clearinghouse makes referrals to national organizations for rare disorders, has programs to help people get medications, and has online communities that share information.

NIH Senior Health

nihseniorhealth.gov

Developed by the National Institute on Aging and the National Library of Medicine, this website is simple to navigate and has basic, easy-to-understand health information for older adults.

HEALTHY AGING

Restart Living

restartliving.org

Created by the National Council on Aging, the site helps seniors manage chronic health conditions, like diabetes or heart disease, and offers referrals to free self-management workshops.

SPRY Foundation

spry.org
301-656-3405

The SPRY (Setting Priorities for Retirement Years) Foundation is an independent, nonprofit research and educational organization that helps people prepare for successful aging. It focuses on physical wellness, mental health, financial security, and engagement in life.

HEARING AND SPEECH

American Tinnitus Association

ata.org
800-634-8978

The association makes referrals to local hearing specialists and self-help groups and has staff and volunteers who can answer individual questions. The website also has general information about tinnitus.

Association of Late-Deafened Adults

alda.org
815-332-1515 (voice/TTY)
866-402-2532

This membership organization provides general information, has an online "email discussion group," and provides referrals to local groups and programs.

Better Hearing Institute

betterhearing.org
800-327-9355

BHI works to erase the stigma associated with hearing loss, and provides information on various aspects of hearing loss.

Hear Now

starkeyhearingfoundation.org/programs/hear-now

The Starkey Hearing Foundation sponsors this program to provide hearing aids and cochlear implants, without charge, to low-income people.

Hearing Loss Association of America
hearingloss.org
301-657-2248

The group distributes information on hearing loss, including tips on coping and help for family members, and provides referrals to local support groups.

National Aphasia Association
aphasia.org
800-922-4622

The association provides information on aphasia (a disorder that interferes with a person's ability to use or comprehend words), and makes referrals to local support groups and services.

National Association of the Deaf
nad.org
301-587-1788

The NAD is a civil rights organization that advocates for deaf and hard-of-hearing people and their families. The website has information about legal rights and referrals to local groups.

NIDCD Information Clearinghouse
www.nidcd.nih.gov
800-241-1044

Part of the National Institutes of Health, the National Institute on Deafness and Other Communication Disorders runs this clearinghouse of information on disorders related to hearing, balance, smell, taste, speech, and language.

HEART DISEASE

American Heart Association
heart.org
800-242-8721

The association provides information on blood pressure, cholesterol, stroke, heart disease, diet, nutrition, exercise, and other topics, and also offers referrals to local CPR courses.

National Heart, Lung, and Blood Institute Information Center
www.nhlbi.nih.gov
301-592-8573

Part of the National Institutes of Health, the center has information on ailments of the heart, lungs, and blood.

HISPANIC SERVICES

National Association for Hispanic Elderly
anppm.org
626-564-1988

The association advocates for the Hispanic elderly, especially those living on low incomes. It has brochures and other information in Spanish and may be able to give referrals.

National Hispanic Council on Aging
nhcoa.org
202-347-9733

This organization educates and advocates for the aging Hispanic community.

HOME CARE AND COMMUNITY PROGRAMS

Alzheimer's Association
communityresourcefinder.org
800-272-3900 (24/7 helpline)

The Alzheimer's Association has put together a database of community programs and resources, from housing options and support groups to lawyers and day care programs.

Eldercare Locator
eldercare.gov
800-677-1116

Run by the U.S. Administration on Aging, this is a good place to start looking for local services. The helpline and website will lead you to the area agency on aging that oversees services in your parent's hometown.

National Adult Day Services Association
nadsa.org
877-745-1440

This website will lead you to adult day programs near your parent.

National Association for Home Care & Hospice
nahc.org
202-547-7424

This professional organization represents a wide range of home care organizations. Click the "Consumers" tab for information on consumer rights and selecting a home care agency, and for referrals to a local home care agency.

National PACE Association
pace4you.org
703-535-1565

Programs of All-inclusive Care for the Elderly (PACE) provide a broad menu of programs and services, from transportation to adult day services to home care, so that elderly people who are eligible for nursing home care can stay in their own homes instead. Only a few areas have PACE programs; they are listed on the website.

HOME MODIFICATION

(See "Accessibility and Home Modification.")

HOSPICE CARE

(See also "Death and End-of-Life Planning.")

Caring Connections
caringinfo.org
800-658-8898

Created by the National Hospice and Palliative Care Organization, this website provides information, referrals, and legal forms.

Hospice Foundation of America
hospicefoundation.org
800-854-3402

The foundation works to improve public policy concerning hospice care. It provides information on hospice, how to choose a hospice agency, and referrals to local hospice services.

HOUSING

(See also "Nursing Homes and Assisted Living.")

National Clearinghouse for Long-Term Care Information
longtermcare.gov
202-619-0724

This clearinghouse, established by the Department of Health and Human Services, has all sorts of information on long-term options, how to pay for LTC, and planning ahead.

National Shared Housing Resource Center
nationalsharedhousing.org

The center provides information about shared housing and referrals to local shared housing organizations.

Village to Village Network
vtvnetwork.org

Village to Village helps communities organize cooperatives in which residents help residents, allowing elderly people to stay in their own homes.

HUNTINGTON'S DISEASE

Huntington's Disease Society of America (HDSA)
hdsa.org
800-345-4372

This society publishes information about all aspects of Huntington's disease and offers referrals to clinics, nursing homes, neurologists, and local chapters that know of local support groups and services.

INCONTINENCE

International Foundation for Functional Gastrointestinal Disorders
aboutincontinence.org
888-964-2001

The foundation has brochures, articles, and other information on irritable bowel syndrome, constipation, diarrhea, fecal incontinence, and other disorders of the bowels.

National Association for Continence
nafc.org
800-252-3337

This organization offers information, a catalog of special products, and a national listing of doctors who specialize in incontinence.

National Kidney and Urologic Diseases Information Clearinghouse
kidney.niddk.nih.gov
800-891-5390

Sponsored by the National Institute of Diabetes and Digestive and Kidney Diseases, the clearinghouse provides up-to-date information on incontinence, as well as disorders and diseases of the kidneys, prostate, and urinary tract.

Simon Foundation for Continence
simonfoundation.org
800-237-4666

A consumer education organization, the foundation publishes books, videos, newsletters, and articles on incontinence.

Urology Care Foundation
urologyhealth.org
800-828-7866

The foundation, part of the American Urological Association, provides information on urinary tract infections, incontinence, diseases and disorders of the prostate and bladder, and other urinary tract and rectal disorders.

INSURANCE

(See "Medicare, Medicaid, and Other Insurance Issues.")

LEGAL ISSUES

American Bar Association
findlegalhelp.org

This ABA site provides a listing of state programs and referrals.

Elder Law Answers
elderlawanswers.com

Started by a Boston lawyer, this site has answers to a variety of legal issues facing the elderly and their families.

National Academy of Elder Law Attorneys
naela.org

This organization will refer you to elder law attorneys (who specialize in issues facing the elderly) in your area.

LONG-TERM CARE

(See also "Nursing Homes and Assisted Living" and "Home Care and Community Programs.")

Medicare.gov
http://longtermcare.gov/medicare-medicaid-more/medicare

This government website provides information on choosing and paying for long-term care.

National Clearinghouse for Long-Term Care
longtermcare.gov

Created by the U.S. Department of Health and Human Services, this website has information and referral services.

National Long-Term Care Ombudsman Resource Center
ltcombudsman.org

Ombudsmen advocate for residents (and their families) of nursing homes, assisted living centers, and other long-term care facilities. They can help you find a facility and resolve problems. The website provides information about long-term care and will direct you to a local ombudsman.

LUNG DISEASE

American Lung Association
lungusa.org
800-586-4872

The association provides information about lung diseases such as asthma, emphysema, tuberculosis, and cancer. It makes referrals for medical care, support groups, smoking cessation programs, and other local services.

National Heart, Lung, and Blood Institute
www.nhlbi.nih.gov
301-592-8573

Part of the National Institutes of Health, this center provides information about ailments of the heart, lungs, and blood.

MEDICARE, MEDICAID, AND OTHER INSURANCE ISSUES

AARP
aarp.org
888-687-2277

AARP has information about Medicare, Medigap, and managed care, among other things.

Center for Medicare Advocacy
medicareadvocacy.org
860-456-7790

This center offers advice and legal help to people struggling with Medicare bureaucracy. The website has information about Medicare, appeals, rights, and litigation.

Federal Long Term Care Insurance Program (FLTCIP)
ltcfeds.com
800-582-3337

This website offers information about the Federal Long Term Care Insurance Program (for federal and U.S. Postal Service employees, active and retired members of the uniformed services, and qualified relatives), downloadable applications, and a calculator that determines how much insurance will cost.

Healthcare.gov
healthcare.gov

This site, part of the U.S. Department of Health and Human Services, has information about insurance and a tool to help you find health insurance specific to your needs and state.

Medicaid.gov
medicaid.gov

This federal website has some very basic state-by-state Medicaid information, but most important, it will direct you to local Medicaid offices, which can help you navigate the system.

Medicare.gov
medicare.gov
800-633-4227

The hotline and website provides extensive information about Medicare, Medigap, and state insurance departments. They also have information on Medicare fraud and other illegal practices.

Medicare Rights Center
medicarerights.org
800-333-4114

This nonprofit organization offers information and free counseling services to people with questions, concerns, and problems regarding Medicare.

My Medicare Matters
mymedicarematters.org

Sponsored by the National Council on Aging, this website has information on Medicare, prescription drug coverage, and staying healthy.

National SHIP Resource Center
shiptalk.org

This national website will direct you to the State Health Insurance Assistance Program (SHIP), which provides one-on-one counseling to people on Medicare and their families.

MENTAL HEALTH

Depression and Bipolar Support Alliance
dbsalliance.org
800-826-3632

This organization offers information on mood disorders and referrals to support groups and local chapters.

Geriatric Mental Health Foundation
gmhfonline.org

The foundation has information on anxiety, phobias, and depression, as well as dementia, addiction, and caregiving. The website also provides referrals to geriatric psychiatrists.

International Foundation for Research and Education on Depression
ifred.org

iFred aims to get people into treatment, as so many people go untreated. The website has information on depression and treatments.

Mental Health America
nmha.org
800-969-6642

Formerly the National Mental Health Association, this group provides information on mental health issues and makes referrals to local organizations.

National Alliance for the Mentally Ill
nami.org
800-950-6264

NAMI provides information on mental illness and referrals to local groups and services.

National Institute of Mental Health
nimh.nih.gov
866-615-6464

NIMH is a federal research institute that provides information to the general public on a wide variety of issues through its website and information line.

National Suicide Prevention Lifeline
suicidepreventionlifeline.org
800-273-8255

If you are thinking about harming yourself, go to the nearest emergency room, call 911, or call this hotline to speak with a trained counselor.

NATIVE AMERICAN SERVICES

National Indian Council on Aging
nicoa.org
505-292-2001

Formed by tribal chairmen in 1976, the NICOA is a nonprofit advocacy group for American Indian and Alaska Native elders. The council offers general information, employment training, and job opportunities.

NURSING HOMES AND ASSISTED LIVING

Assisted Living Consumer Alliance
assistedlivingconsumers.org

The alliance works to protect the rights of residents of assisted living facilities, and has information on choosing a facility and, once in, working with staff.

Medicare's Nursing Home Compare
http://www.medicare.gov/nursinghome
compare/search.html
800-633-4227

This resource, run by the Center for Medicare and Medicare Services (the federal agency that runs the Medicare program), allows users to search for nursing homes across the nation and view quality measures, inspection results, and staff information, along with a star rating system.

National Consumer Voice for Quality Long-Term Care
theconsumervoice.org
202-332-2275

This coalition works to improve nursing homes and other long-term care settings. The website offers help selecting nursing homes and filing complaints, explains laws regulating nursing homes, and provides referrals to local ombudsman programs.

National Long-Term Care Ombudsman Resource Center
ltcombudsman.org
202-332-2275

Operated by the Consumer Voice (above), this website will direct you to a local ombudsman, who can help you find nursing homes, assisted living centers, and other long-term care facilities, apprise you of your rights, and help resolve conflicts within a facility.

NUTRITION AND MEAL SERVICES

Academy of Nutrition and Dietetics
eatright.org

This website offers information on nutrition and referrals to local dietitians.

Food and Nutrition Information Center
nal.usda.gov/fnic
301-504-5414

Part of the National Agricultural Library, this center is run by professional nutritionists and aims to distribute the most current information on food and nutrition. The website offers educational materials, government reports, and research papers.

National Meals on Wheels Association of America
mowaa.org
888-998-6325

The association makes referrals to local meal-delivery programs and congregate or group dining programs.

NutritionGov
nutrition.gov

This website provides access to the U.S. Department of Agriculture's online National Nutrient Database. Nutritional information is offered specifically to senior citizens.

Supplemental Nutrition Assistance Program
fns.usda.gov/snap
800-221-5689

This U.S. Department of Agriculture program, known as SNAP (once known as food stamps), provides financial help to people with very low incomes so that they can buy food.

OCCUPATIONAL THERAPY

(See also "Accessibility and Home Modification.")

American Occupational Therapy Association
aota.org/consumers
301-652-2682

This professional association has consumer information on topics such as making a home safe and accessible, preventing falls, and living with various disabilities.

OSTEOPOROSIS

(See "Arthritis and Osteoporosis.")

PARKINSON'S DISEASE

American Parkinson Disease Association
apdaparkinson.org
800-223-2732

The association provides information on Parkinson's disease and links to local chapters.

National Institute of Neurological Disorders and Stroke
ninds.nih.gov
800-352-9424

Part of the National Institutes of Health, this site provides information about stroke and other brain disorders, such as Parkinson's, Alzheimer's, and epilepsy. It reports on the latest scientific research and makes referrals to local clinical research centers.

National Parkinson Foundation
parkinson.org
800-327-4545

This foundation reports on all aspects of Parkinson's disease and makes referrals to local services and medical experts specializing in the disease.

Parkinson's Disease Foundation
pdf.org
800-457-6676

This organization sponsors research and professional education, educates the public about Parkinson's disease, and makes referrals to specialists.

SKIN

American Academy of Dermatology
aad.org

The academy has information on numerous skin diseases and refers people to dermatologists. Just click on "For the public."

National Institute of Arthritis and Musculoskeletal and Skin Diseases
niams.nih.gov
877-226-4267

Part of the National Institutes of Health, this organization provides information on many disorders and diseases affecting the skin.

SLEEP

American Sleep Apnea Association
sleepapnea.org
888-293-3650

The association website provides information, a "support forum," and referrals to support groups.

American Sleep Association
sleepassociation.org

This organization offers information on an array of sleep disorders.

National Sleep Foundation
sleepfoundation.org
703-243-1697

This foundation has information on sleep disorders and makes referrals to local sleep clinics.

Willis-Ekbom Disease Foundation
rls.org

Formerly the Restless Legs Syndrome Foundation, this group provides information on RLS and clinical trials, and it connects people through chat rooms, discussion boards, and support groups.

SMOKING CESSATION

Quit For Life
quitnow.net

Run by the American Cancer Society, this site will connect you with a "quit coach," and provides tips for quitting smoking.

Quit Tobacco
ucanquit2.org

This is an educational campaign for members of the U.S. military service and veterans.

Smokefree
smokefree.gov
800-784-8669 (QUIT NOW)

Run by the National Cancer Institute of the federal government, Smokefree has a step-by-step guide for quitting and counselors available by phone.

STROKE

American Stroke Association
strokeassociation.org
888-478-7653

ASA offers information on prevention, strokes, and life after a stroke, and referrals to local chapters and support groups.

National Aphasia Association
aphasia.org
800-922-4622

The association has information on aphasia and makes referrals to support groups and other associations.

National Institute of Neurological Disorders and Stroke
ninds.nih.gov
800-352-9424

The institute provides information on stroke and other brain disorders, such as Parkinson's, Alzheimer's, and epilepsy, and makes referrals to local clinical research centers.

National Stroke Association
stroke.org
800-787-6537

The association offers information on strokes and makes referrals to medical experts, support groups, rehabilitation centers, and other services.

VETERANS

Department of Veterans Affairs
va.gov
800-827-1000 (general)
877-222-8387 (health benefits)
800-273-8255 (crisis line)

Contact this office or visit the website for information about benefits and eligibility and for referrals to regional offices and VA medical centers.

VISION

American Foundation for the Blind
afb.org
800-232-5463

The foundation provides referrals to rehabilitation centers, state agencies, low-vision clinics, and other services, and has information on the emotional and practical aspects of coping with vision impairment and loss.

American Macular Degeneration Foundation
macular.org
888-622-8527

This foundation works for the prevention, treatment, and cure for macular degeneration, and offers information about the disease.

Blinded Veterans Association
bva.org
800-669-7079

The association helps veterans get VA benefits, rehabilitation, and other services.

Eye Smart
geteyesmart.org
415-447-0213

Created by the American Academy of Ophthalmology, this website provides information on eye diseases and makes referrals to ophthalmologists, some of whom offer low-cost eye care to people over 65.

Glaucoma Foundation
glaucomafoundation.org
212-285-0080

This foundation offers information about glaucoma and connects sufferers to support groups. Its newsletter, *Eye to Eye*, is available on the website free of charge.

Glaucoma Research Foundation
glaucoma.org
800-826-6693

The foundation provides information and referrals to local glaucoma specialists. Through its Glaucoma Support Network, it provides online chat groups and support.

Lighthouse International Center for Vision and Aging
lighthouse.org
800-829-0500

Contact the Lighthouse for information on every aspect of vision loss and eye disease, as well as for referrals to state agencies, local services, support groups, and low-vision centers.

Macula.org
macula.org
212-605-3719

The website is a collaboration of the Association for Macular Diseases and other groups. It offers emotional support, information, and referrals.

Macular Degeneration Foundation
eyesight.org
888-633-3937

This foundation's website offers the latest news and clinical trials on macular degeneration.

National Eye Institute
nei.nih.gov
301-496-5248

The Institute, which supports research projects, has information on eye disease and the latest research and treatments.

National Federation of the Blind
nfb.org
410-659-9314

The federation runs a number of programs for the blind, provides information on blindness (including medical, social, emotional, legal, and financial issues), and makes referrals to services and support groups.

National Library Service for the Blind and Physically Handicapped
loc.gov/nls
888-657-7323

The library lends out audiobooks and books in Braille (as well as equipment for playing tapes and CDs) to people with vision loss. All of this is free.

Optometry Cares
aoafoundation.org
800-766-4466

The American Optometric Association's VISION USA program provides free eye care to uninsured, low-income people and their families.

VOLUNTEERING, WORKING, AND LEARNING

AARP
aarp.org
888-687-2277

AARP has a lot of information on working and volunteering, and a number of programs to help. For instance, the AARP Foundation Worksearch Information Network (aarpworksearch .org) has tools to help older people find a job. Experience Corps (http://www.aarp .org/experience-corps) gets older adults into classrooms, teaching young children reading and other skills.

ExperienceWorks
experienceworks.org
866-397-9757

This organization offers training and employment programs to low-income, unemployed people over age 55.

Points of Light Foundation
pointsoflight.org
800-865-8683

The foundation can refer you to volunteer centers in your parent's area.

Road Scholar
roadscholar.org
800-454-5768

Road Scholar, formerly known as Elderhostel, offers an array of educational and travel packages to people 55 and older, including those with disabilities.

Senior Corps Corporation for National and Community Service
seniorcorps.org
800-942-2677, press 4

This service runs federal volunteer programs, including the Foster Grandparent Program, the Senior Companion Program, and the Retired Senior Volunteer Program (RSVP).

Senior Job Bank
seniorjobbank.org

This nonprofit referral system helps bring together seniors wishing to work with possible employers or those searching for volunteers.

SeniorNet
seniornet.org

SeniorNet educates adults over 50 about computers and the Internet through online courses and tutorials and through their learning centers.

Service Corps of Retired Executives (SCORE)
score.org
800-634-0245

Through SCORE, retired and working volunteers provide free counseling to small business owners.

Volunteers of America
voa.org
800-899-0089

The national office can link you to one of its local volunteer programs.

WOMEN'S HEALTH AND SERVICES

OWL
owl-national.org
202-567-2606

OWL, which started as the Older Women's League, advocates for economic and social equality of midlife and elderly women. It offers information on issues such as women's health care and economic security, and provides some referrals.

Womenshealth.gov
womenshealth.gov
800-994-9662

This website, run by the Department of Health and Human Services, is dedicated to all aspects of women's health.

Caregiver's Organizer

The following pages are meant to help you gather important information and organize your time so you can care for your parent efficiently and smoothly. They are merely guidelines; adapt them to suit your needs. You can copy or remove these pages, or if you'd rather have electronic copies, go to **careforagingparents.com**.

If a number of people are involved in your parent's care, you might want to put copies of some of these pages into a storage service, such as Dropbox or Evernote, so you and others can access them from anywhere, and update them regularly. The pages provided here are:

- Key Information
- Emergency Identification Cards
- Emergency Medical Information
- Medications List
- Weekly Medications Chart
- Medical Contacts
- Medical Log
- Home Safety Checklist

- Community Services
- Employment Agreement
- Caregiver Contacts
- Daily Log
- Family Caregiver Contract
- Financial/Legal Contacts
- Financial Planner
- Monthly Budget
- End-of-Life Wishes

Key Information

Parent's Full Name _____

Address _____

Phone _____ Cell _____

Date of birth _____ Place of birth _____

Social Security number _____ Passport number _____

Driver's license number _____

Medicare number _____ Medicaid number _____

Military ID_____

Emergency Contacts _____

Religious affiliation/Place of worship _____

Name of clergy person_____ Phone _____

LOCATE THE FOLLOWING:

☐ Certificates of birth, marriage, divorce/separation, citizenship

☐ Will and any codicils (amendments) to the will

☐ Durable power of attorney

☐ Living will and power of attorney for health care

☐ DNR or other medical orders

☐ Insurance policies (life, health, home, etc.)

☐ Keys to house, office, safe-deposit box, post office box, etc.

☐ Combinations to any safe or lock

☐ List of recent employers, dates of employment, terms of employment

☐ Contracts or rental agreements

☐ Titles to real estate, cars, boats, and other vehicles

☐ Jewelry and other valuables

☐ Charge, debit, and banking cards

☐ Check registers, savings passbook

☐ Internet passwords, access codes, PINs

☐ Appraisals of personal property

☐ Copies of federal and state tax returns from the past three to five years

☐ Receipts from property taxes and other large recent payments

☐ Instructions on how to care for a pet, plants, house, or dependent

☐ Burial/cremation and funeral instructions, if any

NOTE: Keep sensitive information (such as Social Security number and passwords) private.

Emergency Identification Cards
(FRONT)

For your parent's wallet:

EMERGENCY MEDICAL ID

NAME: DOB:
ADDRESS:
CITY: STATE:

EMERGENCY CONTACTS:

NAME	PHONE	PHONE
_____	_____	_____
_____	_____	_____
PHYSICIAN	PHONE	PHONE
_____	_____	_____

For yours:

(It's best not to list your parent's name and address here because if your wallet is stolen, you don't want to alert the wrong people that your parent is alone and vulnerable. Instead, list emergency contacts who can then check on your parent.)

IN CASE OF EMERGENCY

I AM THE CAREGIVER OF A DISABLED PERSON.

MY NAME IS:

_____

If I am injured or otherwise detained, please contact
the alternate caregivers listed on the back of this card.

Emergency Identification Cards
(BACK)

For your parent's wallet:

EMERGENCY MEDICAL ID

Medical Conditions: _____

Allergies:_____

Medication: _____

Medication: _____

Medication: _____

Medication: _____

For yours:

IN CASE OF EMERGENCY

NAME	PHONE	PHONE
_____	_____	_____
_____	_____	_____
_____	_____	_____
_____	_____	_____
_____	_____	_____

Emergency Medical Information

Fill this out and place it in a clear plastic bag with a copy of your parent's medications list (see page 640), advance directives, and any medical orders. If more than one elderly person resides in the house, include a photo. Tape the bag to the refrigerator door (or inside of the front door), with "EMERGENCY MEDICAL INFORMATION" clearly visible. Update the information regularly.

Name _____ Nickname _____

Address _____

Phone _____ Cell _____

Date of birth _____ Gender M/F _____ Primary language _____

Primary insurance provider _____ Policy number _____

Secondary insurance provider _____ Policy number _____

Do you have a living will?   Y/N   Health care proxy?   Y/ N

Health care agent: _____ Phone: _____

EMERGENCY CONTACTS:

Name	Cell phone	Home phone	Work phone
_____	_____	_____	_____
_____	_____	_____	_____
_____	_____	_____	_____

Primary physician _____ Phone _____

Secondary physician _____ Phone _____

Preferred hospital _____ Phone _____

MEDICAL CONDITIONS /DISABILITIES:

_____
_____
_____

Allergies _____

Past surgeries (TYPE/ DATE) _____

Height _____ Weight _____ Blood Type _____

Needs: ❏ Glasses ❏ Dentures ❏ Hearing aid ❏ Oxygen ❏ Cane/Walker

Medications List

Keep track of all your parent's medications (including over-the-counter drugs and supplements). Update this list any time prescriptions change.

DRUG (brand and generic) DESCRIPTION (ex.: white, oval)	START / END DATES	PURPOSE	DOSE / INSTRUCTIONS (ex.: 10 mg, 3x/day, with food)	PRESCRIBING DOCTOR / PHONE

Weekly Medications Chart

When multiple medications and/or multiple caregivers are involved, it's wise to have people check off when each pill is taken so there are no mix-ups.

Drug: Dose: Instructions:	TIME	SUN	MON	TUES	WED	THU	FRI	SAT

Drug: Dose: Instructions:	TIME	SUN	MON	TUES	WED	THU	FRI	SAT

Drug: Dose: Instructions:	TIME	SUN	MON	TUES	WED	THU	FRI	SAT

Drug: Dose: Instructions:	TIME	SUN	MON	TUES	WED	THU	FRI	SAT

Drug: Dose: Instructions:	TIME	SUN	MON	TUES	WED	THU	FRI	SAT

Drug: Dose: Instructions:	TIME	SUN	MON	TUES	WED	THU	FRI	SAT

Drug: Dose: Instructions:	TIME	SUN	MON	TUES	WED	THU	FRI	SAT

Drug: Dose: Instructions:	TIME	SUN	MON	TUES	WED	THU	FRI	SAT

Medical Contacts

PRIMARY PHYSICIAN _____

address _____ email _____

phone_____ second phone_____

PHYSICIAN _____

address _____ email _____

phone_____ second phone_____

PHYSICIAN _____

address _____ email _____

phone_____ second phone_____

DENTIST _____

address _____ email _____

phone_____ second phone_____

PHYSICAL / OCCUPATIONAL THERAPIST _____

address _____ email _____

phone_____ second phone_____

PHARMACY _____

address_____

phone _____

HOSPITAL _____

address_____

phone _____

OTHER _____

address _____

phone _____

Medical Log

Keep a log of ailments, symptoms, appointments, test results, and other medical information that you can refer to as your parent's health and medical needs change.

DATE	SYMPTOM / ISSUE	CLINIC / DOCTOR SEEN	NOTES/TESTS / PROCEDURES	INSTRUCTIONS

Home Safety Checklist

- ❏ Program the phone with 911 on speed dial. Be sure it's clearly marked.
- ❏ Post emergency information by the phone or on the refrigerator (whom to call in case of emergency, house street address and cross street, medical information).
- ❏ Lock up or clearly label harsh cleaning agents, insecticides, chemicals, etc.
- ❏ Lock up firearms.
- ❏ Check that smoke and carbon monoxide detectors work.
- ❏ Purchase a backup generator for use in case of a power outage.
- ❏ Store a flashlight by the bed.
- ❏ Set the hot water heater to 120°F (as elderly people are easily scalded).
- ❏ Mark hot and cold taps clearly.
- ❏ Remove or tack down loose rugs (remove throw rugs).
- ❏ Clear pathways of clutter, small furniture, electrical cords, etc.
- ❏ Install handrails along stairs and hallways (one on each side of a stairwell).
- ❏ Install grab bars in the bathroom, but also near the closet or bed, if needed.
- ❏ Fix loose floorboards and remove thresholds at doorways.
- ❏ Get rid of wobbly chairs, three-legged tables, or other unstable furniture.
- ❏ Use nonslip treads and/or mark the edges of steps with bright tape.
- ❏ Check that lighting is adequately bright and evenly distributed.
- ❏ Be sure light switches are easy to locate and use.
- ❏ Reduce glare by aiming lights at walls or ceilings.
- ❏ Use night-lights along any path your parent might use at night.
- ❏ Switch to lever-style handles (which are easier to use).
- ❏ Consider a raised toilet seat.
- ❏ Use rubber mats and nonslip strips on floors that might be wet (in the bathroom and kitchen).
- ❏ Place items your parent uses frequently on shelves that are easily reached.
- ❏ Clearly mark stove dials, epecially the OFF position, with red tape or nail polish.
- ❏ Note food expiration dates and review basic food safety tips.
- ❏ Be sure all medications are clearly labeled so your parent can easily read them.
- ❏ Dispose of medications that are no longer needed.

Community Services

To find services in your parent's community, contact the area agency on aging, which you can find through the Eldercare Locator (eldercare.gov or 800-677-1116).

	PHONE / WEBSITE	CONTACT PERSON	NOTES
Area Agency on Aging			
Senior Center			
Adult Day Services			
Transportation Services			
Meal Programs			
Chores / Home Repair			
Companions / Visitors			
Home Care Agency			
Phone Reassurance			
Geriatric Care Manager			
Hospice			

Employment Agreement

This agreement between _____ (employer) and

_____(employee) _____ (address)

_____(phone) _____ (email)

is effective starting on _____ (date). The employee agrees

to care for _____ (the client) during the following days and

hours: _____

The client has the following limitations and needs: _____

_____

_____

_____

_____

_____

_____

Services to be provided by the employee include, but are not limited to:_____

_____

_____

_____

_____

_____

The employer will pay $_____ /_____ (hour/day/week) for these services.

   The employee understands that despite any physical or mental limitations, this client deserves to be treated with respect, dignity, and compassion. The client should retain as much autonomy as possible. The employee must not take advantage of or coerce the client in any way.
   Changes in the terms of employment must be arranged with the employer in advance. The employee promises to discuss any concerns, problems, changes in symptoms, or mishaps with the employer as soon as they arise. The employee will keep a log and receipts of any approved expenses.
   Likewise, the employer understands that the employee deserves respect, privacy, patience, and compassion. The employer also agrees to discuss any concerns with the employee as they arise.

Signed this day by:

_____(employee) _____ (date)

_____(employer) _____ (date)

Caregiver Contacts

When siblings, therapists, aides, and companions are all providing care, it helps to keep a master list of who's who.

NAME/TITLE	PHONE	EMAIL AND / OR ADDRESS
	(c)_____ (h)_____ (w)_____	
	(c)_____ (h)_____ (w)_____	
	(c)_____ (h)_____ (w)_____	
	(c)_____ (h)_____ (w)_____	
	(c)_____ (h)_____ (w)_____	
	(c)_____ (h)_____ (w)_____	
	(c)_____ (h)_____ (w)_____	
	(c)_____ (h)_____ (w)_____	
	(c)_____ (h)_____ (w)_____	

Daily Log

When multiple caregivers are involved, you may want to keep a log of who's doing what. Circle or highlight the boxes to indicate what needs to be done on each day, and then ask caregivers to check off each item when it's done. Here's an example:

	SUN	MON	TUES	WED	THU	FRI	SAT
Shower							
Shampoo							
Oral care							
Nail care							
Shave							
Get dressed							
Breakfast							
Toileting							
Morning meds							
Wound care							
Skin care							
Laundry							
Clean kitchen							
Change linens							
Vacuum/Dust							
Lunch							
Afternoon meds							
Emails/Calls							
Groceries							
Exercises							
Dinner							
Dress for bed							
Night meds							
Other							

Family Caregiver Contract

When one family member does most of the caregiving, compensation for the work can ease family tensions and reduce stress on the primary caregiver. However, the details need to be carefully ironed out. It's wise to consult an attorney when drafting such a document, because taxes and Medicaid eligibility can be affected. This provides a starting point as you write your own agreement:

This agreement between _____ (caregiver) and

_____

_____(family members)
is effective starting on _____ (date).

The caregiver agrees to care for _____ (parent's name) during

the following days and hours: _____

The duties will include, but are not limited to [be as specific as possible]:

_____

_____

_____

_____

As compensation, the caregiver will receive _____
[This might be a weekly fee comensurate to what local home care agencies charge, a lump sum, or some other compensation, such as free rent or proceeds from a life insurance policy.
Note: Compensation is considered income and is subject to taxes.]
The caregiver will get vacation and personal days as follows:_____

_____.

When a sibling steps in to provide respite, he or she will not be paid, as assisting temporarily is a filial duty and not a full-time arrangement. If the caregiver is sick, the backup plan is _____

_____.

We, the other siblings and family members, understand that compensation is the right thing to do and we fully support it. We bear no grudges or reluctance in endorsing this agreement. We will continue to help our parent and the primary caregiver in any way we can.

Signed by:

_____ (date)_____

_____ (date)_____

_____ (date)_____

_____ (date)_____

Financial/Legal Contacts

Account information and passwords are extremely private, so store this in a safe place.

PRIMARY BANK _____

contact _____ phone _____

account #/description _____

website _____ login/password _____

SECONDARY BANK _____

contact _____ phone _____

account #/description_____

website _____ login/password _____

ACCOUNTANT_____

firm _____ phone _____

email _____

LAWYER _____

firm _____ phone _____

email _____

FINANCIAL ADVISOR _____

firm _____ phone _____

email _____

INSURANCE AGENT _____

firm _____ phone _____

email _____

Financial Planner

If you are (or one day might be) helping with your parent's finances, you will need a list of assets and liabilities. Gather records, contracts, bills, agreements, trusts, account numbers, and so forth, or know where that information is kept. Update these records as needed.

ASSETS	ACCOUNT #	BALANCE
Savings account	_____	_____
Checking account	_____	_____
Investment account	_____	_____
Other securities/funds	_____	_____
Retirement accounts (IRA, 401k)	_____	_____

	DESCRIPTION	VALUE
Real estate	_____	_____
Cars, boats, and other vehicles	_____	_____
Valuables (jewelry, paintings, etc.)	_____	_____
Business and partnership agreements	_____	_____
Profit-sharing and pension plans	_____	_____
Annuities	_____	_____
Life insurance	_____	_____
Other	_____	_____

DEBTS	DESCRIPTION	AMOUNT
Mortgage	_____	_____
Car loan	_____	_____
Other outstanding loans	_____	_____
Credit card debt	_____	_____
Other	_____	_____

ESTIMATED FUTURE EXPENSES	COST
Home renovations (to make it more accessible)	_____
Assisted living devices (automatic door openers, stair lift, hearing/vision aids, walkers, etc.)	_____
Medical bills, copays	_____
Home health care	_____
Assisted living and/or nursing home	_____
Legal/financial fees	_____
Funeral expenses	_____

Monthly Budget

If you are helping your parent create a budget, make a list of all income and expenses, so you know where the money is going and what can be trimmed if necessary.

MONTHLY INCOME

Salary/Wages _____

Other business income _____

Retirement benefits (pension, IRA, Keogh, etc.) _____

Social Security _____

Dividends _____

Interest (from investments) _____

Rental income _____

SSI, food stamps, or other entitlements _____

Other _____

MONTHLY BILLS

Mortgage/Rent _____

Taxes _____

Utilities

   (Gas/Electric/Oil/Phone/Cable/TV/Water) _____

Insurance premiums

   (Home/Car/Health/Life/Disability/Long-term care) _____

Food _____

Transportation

   Car payments/garage fees/gas and upkeep _____

   Public transportation _____

Clothing _____

Medical

   (medications, copays, etc.) _____

Home and yard upkeep _____

Interest payments

   (credit cards, outstanding loans) _____

Hobbies and pastimes _____

Pet care _____

Entertainment _____

Gifts/Donations _____

Other _____

_____

End-of-Life Wishes

Your parent needs advance directives (a living will and health care proxy) that are particular to his state. It's essential that he also discuss his views at length because the issues that arise are extremely complicated. Here's a starting point for these conversations:

YOUR PROXY

- Who will make medical decisions on your behalf if you cannot make them yourself?
- Will this person be able to confer with doctors and make hard choices at an emotional time?
- Who, beyond your doctors and your proxy, should be consulted?
- Do family members know and accept that your proxy will be making decisions?

IMMEDIATE GOALS

- What are your goals at this point in your life?
- Is there anything left undone or unsaid?
- If there is something you want to accomplish or do, can that happen now?

GENERAL VIEWS

- What do you fear about illness and death?
- What disability or situation do you think would be intolerable?
- How do your religious or personal beliefs affect your views on the end of life?
- How would you describe a "good" death?
- How important is it to you where you die (e.g., at home or in a hospital)?

MEDICAL DECISIONS

- How direct should your doctor be with you? Do you want to know everything?
- What should be the goal of treatment? More time? Comfort? Mobility? Lucidity?
- How might those goals change if you were extremely ill and in pain?
- How aggressively should doctors act to keep you alive?
- If you were extremely ill and the prognosis bleak, would you want:

Hospitalization _____ Artificial hydration _____

Surgery _____ Resuscitation _____

Artificial nutrition _____ Ventilator _____

- Do you have/want medical orders (such as a DNR or POLST) that protect you from any of the above?

COMFORT

- What do you think of hospice care and would you like that for yourself?
- Would you like to talk with a hospice provider to learn more about it?
- What might bring you comfort if you were at the end of life? For example:

Music _____ Visitors _____

Massage/touch _____ People talking _____

Prayer, stories, or music _____ Silence _____

A particular pet_____ Solitude _____

Index

A

Abuse, 39–40, 50, 175, 325–36, 380, 448–49, 490
Accessibility, 128, 610. *See also* Home, modification of
Accessory dwelling units (ADUs), 398, 399–400, 408–9
Accountants, 322
Accusations, 515–16
Acid reflux, 253–54
Activities of daily living (ADL), definition of, 163. *See also* Bathing and grooming; Dressing; Food and eating
Activities/staying active, 104–8
Acupuncture, 95, 193, 267
Adaptability, 601–2
Addiction, 39–40
Adult day services/adult day care, 106, 155–56, 168, 610. *See also* Senior centers
Adult Protective Services, 27
Advance directives
discussion of, 367–71
doctors' copies of, 188–89
following parent's wishes and, 280, 526–28
forms for, 361
health care proxies, 10, 188–89, 280, 368, 587
living wills, 10, 280, 367–68, 526, 587
see also End-of-life care
Advocate, acting as, 188–192, 440–43
Aerobic exercise, 84–85
African American services, 611
Agencies on aging, 14–15, 29, 39, 157

Age-related macular degeneration (AMD), 206–7
Aggression, 474, 518–19
Aging
acceptance of, 602–3
general resources on, 619–20
healthy, 82–95, 621
Agitation, 512–13
Aides, 160–61, 162–63, 165
Alarm systems, 119, 213, 514. *See also* Monitors and alert systems
Alcohol
delirium and, 268
dementia and, 459, 471
depression and, 265
falls and, 125
grief and, 570
heartburn and, 254
incontinence and, 245
memory loss and, 457
osteoporosis and, 235
overview of, 92–94
services for, 611
sleep and, 218, 220
ulcers and, 255
weight and, 134
Alcoholism, 92–94, 134, 459, 594, 611
Alert systems. *See* Monitors and alert systems
Alternative medicine, 192–95, 267
Alzheimer's disease, 243, 261, 458, 465–68, 482, 611–12. *See also* Dementia
Ambulances, 546
Anemia, 235, 256–57
Anger
of caregiver, 34–35, 48–50, 573
dementia and, 489–490
grief and, 569
of parent, 26, 538

Antacids, 254, 255
Antiaging miracles, 598
Anticholinergic drugs, 200, 456
Antidepressants, 265–66, 268, 271,
    474, 475
Antipsychotic medications, 474, 475
Anxiety, 83, 194–95, 457, 474
Anxiety disorders, 261, 269–71
Apartments
    accessory, 398, 399–400
    senior, 406, 408–9
Apathy, 474
Appetite loss, 134, 136. See also Diet; Food
    and eating
Arbitration, 431
Art/art therapy, 105, 485
Arthritis, 85, 89–90, 140, 238–41, 261, 612
Asian services, 613
Assessing the situation, 2, 28–29
Asset protection, 109, 310–11, 334,
    336, 338, 354–55, 358, 372. See also
    Financial issues; Medicaid; Trusts
Assisted living, 408–9, 410–12, 613, 628.
    See also Nursing homes
Assistive devices, 144–46, 212–13, 239, 510
Audiobooks, 105, 106, 208, 287, 480, 508
Audiologists, 214
Autopsy, 556

B

Bad breath, 231
Balance, exercise and, 84–85, 86
Banks
    gathering information from, 14
    joint accounts at, 306, 377
    see also Financial issues
Bathing and grooming, 130–31, 495–99
Bathrooms, 128
Bedpans/commodes, 128, 245–46, 501
Beds, 127, 130
Bedsores, 226, 293–94
Behavioral changes, 479, 480, 516–17.
    See also Personality changes
Benefits, accelerated, 357
Benefits and discounts, 153, 303, 308,
    314–17, 349

Bills
    automatic payments for, 307
    from hospitals, 299. See also Financial
        issues
Biofeedback, 245, 248–49, 267
Biologic response modifiers, 240
Bladder training, 244. See also Incontinence
Blindness, hypertension and, 220. See also
    Vision problems
Blood pressure
    Alzheimer's disease and, 468
    dementia and, 468
    exercise and, 85
    memory loss and, 457
    peripheral artery disease (PAD) and, 230
    sleep apnea and, 220
Body manipulation, 193–94
Bones and joints
    arthritis, 238–41
    bone density tests, 235
    exercise and, 84
    osteoarthritis, 84, 235, 238
    osteoporosis, 83, 85, 89–90, 234–38,
        254, 612
Boundaries. See Limits, establishing
Bowel function
    dehydration and, 224
    exercise and, 84
    fecal incontinence, 247–49
    obstruction and, 251–52
Brain
    exercising, 599
    mild cognitive impairment (MCI) and,
        456–58
    normal aging of, 455–56
Brain death, 536
Breathing exercises, 267
Brokers, 323
Bruising, 228
Budget, monthly, form, 652
Burials, 557–59, 561, 602
Bypass trusts, 374–75

C

Caffeine, 216, 218, 219, 225, 245, 254, 255
Calcium, 234, 235, 236–37

Cancer
anemia and, 257
constipation and, 250
depression and, 261
diarrhea and, 252
dysphagia and, 137, 252
estrogen therapy and, 237
exercise and, 83, 596
incontinence and, 247
oral, 231, 232
resources on, 95, 191, 613
skin, 227
swallowing problems and, 252
tobacco use and, 95
ulcers and, 254
weight and, 90, 134
Carbon monoxide detectors, 118
Cardiopulmonary resuscitation (CPR), 11, 527
Cardiovascular disease. See Heart disease
Careers and caregiving, 78–80
Caregiver Action Network, 54
Caregiver websites, 18, 613, 614
Caregivers
as advocates, 188–92, 440–43
careers and, 78–80
caring for, 41–59
compensation for, 44, 66–69, 310, 391, 392
contact information for, 647
contract for, 646, 649
coordination resources for, 614–15
coping with dementia and, 485–492
depression and, 264, 571
grief of, 572–75
hiring, 166–69
interviewing, 169–70
live-in, 161
medications and, 202–3
planning and, 44–45
primary, 62–64
reimbursement for, 308–9
secondary, 64–65
sleeplessness and, 221
support services for, 613–14
use of personal funds by, 308–10
See also Self-care, for caregiver
Cars, 139–44
Caskets, 557–58
Cataracts, 141, 204–5
Catheters, 246–47, 294, 501

CCRCs (continuing care retirement communities), 403, 405, 408–9, 412–14
Cell phones, 121. See also Telephones
Cellulitis, 228
Cemeteries, 559, 560–61
Centers for Disease Control and Prevention, 14
Central sleep apnea, 220
Charitable remainder trust, 376
Children
aging without, 596
explaining dementia to, 514
funerals and, 560
grief and, 579–81
making time for, 75–77
visits and, 288, 439
working with, 104
Chiropractic medicine, 193–94
Choking, 253
Cholesterol, 468
Cholinesterase inhibitors, 473, 475
Chondroitin sulfate, 241
Chore services, 151–52
Chronic inflammation, anemia and, 257
Cigarettes. See Tobacco use
Circadian rhythm, cataracts and, 204–5
Citizen advocacy groups, 422–23, 446
Clothing, 132–33, 499–500
Cochlear implants, 215–16
Cognitive behavioral therapy (CBT), 273
Cognitive training, 142
Colostomy, 249
Comas, 535–36
Comfort Only orders, 546
Commodes, 128, 245–46, 501
Communication
about death and dying, 10–11, 368–70, 526–27, 539–540
about medical care, 9, 10–11, 368–70
with bosses, 80
with children, 75–77
dementia and, 469, 505–6
difficulties with, 439
with doctors, 526, 532–33
end-of-life care and, 368–70, 526–27
at family meetings, 71–72
during final moments, 550
financial issues and, 8–9, 303–5
fraud and, 334–35
guidelines for, 5–8

importance of, 4, 585
in-home aides and, 174
Internet and, 99–100
parent's denial and, 11–12
with siblings, 63
with spouses, 72–74
Community groups, 15
Community services
adult day services, 155–56, 168
chore services, 151–52
companions and homemakers, 151
finding, 14–16, 157, 308
form for recording, 645
free and discounted, 153
meal programs. *see* Meal programs
resistance to, 154
resources on, 157, 623
senior centers, 153–55
telephone calls and visitors,
150–51
transportation services, 153
Community Spouse Resource Allowance
(CSRA), 356
Companions, 151, 160–61, 165, 290
Compensation for caregivers, 66–69, 309,
310, 391, 392
Competency issues, 28, 378–81
Complaints
dealing with, 37–39
funeral homes and, 553–54
Complementary and alternative medicine
(CAM), 192–95, 267
Computers, 99–100, 106
Conflicts, resolving, 29, 32
Confusion, 141, 456, 459
Congregate housing, 404–5, 408–9
Congregate meals, 137, 152
Conservators. *See* Guardians/guardianship
Constipation, 91, 242, 247, 248, 249–52
Contingency plans, 16
Continuing care retirement communities
(CCRCs), 403, 405, 408–9, 412–14
Contracts, 68, 646, 649
Conversations with parent, 4–12. *See also*
Communication
Cooking, 129, 135–36, 503–4. *See also*
Food and eating
Corns, 230
Corticosteroids, 240
Cortisol, 218
Counseling, 266, 288

CPR (cardiopulmonary resuscitation),
11, 527
Creativity, 105, 265
Credit cards, 311, 331
Cremation, 556–57
Crime precautions, 119
Criticism, dealing with, 37–39
CT scans, 465
Culture change, 420

D

Daily living
assistive devices for, 144–46
bathing and grooming, 130–31, 495–99
conversations about, 8
dressing, 132–33, 499–500
driving, 139–44, 204, 508–9, 616
food, 133–39
home modifications and, 125–130, 148,
387, 391, 544, 610
monitors and alert systems, 120–23
safety concerns, 115–19
see also Falls
Daily log, 648
Daily money manager, 299
Dating, 108–9
Death and dying
actions required after, 561–66
care during, 540–42
communication about, 10–11, 368–70,
526–27, 539–40
description of, 548–51
five stages of, 537–39
handling the body, 556–57
home care and, 543–44
in the hospital, 547–48
parent's perspective on, 536–39
planning ahead for, 10–11, 368–70,
525–36
planning resources for, 615
thoughts of, 49
Death certificates, 562
Death rattle, 549
Dehydration, 223–24, 242, 243, 252, 268,
272, 457, 535
Delegating chores, 45

Delirium, 224, 261, 268–69, 272, 276,
    290–92, 471, 511
Delusions, 272, 519–20
Dementia
    anxiety disorders and, 270
    bathing and, 495–98
    brain exercise and, 599–600
    causes of, 458–59
    communication and, 505–6
    complicating factors for, 471
    day-to-day management of,
        493–521
    dealing with diagnosis of, 469–72
    delusions and, 272
    depression and, 261, 263
    dressing and, 498–500
    driving and, 140, 508–9
    dysphagia and, 252
    eating and, 501–4
    exercise and, 83
    grooming and, 499
    helping parent with, 478–85
    identification card and, 118
    incontinence and, 242, 247, 500–501
    late-stage, 520–21
    living with, 477–92
    mail and, 510
    medications and, 456, 473–76, 509
    money and, 509–10
    nursing homes and, 416, 427
    oral hygiene and, 498–99
    planning ahead and, 471–72
    problem behaviors and, 511–17
    psychotic symptoms and, 518–20
    resources on, 611–12
    restraints and, 446–47
    safety checklist for, 494–95
    sex and, 110
    signs of, 38, 102
    sleeplessness and, 216, 218, 507–8
    supervision and, 483
    support groups for, 482
    symptoms of, 261, 459–61
    telephones and, 510
    temperature regulation and, 223
    testing for, 462–65
    time sense and, 506–7
    treating, 472–76
    types of, 458–59, 468–69
    visits and, 441
    weight and, 90

Denial, 11–12, 538, 540
Dental problems, 231–32, 615–16.
    See also Oral hygiene
Dentures, 137, 231
Department of Veterans Affairs, 14
Depression
    caregivers and, 264, 488, 571
    cataracts and, 205
    delusions and, 272
    dementia and, 263, 471, 474, 511
    discussing, 263–64
    driving and, 140
    end-of-life care and, 538
    exercise and, 83, 85
    grief and, 262–63, 571
    medications for, 474
    memory loss and, 457
    nursing homes and, 441
    overview of, 260–62
    pets and, 107
    precursors of, 259
    resources on, 627
    signs of, 38, 52, 102
    sleep problems and, 216, 220
    symptoms of, 261, 265
    tinnitus and, 212
    treating, 264–67
    weight and, 90, 134
Detaching, 545
Diabetes, 83–84, 89–90, 207, 223, 230, 235,
    243, 250, 257–58, 468, 616
Diabetic retinopathy, 207
Diapers, 246, 249, 501
Diarrhea, 247, 248, 252
Diet
    constipation and, 250
    dementia and, 599
    depression and, 265
    guidelines for, 88–92
    importance of, 598
    incontinence and, 245, 248
    see also Cooking; Food and eating
Dietary supplements, 192–93
Dietician/nutritionist, 90, 163
Digestive disorders, 252–56, 616.
    See also Constipation; Incontinence
Dignity, 25, 288–89, 442, 482–83, 541
Disability products, 144–46
Discharge planners, 15, 167, 278–79, 290,
    297–98, 419
Discounts. See Benefits and discounts

Disease-modifying anti-rheumatic drugs
    (DMARDs), 240
Disgust, 50–51
Disorientation, 459
Disputes, resolving, 296–97
Diverticular disease, 255
Dizziness, 141, 209, 237
Do Not Resuscitate (DNR) order, 10, 280,
    370, 527–28, 546
Doctors
    communication with, 526, 532–33
    finding, 182–84
    information gathering for, 184
Documents
    checklist for, 12–13
    crucial, 10
    gathering, 13–14
    see also Advance directives
Donut hole, 348
Double effect, 535
Dressing, 132–33, 499–500
Drinking. See Alcohol
Driving, 139–44, 204, 508–9, 616
Drug abuse, 611
Dry mouth, 197, 232, 252
Durable power of attorney, 10, 12, 306,
    363–67, 376, 379, 587
Dyspepsia, 254
Dysphagia, 137–38, 252–53

E

Eating. See Food and eating
Elder Cottage Housing Opportunity
    (ECHO) homes, 399–400, 408–9
Elder law attorneys, 323, 355, 382
Eldercare Locator, 15, 17
Electrical outlets, 129
Electroconvulsive therapy (ECT),
    266–67
Electronic health or medical record
    (EHR), 188
Embalming, 556–57
Emergencies
    call buttons, 121
    identification cards for, 637–38
    information for, 173

    living far away and, 19–20
    medical information for, 639
    monitors and, 120–21
    planning ahead for, 115–18, 546
    preparation for, 11
    response systems and, 20, 120–21
Employee assistance plans, 15, 157
Employment
    parent's, 103–4
    resources for, 632–33
    sample agreement for, 646
End-of-life care
    advance directives and, 367
    conversations about, 10, 368
    dementia and, 520
    disagreements regarding, 531
    planning ahead for, 525–36, 615, 653
    see also Hospice care
Energy assistance programs,
    315–16
Entombment, 556
Erysipelas, 228
Escape routes, 118
Estate attorneys, 323
Estate planning, 359
Estate taxes, 372–73, 374–77
Estrogen therapy, 237
Ethics committees, 297, 531
Exercise
    arthritis and, 239
    benefits of, 83–84
    for caregiver, 55–56
    constipation and, 250
    dementia and, 484–85, 599–600
    depression and, 265
    driving and, 141
    falls and, 124
    finding right program of, 84–86
    guidelines for, 86–88
    importance of, 598
    osteoporosis and, 236
    peripheral artery disease (PAD) and,
        230
    resources on, 616–17
    sleep disorders and, 217, 219
    videos for, 86
Exploitation, 109, 119, 171, 351,
        447–48. See also Fraud; Scams and
        scammers
Eye diseases, 204–8
Eyesight. See Vision problems

F

Fainting, 237
Falls
  cataracts and, 204
  monitors and, 120–23
  osteoporosis and, 234–38
  prevention, 123–30
  restraints, 293, 447
Family and Medical Leave Act (1993), 80
Family caregiver contract, 649
Family meetings, 3, 5, 65, 69–72, 73, 335,
  527. *See also* Communication
Fatigue, 141
Fear. *See* Phobias
Fecal disorders, delirium and, 268–69
Fecal incontinence, 247–49
Federally qualified health centers
  (FQHCs), 338
Feeding tubes, 134
Fiber, 250, 251
Filial responsibility laws, 309
Financial issues
  after death, 562, 564
  benefits and discounts, 153, 303, 308,
    314–17, 349
  caregiver compensation and, 66–69, 310
  caregiver's funds and, 308–10
  communication about, 8–9, 303–5, 306
  contact information for, 650
  dementia and, 509–10
  first steps regarding, 306–7
  funeral costs and, 312, 555–56
  gathering information about, 13–14
  home and, 317–20
  inheritances, 313
  marriage and, 111–12
  monthly budget form, 652
  moving out of home and, 387
  "payable on death" account, 312
  paying for old age, 586–95
  planning for, 310–14
  professional help for, 322–24
  resources on, 617
  retirement and, 586–87
  simplifying, 306–7
  taxes, 317, 320–22, 372–73, 374–77, 399,
    400, 564

  see also Exploitation; Fraud; Scams and
    scammers
Financial planners, 304–5, 322, 651
Flexibility, 85–86, 496
Flu shots, 257
Food and eating
  benefits for, 315
  dementia and, 501–4
  disinterest in, 548
  end-of-life care and, 535
  in hospitals, 285
  meal programs, 152–53
  overview of, 133–39
  resources on, 628–29
  swallowing problems and, 137–38,
    252–53
Food stamps (SNAP), 135, 152, 315, 316,
  629
Food-borne illness, 138–39
Foot care, 229, 618. *See also* Legs and feet
Forgetfulness/memory loss. *See* Dementia
Forms for organizing information,
  635–53
Foster homes, 407, 408–9
Fraud, 9, 325–336, 618. *See also*
  Exploitation; Scams and scammers
Friends, 98–99
Funeral directors, 553–54
Funerals, 312, 328, 555–61, 562–63, 618
Fungal infections, 227
Furniture, 127. *See also* Beds

G

Gas, 255–56
Gay and lesbian issues, 112, 428, 619
Generalized anxiety disorder, 269–70
Geriatric assessments, 186–87
Geriatric care managers, 16, 20, 39, 78,
  157–58
Gifts, 288, 374
Glaucoma, 205
Glucosamine, 241
Goals, parent's, 4, 7–8, 9–10, 182
Gout, 238–39, 241
Grab bars, 124, 126, 128, 130, 225, 248,
  319, 399, 429, 441, 494, 497, 501

Granny cams, 444. *See also* Monitors and alert systems
Granny pods, 399–401
Green burials/cemeteries, 559
Grief
  of caregiver, 572–75
  children and, 579–81
  dementia and, 470, 488
  depression and, 262–63, 571
  drugs and, 570
  facets of, 568–72
  growing from, 575–77
  of parent, 538
  of surviving parent, 578–79
Grooming. *See* Bathing and grooming
Guardians/guardianship, 328, 336, 363–64, 366, 372, 379–81
Guilt, 4, 19, 48, 278, 419, 470, 569, 572

H

Halitosis, 231
Hallucinations, 272, 469, 475, 519–20
Handrails, 125, 126, 127
Happiness, importance of, 96–97
Health and medicine resources, 620–21
Health care proxies, 3, 9, 10, 188–89, 280, 368, 587
Health Insurance Portability and Accountability Act (HIPAA), 189
Health maintenance organizations (HMOs), 342
Healthy body, importance of, 82
Hearing aids, 212, 213–14
Hearing loss, 125, 197, 208–16, 268, 272, 457, 471, 621–22
Heart attack, 220
Heart disease
  anxiety disorders and, 269
  cataracts and, 205
  depression and, 261
  diabetes and, 257
  estrogen therapy and, 237
  exercise and, 83–84
  gum disease and, 231
  hypertension and, 220
  resources on, 622
  sleeplessness and, 216
  temperature regulation and, 223
  weight and, 89–90, 134
Heart failure, 268
Heartburn, 253–54
Heat exhaustion, 222
Heatstroke, 222
Help
  accepting, 553
  asking for, 149
  for caring for parent with dementia, 491–92
  signs of need for, 148
  where to find, 157
  see also Community services; In-home care; Support networks/services
Helplessness, 48
Hemorrhoids, 250, 255
Herpes zoster (shingles), 227–28
Hip fractures, 234
HIPAA, 189
Hispanic services, 622
HIV, 111
Hoarding, 270, 460, 511–12
Hobbies, 56, 107
Home
  conversations about, 8, 385–6
  costs of, 387
  maintenance of, 3
  Medicaid and, 354
  modification of, 125–30, 148, 387, 391, 544, 610
  mortgages on, 317
  moving out of, 387–89
  moving into yours, 390–98
  repair loans, 319–20
  safety checklist for, 644
  sale-leaseback plans, 320
  see also Housing options; In-home care
Home and Community Based Services (HCBS), 353. *See also* Community services; In-home care
Home care agencies, 166–69. *See also* In-home care
Home health aides, 162–63, 165. *See also* In-home care
Homemakers, 151, 162, 165
Homosexuality, 112, 428, 619
Hope, 531–32, 538
Hormonal changes, 242, 249

Hospice care, 429, 526–27, 533, 544–46,
    623. *See also* End-of-life care
Hospital committees, 296–97
Hospital-acquired infections (HAI), 294
Hospitalists, 279, 284
Hospitals
    admission to, 277–280
    avoiding, 275
    bedsores and, 293–94
    bills from, 299
    choosing, 275–77
    coping with stay at, 285–89
    costs of, 276–77, 279–80, 299
    dangers of, 290–96
    delirium and, 290–92
    discharge from, 297–99, 418
    discharge planners at, 15, 297
    disputes and, 296–97
    falls and, 293
    following parent's wishes and, 280
    hospital-acquired infections and, 294
    managing from far away, 289–90
    medical mishaps in, 292–93
    nurses and, 282–84
    packing for, 278
    pain relief in, 294–96
    recovery and, 295
    restraints and, 293
    treatments at, 281–82
    visiting at, 285–88
House. *See* Home; Housing options
Housemates, 402–4
Housing options
    assisted living, 408–9, 410–12, 613, 628
    benefits for, 316–17
    congregate housing, 404–5
    foster homes, 407
    at a glance, 408–9
    living together, 390–98
    moving out, 387–89
    resources on, 624
    retirement communities, 403, 405–6,
        408–9, 412–14
    roommates, 402–4
    senior apartments, 406
    shared housing, 402–4
    talking to parent about, 8, 385
    see also Home; Nursing homes
Human service information lines (211), 16
Humor and laughter, 37, 57–58, 74,
    490–91, 496, 543, 601

Huntington's disease, 624
Hygiene, 3, 130–31, 148, 459, 495–99.
        See also Bathing and grooming;
        Oral hygiene
Hypertension, 220. *See also* Blood pressure
Hyperthermia, 197, 222, 223
Hyperthyroidism, 269
Hypochondria, 272–73
Hypothermia, 197, 222, 223

I

Iatrogenic disease, 292
ICE (In Case of Emergency), 117
ICU (intensive care unit), 276, 286, 287,
    290, 291, 547
Identification, 116–17, 515, 637
Imagery, 485
Inactivity, falls and, 124
Incontinence, 51, 91, 224, 235, 241–49,
    500–501, 624–25
Independence, 25, 83, 85
Independent living communities,
    405–6
Indigestion, 254. *See also* Digestive
    disorders
Industrial fraud, 327–28
Infections
    fungal, 227
    hospital-acquired, 294
    hospital-acquired, 294
    nosocomial, 294
    skin, 228
    urinary tract, 224, 242, 294
Ingrown nails, 230
In-home care
    agencies providing, 166–69
    costs of, 159–60
    defining responsibilities,
        171–72
    hiring process for, 166–70
    managing, 172–76
    overview of, 165
    resistance to, 176
    resources on, 623
    types of, 160–65
In-law apartments, 398, 399–400

Insomnia/sleeplessness, 85, 140, 197, 216–21, 457, 474. *See also* Sleep disorders
Instrumental activities of daily living (IADL), 163
Insults, 515–16
Insurance
    early pay-outs on, 357
    evaluating, 312
    long-term care, 358, 432, 588–95
    resources on, 626–27
    trusts and, 375
    see also Medicaid; Medicare
Integrative medicine, 192–95
Intensive care unit (ICU), 276, 286, 287, 290, 291, 547
Intergenerational living, 390–98
Internal Revenue Service, 317. *See also* Financial issues; Taxes
Internet
    caution regarding, 15
    legal forms available on, 361
    Medicare and, 350
    purchasing drugs on, 349
    resources on, 191, 608–9
    socializing via, 99–100
Internment, 556
Intertrigo, 228
Intimacy, 108–12
Investors, 323
Irrevocable life insurance trust, 375
Irrevocable living trusts, 373
Irritable bowel syndrome, 249
Isolation, 53, 208, 327, 331, 334–35, 388, 457

J

Joint tenancy, 377

K

Kegel exercises, 244
Keys, 19

Kidney problems, 220, 224, 257, 268
Kitchens, 128–29, 135–36, 503–4. *See also* Food and eating
Kübler-Ross, Elisabeth, 537

L

Lactose intolerance, 252, 256
Language difficulties, 459
Laughter and humor, 37, 57–58, 74, 490–91, 496, 543, 601
Lawyers, 322–23. *See also* Legal issues
Laxatives, 251
Legal issues
    advance directives, 367–71
    assistance with, 382
    competency issues, 378–81
    contact information for, 650
    conversations about, 8–9
    letters of instruction, 362–63
    power of attorney, 363–67
    probate, 377–78
    reducing estate taxes, 374–77
    resources on, 625
    terms, 364
    trusts, 371–74
    wills, 360–62
Legs and feet, 229–30
Letters of instruction, 362–63. *See also* Advance directives; Wills
Lewy body dementia, 458–59, 469, 475
LGBT issues, 112, 428, 619
Life review, 571, 577
Life support, 534–35
Life care centers, 412–14
Lifeline, 316
Lifting, 130
Lighting, 129
Limits, establishing, 29, 40, 42–47, 79
Liners, 559
Listening
    importance of, 6–7
    when parent won't, 27–31
    see also Communication
Liver disease, anemia and, 257
Living wills, 10, 280, 367–68, 526, 587

Living with parent, 390–98
Loans, 318–20. *See also* Financial issues
Loneliness, 134, 574
Long-distance caregiving, 443–44
Long-term care
    costs of, 9, 357–58, 587–88
    financial planning and, 312–13
    insurance for, 358, 432, 588–95
    resources on, 625
    talking about, 4–12, 304
Long-term care ombudsmen, 15, 334, 403,
        410, 422, 430, 431, 443, 446, 450, 451,
        608
Long-term services and supports (LTSS),
        163
Low Income Home Energy Assistance
        Program (LIHEAP), 315–16
Low vision aids, 207–8. *See also* Vision
        problems
Lung disease, 216, 261, 269, 625–26

M

Macular degeneration, 206–7
Mail, dementia and, 510
Male caregivers, 58–59
Malnutrition, 88–89, 285
Manipulation, 39
Marriage, 111–12. *See also* Spouse
Massage, 193, 267
Meal programs, 152–53, 315, 503, 628–29.
        See also Food and eating
Mediation, 29, 69, 380
Medicaid
    assisted living and, 411
    caregiver compensation and,
        67–68
    day services and, 156, 168
    doctors and, 182
    eligibility for, 308, 312, 317, 400, 588
    exploitation and, 351
    foster homes and, 407
    hearing aids and, 214
    home ownership and, 394
    hospitals and, 279
    in-home care and, 159, 162, 164,
        166, 393

insurance partnerships and, 593
look-back period, 355–56
nursing homes and, 416, 423, 428,
        430–33, 449
overview of, 352–57
protecting assets and, 354–57
resources on, 626–27
trusts and, 372
use of, 310
Medical care
    age and, 181–82
    alternative, 192–95
    conversations about, 9
    geriatric assessments and, 186–87
    personal health records (PHRs) and,
        187–88
    wellness visits and, 185–86
    see also Doctors; End-of-life care;
        Hospitals; Medications; *individual
        ailments*
Medical contacts, 642
Medical emergency identification, 11,
        116–17, 637–38
Medical expenses, deductions for, 321
Medical history, 17
Medical log, 643
Medical mishaps, 292–93
Medical power of attorney. *See* Health care
        proxies
Medical savings accounts, 343
Medicare
    appealing a decision, 351–52
    assisted living and, 411
    billing questions and, 299
    cost plans, 343
    day services and, 156
    discharge and, 298
    doctors and, 182
    explanation of, 15, 339–44
    exploitation and, 351
    flu shots and, 257
    fraud and, 328
    hearing aids and, 214, 215
    hospice care and, 545
    hospitals and, 275, 277, 279
    in-home care and, 159, 163, 166,
        175–76, 358
    nursing homes and, 419–20, 423, 430,
        431, 432, 437
    online registration and, 350
    Part A, 339, 340

Part B, 339, 341
Part D, 347–350
PHRs and, 188
prescription drug coverage, 347–50
preventive services and, 185
Quality Improvement Organizations (QIO) and, 297
records access, 343
resources on, 344, 626–27
respite care and, 177
Savings Programs, 350–51
second opinions and, 281
Summary Notice (MSN), 348
wellness visits and, 185
Medicare Advantage, 342–43, 345, 347, 348
Medicare Supplement Insurance (Medigap), 338, 344, 345–47
Medications
alcohol and, 93
appetite and, 90
arthritis and, 240–41
compliance and, 201
constipation and, 250
costs of, 201, 348–50
dangerous, 200
delirium and, 268, 291–92
delusions and, 272
dementia and, 471, 473–76, 509, 600
dental care and, 231, 232
depression and, 261, 265–66
discount programs for, 348–50
dizziness and, 209
donut hole and, 348
driving and, 140, 141
Extra Help for, 348
falls and, 124
grief and, 570
heartburn and, 254
hypertension and, 220
incontinence and, 242, 245, 247
keeping track of, 198–99, 640–41
list of, 640, 641
Medicare and, 347–50
memory loss and, 456, 457
nursing homes and, 202
nutritional supplements and, 91
online purchasing of, 349
osteoporosis and, 234–35, 237–38
overmedication and, 198
questions to ask about, 199–201

review of, 185
saving on, 348–50
sexual dysfunction and, 110
signs of problems with, 197
skin care and, 228–29
sleeplessness and, 217, 218
temperature regulation and, 223
ulcers and, 254
weekly chart for, 641
weight and, 134
Medigap (Medicare Supplement Insurance), 338, 344, 345–47
Meditation, 37, 195, 267
Melatonin, 217, 218
Memantine, 475
Memorial services. See Funerals
Memory loss/forgetfulness, 3, 84, 220, 459, 513, 600. See also Dementia
Mental illness, 259–73, 627
Mental status test, 464
Mild cognitive impairment (MCI), 456–58, 482
Mind, exercising, 104–5, 599
Mind-body connection, 55, 194–95
MOLST (Medical Orders for Life Sustaining Treatment). See POLST (Physician Orders for Life Sustaining Treatment)
Money. See Financial issues
Money managers, 323. See also Financial planners
Monitors and alert systems, 120–23, 444
Mortgages, 317, 318–19
Mourning. See Grief
Mouth ailments, 197, 231–32. See also Dental problems; Oral hygiene
Moving out of home
into accessory dwelling units, 398–400
to be closer, 389
day of, 435–37
deciding to, 387–89
discussing, 385–86
into your home, 390–98
MRIs, 465
Multi-infarct dementia (MID), 468
Multiple Support Declaration, 320, 321
Music, 105, 485

N

Naps, sleeplessness and, 217
Native American services, 627
Naturally Occurring Retirement
    Community (NORC), 405, 597
Needs assessments, 148, 437
Negativity, 102
Neglect, 39–40, 175, 447–48
Nerve damage, diabetes and, 257
Nerve deafness, 211
Nicotine replacement therapy, 95
Nonsteroidal anti-inflammatory drugs
    (NSAIDs), 240, 254–55
Nosocomial infections, 294
NSAIDs (nonsteroidal anti-inflammatory
    drugs), 240, 254–55
Nurses, 164–65, 282–84. See also Home
    health aides
Nurse's aides, 162–63
Nursing homes
    admissions process, 429–31
    certification and licensing of, 423
    costs of, 423–24, 431–33
    deciding to move to, 415–18
    discharges, unwanted, 449–50
    easing transition to, 435–37, 450
    evaluating placement, 450–51
    food at, 427–28
    gathering information about, 15
    inspections of, 420–21, 446
    looking for, 418–29
    Medicaid and, 389, 416
    person-directed care and, 420
    plans of care at, 424, 437–38
    preparing for move to, 435–37
    problems in, addressing, 445–50
    quality measures for, 421
    reactions to, 419
    resources on, 628
    room changes, 449–50
    services provided by, 417–18
    staffing of, 421, 425
    timing of move to, 416
    visits with parent at, 438–40
    when you live far away, 443–44
Nutrition, resources on, 628–29.
        See also Diet; Food and eating

Nutritional supplements, 90, 91, 125, 135,
    192–93, 236–37. See also Diet; Food
    and eating
Nutritionist/registered dietician, 90, 163

O

Obesity, 230, 245
Obituaries, 554
Obsessive-compulsive disorder, 270
Obstructive sleep apnea, 220
Occupational therapy, 164, 239–40, 629
Ombudsmen, 296, 298, 344, 422, 446,
    449, 531. See also Long-term care
    ombudsmen
Omega-3 fatty acids, 476
Only children, 62
Oral hygiene, 231–32, 498–99.
        See also Dental problems
Organ donation, 556
Organization, 2, 14, 16–20, 75, 635–53
Osteoarthritis, 84, 235, 238
Osteoporosis, 83, 85, 89–90, 234–38, 254,
    612
Overmedication, 197, 198–203, 227,
    446–48, 456

P

Pads for incontinence, 246
Pain relief, 84, 85, 294–96, 535, 536, 541,
    548
Palliative care, 526, 532–33, 536, 544
Parent, healthy, 59. See also Spouse,
    surviving
Parent-child relationship
    adapting to new roles in, 23–27
    claiming parent as dependent, 320–21
    coping day to day in, 34–37
    defusing old struggles in, 31–34
    exceptionally difficult parent and, 37–40
    intervention in parent's situation and,
        27–31

Parenting your parent, 23–24
Parkinson's disease, 140, 223, 243, 250, 261, 459, 629
Participant-directed services, 353
Patient advocates, 296, 298
Pelvic muscle exercises (PMEs), 244
Periodic limb movement, 219
Peripheral artery disease (PAD), 229–30
Persistent vegetative states, 535–36
Personal connections, importance of, 96–100
Personal health records (PHRs), 187–88
Personal hygiene. *See* Bathing and grooming; Hygiene; Oral hygiene
Personal sound amplifiers (PSAPs), 212
Personality changes, 3, 459. *See also* Behavioral changes
Person-directed care, xiv–xv, 420
PET scans, 465
Pets, 107–8, 265, 485
Phishing, 328
Phobias, 270
Phones. *See* Telephones
Physical aid, 498
Physical contact, importance of, 287
Physical therapy, 124, 163–64, 239–40, 616–17
Physician-assisted suicide, 534
Physicians, participating, 342
Pilates, 88
Pill reminders, 202–3. *See also* Medications
Pilot programs, 343
Planning ahead
    community services and, 14–16
    contingency plans and, 16
    conversations with parent and, 4–12
    information gathering and, 13–16
    living far away and, 19–20
    organization and, 14, 16–19
    parent's denial and, 11–12
Plan of care, 424, 437–38
Pneumonia vaccine, 257
Point of service plans, 343
POLST (Physician Orders for Life Sustaining Treatment), 10, 280, 370, 527–28
Possessions, dividing, 564–66
Power of attorney, 10, 188–89, 336, 363–67, 372, 526, 587

Powerlessness, 48
Preferred provider organizations (PPOs), 342–43
Prenuptial agreements, 112
Presbycusis, 211
Prescription drug coverage, 347–50
Prevention, 182
Preventive services, 185
Primary caregiver, siblings and, 62–64
Primary physician, importance of, 180
Privacy, 122, 123, 286, 394, 396, 442, 444
Private fee-for-service (PFFS), 343
Probate, 364, 371–72, 377–78, 562
Promises, 8, 417
Property tax deferral loans, 320
Prostrate problems, incontinence and, 242, 243
Prunes, 250
Pruritus, 225
Pseudogout, 238–39, 241
Psychiatry, geriatric, 266
Psychosis, 474
Psychotherapy, 266
Psychotic symptoms, 518–20

Q

Qualified Personal Residence Trust, 375–76
Quality Improvement Organization (QIO), 297, 299

R

Real estate. *See* Home; Housing options
Records, vital, 14, 436. *See also* Documents
Registered nurses (RNs), 165
Regret, 572–73
Rehab facilities, 276
Relationships, importance of, 600–601
Relaxation, 57, 212, 218, 219

Religion
  cremation and, 556
  end-of-life care and, 537, 538
  grief and, 570
  nursing homes and, 428–29
  spiritual fulfillment and, 100
  see also Spiritual support
Religious organizations, 15, 157
Remembering/reminiscing, 24, 37, 101
Repetition, 515
Resentment, 48–50
Respect, 4, 25–27, 442–43, 482–83, 541
Respirators, 534–35
Respite care, 52–53, 165, 176–77, 542
Restless leg syndrome (RLS), 219
Restraints, 293, 424, 427, 446–48, 534
Retinol, 237
Retirement
  costs of, 586–87
  location for, 595–97
  timing of, 589
Retirement communities, 405–6, 408–9,
    412–14, 597
Reverse mortgages, 318–19
Revocable living trusts, 373
Rewards, 35, 36
Rheumatoid arthritis, 238
Roommates
  in the hospital, 289
  as housing option, 402–4

S

Safety issues
  checklist for, 644
  daily living and, 115–19
  dementia and, 494–95
  driving and, 141–43
  falls and, 124–30
  food and, 138–39
  moving out of home and, 387
Sale-leaseback plans, 320
Sandwich generation, 75, 77–78
Savings, 586–87
Scalding risk, 118
Scams and scammers, 109, 119, 327–36,
    509. *See also* Exploitation; Fraud

Scans, 281, 465
Seat belts, 142
Second opinions, 281
Security systems. *See* Alarm systems;
    Monitors and alert systems
Sedatives, 293, 476
Self-care, for caregiver
  dementia and, 472, 477, 485–86
  difficult parent and, 40
  during final stages, 542–43
  hospital stays and, 289
  importance of, 20, 41–42
  mind-body connection, 55
  planning ahead and, 3
  signs you need help, 17
  support networks and, 37
  12 steps to a healthy mind-set, 52–58
Senior centers, 15, 107, 153–55
Sensorineural hearing loss, 211
Sex, 109–11
Sexual behavior and dementia, 516–17
Sexually transmitted diseases, 111
Shared housing, 402–4, 408–9
Shingles, 227–28, 257
Shoes, 125, 230, 239
Shopping, for food, 133–35
Showers, 128, 131
Siblings
  anger and, 573
  coordinating care with, 66
  denial and, 463
  dividing possessions among,
    565–66
  family meetings and, 65
  help from, 40, 45
  jealousy and, 573
  long-distance, 65
  refusing to help, 65–66
  sharing costs with, 392
  working with, 61–66, 397
Significant others, 72–74
Signs of trouble, 3
Simplicity, 496, 502, 503
Skin care, 197, 224–29, 498, 629–30
Skype, 20
Sleep
  for caregiver, 56, 221
  depression and, 265
  exercise and, 84
  in hospitals, 285
  for parent, 216–20

Sleep apnea, 219–20
Sleep disorders, 218–220, 457, 507–8, 630.
　　See also Insomnia/sleeplessness
Smell, sense of, 136
Smoke detectors, 118
Smoking. See Tobacco use
Snoring, 219–20
Social isolation. See Isolation
Social needs, 54, 98–100, 107
Social Security Administration, 14,
　　561–62, 563
Social workers, 163
Socializing, dementia and, 486
Special needs plans (SNPs), 343
Speech issues, resources on, 621–22
Speech therapy, 164, 253
Spending down, 308, 310, 312, 355, 357,
　　602
Spiritual support, 56–57, 100, 288, 601.
　　See also Religion
Sponge baths, 131
Sports, 107
Spouse
　　of caregiver, 72–74
　　surviving, 564, 578–79
　　well, 59
Stairs, 29, 127, 129, 145, 206, 237, 305, 391
Stasis dermatitis, 229
State boards and agencies, 297
State Health Insurance Counseling and
　　Assistance Program (SHIP), 299
State long-term-care ombudsman, 15
Strength exercises, 84–85, 236
Stress, 57, 457
Stroke
　　delirium and, 268
　　dementia and, 458, 468
　　depression and, 261
　　diabetes and, 257
　　dysphagia and, 252
　　gum disease and, 231
　　hypertension and, 220
　　incontinence and, 242, 243, 247
　　resources on, 630–31
　　sleep apnea and, 220
　　temperature regulation and, 223
Suicide, 262, 534
Sundowning, 484, 496
Sunscreen, 229
Supplemental Nutrition Assistance
　　Program (SNAP; food stamps), 135,
152, 315, 316, 629
Supplemental Security Income (SSI), 315,
　　400, 407
Support groups, 53–54, 265, 577, 579
Support hose, 229
Support networks/services, 17, 19–20, 37,
　　45, 49–50, 53
Surgery, 241, 245, 275, 282, 291
Survival tips, 2–4
Swallowing problems, 137–38, 252–53
Swimming and water exercises, 84

T

Tai chi, 85, 124, 195, 239, 267
Taxes
　　after death, 564
　　capital gains, 321, 373, 375, 376
　　estate, 374–77
　　help with, 317
　　property, 399, 400
　　tips regarding, 320–22
　　trusts and, 372–73
　　See also Financial issues
Teenagers, 76
Teeth and mouth, 231–32
Telehealth devices, 144
Telephone numbers
　　for emergencies, 173
　　gathering and organizing, 17, 19, 20
Telephone reassurance programs,
　　150–51
Telephones
　　bills, 316
　　cell phones, 121
　　dementia and, 510
　　Do Not Call registry, 330
　　emergencies and, 117, 173
　　hearing loss and, 213, 214
Temperature, in home, 129
Temperature regulation, 221–23
Tenants in common, 377
Testamentary trusts, 373
Tests, medical, 281–82
Theft, 171, 175. See also Fraud
Therapeutic fibbing, 481
Therapeutic touch, 194

Therapists, 163–64, 165.
  See also Occupational therapy;
  Physical therapy; Psychotherapy;
  Speech therapy
Thirst, sense of, 86, 87, 91.
  See also Dehydration
Thrush, 253
Thyroid disorders, 223, 257, 268, 269,
  457
Time, confusion of, 459–60, 506–7
Tinnitus, 211–12
Tobacco use
  dementia and, 468
  dry skin and, 225
  heartburn and, 254
  memory loss and, 457
  osteoporosis and, 235, 237
  peripheral artery disease (PAD) and,
    230
  quitting, 94–95, 630
  sleep disorders and, 219, 220
  sleeplessness and, 218
  ulcers and, 255
Toilets, 128, 248, 501. *See also* Commodes;
  Incontinence
Transfer belts, 130, 498
Transportation options, 143, 153, 317
Travel, 105–6
Trusts, 306, 336, 355, 371–76
211 (human service information line),
  16, 157

U

Ulcers, 254–55
Undifferentiated somatoform disorder,
  272–73
Undue influence, 333, 379–80
Unsteadiness, 3. *See also* Falls
Uric acid, 238–39, 241
Urinary disorders, delirium and,
  268–69
Urinary incontinence, 241–47
Urinary tract infections, 224, 242,
  294
Urns, 559

V

Vaccinations, 182, 228, 257
Varicose veins, 229
Vascular dementia, 458, 468, 473
Vaults, 559
Ventilators, 534–35
Veterans
  benefits for, 14, 153, 157, 308, 338, 344,
    355
  burials of, 360, 557
  death benefits for, 563
  Home and Community Based Services
    (HCBS) for, 353
  in-home care and, 164
  hospitals for, 276
  personal health records (PHRs) for,
    188
  resources for, 610, 614, 630, 631
  respite care and, 177
  taxes and, 320
Vial of life, 115–16
Viewings, 560
Villages, 596–97
Violence, 518–19
Vision problems
  coping with, 206, 207–8
  delirium and, 268
  delusions and, 272
  dementia and, 471
  driving and, 141
  eye diseases, 204–8
  falls and, 125
  memory loss and, 457
  overview of, 203–8
  resources for, 631–32
  signs of, 197
Visits with parent, 36, 63, 285–88,
  438–40
Visualization, 195
Vitamin A, 237
Vitamin B12, 257, 261, 471
Vitamin D, 125, 236–37
Vitamin deficiencies, 457
Vitamin E, 476
Vitamin K, 237
Volunteering, 102–3, 632–33

W

Wakes, 560
Walkers, 130, 239
Walking, 87
Wandering, 513–15
Water, end-of-life care and, 535, 548.
    See also Dehydration
Water filter, 139
Webcams, 444
Weight changes, 3, 84, 89–90, 134, 148.
    See also Obesity
Weight loss, 90, 134
Weight training, 84–85, 236
Well Spouse Foundation, 59
Wellness visits, 185–86
Wills, 10, 360–62, 376, 587
Withdrawal, 94
Women's health and services, 633

Working caregivers. *See* Employee
    assistance plans
Working parents, 103–4
Worry, 48, 538

Y

Yellow pages, 20
Yoga, 88, 267

Z

Zoning regulations, 399–400, 405

We Welcome
Your Views

How to Care for Aging Parents has tried to address the wide range of concerns and questions that caregivers face in as much detail as possible. But there is always room for improvement. Please let us know your thoughts on the book—advice that was helpful, questions that weren't addressed, facts we might have missed—so that we can make adjustments and include your views in any future editions. You can reach us at careforagingparents.com. We look forward to hearing from you.

VIRGINIA MORRIS is an award-winning author and journalist and a nationally recognized authority on eldercare. She testified before the Joint Economic Committee of the U.S. Congress. She has also appeared on *Oprah*, *The Today Show*, *Good Morning America*, *CBS This Morning*, *Primetime*, *ABC World News with Diane Sawyer*, NPR's *The Diane Rehm Show*, *Katie*, and a host of other national media. Her previous book is *Talking About Death*. Morris lives in Sag Harbor, NY, with her family.

She is available for speaking engagements, media appearances, and consulting. She regularly gives keynote addresses and joins panel discussions addressing the needs of family caregivers, professionals, businesses, and employees. For more information, visit careforagingparents.com.